Surgical Procedures in Orthopedics

Surgical Procedures in Orthopedics

Edited by Marlow Coffey

hayle medical
New York

Hayle Medical,
750 Third Avenue, 9th Floor,
New York, NY 10017, USA

Visit us on the World Wide Web at:
www.haylemedical.com

ISBN: 978-1-63241-521-9

The publisher's policy is to use permanent paper from mills that operate a sustainable forestry policy. Furthermore, the publisher ensures that the text paper and cover boards used have met acceptable environmental accreditation standards.

Printed in China.

Cataloging-in-Publication Data

Surgical procedures in orthopedics / edited by Marlow Coffey.
p. cm.
Includes bibliographical references and index.
ISBN 978-1-63241-521-9
1. Orthopedic surgery. 2. Orthopedics. I. Coffey, Marlow.

RD731 .S87 2018
617.47--dc23

Table of Contents

Preface

Every book is a source of knowledge and this one is no exception. The idea that led to the conceptualization of this book was the fact that the world is advancing rapidly; which makes it crucial to document the progress in every field. I am aware that a lot of data is already available, yet, there is a lot more to learn. Hence, I accepted the responsibility of editing this book and contributing my knowledge to the community.

The surgical procedures in orthopedics treat the diseases and disorders related to the musculoskeletal system of living organisms. The most significant function of the musculoskeletal system is to support the body and facilitate its motion. It consists of the skeleton, ligaments, joints, muscles and connective tissues. This book provides significant information about orthopedics to help develop a good understanding of the subject and its related fields. The topics covered in this extensive text deal with the core aspects of orthopedic surgery and implants. Those in search of information to further their knowledge will be greatly assisted by the text.

While editing this book, I had multiple visions for it. Then I finally narrowed down to make every chapter a sole standing text explaining a particular topic, so that they can be used independently. However, the umbrella subject sinews them into a common theme. This makes the book a unique platform of knowledge.

I would like to give the major credit of this book to the experts from every corner of the world, who took the time to share their expertise with us. Also, I owe the completion of this book to the never-ending support of my family, who supported me throughout the project.

Editor

1

Minimally Invasive Surgical Approaches and Traditional Total Hip Arthroplasty: A Meta-Analysis of Radiological and Complications Outcomes

Baohui Yang, Haopeng Li*, Xijing He, Guoyu Wang, Siyue Xu

Department of Orthopaedic Surgery, The 2nd Affiliated Hospital of Medical College, Xi'an Jiaotong University, Xi'an, Shaanxi Province, People's Republic of China

Abstract

Background: Minimally invasive total hip arthroplasty (MITHA) remains considerably controversial. Limited visibility and prosthesis malposition increase the risk of post-surgical complications compared to those of the traditional method.

Methods: A meta-analysis was undertaken of all published databases up to May 2011. The studies were divided into four subgroups according to the surgical approach taken. The radiological outcomes and complications of minimally invasive surgery were compared to traditional total hip arthroplasty (TTHA) using risk ratio, mean difference, and standardized mean difference statistics.

Results: In five studies involving the posterolateral approach, no significant differences were found between the MITHA groups and the TTHA groups in the acetabular cup abduction angle ($p = 0.41$), acetabular anteversion ($p = 0.96$), and femoral prosthesis position ($p = 0.83$). However, the femoral offset was significantly increased (WMD = 3.00; 95% CI, 0.40–5.60; $p = 0.02$). Additionally, there were no significant differences among the complications in both the groups (dislocations, nerve injury, infection, deep vein thrombosis, proximal femoral fracture) and revision rate ($p > 0.05$). In three studies involving the posterior approach, there were no significant differences in radiological outcomes or all other complications between MITHA or TTHA groups ($p > 0.05$). Three studies involved anterolateral approach, while 2 studies used the lateral approach. However, the information from imaging and complications was not adequate for statistical analysis.

Conclusions: Posterior MITHA seems to be a safe surgical procedure, without the increased risk of post-operative complication rates and component malposition rates. The posterolateral approach THA may lead to increased femoral offset. The current data are not enough to reach a positive conclusion that lateral and anterolateral approaches will result in increased risks of adverse effects and complications at the prosthesis site.

Editor: Joel Joseph Gagnier, University of Michigan, United States of America

Funding: The authors have no support or funding to report.

Competing Interests: The authors have declared that no competing interests exist.

* E-mail: LHP-3993@163.com

Introduction

Total hip arthroplasty (THA) is considered one of the most successful operations in orthopedic surgery for over 40 years, during which improvements in the design of implants and biological materials have resulted in positive clinical outcomes. However, for the past decade, considerable interest has been devoted to the development of minimally invasive surgical techniques [1]. Minimally invasive total hip arthroplasty (MITHA) has now become popular around the world. It is defined as the use of a 10 cm or even smaller incision to complete the total hip joint replacement [2,3,4].

The advantages of minimally invasive surgeries include less soft-tissue trauma (smaller skin incision and less muscle damage), reduced blood loss and fewer blood transfusion requirements. Postoperative benefits include less pain, shorter hospital stay, quicker return to function and a better cosmetic appearance [2,4,5].

Despite the increase in adopting MITHA, its risks and benefits still generate debates among orthopedic surgeons. Many of them believe that MITHA introduces additional risks due to the limited visibility of anatomical landmarks and vital structures [6]. Higher risks for thromboembolism, infection, neurovascular injury, femoral fracture and component malposition leading to increased prosthetic wear, are the various complications that have been documented [7]. Bradley P et al [8] retrospectively reviewed 46 revision THAs performed during a 3-year period and concluded that MITHA may be a risk factor for early revision surgery and the long-term survival therefore may be lower than that for non-minimal invasive surgery. Another drawback seems to be the learning curve, which tends to be longer for surgeons with little experience of hip prosthetic surgery. Some other randomized, case-control studies also reveal inconsistent results regarding these issues [9–12]. Therefore, it remains controversial whether MITHA increases post-operative complications and prosthesis malposition.

There have been several related meta-analysis studies [13,14]. These analyses seem to have simply pooled the results together without an explicitly defined sub-group analysis of the surgical approach. Clearly, a 12 cm posterior approach would have very different risks and complications than an 8 cm direct anterior, or two incision approach. A very recent study [15] also pointed this issue. Therefore, to group all MITHA approaches together and make comparisons in a pooled analysis is unsound since differences in technique (e.g. between the mini-anterior, mini-posterior, mini-anterolateral approaches) are significant and need to be analyzed separately. The purpose of this meta-analysis was to compare the MITHA with conventional, or traditional total hip arthroplasty (TTHA) with respect to complications and post-operative results through imaging, of subgroups formed by the surgical approaches taken.

Materials and Methods

We conducted a meta-analysis using the guidelines of the Cochrane Collaboration [16], and our findings were reported according to the Quality of Reporting of Meta-analyses statement [17].

Types of studies included

Any randomized controlled trials comparing MITHA and TTHA for the treatment of hip disease.

Types of Participants

Participants of the 2 treatment groups were similar demographically, and there were no statistically significant differences with respect to the variables of age, gender, body mass index (<35.0).

Types of interventions

We focused on comparing MITHA and TTHA with a common operation approach that is, posterior, posterolateral:, anterolateral, lateral, so that there would be a consistency between the two groups.

We excluded studies in which the surgical approach was inconsistent (for example, if the minimally invasive group used the anterolateral approach, and the traditional group used the posterior approach, etc.). In addition, we also excluded studies that examined the double incision surgical approach.

Types of outcome measures

The primary outcomes were:

1. Imaging outcomes (acetabular abduction angle, acetabular anteversion, femoral prosthesis position (varus or valgus), and femoral offset.
2. Postoperative complications (dislocation, iatrogenic nerve injury, infection, deep vein thrombosis, proximal femoral fracture, and revision rate).

Search strategy

The following search terms were used: total hip arthroplasty (or THA), total hip replacement (or THR), prosthesis (or prostheses or implant), minimally invasive (or less invasive), mini-incision (or MIS or minimal incision or small incision). The literature range was defined as between February 1990 and May 2011. The databases searched included PubMed, Cochrane Central Register of Controlled Trials, Embase, and CBMdisc. A manual search was performed for relevant publications from European Federation of National Associations of Orthopaedics and Traumatology and British Hip Society.

Data collection and analysis

Both review authors (BaoHui Yang and HaoPeng LI) assessed potentially eligible trials for inclusion, any disagreement were resolved through discussion. Titles of journals, names of authors or supporting institutions were not masked at any stage.

Data extraction and management

Data were extracted independently by both authors using piloted forms. The data included the general characteristics of each study and the outcomes measured. General characteristics included study design, first author, year of publication, sample size, and interventions. Only the primary outcomes were measured.

Assessment of risk of bias in included studies

To avoid inherent problems with scale validity [17], we did not use a quality scale or a checklist. We assessed the methodological quality as described by the Cochrane Reviews Handbook 5.0.2 [17], Methodological quality assessment scheme (Table S1). The studies were classified into A: low risk of bias and each of the criteria was appropriate, B: medium risk of bias and most of the criteria were appropriate, and C: high risk of bias and most of the criteria were not appropriate.

Measures of treatment effect

For continuous data such as acetabular cup abduction angle, the mean and standard deviation were used to calculate the weighted mean difference (WMD) and 95% confidence interval (CI); for count data such as post-operative complications, the odds ratio (OR) or relative risk (RR) and 95% CI were used. Data processing was performed using Review Manager 5.0 software (the Cochrane Collaboration).

Assessment of heterogeneity. The heterogeneity test P values revealed by the forest plot were used to determine the heterogeneity of the included studies. I^2 was used to estimate the size of the heterogeneity. $I^2>50\%$ indicated considerable heterogeneity among the included studies.

Subgroup analysis and investigation of heterogeneity

We planned separate outcome analyses according to the different surgical approaches, and if there is no heterogeneity internal each groups, data were pooled using the fixed-effect model and 95% confidence intervals. Where there was clear or significant heterogeneity, we viewed the results of the random-effects model, but in such cases opted not to pool data where the outcome measures were clearly different.

Results

Description of studies

A total of 552 citations were identified from the search strategy. Twelve studies were deemed appropriate (Figure 1). Eleven were written in English, one was in Chinese, and a total of 1077 cases were reported in the included studies. The basic characteristics of the 12 included studies are summarized in Table S2. The diseases included: osteoarthritis, rheumatoid arthritis, traumatic arthritis, congenital dislocation of the hip, femoral head necrosis, femoral neck fracture and other types. Consistent baselines were observed for all patients.

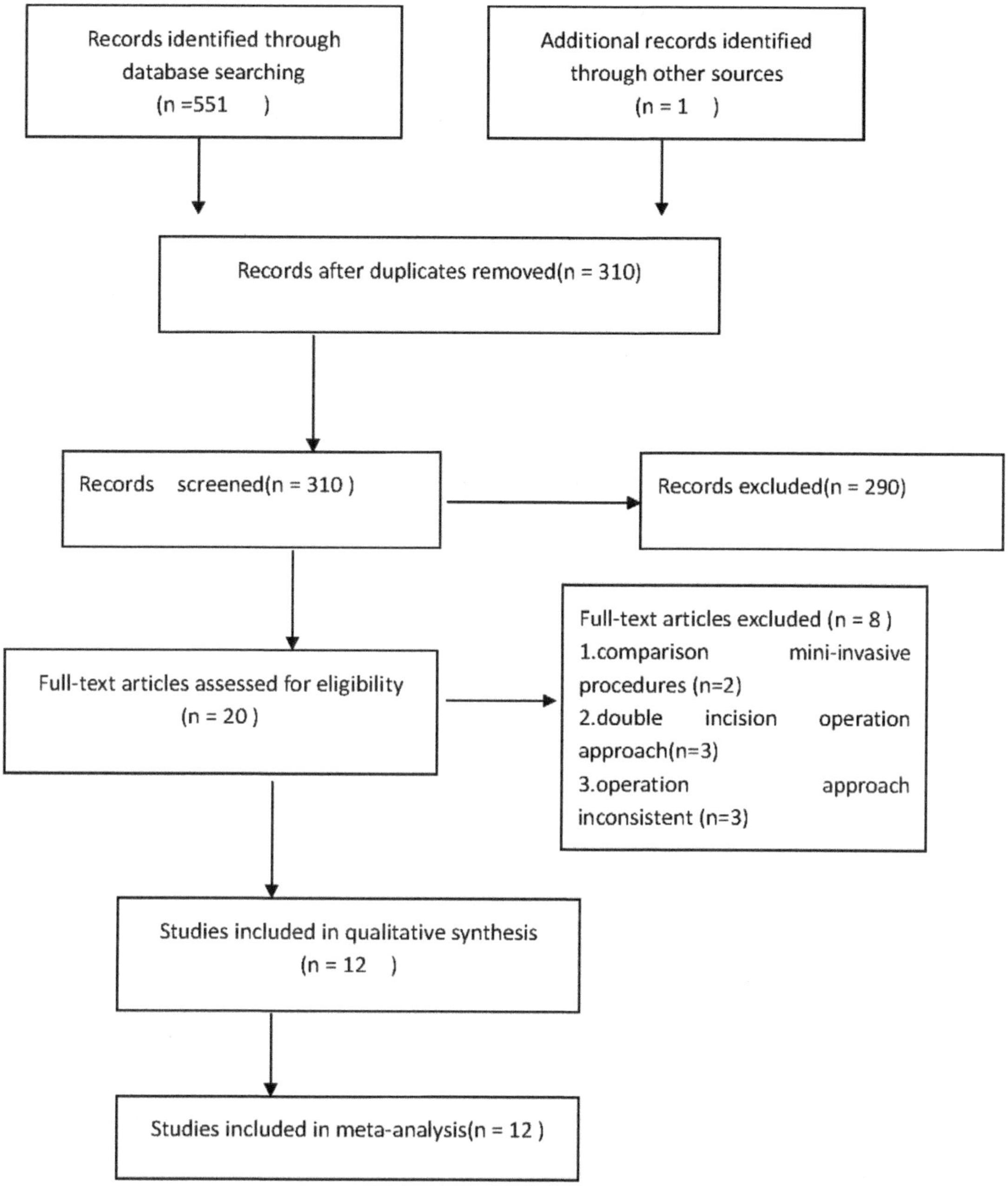

Figure 1. The process of identifying relevant studies is summarized.

The surgical interventions included 4 studies that used the lateral approach [18,19,20,21], 3 studies applied a posterior approach [22,23,24], 6 cases utilized the posterolateral approach [10,11,12,18,25,26], and one case adopted the anterolateral approach [23]. mong them, the study by Goosen et al exercised both, the anterolateral approach and the posterior approach; Shitama et al also employed the posterolateral approach and the lateral approach; and 3 cases make use of the bone cement approach [10,25,23]. Follow-up studies of clinical outcomes and complications ranged between 6 weeks and 80 months.

Risk of bias in included studies

A summary of methodological domain assessment for each study is detailed in figure 2. Overall, the methodological quality of all the trials were found to be of medium risk of bias, The randomization technique was mentioned in 9 trials, which the randomized cohort picked a card, randomization number, or a randomization scheme. Six trials mentioned allocation concealment, 3 studies were single-blinded to the observers [10,11,25], and 2 studies were double-blinded to both the observers and the patients [22,23]. All the studies could result in a potential selection bias. A variety of different THA prostheses were used in the studies reviewed which might result in a performance bias.

Although there were 'lost to follow-up' phenomenon in some studies, missing outcome data balanced in numbers across intervention groups, with similar reasons for missing data across groups, so attrition bias was considered as a low risk of bias.

	Adequate sequence generation?	Allocation concealment?	Blinding?	Incomplete outcome data addressed?	Free of selective reporting?	Free of other bias?
Chimento GF2005	+	?	+	+	+	+
Dorr2007	?	?	+	+	+	?
Farhad2009	?	?	-	+	?	+
Goosen JH2011	+	+	+	+	+	?
Hart R2005	+	?	+	?	?	?
Kim2006	?	+	+	?	+	+
ogonda L2005	?	+	+	+	+	+
Roy2010	?	+	-	?	+	?
Shitama2009	+	?	?	?	+	+
Varela2010	+	+	-	+	+	+
Wohlrab2008	+	?	-	?	+	?
Yang YH2008	+	?	-	?	+	?

Figure 2. Risk of bias summary. A review of the authors' judgments about each risk of bias item for each included study. + is "yes", – is "no",?is "unclear".

Publication bias analysis

Abduction angle of the acetabular cup was again used for the funnel plot analysis of publication bias (Figure 3), which revealed there was publication bias evident for the primary outcome frequency of the abduction angle.

Primary outcomes: Imaging results

Posterolateral approach. No significant differences were found between the MITHA and the TTHA groups in the imaging data of the acetabular cup abduction angle (p = 0.41), acetabular anteversion (p = 0.96), femoral prosthesis position (p = 0.83). The average femoral offset was significantly increased in the MITHA group than in the TTHA group (WMD = 3.00; 95% CI, 0.40–5.60; p = 0.02) (Tables S3, S4 and Figures 4).

No significant differences were noticed in the complications that occurred [dislocations (p = 0.24), nerve injury (p = 0.57), infection (p = 0.5), deep vein thrombosis (p = 1.00)], and revision rate (p = 0.44) (Tables S3 and S4).

Posterior approach. No significant differences were found between the MITHA and the TTHA groups in the imaging data of the acetabular cup abduction angle (p = 0.46), acetabular anteversion (p = 0.67), femoral prosthesis position (p = 0.25), and femoral offset (p = 0.16) (Tables S3 and S4).

No significant differences were found between the two groups in the complications that occurred [dislocations (p = 0.50), nerve injury (p = 0.50), infection (p = 0.46), deep vein thrombosis (p = 0.10), proximal femoral fracture (p = 0.73)], and revision rate (p = 0.41) (Tables S3 and S4).

Anterolateral approach. No significant differences were found between the two groups in the acetabular cup abduction angle (p = 1.00) and proximal femoral fracture (p = 0.16). However, data on acetabular anteversion, femoral prosthesis position, femoral offset, dislocations, nerve injury, infection, deep vein thrombosis, and revision rate were not adequate for analysis (Tables S3 and S4).

Lateral approach. No significant differences were found in the imaging data of the acetabular cup abduction angle (p = 0.88) and femoral prosthesis position (p = 0.30). Acetabular anteversion and femoral offset were not evaluated (Tables S3 and S4).

No significant differences were found among complications such as dislocations (p = 1.00), infection (p = 1.00), and deep vein thrombosis (p = 0.33). Nerve injury, proximal femoral fracture, and revision rate were not evaluated (Tables S3 and S4).

Discussion

Minimally invasive total hip arthroplasty has often been the subject of debate in recent years. No clear definition exists for what constitutes MITHA, but there is a relative consensus that hip arthroplasties performed with any incision less than 10 centimeters can be included. Proponents of MITHA believe that this approach leads to a faster functional recovery, quicker hospital discharge, and increased patient satisfaction. Opponents believe that compared with TTHA, MITHA leads to increased iatrogenic nerve injury, prosthesis malposition, and revision rate, because of the limited field of vision during the surgery [6–8].

During THAs, the position of prosthesis is directly related to the efficacy of the procedure, and malposition of the prosthesis can cause dislocation, impaction, and pain post-operatively. The bony marks can be clearly visualized in TTHA. In contrast, any approach that is taken in MITHA, is plagued by limited surgical vision and inadequate exposure, thus resulting in difficult, and often, a malpositioning of the prosthesis. Hence, in our study, X-ray assessment of the acetabular abduction angle, anteversion, femoral prosthesis positions were generally considered reliable indicators of successful MITHA.

Total hip arthroplasty -related complications can severely compromise the efficacy of the surgery, such as infection, deep vein thrombosis, fracture adjacent to the prosthesis, and dislocation. The commonly seen complications after THA include dislocation (3.9%), pulmonary embolism (0.9%), and deep infection (0.2%) [27]. Woolson et al [7] described a retrospective cohort study of 135 hip arthroplasties and reported that their mini-incision group had a significantly higher risk of wound complications.

Minimally invasive surgeries for THAs can be divided into five categories: posterior, anterolateral (OCM: a modified Watson-Jones approach) [28], lateral and single anterior minimally

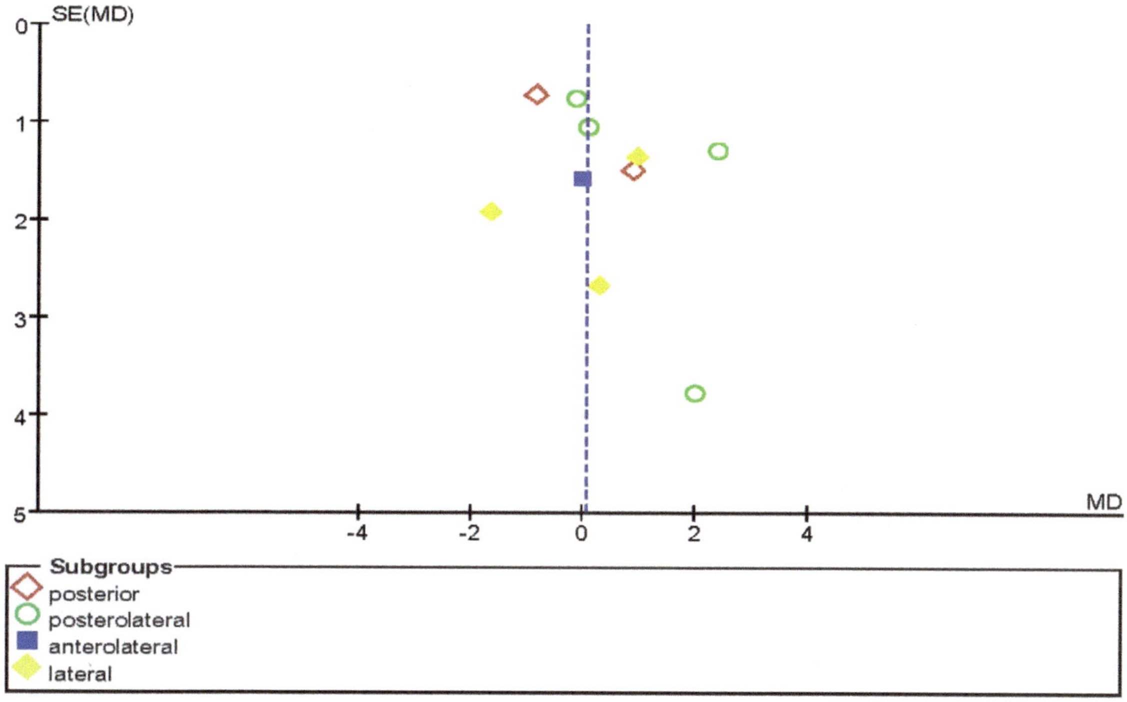

Figure 3. The funnel plot showing the publication bias of the subgroups of different surgical approaches for the most frequently reported outcome—acetabular cup abduction angle. SE (MD) standard error (mean difference).

invasive approach [29], two-incision muscle sparing approach [30] and posterior-lateral minimally invasive approach [31]. Surgical approaches can cause injuries to different soft tissues as they go through different tissue layers. In the past decade, the best surgical approach for THA has been controversially debated. Therefore, previous meta-analyses data of different approaches were not included in our analysis. In contrast, we divided the studies by the surgical approaches to gain a more objective result.

Minimally invasive posterolateral approach

This approach can spare the gluteus medius and the hip flexors. In addition, this approach is a modification of the conventional posterolateral one and is easy for surgeons to master.

In this meta-analysis, no significant differences were found in the acetabular cup abduction angle (p = 0.41), acetabular anteversion (p = 0.96), and femoral prosthesis position (p = 0.83). In addition, there were no significant differences observed with respect to complications. However, one study found that the average femoral offset was significantly increased in the MITHA group (1.6±0.76 cm) than in the TTHA group (1.3±0.81 cm) (WMD = 3.00; 95% CI, 0.40–5.60; p = 0.02). Femoral offset is the distance from the center of rotation of the femoral head to a line bisecting the long axis of the femur. A decrease in the femoral offset moves the femur closer to the pelvis, which can result in impingemen at the extremes of movement. Moving the femur medially results in soft tissue laxity. Both of these problems can cause instability and possible dislocation [32,33]. An increase in

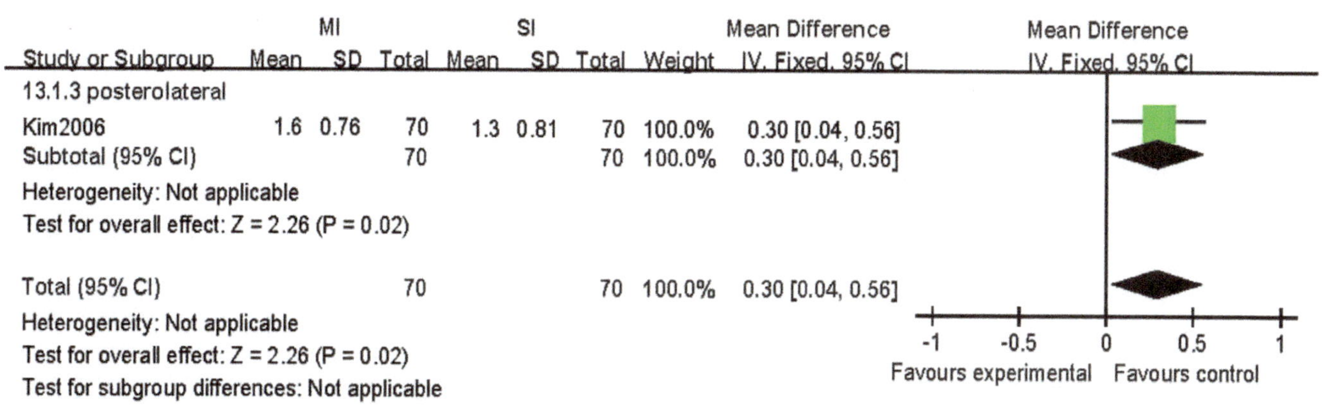

Figure 4. Forest plot of the differences in the increase of post-operative femoral offset in the MITHA and TTHA groups. The MITHA groups had significantly increased femoral offset than the TTHA groups (p = 0.02).

the femoral offset will move the femur laterally and will decrease impingement and improve soft tissue tension resulting in better stability without lengthening of the leg. However, excessive femoral offset can result in unevenly distributed stress, increased micromovement, thus increasing the risk of loose, osteolysis, and synovitis [34,35]. This suggests a posterolateral minimally invasive approach may lead to better hip stability. At the same time, it must be pointed out, this result is only a research report with 140 patients and the results still need to be treated with caution.

Minimally invasive posterior approach

In our meta-analysis, the results showed the radiological outcomes [acetabular cup abduction angle ($p = 0.46$), acetabular anteversion ($p = 0.67$), femoral prosthesis position ($p = 0.25$), femoral offset ($p = 0.16$)] and complications [dislocations ($p = 0.50$), nerve injury ($p = 0.50$), infection ($p = 0.46$), deep vein thrombosis ($p = 0.10$), proximal femoral fracture ($p = 0.73$), revision rate ($p = 0.41$)] were not statistically significant between the two treatments by the posterior approach. The possible reason might be that the posterior approach is well-established and the anatomical structures are well understood. The minimally invasive incision can easily be determined in THA through the posterior approach. Additionally, the correct use of retractors can increase the operation field. Particularly, this approach can clearly expose the medullary cavity of the femur at the proximal end of the incision, and expose the acetabulum side at the distal end of the incision. The long-term effects, however, still need further observation.

Minimally invasive anterolateral and lateral approach

The minimally invasive anterolateral and lateral approach was thought to be difficult to perform as the acetabular cup installation was prone to excessive anteversion and abduction, causing post-operative anterior dislocation [36]. Siguier et al. summarized 1037 cases of total hip replacements performed by the anterolateral approach and concluded that this procedure can best spare the external rotators of the hip, fascia lata, great trochanter, and gluteal muscles, thus minimizing the damage to soft tissues adjacent to the hip and maintaining the balance in soft tissues, without increasing the risk of dislocation.

In our meta-analysis, only the acetabular cup abduction angle ($p = 1.00$) and proximal femoral fracture ($p = 0.16$) were analyzed and no statistical significance was found ($p > 0.05$). However, no adequate data was available to effectively evaluate the acetabular anteversion, femoral prosthesis position, femoral offset, dislocations, nerve injury, infection, deep vein thrombosis, and revisions. Therefore, no positive conclusion can be drawn from the current study until more high-quality randomized controlled studies are available.

The lateral approach also has a relatively lower risk of postoperative dislocation. he acetabulum can be adequately exposed and the prosthesis can be easily implanted. Nevertheless, the major shortcoming of this procedure is that part of the gluteus medius and gluteus minimus is spliced, causing weakness of the abductor, damage to the superior gluteal nerve, ipsilateral post-operative lameness, and increased risk of heterotopic ossification around the hip [37]. In addition, this procedure has poor exposure when manipulating the prosthesis and the retractor often causes severe damage to the skin. In this study, acetabular anteversion, femoral offset, nerve injury, proximal femoral fracture, and revision were not evaluated and therefore the safety profile is not confirmed yet.

Our findings are mainly limited by the quality and the low number of included studies. This limited our assessment of potential publication bias and unpublished research having negative results that cannot be identified. Therefore, publication bias may exist, which could result in the overestimation of the effectiveness of interventions. Third, the methodological quality of the all trials was found to be medium risk of bias. Due to these limitations, the combined results of this meta-analysis should be cautiously accepted, and more independent high-quality RCTs with effectiveness analyses are needed.

Conclusion

Our meta-analysis indicates that the posterior approach in MITHA is a safe surgical procedure, without increased operative complication rates and component malposition rates. The posterolateral approach may lead to increased femoral offset. No thorough conclusion can be drawn from the lateral or anterolateral approach as the risks of adverse effects and complications are increased at the site of prosthesis. It must be pointed out, that this result is only a research report from140 patients and the results need to be treated with caution. More high-quality studies are needed to assess the best surgical approach in minimally invasive hip arthroplasties.

Supporting Information

Table S1 The Cochrane Collaboration's tool for assessing risk of bias.

Table S2 Characteristics of included randomized controlled trials (RCTs).

Table S3 Minimally invasive versus traditional total hip arthroplasty (radiological outcomes).

Table S4 Minimally invasive versus traditional total hip arthroplasty (complications outcomes).

Author Contributions

Conceived and designed the experiments: HL. Performed the experiments: BY. Analyzed the data: XH. Contributed reagents/materials/analysis tools: GW. Wrote the paper: SX.

References

1. Berry DJ, Berger RA, Callaghan JJ, Dorr LD, Duwelius PJ, et al. (2003) Minimally invasive total hip arthroplasty. Development, early results, and a critical analysis. J Bone Joint Surg Am 85-A(11): 2235–2246.
2. Sculco TP, Jordan LC, Walter WL (2004) Minimally invasive total hip arthroplasty : the Hospital for Special Surgery experience. Orthop Clin North Am 35: 137–142.
3. Szendroi M, Sztrinkai G, Vass R, Kiss J (2006) The impact of minimally invasive total hip arthroplasty on the standard procedure. Int Orthop 30: 160–71.
4. Wall SJ, Mears SC (2008) Analysis of published evidence on minimally invasive total hip arthroplasty. J Arthroplasty 23: 55–58.
5. Pagnano MW, Hebl J, Horlocker T (2006) Assuring a painless total hip arthroplasty: a multimodal approach emphasizing peripheral nerve blocks. J Arthroplasty 21: 80–84.
6. Nakamura S, Matsuda K, Arai N, Wakimoto N, Matsushita T (2004) Mini-incision posterior approach for total hip arthroplasty. Int Orthop 28: 214–217.

7. Woolson ST, Mow CS, Syquia JF, Lannin JV, Schurman DJ, et al. (2004) Comparison of primary total hips replacements performed with standard incision or mini-incision. J Bone Joint Surg 86-A: 1353–8.
8. Bradley P, Graw MD, Steven T, Woolson MD, Heather G, et al. (2010) Minimal Incision Surgery as a Risk Factor for Early Failure of Total Hip Arthroplasty. Clin Orthop Relat Res 468: 2372–6.
9. Bennett D, Ogonda L, Elliot D, Humphreys L, Lawlor M, et al. (2007) Comparison of immediate postoperative walking ability in patients receiving minimally invasive and standard-incision hip arthroplasty: a prospective blinded study. J Arthroplasty 22: 490–495.
10. Chimento GF, Pavone V, Sharrock N, Kahn B, Cahill J, et al. (2005) Minimally invasive total hip arthroplasty: a prospective randomized study. J Arthroplasty 20: 139–144.
11. Kim YH (2006) Comparison of primary total hip arthroplasties performed with a minimally invasive technique or a standard technique: a prospective and randomized study. J Arthroplasty 21: 1092–1098.
12. Ogonda L, Wilson R, Archbold P, Lawlor M, Humphreys P, et al. (2005) A minimal-incision technique in total hip arthroplasty does not improve early postoperative outcomes: a prospective, randomized, controlled trial. J Bone Joint Surg Am 87: 701–710.
13. Cheng T, Feng JG, Liu T, Zhang XL (2009) Minimally invasive total hip arthroplasty: a systematic review. Int Orthop 33: 1473–1481.
14. Smith TO, Blake V, Hing CB (2011) Minimally invasive versus conventional exposure for total hip arthroplasty: a systematic review and meta-analysis of clinical and radiological outcomes. Int Orthop 35: 173–184.
15. Khan RJ (2011) Comments on Smith et al: Comments on Smith et al.: minimally invasive versus conventional exposure for total hip arthroplasty: a systematic review and meta-analysis of clinical and radiological outcomes. Int Orthop 35: 299.
16. Higgins J, Green S (2008) Cochrane Handbook for Systematic Reviews of Interventions Version 5.0.0. The Cochrane Collaboration. Available from www.cochrane-handbook.org.
17. Moher D, Cook DJ, Eastwood S, Olkin I, Rennie D, et al. (1999) Improving the quality of reports of meta-analyses of randomized controlled trials: the QUOROM statement. Quality of reporting of meta-analyses. Lancet 354: 1896.
18. Shitama T, Kiyama T, Naito M, Shiramizu K, Huang G, et al. (2009) Which is more invasive-mini versus standard incisions in total hip arthroplasty? Int Orthop 33: 1543–1547.
19. Varela-Egocheaga J R, Suárez-Suárez M A, Fernandez-Villan M (2010) Minimally invasive lateral approach in total hip replacement: a prospective randomised study. Rev Esp Cir Ortop Traumatol 54: 27–33.
20. Mazoochian F, Weber P, Schramm S, Utzschneider S, Fottner A, et al. (2009) Minimally invasive total hip arthroplasty: a randomized controlled prospective trial. Arch Orthop Trauma Surg 129: 1633–1639.
21. Wohlrab D, Droege JW, Mendel T, Brehme K, Riedl K, et al. (2008) Minimally invasive vs. transgluteal total hip replacement. A 3-month follow-up of a prospective randomized clinical study. Orthopäde 37: 1121–1126.
22. Dorr LD, Maheshwari AV, Long WT, Wan Z, Sirianni LE, et al. (2007) Early pain relief and function after posterior minimally invasive and conventional total hip arthroplasty. A prospective, randomized, blinded study. J Bone Joint Surg Am 89: 1153–1160.
23. Goosen JH, Kollen BJ, Castelein RM, Kuipers BM, Verheyen CC, et al. (2011) Minimally invasive versus classic procedures in total hiparthroplasty: a double-blind randomized controlled trial. Clin Orthop Relat Res 469: 200–208.
24. Roy L, Laflamme GY, Carrier M, Kim PR, Leduc S (2010) A randomised clinical trial comparingminimally invasive surgery to conventional approach for endoprosthesis in elderly patients with hip fractures. Injury 41: 365–369.
25. Hart R, Stipcák V, Janecek M, Visna P (2005) Component position following total hip arthroplasty through a miniinvasive posterolateral approach. Acta Orthop Belg 71: 60–64.
26. Yang YH, Gao ZL, Wang JC (2008) Mini—incision Total Hip Replacement for Femoral Neck Fracture in Senile Patients. Chinese Journal of bone and joint injury 23: 110–112.
27. Phillips CB, Barrett JA, Losina E, Mahomed NN, Lingard EA, et al. (2003) Incidence rates of dislocation, pulmonary embolism, and deep infection during the first six months after elective total hip replacement. J Bone Joint Surg (Am) 85: 20–26.
28. Bertin KC, Röttinger H (2004) Anterolateral mini-incision hip replacement surgery: a modified Watson-Jones approach. Clin Orthop Relat Res 429: 248–255.
29. Siguier T, Siguier M, Brumpt B (2004) Mini-incision anterior approach does not increase dislocation rate: a study of 1037 total hip replacements. Clin Orthop Relat Res 426: 164–173.
30. Berger RA (2004) The technique of minimally invasive total hip arthroplasty using the two-incision approach. Instr Course Lect 53: 149–155.
31. Goldstein WM, Branson JJ (2004) Posterior-lateral approach to minimal incision total hip arthroplasty. Orthop Clin North Am 35: 131–136.
32. Morrey BF (1997) Dificult complications after hip replacem. Clin Orthop 344: 179–187.
33. Dorr LD, Wan Z (1998) Causes of and treatment protocol for instability of total hip replacement. Clin Orthop Relat Res 355: 14–51.
34. Cannestra VP, Berger RA, Quigley LR, Jacobs JJ, Rosenberg AG, et al. (2000) Total hip arthroplasty with a precoated ofset stem. Four to nine—year results. J Bone Joint Surg Am 82: 1291–9.
35. Kleemann RU, Heller MO, Stoeckle U, Taylor WR, Duda GN (2003) THA loading arising from increased femoral an terversion and ofset may lead to critical cement stresses. Onhop Res 21: 767–774.
36. Yang CF, Zhang DW, Niu S, Kong LZ, Zhu JY, et al. (2009) Curative Effect of Minimally-invasive Total Hip Arthroplasty. Chinese Journal of bone and joint injury 24: 385–388.
37. Archibeck MJ, Berger RA, Jacobs JJ, Quigley LR, Gitelis S, et al. (2001) Second-generation cementless total.hip arthroplasty. Eight to eleven- year results 83: 1666–1673.

2

Postoperative Admission to a Dedicated Geriatric Unit Decreases Mortality in Elderly Patients with Hip Fracture

Jacques Boddaert[1,2]*¶, Judith Cohen-Bittan[1], Frédéric Khiami[3], Yannick Le Manach[4], Mathieu Raux[1,5,8], Jean-Yves Beinis[6], Marc Verny[1,2], Bruno Riou[1,7,8]

1 Université Pierre et Marie Curie (UMRS 956, UMRS 1158), Paris, France, **2** Department of Geriatrics, Groupe hospitalier (GH) Pitié-Salpêtrière, Assistance Publique Hôpitaux de Paris (APHP), Paris, France, **3** Department of Orthopedic Surgery and Trauma, GH Pitié-Salpêtrière, APHP, Paris, France, **4** Departments of Anesthesia & Clinical Epidemiology and Biostatistics, Michael DeGroote School of Medicine, Faculty of Health Sciences, McMaster University, Hamilton, Ontario, Canada, **5** Department of Anesthesiology and Critical Care, GH Pitié-Salpêtrière, APHP, Paris, France, **6** Department of Rehabilitation, Groupe Hospitalier Charles Foix, APHP, Ivry-sur-Seine, France, **7** Department of Emergency Medicine and Surgery, GH Pitié-Salpêtrière, APHP, Paris, France, **8** Institut national de la santé et de la recherche médicale (UMRS 956, UMRS 1158, UMR 689), Paris, France

Abstract

Background: Elderly patients with hip fracture have a 5 to 8 fold increased risk of death during the months following surgery. We tested the hypothesis that early geriatric management of these patients focused on co-morbidities and rehabilitation improved long term mortality.

Methods and Findings: In a cohort study over a 6 year period, we compared patients aged >70 years with hip fracture admitted to orthopedic versus geriatric departments in a time series analysis corresponding to the creation of a dedicated geriatric unit. Co-morbidities were assessed using the Cumulative Illness Rating Scale (CIRS). Each cohort was compared to matched cohorts extracted from a national registry (n = 51,275) to validate the observed results. Main outcome measure was 6-month mortality. We included 131 patients in the orthopedic cohort and 203 in the geriatric cohort. Co-morbidities were more frequent in the geriatric cohort (median CIRS: 8 vs 5, $P<0.001$). In the geriatric cohort, the proportion of patients who never walked again decreased (6% versus 22%, $P<0.001$). At 6 months, re-admission (14% versus 29%, $P = 0.007$) and mortality (15% versus 24%, $P = 0.04$) were decreased. When co-morbidities were taken into account, the risk ratio of death at 6 months was reduced (0·43, 95%CI 0·25 to 0·73, $P = 0.002$). Using matched cohorts, the average treatment effects on the treated associated to early geriatric management indicated a reduction in hospital mortality (−63%; 95% CI: −92% to −6%, $P = 0.006$).

Conclusions: Early admission to a dedicated geriatric unit improved 6-month mortality and morbidity in elderly patients with hip fracture.

Editor: Darwin Ang, University of South Florida, United States of America

Funding: All authors declare that no authors have support from any company for the submitted work; no authors have relationships with any company that might have an interest in the submitted work in the previous 3 years; their spouses, partners, or children have do not have any financial relationships that may be relevant to the submitted work; and no authors have any-financial interests that may be relevant to the submitted work.

Competing Interests: The authors have declared that no competing interests exist.

* E-mail: jacques.boddaert@psl.aphp.fr

¶ Pr J. Boddaert is the designated author signing on behalf of all co-authors of the contribution.

Introduction

Worldwide 1.6 million patients suffer a hip fracture each year [1] and as the population continues to age this figure has increased by 25% each decade [2]. In the elderly patient hip fracture has devastating consequences. The hospital mortality of the condition ranges from 2.3% to 13.9% [3–7], with patients discharged home having a 5 to 8 fold increased risk of death in the months immediately following surgery [8]. This risk persists well beyond the immediate surgical period with 6 month mortality rates ranging from 12 to 23 % [7,9–12], and it is estimated that hip fractures account for more than 1.5% of all deaths in patients aged 50 years or more [13].

When compared to elective total hip replacements, patients presenting with hip fracture have a 6 to 15 fold mortality risk [14]. This can largely be explained by the high prevalence of pre-existing medical conditions seen in this population: 75% of patients are older than 70 years [1], and 95% of them present with at least one major preoperative comorbidity [15]. However studies suggest that only 1 in 4 of hip fracture associated deaths may be causally related to the fracture itself rather than due to pre-existing medical conditions [13]. This suggests that the insult of the hip fracture destabilizes an elderly population with a high burden of pre-existing morbidities thereby resulting in excess mortality.

Despite the magnitude of this problem there are no established effective strategies to prevent mortality after hip fracture. Approaches that combine both orthopedic and geriatric management have been studied but these have provided conflicting results

[16–20] and few studies report an improvement in short and long term clinical outcomes [21].

To address this significant public health problem, we formed a multi-disciplinary management team and created a dedicated care unit with the aim of providing integrated postoperative orthopedic and geriatric care for elderly patients with hip fracture. We hypothesized that the provision of early care with specific management of these patients focused on co-morbidity management and rehabilitation would significantly impact long term mortality. To evaluate the impact of this strategy we conducted an interrupted time series study. In addition, we used a national registry to provide external validation of our results.

Methods

Ethics statement

Our hospital ethics committee (CPP Ile de France VI, Paris, France) approved this study and authorized waived informed consent since the study was observational. The database was declared to the French National Commission on Computing and Liberty (CNIL, Paris, France).

Patients

From September 2005 to March 2012 all consecutive patients admitted to our Emergency Department (ED) were evaluated for eligibility. Patients were included if their primary presentation was due to hip fracture and if they were ≥70 years of age. Patients were excluded if they presented with multiple fractures, a metastatic fracture, a fracture complicated by a previous hip prosthesis or osteosynthesis, if they had been transferred to another hospital before surgery, or were already hospitalized at the time of diagnosis.

Intervention

In June 2009, we created a new geriatric unit (Unit for Post-Operative Geriatric Care, UPOG) devoted to the post-operative care of elderly patients with hip fracture. Before its opening, the medical staff from the emergency, anesthesiology and critical care, geriatric, orthopedic surgery, and rehabilitation departments met to define priorities for patients who would be admitted. Four key factors were identified: (1) early alert from the ED; (2) consideration of hip fracture as an emergency case requiring emergency surgery as soon as feasible (*i.e.* 24 hours a day); (3) rapid transfer to the UPOG after surgery (<48 h); and (4) rapid transfer of stable patients to a dedicated rehabilitation unit. Management strategy focused on early mobilization -with the aim of chair-sitting and walking (first steps) within 24 and 48 hours after arrival respectively, pain management -using acetaminophen and morphine, the provision of air-filled mattresses for patients with pressure ulcers or a high risk of pressure ulcers as evaluated by the Braden scale [22], swallowing disorders detected using a systematic medical survey, detection of stool impaction and urinary retention using ultrasound, the presence of anemia and liberal transfusion of packed red blood cells (usually when the hemoglobin level was <10 g.L^{-1}), detection of delirium using the Confusion Assessment Method [23], and malnutrition detection and management in conjunction with a nutritionist. All skills are regrouped in the same ward, allowing a common plan of care for all patients, implicating physicians, nurses, physiotherapists, speech therapist and nutritionist.

Data collection

Data were collected from computerized ED medical charts (instituted September 1st, 2005) and from hand-written medical charts of other departments. Since the opening of the UPOG in June 2009, data were prospectively entered in the database. The following variables were collected: age, sex, home or nursing home living conditions, walking ability, previous medical history, type of fracture and surgical treatment, delay and duration of surgery. Co-morbidity severity was assessed using the Cumulative Illness Rating Scale (CIRS) in which co-occurring medical conditions are weighted from 0 to 4 in 13 main systems [24]. We recorded the preoperative hemoglobin level and its lowest value during the acute care period. Anemia was defined following WHO guidelines [25]. We measured serum creatinine and estimated creatinine clearance [26]. All complications during the acute care period were recorded including delirium, need for physical restraints, stool impaction, urinary retention requiring drainage, morphine administration, pressure ulcer, infection, thromboembolic event, need for blood transfusion, aspiration related to swallowing disorders, cardiac insufficiency (*i.e.* acute cardiac failure or acute pulmonary edema), and admission into an intensive care unit (ICU).

Patients were followed until death or 6 months after admission. Surviving patients or their family were contacted and interviewed by telephone. Missing patients were tracked through health care providers, particularly general practitioners, or any identified acquaintances.

Study cohort

We compared the intervention cohort of patients admitted to the UPOG (*geriatric cohort*) to a control cohort of patients admitted to the orthopedic surgery department (*orthopedic cohort*). All patients transferred >48 h after surgery to the UPOG were assigned to the orthopedic cohort. After the opening of the UPOG, the proportion of patients admitted to the orthopedic department rapidly decreased as did the proportion of transfers to other hospitals (Figure 1), providing a nearly perfect time series analysis [27]. There was no selection of the patients admitted into the UPOG. Nevertheless, before the opening of the UPOG, a selection of patients admitted to the orthopedic department (versus transfer) was very likely. Thus it was expected that the co-morbidities of the cohorts may differ, the patients in the orthopedic cohort being expected to be less severe.

External validation cohort

We identified all patients admitted to French private or public health institutions in 2010 (n = 7,051,113) (See Table S1 in File S1). To create a hip fracture validation cohort we identified all patients undergoing surgery for hip/femur fracture related to a recent trauma, and then excluded patients <70 years of age and those from our institution. We then extracted patient age, sex, length of acute care stay and presence of pre-existing medical conditions (See Table S2 in File S1) and in-hospital mortality.

End points

The primary end point was 6-month mortality. The main secondary endpoints were re-hospitalization, re-fracture, new admission into a nursing home, and ability to walk 6 months after admission. We also considered length of stay and mortality while in acute care and rehabilitation facilities, admission into an ICU, delay to first sitting and first walking, and the ability to walk after the acute care and/or rehabilitation period. For the comparison with the external national validation cohort, only hospital mortality was available and this was used as the primary endpoint.

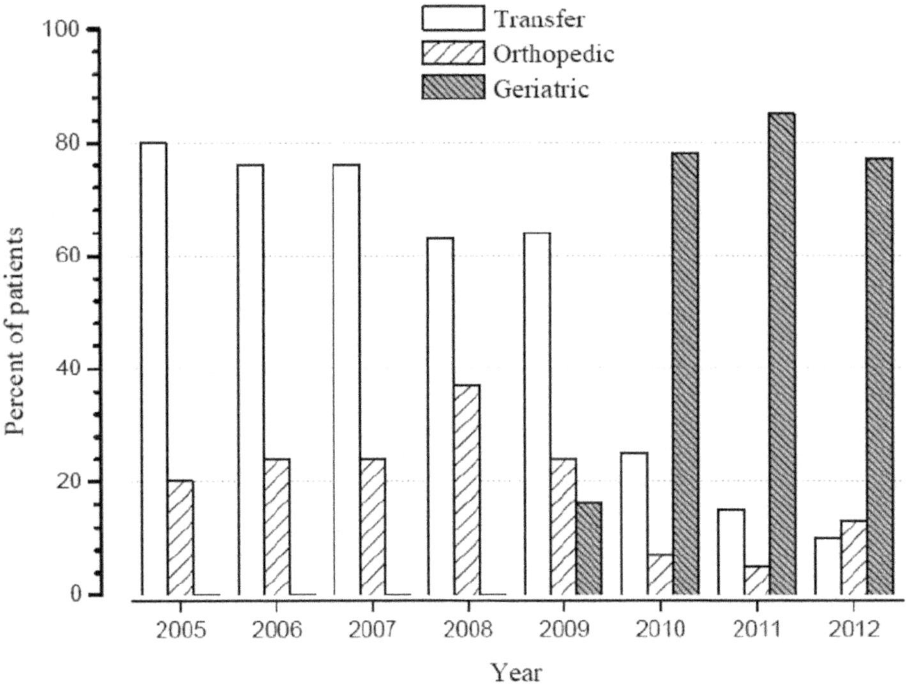

Figure 1. Transfers and allocation of patients. Evolution of transfers out of the hospital (n = 392) and allocation to the orthopedic (n = 131) and geriatric (n = 203) cohorts during the study period. There were only 4 months (September to December) in 2005 and 3 months (January to March) in 2012.

Sample size calculation

Assuming a baseline 6 month mortality rate of 20% [7] and a mortality reduction of 40% (*i.e.* from 20% to 12%) in the geriatric cohort, we estimated that we would require 298 patients to obtain a 80% power with a two-tailed *P* value of 0·05. This estimation hypothesized a weak relationship between the predictors of the primary endpoint and the strategy tested, which was sustained by the design of the study and by the absence of major change in the recruitment of these patients. A study period of at least 30 months after the opening of the UPOG was planned.

Statistical analysis

Data are presented as mean ± SD, median [25–75 interquartile] for non-Gaussian variables, or number (percentages). Comparison between cohorts was performed using the unpaired Student t test, Mann-Whitney test, Fisher's exact method, and multivariate analysis of variance when appropriate. Survival was estimated by the Kaplan-Meier method and differences were assessed by the log-rank test. In a preliminary analysis (n = 100) using a multivariate Cox proportional-hazards model we determined that three variables (age, sex, CIRS) were associated with 6-month mortality. We tested the impact of the intervention by calculating the hazard ratio and its 95 percent confidence interval (CI) in association with these prognostic variables.

To provide external validation all patients in the geriatric and orthopedic cohorts were matched with patients drawn from the external national validation cohort. Logistic models using all variables specified in Table S2 in File S1 were developed to determine the probabilities to be in the geriatric or in the orthopedic cohorts. These probabilities (*i.e.* propensity scores) were used to match the patients of the geriatric cohort and those of the orthopedic cohort to patients from the national cohort. Matching was performed using a nearest neighbor matching method with a caliper of 20% of the *logit* of these probabilities. Each patient from the geriatric and orthopedic cohorts was matched to 3 patients from the national cohort using this probability [28]. The absolute standardized difference (ASD) was used to assess balance between the groups. An ASD above 10 to 15% is considered to represent meaningful imbalance [29]. The average treatment effect on the treated (ATT) was estimated in these two cohorts, which represents the average impact of the care program among those who have been exposed to it, was estimated in these two cohorts. We also conducted a sensitivity analysis without caliper use.

All P values were two-sided and P<0.05 was considered significant. R 2.14 software (www.cran.r-project.org last date accessed February 2, 2013) was used for statistical analyses.

Results

Among the 726 elderly patients with hip fracture admitted to the ED, 334 were selected, 131 in the orthopedic cohort and 203 in the geriatric cohort (Figure 2). Only 3 patients were transferred to UPOG more than 48 hours after surgery and so were assigned to the orthopedic cohort.

Patients from the two cohorts differed slightly in the prevalence of co-morbidities and the proportion who received gamma nail and dynamic screw fixation (Table 1). Patients in the geriatric cohort underwent surgery 1 hour before the orthopedic cohort, a clinically insignificant difference but the proportion of patients delayed for >48 h did not. Surgery duration was shorter in the geriatric cohort, probably as a result of the higher proportion of gamma nails (effect of surgical treatment: F = 11.92, $P<0{\cdot}001$; effect of cohort: F = 0·09, $P = 0{\cdot}78$) (Table 1). The observed difference in surgery duration (10 min) was not considered to be clinically relevant.

During the acute care period, patients in the geriatric cohort received more morphine, less physical restraint, were transfused

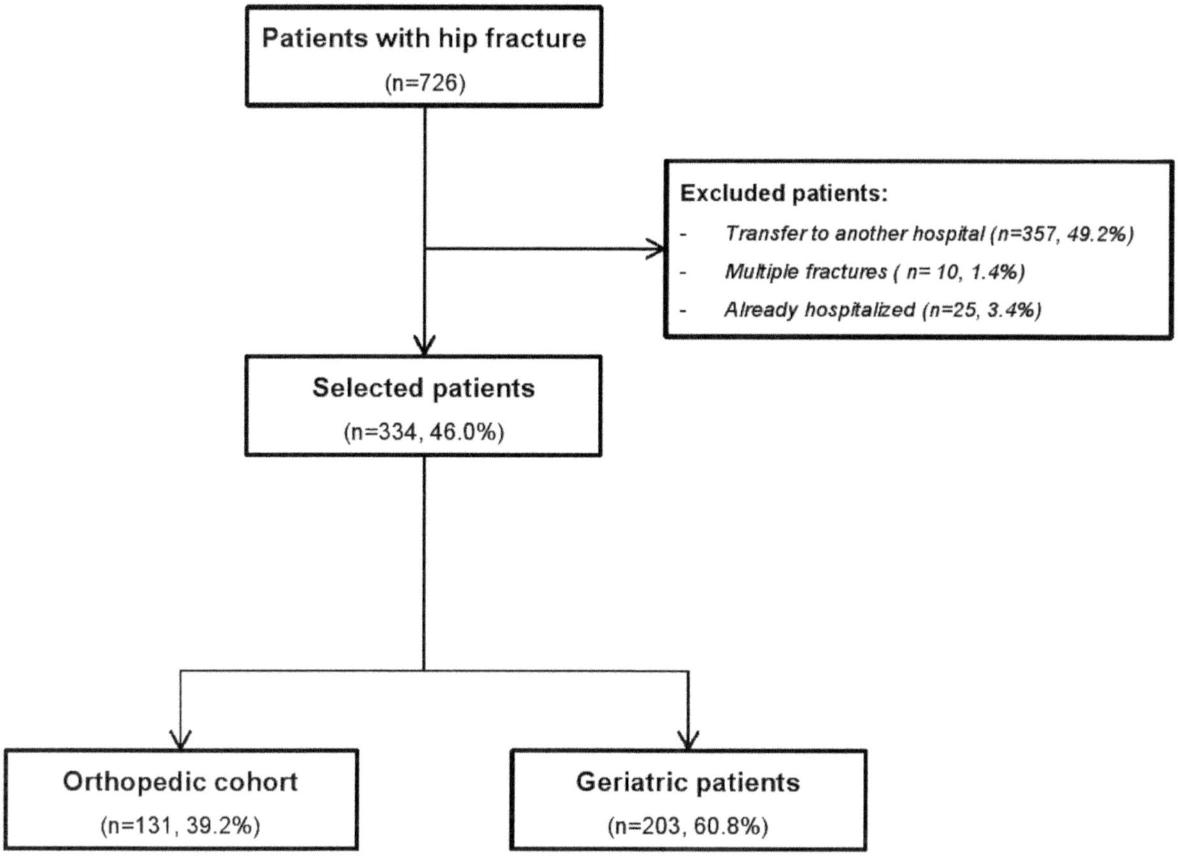

Figure 2. Study flow chart.

more frequently, and were diagnosed with stool impaction and swallowing disorders more frequently. They were less frequently admitted into an ICU and suffered fewer pressure ulcers. However episodes of cardiac insufficiency occurred more frequently. Patients in the geriatric cohort had a markedly reduced time to first sitting and first walking, a much shorter stay in acute care, and a greater proportion of walking patients at the end of the intervention period (Table 2).

Only 3 (0.9%) patients were lost to follow-up, 2 in the geriatric cohort and 1 in the orthopedic cohort (all due to transfer to foreign countries). During the follow up period, both mortality and re-hospitalization risks were significantly reduced in the geriatric cohort (Figure 3). When taking into account age, sex, and co-morbidities (using the CIRS), patients in the geriatric cohort showed a profound reduction in both risks of mortality and re-hospitalization. No significant difference was observed for the risk of re-fracture or new admission to a nursing home (Table 3).

In the unmatched cohorts, hospital mortality was 7.6 % in the orthopedic cohort (n = 131), 3·0 % in the geriatric cohort (n = 203), and 3.9 % in the external national validation cohort (n = 51,275) but large imbalances were observed between these cohorts (See Table S2 in File S1). After matching, the highest ASD was 9.8% in the geriatric cohort (23 discarded patients) and 13.5% in the orthopedic cohort (18 discarded patients). In the matched populations, hospital mortality was significantly lower in the geriatric cohort compared to the external national validation cohort (2.5% versus 5.4%, log rank test P = 0·04), but not significantly different in the orthopedic cohort (6.3% versus 5.4%, log rank test P = 0.72) (Figure 4). The relative ATT associated to the geriatric cohort indicated a significant reduction in mortality (−63%; 95% CI: −92% to −6%; *P* = 0.006) whereas the relative ATT associated with the orthopedic cohort was not significantly different from zero (32%; 95% CI: −2 to +67%; *P* = 0.57).

In the matching procedure conducted without calipers (*i.e.*, no discarded patients in geriatric and orthopedic cohorts) the population characteristics were not similar with most variables showing an AST>15%. However the relative ATT was −70% (95%CI: −98% to −3%; P<0.001) in the matched geriatric cohort and 51% (95%CI: −12% to 111%; P = 0.83) in the matched orthopedic cohort.

Lastly, we compared the key management factors previously identified (*vide supra*) between patients who were alive at 6 month and those who died. There was no significant difference between groups swallowing disorders (19 vs 26%, P = 0.20), physical restraint (5 vs 10%, P = 0.12), stool impaction (31 vs 39%, P = 0.28), morphine administration (59 vs 62%, P = 0.65), blood transfusion (62 vs 74 %, P = 0.08), and delay for surgery (22 [13–34] vs 23 [15–44] hours, P = 0.23). In contrast, we observed significant differences in pressure ulcers (16 vs 28 %, P = 0.037), delirium (33 vs 61 %, P<0.001), urinary retention (23 vs 37 %, P = 0.04), delay to first sitting (2 [1–3] vs 2 [1–5] days, P = 0.015), delay to first walking (3 [1–5] vs 5 [2–8] days, P<0.001), and proportion of patients who never walked (3 vs 52 %, P<0.001).

Discussion

In this study, we observed that elderly patients with hip fracture, admitted early into a dedicated geriatric unit and managed with a

Table 1. Comparison of the main characteristics of the two study cohorts.

	Orthopedic cohort	Geriatric cohort	All patients
	(n = 131)	(n = 203)	(n = 334)
Age (years)	85±6	86±6	86±6
Male	44 (34)	50 (25)	94 (28)
Medical history			
Obesity[a]	3 (2)	20 (10)	23 (7)
Dementia	32 (24)	78 (38)*	110 (33)
Diabetes	16 (12)	27 (13)	43 (13)
Hypertension	74 (56)	138 (68)*	212 (63)
Cardiac failure	18 (14)	33 (16)	51 (15)
Coronary artery disease	22 (17)	27 (13)	49 (15)
Heart valve disease	9 (7)	17 (8)	26 (8)
Atrial fibrillation	28 (21)	47 (23)	75 (22)
Peripheral vascular disease	5 (4)	12 (6)	17(5)
Stroke	17 (13)	33 (16)	50 (15)
Hemiplegia/paraglegia	1 (1)	8 (4)	9 (3)
Cancer	24 (18)	37 (18)	61 (18)
COPD	10 (8)	15 (7)	25 (7)
Pulmonary hypertension	0 (0)	2 (1)	2(1)
Alcohol abuse	2 (2)	10 (5)	12 (4)
Chronic renal insufficiency	16 (12)	31 (15)	47 (14)
Creatinine clearance ($ml.min^{-1}$)[b]	53±25	53±22	53±23
CIRS 52	5 [3–8]	8 [6–11]	7[4–10]
Hemoglobin ($g.dL^{-1}$)	12.0±1.8	12.1±1.4	12.1±1.5
Anemia	70 (53)	98 (48)	168 (50)
Living status			
Living at home	117 (89)	182 (90)	299 (90)
Living in institution	14 (11)	21 (10)	35 (10)
Unknown	0	0	0
Live alone	42 (37)	28 (14)*	70 (21)
Unknown	19	0	19
Walking ability			
No walking disability	118 (90)	187 (92)	305 (91)
Moderate walking disability	11 (8)	14 (7)	25 (7)
Does not walk	2 (2)	2 (1)	4 (1)
Unknown	0	0	0
Fracture			
Femoral neck fracture	59 (45)	112 (55)	171 (51)
Intertrochanteric fracture	72 (55)	91 (45)	163 (49)
Surgery			
Delay to surgery (h)	23 [15–40]	22 [12–34]	22 [14–35]
Delay to surgery >48 h	25 (19)	26 (13)	51 (15)
Duration of surgery (min)	150 [120–175]	140 [110–160]*	140 [120–170]
Gamma nail	33 (25)	102 (50)*	135 (40)
Dynamic hip screw	39 (30)	24 (12)*	63 (19)
Unipolar prosthesis	52 (40)	70 (34)	122 (36)
Bipolar prosthesis	7 (5)	7 (3)	14 (4)

Data are mean ± SD, median [25–75 interquartile], or number (percentage). COPD: chronic obstructive pulmonary disease; CIRS: cumulative illness rating scale;
[a]: defined as body mass index >30 $kg.m^{-2}$;
[b]: creatinine clearance could be calculated in 99 (76%) and 200 (98%) patients in the orthopedic and geriatric cohorts respectively.
*: $P<0.05$ vs Orthopedic cohort.

Table 2. Acute care, rehabilitation, and walking ability.

	Orthopedic cohort (n = 131)	Geriatric cohort (n = 203)	P value
Delay to first sitting (days)	3 [2–4]	1 [1–2]	<0.001
Delay to first walking (days)	5 [3–9]	2 [1–4]	<0.001
Walking initially contra-indicated	8 (6)	9 (4)	0.61
Acute care complications			
Delirium	49/118 (41)	72/203 (35)	0.29
Physical restraint	18/121 (15)	1/203 (0.5)	<0.001
Morphine administration	37/116 (32)	152/203 (75)	<0.001
Swallowing disorders	8/120 (7)	56/203 (28)	<0.001
Lowest hemoglobin (g.dL^{-1})	9.3±1.7	9.2±1.3	0.54
Blood transfusion	72/131 (55)	141/203 (69)	0.008
Stool impaction	23/120 (19)	83/203 (41)	<0.001
Urinary retention	26/120 (22)	57/203 (28)	0.24
Pressure ulcer	40/121 (33)	18/203 (9)	<0.001
Acute heart failure	6/120 (5)	33/203 (16)	0.002
Infection	31/123 (25)	40/203 (20)	0.27
Venous thromboembolism	1/122 (1)	10/203 (5)	0.06
Fall	9/120 (7)	9/203 (4)	0.32
Admission into ICU	17/131 (13)	8/203 (4)	0.005
LOS acute care (days)	13 [10–20]	11 [8–16]	0.001
Admission to rehabilitation care[a]	91/121 (75)	167/197 (85)	0.04
LOS rehabilitation care (days)	41 [25–71]	42 [30–62]	0.78
Total LOS (acute and rehabilitation care) (days)	43 [22–70]	49 [30–68]	0.41
Death during acute care	10/131 (8)	6/203 (3)	0.07
Death during rehabilitation	10/91 (11)	14/166 (8)	0.51
Death during acute care and/or rehabilitation	20/130 (15)	20/202 (10)	0.17
Return to home[b]	92/129 (71)	149/202 (74)	0.70
New admission into nursing home[c]	14/97 (14)	25/163 (15)	1.00
Unknown	2	1	
Readmission within 30 days[d]	19/111 (17)	10/183 (5)	0.002
Redo surgery within 30 days	6/130 (5)	3/201 (1)	0.16
Unknown	2	1	
Walking ability			
After acute care/rehabilitation			
No walking disability	41/111 (37)	88/182 (48)	0.07
Moderate walking disability	55/111 (50)	88/182 (48)	0.90
Does not walk	15/111 (14)	6/182 (3)	0.002
Missing data	0	1	
After 6 months			
No walking disability	33/99 (33)	57/172 (33)	1.00
Moderate walking disability	56/99 (57)	107/172 (62)	0.37
Does not walk	10/99 (10)	8/172 (5)	0.13
Missing data	1	2	
Never walked	29/131 (22)	12/203 (6)	<0.001

Data are mean ± SD, median [25–75 interquartile], or number (percentage). LOS: length of stay; ICU: intensive care unit;
[a]: excluding death during acute care;
[b]: institution was considered as "home" in patients previously living in an institution;
[c]: excluding patients previously living in an institution;
[d]: excluding patients who died in acute care and/or rehabilitation.

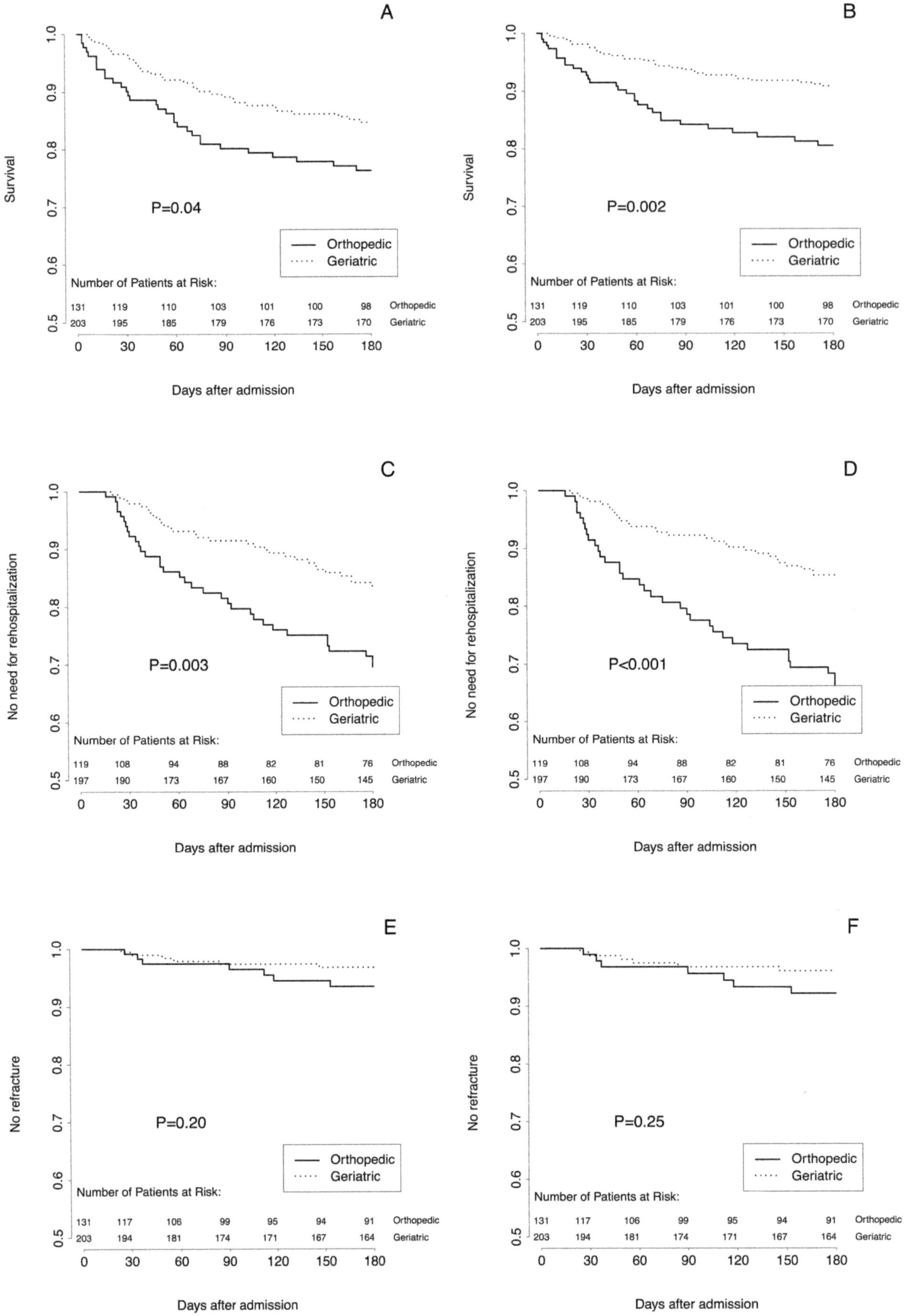
A
Survival
P=0.04
Orthopedic
Geriatric
Number of Patients at Risk:
131 119 110 103 101 100 98 Orthopedic
203 195 185 179 176 173 170 Geriatric
Days after admission
B
Survival
P=0.002
Orthopedic
Geriatric
Number of Patients at Risk:
131 119 110 103 101 100 98 Orthopedic
203 195 185 179 176 173 170 Geriatric
Days after admission
C
No need for rehospitalization
P=0.003
Orthopedic
Geriatric
Number of Patients at Risk:
119 108 94 88 82 81 76 Orthopedic
197 190 173 167 160 150 145 Geriatric
Days after admission
D
No need for rehospitalization
P<0.001
Orthopedic
Geriatric
Number of Patients at Risk:
119 108 94 88 82 81 76 Orthopedic
197 190 173 167 160 150 145 Geriatric
Days after admission
E
No refracture
P=0.20
Orthopedic
Geriatric
Number of Patients at Risk:
131 117 106 99 95 94 91 Orthopedic
203 194 181 174 171 167 164 Geriatric
Days after admission
F
No refracture
P=0.25
Orthopedic
Geriatric
Number of Patients at Risk:
131 117 106 99 95 94 91 Orthopedic
203 194 181 174 171 167 164 Geriatric
Days after admission

Figure 3. Survival curves for mortality, re-hospitalization, and re-fracture. Survival curves for mortality, re-hospitalization, and re-fracture for patients in the orthopedic (solid lines) and geriatric (dotted line) cohorts. Survival is non-adjusted (panels A, C, and E) and adjusted (panels B, D, and F) for age, sex and Cumulative Illness Rating Scale (CIRS) calculated with a Cox regression analysis. For re-hospitalization and re-fracture, death was considered as a censored observation. *P* values refer to log-rank test.

multidisciplinary approach, had reduced long term mortality and improved walking ability. These observations were externally validated against a matched cohorts derived from a national hospital database.

Various approaches have been taken to integrate orthopedic and geriatric care, also known collectively as orthogeriatrics, for hip fracture patients. As in our study, some of these measures have included admission into a geriatric ward under the specialist care of an orthopedic consultant [16,17]. However, no previous studies have demonstrated a clear mortality benefit with this approach. Alternative approaches have included using an orthopedic ward with geriatric consultation [30], or an orthopedic ward with daily geriatric management [31–33]. When these approaches have shown mortality reduction, it was transient or without reduction in detailed patient morbidity. To our knowledge, this is the first orthogeriatric study that has shown sustained mortality reduction, together with improved walking ability and less morbidity.

We observed a marked reduction (risk ratio 0.43) in the risk of death at 6 months (Table 3). This treatment effect is approximately twice that observed in randomized trials conducted to demonstrate the benefit of early surgery in hip fracture patients [34]. In the geriatric cohort we observed a significant reduction in the length of stay in acute care facilities, but this was not observed when taking into account the rehabilitation period. We believe that some patients in the orthopedic cohort may have been discharged prematurely and that this may at least partially explain the higher proportion of readmitted patients. However, we cannot rule out the possibility that these differences may be due to the lower number of co-morbidities in the orthopedic cohort. When comparing patients who survived at 6 months and those who did not, it seems that early sitting and walking, prevention of pressure ulcer, early identification of urinary retention and delirium, may be the most important management factors associated with survival improvement. Irrespective of the reasons behind this difference our results emphasize the role played by the rehabilitation facilities as well as the importance of the cooperation between acute care and rehabilitation facilities.

Despite considering geriatric hip fracture as an emergency requiring surgery as soon as feasible (i.e. 24 hours a day) [34,35], we were unable to observe any significant reductions in the time delay until surgery (Table 1). However, in both cohorts, the proportion of patients with delayed surgery was lower than that reported in previous studies [19,30,35], suggesting that this goal had already been appropriately implemented in our hospital. Moreover, surgery must sometimes be postponed in some patients due to their pre-existing conditions, including drugs that interfere with hemostasis. The delays to surgery reported in previous orthogeriatric studies were usually longer [19,30,35].

Some events in the geriatric cohort such as stool impaction, swallowing disorders, venous thromboembolism, and acute heart failure were more frequently reported. Although these differences may be due to the retrospective recording of data in the orthopedic cohort, we believe that they were detected more frequently in the UPOG due to improved surveillance. Swallowing disorders are a strong risk factor for the development of aspiration pneumonia, and their detection has led to food consistency being thickened and heightened pneumonia surveillance. Despite this we did not observe a significant difference in infection rates. Stool impaction represents a source of discomfort for patients, with increased risk of urinary retention, which may delay rehabilitation and result in life-threatening complications [35]. We cannot rule out the hypothesis that increased morphine consumption in the geriatric cohort may have lead to higher rates of stool impaction. Improved surveillance probably explains the increased venous thromboembolism detection while the increased incidence of acute heart failure could be related either to better clinical detection or intolerance to blood transfusion. However, these differences probably had a limited influence on outcome.

Patients in the geriatric cohort received more blood transfusions and this is explained by our strict adherence to French national transfusion guidelines [36]. These recommend maintaining a hemoglobin >10 g/dL in geriatric patients who are unable to tolerate anemia. This goal was modified in 2011 after Carson et al. [37] showed no benefit of a liberal transfusion regimen as compared to a restrictive one.

Our study has several limitations. First, it was an observational study and the orthopedic cohort data were collected retrospectively. However, we validated our results externally against matched cohorts derived from a national hospital database, used mortality as our primary endpoint, and successfully followed-up

Table 3. Multivariate cox proportional-hazards analysis predicting death, re-fracture, and re-hospitalization.

Variables	Risk Ratio[95% CI]	P value
Prediction of death (n = 334)		
Age	1.04 [1.00–1.08]	0.047
Male sex	1.88 [1.11–3.18]	0.02
CIRS	1.17 [1.10–1.25]	<0.001
Geriatric cohort	0.43 [0.25–0.73]	0.002
Prediction of re-fracture (n = 334)		
Age	0.98 [0.90–1.06]	0.58
Male sex	0.22 [0.03–1.76]	0.16
CIRS	1.00 [0.85–1.17]	0.97
Geriatric cohort	0.50 [0.15–1.65]	0.26
Prediction of re-hospitalization (n = 294)[a]		
Age	0.99 [0.95–1.03]	0.68
Male sex	0.76 [0.41–1.41]	0.39
CIRS	1.08 [1.00–1.16]	0.04
Geriatric cohort	0.40 [0.23–0.70]	0.001
Prediction of admission into a new institution (n = 296)[b]		
Age	1.08 [1.03–1.14]	0.003
Male sex	1.71 [0.86–3.41]	0.13
CIRS	1.06 [0.97–1.15]	0.21
Geriatric cohort	0.98 [0.47–2.00]	0.95

CI: confidence interval; CIRS: cumulative illness rating scale;
[a]: only patients who survived to acute care and rehabilitation were considered;
[b]: only patients who were not previously living in an institution were considered. For re-hospitalization and re-fracture, death was considered as a censored observation.

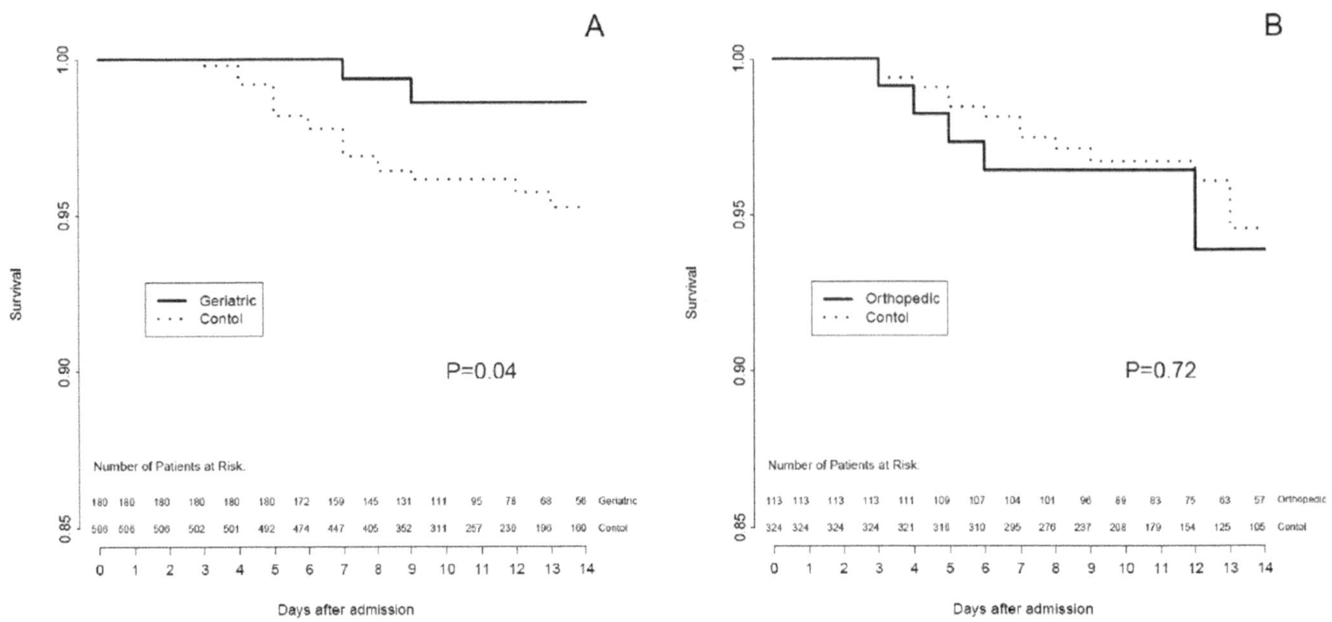

Figure 4. Survival curves for in-hospital mortality. Survival curves for in-hospital mortality in the geriatric (Panel A) and orthopedic (Panel B) cohorts, and their respective matched cohorts from the national registry. *P* values refer to log-rank test.

99% of enrolled patients. When comparing complex health procedures, randomized trials are difficult to conduct and interrupted time series analysis are often used. A multicenter cluster randomized study may also be an appropriate methodology. Second, we were unable to compare our results to other models of orthogeriatric reported in the literature [15–19]. Comparisons of this nature are difficult due to differences between health care systems and/or local hospital organization, varying study end points, and a lack of reported long term outcomes [30–33]. However, our results suggest that an alignment of multidisciplinary hospital teams (physicians and nurses) and hospital care paths (from ED admission to rehabilitation care) toward optimal care of the geriatric hip fracture patient is key factor in successful patient management. Lastly, our results may in part be attributable to certain characteristics of the French health care system and may not be appropriate in countries with different health systems.

Conclusion

We observed that elderly patients with hip fracture, admitted early into a dedicated geriatric unit and managed with a multidisciplinary approach, had reduced long term mortality and an improved walking ability.

Supporting Information

File S1 Contains the following: Table S1. Classification of ICD-10 codes into disease groups. Table S2. Comparison of the main characteristics of the matched populations.

Acknowledgments

We thank Dr. David Baker, DM, FRCA, (Department of Anesthesiology and Critical Care, Hôpital Necker-Enfants Malades, Paris) and Dr. Reitze Rodseth, MB ChB, FRCA (Lecturer, Perioperative Research Group, Department of Anaesthetics, University of KwaZulu-Natal, Durban, South Africa & Research Fellow, Population Health Research Institute, Hamilton, Canada) for reviewing the manuscript.

Author Contributions

Conceived and designed the experiments: JB BR YLM. Performed the experiments: JB JCB FK MR JYB. Analyzed the data: JB BR YLM. Contributed reagents/materials/analysis tools: YLM BR. Wrote the paper: JB YLM BR. Critical revision of the manuscript for important intellectual content: JB JCB FK MR JYB MV BR.

References

1. Johnell O, Kanis JA (2006) An estimate of the worldwide prevalence and disability associated with osteoporotic fractures. Osteoporosis Int 17: 1726–33.
2. Johnell O, Kanis JA (2004) An estimate of the worldwide prevalence, mortality and disability associated with hip fracture. Osteoporosis Int 15: 897–902.
3. Rapp K, Becker C, Lamb SE, Icks A, Klenk J (2008) Hip fractures in institutionalized elderly people: incidence rates and excess mortality. J Bone Mineral Res 23: 1825–31.
4. Jiang HX, Majumdar SR, Dick DA, Moreau M, Raso J, et al. (2005) Development and initial validation of a risk score for predicting in-hospital and 1-year mortality in patients with hip fractures. J Bone Mineral Res 20: 494–500.
5. Myers AH, Robinson EG, Van Natta ML, Michelson JD, Collins K, et al. (1991) Hip fractures among the elderly: factors associated with in-hospital mortality. Am J Epidemiol 134: 1128–37.
6. Endo Y, Aharonoff GB, Zuckerman JD, Egol KA, Koval KJ (2005) Gender differences in patients with hip fracture: a greater risk of morbidity and mortality in men. J Orthop Trauma 19: 29–35.
7. Abrahamsen B, van Staa T, Ariely R, Olson M, Cooper C (2009) Excess mortality following hip fracture: a systematic epidemiological review. Osteoporosis Int 20: 1633–50.
8. Haentjens P, Magaziner J, Colón-Emeric CS, Vanderschueren D, Milisen K, et al. (2010) Meta-analysis: excess mortality after hip fracture among older women and men. Ann Intern Med 152: 380–90.
9. Penrod JD, Litke A, Hawkes WG, Magaziner J, Doucette JT, et al. (2008) The association of race, gender, and comorbidity with mortality and function after hip fracture. J Gerontol A Biol Sci Med Sci 63: 867–72.

10. Bentler SE, Liu L, Obrizan M, Cook EA, Wright KB, et al. (2009) The aftermath of hip fracture: discharge placement, functional status change, and mortality. Am J Epidemiol 170: 1290–9.
11. Hannan EL, Magaziner J, Wang JJ, Eastwood EA, Silberzweig SB, et al. (2001) Mortality and locomotion 6 months after hospitalization for hip fracture: risk factors and risk-adjusted hospital outcomes. JAMA 285: 2736–42.
12. Bass E, French DD, Bradham DD, Rubenstein LZ (2007) Risk-adjusted mortality rates of elderly veterans with hip fractures. Ann Epidemiol 17: 514–9.
13. Kanis JA, Oden A, Johnell O, De Laet C, Jonsson B, et al. (2003) The components of excess mortality after hip fracture. Bone 32: 468–73.
14. Cram P, Lu X, Kaboli PJ, Vaughan-Sarrazin MS, Cai X, et al. (2011) Clinical characteristics and outcomes of Medicare patients undergoing total hip arthroplasty, 1991–2008. JAMA 305: 1560–7.
15. Nikkel LE, Fox EJ, Black KP, Davis C, Andersen L, et al. (2012) Impact of comorbidities on hospitalization costs following hip fracture. J Bone Joint Surg Am 94: 9–17.
16. Gilchrist WJ, Newman RJ, Hamblen DL, Williams BO (1988) Prospective randomised study of an orthopaedic geriatric inpatient service. BMJ 297: 1116–8.
17. Adunsky A, Lusky A, Arad M, Heruti RJ (2003) A comparative study of rehabilitation outcomes of elderly hip fracture patients: the advantage of a comprehensive orthogeriatric approach. J Gerontol A Biol Sci Med Sci 58: 542–7.
18. Kennie DC, Reid J, Richardson IR, Kiamari AA, Kelt C (1988) Effectiveness of geriatric rehabilitative care after fractures of the proximal femur in elderly women: a randomised clinical trial. BMJ 297: 1083–6.
19. Naglie G, Tansey C, Kirkland JL, Ogilvie-Harris DJ, Detsky AS, et al. (2002) Interdisciplinary inpatient care for elderly people with hip fracture: a randomized controlled trial. CMAJ 167: 25–32.
20. Friedman SM, Mendelson DA, Bingham KW, Kates SL (2009) Impact of a comanaged geriatric fracture center on short-term hip fracture outcomes. Arch Intern Med 169: 1712–7.
21. Kammerlander C, Roth T, Friedman SM, Suhm N, Luger TJ, et al. (2010) Ortho-geriatric service–a literature review comparing different models. Osteoporosis Int 21: S637–46.
22. Bergstrom N, Demuth PJ, Braden BJ (1987) A clinical trial of the Braden Scale for predicting pressure sore risk. Nurs Clin North Am 22: 417–28.
23. Inouye SK, van Dyck CH, Alessi CA, Balkin S, Siegal AP, et al. (1990) Clarifying confusion: the confusion assessment method. A new method for detection of delirium. Ann Intern Med 113: 941–8.
24. Linn BS, Linn MW, Gurel L (1968) Cumulative illness rating scale. J Am Geriatr Soc 16: 622–6.
25. McLean E, Cogswell M, Egli I, Wojdyla D, de Benoist B (2009) Worldwide prevalence of anaemia, WHO Vitamin and Mineral Nutrition Information System, 1993–2005. Public Health Nutr 12: 444–54.
26. Cockcroft DW, Gault MH (1976) Prediction of creatinine clearance from serum creatinine. Nephron 16:31–41.
27. Ramsay CR, Matowe L, Grilli R, Grimshaw JM, Thomas RE (2003) Interrupted time series designs in health technology assessment: lessons from two systematic reviews of behavior change strategies. Int J Technol Assess Health Care 19: 613–23.
28. Austin PC (2011) Optimal caliper widths for propensity-score matching when estimating differences in means and differences in proportions in observational studies. Pharm Stat 10: 150–61.
29. Austin PC (2009) Balance diagnostics for comparing the distribution of baseline covariates between treatment groups in propensity-score matched samples. Stat Med 28: 3083–107.
30. Leung AH, Lam TP, Cheung WH, Chan T, Sze PC, et al. (2011) An orthogeriatric collaborative intervention program for fragility fractures: a retrospective cohort study. J Trauma 71: 1390–4.
31. Fisher AA, Davis MW, Rubenach SE, Sivakumaran S, Smith PN, et al. (2006) Outcomes for older patients with hip fractures: the impact of orthopedic and geriatric medicine cocare. J Orthop Trauma 20: 172–8.
32. Koval KJ, Chen AL, Aharonoff GB, Egol KA, Zuckerman JD (2004) Clinical pathway for hip fractures in the elderly: the Hospital for Joint Diseases experience. Clin Orthop Relat Res 425: 72–81.
33. Vidan M, Serra JA, Moreno C, Riquelme G, Ortiz J (2005) Efficacy of a comprehensive geriatric intervention in older patients hospitalized for hip fracture: a randomized, controlled trial. J Am Geriatr Soc 53: 1476–82.
34. Simunovic N, Devereaux PJ, Sprague S, Guyatt GH, Schemitsch E, et al. (2010) Effect of early surgery after hip fracture on mortality and complications: systematic review and meta-analysis. CMAJ 182: 1609–16.
35. Vidan MT, Sanchez E, Gracia Y, Maranon E, Vaquero J, et al. (2011) Causes and effects of surgical delay in patients with hip fracture: a cohort study. Ann Intern Med 155:226–33.
36. Agence Nationale de Sécurité du Médicament (ANSM) (2002) Recommandations pour la transfusion de globules rouges homologues: produits, indications, alternatives. http://ansm.sante.fr/var/ansm_site/storage/original/application/3a08e904ce75401d27f52e600d53a0cc.pdf (last access March 21, 2013).
37. Carson JL, Terrin ML, Noveck H, Sanders DW, Chaitman BR, et al. (2011) Liberal or restrictive transfusion in high-risk patients after hip surgery. N Engl J Med 365: 2453–62.

3

Can Particulate Air Sampling Predict Microbial Load in Operating Theatres for Arthroplasty?

Maria Luisa Cristina*, Anna Maria Spagnolo, Marina Sartini, Donatella Panatto, Roberto Gasparini, Paolo Orlando, Gianluca Ottria, Fernanda Perdelli

Department of Health Sciences, University of Genoa, Genoa, Italy

Abstract

Several studies have proposed that the microbiological quality of the air in operating theatres be indirectly evaluated by means of particle counting, a technique derived from industrial clean-room technology standards, using airborne particle concentration as an index of microbial contamination. However, the relationship between particle counting and microbiological sampling has rarely been evaluated and demonstrated in operating theatres. The aim of the present study was to determine whether particle counting could predict microbiological contamination of the air in an operating theatre during 95 surgical arthroplasty procedures. This investigation was carried out over a period of three months in 2010 in an orthopedic operating theatre devoted exclusively to prosthetic surgery. During each procedure, the bacterial contamination of the air was determined by means of active sampling; at the same time, airborne particulate contamination was assessed throughout the entire procedure. On considering the total number of surgical operations, the mean value of the total bacterial load in the center of the operating theatre proved to be 35 CFU/m^3; the mean particle count was 4,194,569 no./m^3 for particles of diameter $\geq$0.5 µm and 13,519 no./m^3 for particles of diameter $\geq$5 µm. No significant differences emerged between the median values of the airborne microbial load recorded during the two types of procedure monitored. Particulates with a diameter of $\geq$0.5 µm were detected in statistically higher concentrations ($p<0.001$) during knee-replacement procedures. By contrast, particulates with a diameter of $\geq$5 µm displayed a statistically higher concentration during hip-replacement procedures ($p<0.05$). The results did not reveal any statistically significant correlation between microbial loads and particle counts for either of the particle diameters considered ($\geq$0.5 µm and $\geq$5 µm). Consequently, microbiological monitoring remains the most suitable method of evaluating the quality of air in operating theatres.

Editor: Herman Tse, The University of Hong Kong, Hong Kong

Funding: The authors have no support or funding to report.

Competing Interests: The authors have declared that no competing interests exist.

* E-mail: cristinaml@unige.it

Introduction

All surgical procedures carry a risk of post-operative infection, which can be particularly serious in orthopedic surgery such as joint replacement [1]. The prevention of surgical site infection (SSI) after orthopedic implant surgery is a hot topic for politicians, hospital administrators and clinicians, given the enormous amount of resources these infections consume in terms of extra costs of medications, reoperations, and prolonged hospitalization [2]. Prevention involves identifying and controlling potential sources of microbial contamination.

Factors causing surgical site infections are multivarious [3], including surgical characteristics (e.g. type of procedure, duration of the operation etc), the appropriateness of staff behaviors (limited number of personnel and restricted movements) and microbial contamination of the air (especially in clean surgery) [4], [5]. In turn, the latter factor can be, at least partially, determined by factors linked to the surgical characteristics and staff behaviors.

Several studies have proposed that the microbiological quality of the air in operating theatres be indirectly evaluated by means of particle counting, a technique derived from industrial clean-room technology standards [6], using airborne particle concentration as an index of microbial contamination [6], [7]. One of the sources of airborne particulates in operating theatres may be the surgical smoke produced by particular instruments or techniques, such as the ultrasonic scalpel, electrocautery etc, during surgical procedures.

However, the relationship between particle counting and microbiological sampling has rarely been evaluated and demonstrated in operating theatres. Seal and Clark [8] compared airborne particle counting in eight size-ranges with the numbers of bacteria-carrying particles, in ultra-clean and turbulently ventilated operating theatres. They found that the number of particles in the 5–7 µm size-range correlated significantly with microbiological contamination. Landrin et al [6] compared these two methods in empty operating theatres equipped with conventional ventilation through HEPA filters. No correlation was observed between the two methods (Spearman correlation coefficient = 0.06, P = 0.6). These authors concluded that there was no reason to replace microbiological sampling with particle counting for the routine evaluation of microbiological contamination in conventionally ventilated operating theatres.

Another study that investigated whether the density of airborne particulates could predict the density of viable airborne bacteria was conducted by Stocks et al [9] during 22 arthroplasty procedures in operating rooms with a conventional ventilation system (turbulent air flow). They found a correlation between the presence of larger particles (>5 μm) and microbial contamination, which was attributed to the capability of larger particles to carry bacteria. Thus, given the inhomogeneity of the results obtained, the literature regarding the relationship between airborne particulates and airborne microbes remains controversial.

The aim of the present study was to determine whether particle counting could predict microbiological contamination of the air in an operating theatre during 95 surgical arthroplasty procedures (hip and knee). In addition, we examined the possible correlations among the microbial load, particle counting and other variables: i.e. the frequency of use of instruments that generate particulates, door-opening rates, the number of persons present in the operating theatre and the duration of the surgical procedure.

Methods

This investigation was carried out over a period of three months in 2010 in an orthopedic operating theatre devoted exclusively to prosthetic surgery and situated within a hospital facility in the north-west of Italy. About 1,200 hip- and knee-replacement procedures (ICD9-CM: 81.51–81.54) are performed per year in this operating theatre, which has a surface area of 35.51 m^2 and is part of a complex that provides adequate space for reception, anesthesia, surgery, recovery and observation.

We monitored 95 surgical arthroplasty procedures: 59 hip replacements (ICD9-CM 81.51) and 36 knee replacements (ICD9-CM 81.54). During each procedure, the bacterial contamination of the air was determined by means of active sampling; at the same time, airborne particulate contamination was assessed throughout the entire procedure. Moreover, particle counts were recorded during the use of instruments able to produce surgical smoke. Figure 1 shows the floor plan of the operating theater and the positions of the air and particulate samplers.

During each operation, detailed information on the surgical procedure was collected, including the length of the procedure, the number of people present in the theatre, the door-opening rate per procedure, and the duration of use of instruments that produce surgical smoke.

At the beginning of the study, when the operating theatre was at rest, we recorded the number of air exchanges provided by the air-conditioning system and checked for any microbial contamination of the airflow from the inlet ports of the system. The operating theatre has a turbulent-flow ventilation system equipped with HEPA filters, which are 99.97% efficient in removing airborne particles of 0.3 μm or larger; the filters are replaced every 6 months and maintenance work on the system is carried out periodically. The operating room is under positive pressure in relation to the adjacent rooms (≥5 Pa); air temperature and humidity are set respectively at 17°C ±1°C and 50% ±5%.

Determining Bacterial Contamination of the Air from the Inlet Ports and in the Centre of the Room

To determine the total airborne bacterial load, we used an SAS SUPER 100 (PBI International®) impactor equipped with RODAC plates (Ø = 55 mm) containing γ-irradiated TSA (Tryptone Soy Agar) culture medium (Biotest Italia s.r.l.). In order to sample the air in the centre of the room, the instrument was positioned in the immediate vicinity of the operating table, at a height of 1.5 m. During each procedure, a 1000 L volume of air was aspirated by means of a multi-aspiration modality; the impactor was switched on by remote control just as the skin was incised, and was switched off on completion of suturing.

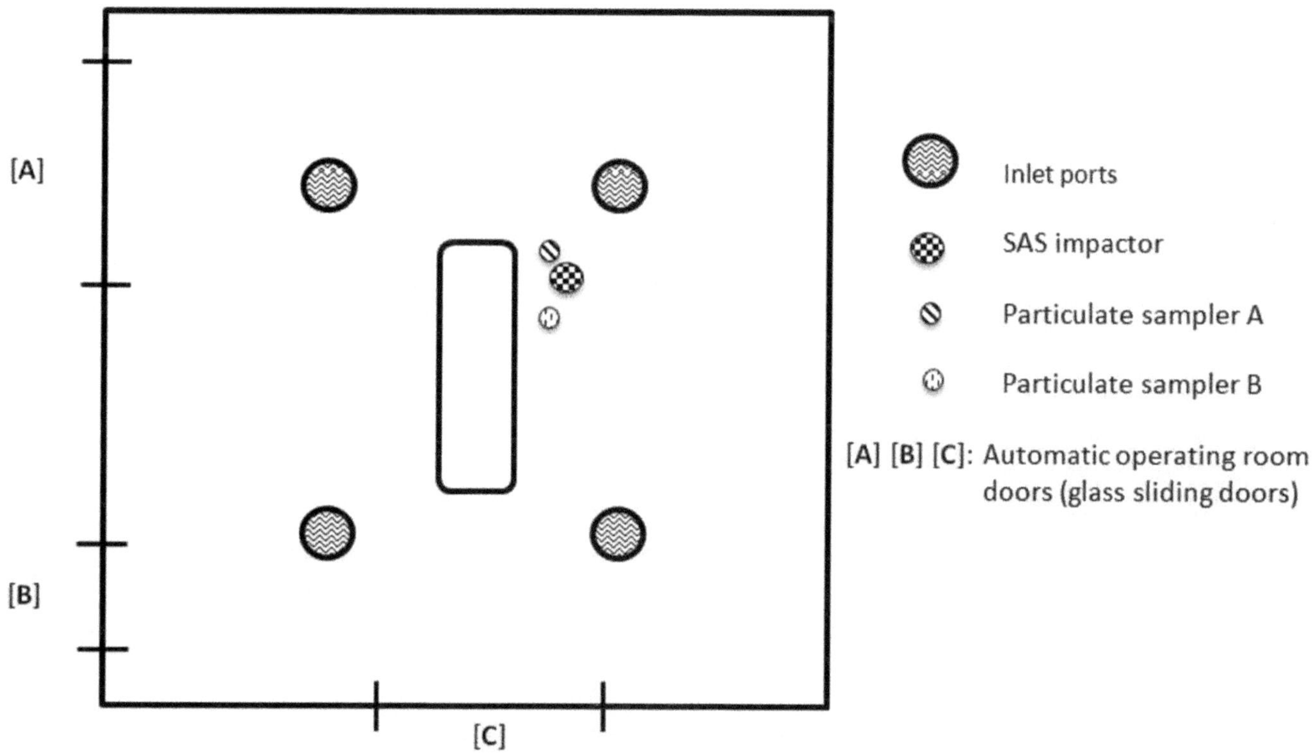

Figure 1. Floor plan of the operating theater, showing the positions of the samplers.

To determine the bacterial load of the airflow from the inlet ports of the ventilation system in at-rest conditions, the sampler was positioned in proximity to the flow-regulators. The total volume of air sampled was 1000 L.

Plates were incubated at 37°C for 48 h before the total aerobic bacterial count was measured. Microbiological results are expressed as CFU (Colony Forming Units)/m^3.

Determining Contamination by Airborne Particulates

Airborne particulates (particles ≥0.5 μm and particles ≥5 μm in size) were counted by means of two light-scattering particle analyzers (Met One, Pacific Scientific Instruments, Grants Pass, OR, USA) at a flow rate of 2.8 L/min., and expressed as numbers of particles per m^3. Both apparatuses were placed in the same position as the SAS impactor; one (Sampler A) was activated by remote control in parallel with the impactor, i.e. for the entire duration of the procedure, while the other (Sampler B), again activated by remote control, recorded the particle count both on each occasion when surgical smoke-producing instruments were used and when such instruments were not used.

Determining the Number of Efficacious Air Exchanges

The efficacy of the air-conditioning system was assessed in at-rest conditions by measuring the decay of the concentration of tracer gas by means of a portable GA301 meter (Eco-CONTROL, Milan) connected to a computer for the collection and analysis of data, as described by Sartini et al [10].

Statistical Analysis

Statistical analysis was carried out by means of STATA SE9^{TM} software (Stata Corp LP - USA). The results were analyzed in terms of descriptive statistics, and the relationships between data were examined by using the non-parametric Mann-Whitney-Wilcoxon ranksum test. The rho Spearman rank correlation was used to assess the degree of association among particulate diameter ≥5 μm, particulate diameter ≥0.5 μm, bacterial load, procedure duration, percentage frequency of ultrasonic scalpel use, number of persons present and door-opening rate.

Moreover, the sensitivity and specificity of particle counting in discriminating between microbiological counting values were evaluated by means of receiver-operating characteristic (ROC) analysis.

Ethics Statement

We didn't need ethics approval because the study was carried out as part of routine control tests that we conduct in the operating theatres of the Hospital. As is the case of all studies conducted in the hospital environment, the General Management of the hospital approved the study protocol. The General Management is responsible for ensuring the ethical aspects of all activities of the hospital. Furthermore, the entire study was organised in accordance with a protocol agreed upon with the operating theatre teams. On entering the hospital, all patients sign an informed consent form regarding treatments in the hospital and the conditions of those treatments. Finally, the research was carried out in full respect of the Italian law on the privacy (Decreto legislativo 30 giugno 2003, n. 196).

Results

With regard to the characteristics of the air-conditioning system, 20 efficacious air exchanges were carried out per hour. The microbial load of the airflow through the inlet ports proved to be <1 CFU/m^3.

On considering the total number of surgical operations, the mean value of the total bacterial load in the center of the operating theatre proved to be 35 CFU/m^3; the mean particle count measured by Sampler A was 4,194,569 no./m^3 for particles of diameter ≥0.5 μm and 13,519 no./m^3 for particles of diameter ≥5 μm (Table 1).

Table 1 also reports the data on the microbial load and on the counts of particles of the 2 diameters (≥0.5 and ≥5 μm), subdivided by type of procedure. No significant differences emerged between the median values of the airborne microbial load (hip replacement median value: 35 CFU/m^3; knee replacement median value: 40 CFU/m^3) recorded during the two types of procedure monitored (p = 0.4558).

Particulates with a diameter of ≥0.5 μm were detected in statistically higher concentrations (z = −6.013; p = 0.0000) during knee-replacement procedures (median value 6,468,327 no./m^3). By contrast, particulates with a diameter of ≥5 μm displayed a statistically higher concentration (z = 2.013, p = 0.0441) during hip-replacement procedures (median value 14,520 no./m^3).

Table 2 reports the data on the duration of the procedures, the number of persons present in the room and door-opening rates. The difference in the median duration of the two types of procedure (hip-replacement : 40 min; knee-replacement: 45 min) proved to be statistically significant (z = −3.569; p = 0.0004).

Table 1. Mean values, standard deviations (SD), minimum and maximum values, median and quartiles (Q1–Q3) of the total bacterial load (CFU/m^3) and counts of particles (Sampler A) of diameter ≥0.5 μm and diameter ≥5 μm (no./m^3) in all the procedures monitored and in each of the two types of procedure.

	Total airborne bacterial load (CFU/m^3)		
	Hip replacement	**Knee replacement**	**All procedures**
Mean ± SD	35±16	34±11	35±15
Min-max	10–70	20–45	10–70
Median	35	40	40
Q1–Q3	25–40	22–45	25–45
	Count of airborne particles of diameter ≥0.5 μm (no./m^3)		
	Hip replacement	**Knee replacement**	**All procedures**
Mean ± SD	2,538,425±1,480,054	6,908,804±3,269,100	4,194,569±3,142,263
Min-max	600,353–5,164,279	2,925,281–11,219,627	600,353–11,219,627
Median	2,418,086	6,468,327	3,127,466
Q1–Q3	1,294,603–3,586,316	3,760,520–9,683,440	1,630,903–5,164,279
	Count of airborne particles of diameter ≥5 μm (no./m^3)		
	Hip replacement	**Knee replacement**	**All procedures**
Mean ± SD	13,915±3,592	12,868±3,488	13,519±3,571
Min-max	5,879–19,756	8,352–17,764	5,879–19,756
Median	14,520	12,207	14,520
Q1–Q3	12,657–16,608	9,926–16,046	11,500–16,608

Table 2. Mean, standard deviation (SD), median and range of the values of procedure length (min), number of persons present in theatre, and door-opening rate (no./min) for all surgical procedures and for hip and knee replacements.

	Mean±SD	Median (range)
All surgical procedures		
Operation length (min)	45±10	40 (35–70)
N° persons present	8±1	7 (6–10)
Door-opening rate (no./min)	0.20±0.03	0.20 (0.12–0.26)
Hip replacement (ICD9-CM 81.51)		
Operation length (min)	41±6	40 (35–50)
N° persons present	8±1	8 (6–10)
Door-opening rate (no./min)	0.20±0.03	0.20 (0.12–0.26)
Knee replacement (ICD9-CM 81.54)		
Operation length (min)	50±12	45 (40–70)
N° persons present	6±1	6 (6–7)
Door-opening rate (no./min)	0.20±0.04	0.18 (0.16–0.25)

During each operation, doors were opened a mean of 0.20 times per minute, with no statistically significant difference emerging between the two types of procedure ($p = 0.2334$).

All operating theatre staff wore nonwoven fabric suits; surgeons also wore highly effective isolation helmets, and instrument-handlers wore semi-integral masks, while the anesthetist and circulating nurses wore surgical masks and hair covering.

Evaluation of the surgical instruments able to release surgical smoke revealed that the ultrasonic scalpel was the instrument most frequently used in both types of procedure. Figure 2 reports the duration of the use of the ultrasonic scalpel as a percentage of procedure time (calculated as minutes of use/procedure duration x 100), subdivided by type of procedure. In this regard, statistically significant differences ($z = -3.145$; $p = 0.0017$) emerged between the two types of procedure.

Airborne particulate concentration as a function of the use of the ultrasonic scalpel was evaluated by means of Sampler B. This evaluation revealed that the median concentration of particulates with a diameter of ≥0.5 μm was significantly higher ($z = -4$–432; $p = 0.000$) when this instrument was used (8,014,873 no./m^3) than when it was not used (2,958,536 no./m^3). A similar pattern was seen in the concentration of ≥5 μm diameter particles (13,965 no./m^3 vs. 12,878 no./m^3), though the difference was not statistically significant ($p = 0.2019$).

A highly significant correlation emerged between the percentage use of the ultrasonic scalpel and the duration of the procedures (rho = 0.8254 $p<0.001$). Table 3 reports of the Spearman correlation coefficients (rho) and significances (p) of the mean concentrations of particulates (≥0.5 μm and ≥5 μm) recorded by Sampler A in relation to procedure duration (min), percentage use of the ultrasonic scalpel, number of persons present and door-opening rate, both for the total number of procedures and for each procedure type (hip and knee replacement).

The results did not reveal any statistically significant correlation between microbial loads and particle counts for either of the particle diameters considered (≥0.5 μm and ≥5 μm).

A statistically significant correlation (rho = 0.2344 $p<0.05$) emerged between the number of persons present in the operating theatre and the airborne microbial load during both types of procedure.

On the basis of ROC analysis, no particulate count value for the diameters of ≥0.5 and ≥5 μm can predict a microbiological count higher than 20 CFU/m^3 (ROC area = 0.4661 and 0.1080, respectively). The choice of this cut-off was determined by the fact that the national standard reference value for operating theatres with turbulent-flow ventilation (180 CFU/m^3) has never been reached; the most suitable cut-off value for our data proved to be the Italian and British standard value indicated for operating theatres in which ultraclean surgery is performed, despite the fact that laminar-flow ventilation is recommended.

Discussion

During surgical procedures, dust particles, textile fibers, skin scales and respiratory aerosols loaded with viable microorganisms are released from the surgical team and patient into the surrounding air of the operating room [11]. Moreover, the use of some particular instruments during surgical procedures increases the dispersion of particulates in the air. The size of such particles closely depends on the particular instruments used. Indeed, various investigations have revealed that the electrocautery releases the smallest particles, with a mean aerodynamic size of 0.07 μm, whereas laser tissue coagulation produces larger particles (0.31 μm) and the largest particles are generated by the ultrasonic scalpel (0.35–6.5 μm) [12].

The aim of the present study was to determine whether the concentration of the airborne particulates could predict microbial contamination during surgical operations. Particle counting could offer several advantages over microbiological sampling. Indeed, microbiological sampling is time-consuming and the results may only be available after several days [6]. Another critical point concerning microbiological sampling is the absence of uniform standardized sampling procedures, which prevents data collected in different countries from being compared. In addition, a range of instruments are used in volumetric air-sampling, which hampers the correlation of results on account of their variability [3].

Conversely, particle counting is less demanding and yields immediate results. However, the information obtained is indirect [6]. This method enables results to be compared with reference values applicable to classes of maximum particle concentration. Most industrialized countries have set their own standards, based on measuring the presence of particles of varying sizes and number; many of these standards have been amended to conform to the International Standards Organization (ISO) 14644 [3], [13].

Some similar studies [6], [8], [9] have yielded results which conflict with one another, thus leaving the question unresolved.

With regard to microbial contamination in operating theatres, it is well known that the number of airborne bacteria depends on several factors, such as the number of people present in the room and their activities and behavior.

Few countries have set bacterial threshold limits in conventionally-ventilated operating theatres, although most recommend 20 air exchanges per hour, so as not to exceed values of 50–150 colony forming units (CFU)/m^3 of air during surgical operations.

In some countries, the concentration should not exceed 180 CFU/m^3 for an average 5-min period during activity [3].

In France [14], the microbiological limits are more restrictive than in Italy [15] and the UK, with values of ≤20 CFU/m^3 and ≤5 CFU/m^3 being indicated for turbulent and unidirectional airflows, respectively [16].

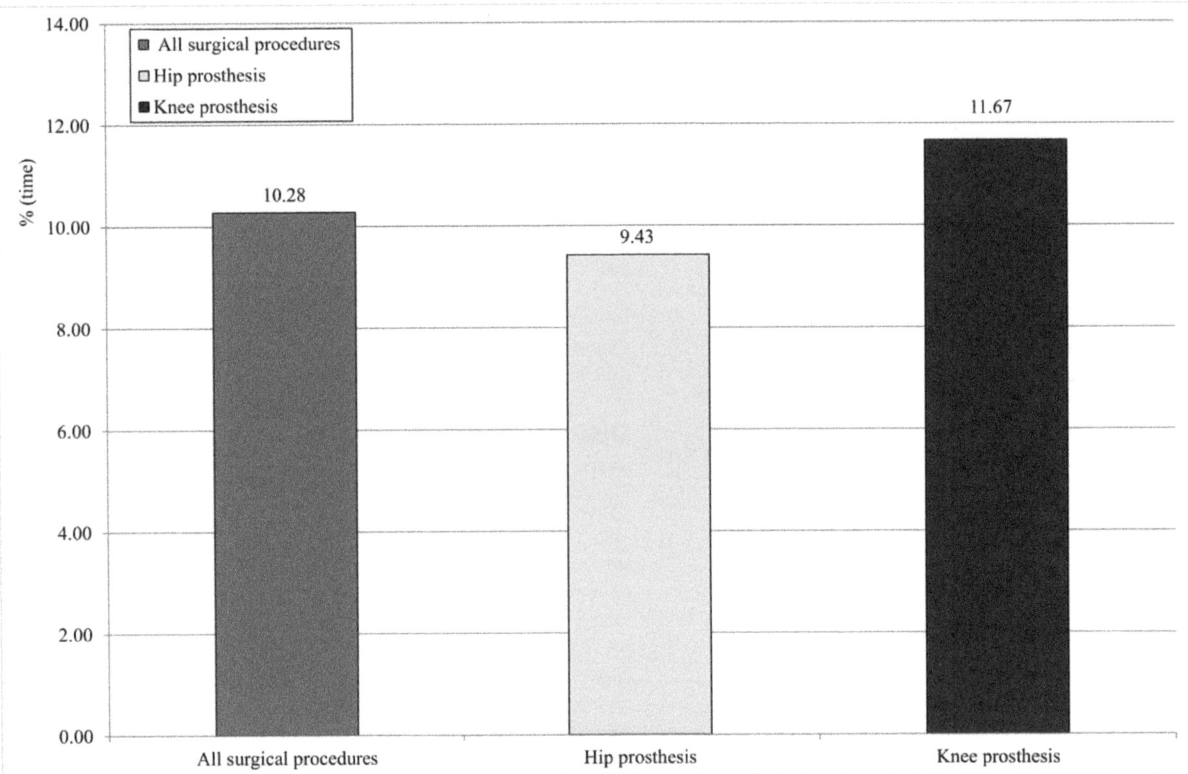

Figure 2. Duration of use of the ultrasonic scalpel as a percentage of operating time, subdivided by type of procedure.

In the present study, the mean values of the airborne microbial load (35 CFU/m^3) proved to be below the standard values for conventionally-ventilated [15] operating theatres in Italy. However, they exceeded the values proposed in some countries, such as France, and the generally accepted level of airborne microbial contamination during arthroplasty (10 CFU/m^3) [10]. The values that we recorded prove to be higher than those reported in other studies of the same types of surgical procedure [9], [17].

Our analysis of the quality of the air provided by the ventilation system revealed the microbial load of <1 CFU/m^3; it can

Table 3. Spearman's correlation coefficients (Rho) and significances (p) between the mean concentration of particulate measured by Sampler A (≥5 and ≥0.5 μm) and data on procedure duration (min), ultrasonic scalpel use, number of persons present in theatre and door-opening rates, referred to all procedures and broken down by procedure type (hip and knee replacement).

	Mean concentration of particulate ≥5 μm	**Mean concentration of particulate ≥0.5 μm**
Procedure length (min)°°	rho = 0.1706; p = 0.0984 (*)	rho = 0.6865; **p<0.001** (*)
	rho = 0.2418; p = 0.0650 (°)	rho = 0.1888; p = 0.1521 (°)
	rho = 0.1343; p = 0.4350 (§)	rho = 0.7622; **p<0.001**(§)
% use of ultrasonic scalpel	rho = 0.1460; p = 0.1581 (*)	rho = 0.7082; **p<0.001** (*)
	rho = 0.2347; p = 0.0736 (°)	rho = 0.8612; **p<0.001** (°)
	rho = 0.5881; **p<0.001** (§)	rho = 0.7933; **p<0.001** (§)
N° persons present	rho = 0.2854; **p<0.01** (*)	rho = 0.1624; p = 0.1158 (*)
	rho = 0.4723; **p<0.001** (°)	rho = 0.2104; p = 0.1097 (°)
	rho = 0.3199; p = 0.0571 (§)	rho = 0.1464; p = 0.3943 (§)
Door-opening rate (no./min)	rho = 0.1184; p = 0.2530 (*)	rho = 0.0378; p = 0.7159 (*)
	rho = 0.2418; p = 0.0650 (°)	rho = 0.0645; p = 0.6275 (°)
	rho = 0.6895; **p<0.001** (§)	rho = 0.1389; p = 0.4192 (§)

°° skin - skin.
(*) all procedures.
(°) hip replacement.
(§) knee replacement.

therefore be supposed that the contamination detected was produced during surgical activity.

With regard to particle counting, the results obtained revealed mean values that exceeded the European ISO 14644 Standard limits for ISO 7 clean-rooms ($352 \times 10^3 \geq 0.5$ μm particles/m^3 and 2,930≥5 μm particles/m^3) [13]. Moreover, the concentration values recorded in the present study, with regard to both sizes of particulates, differed from those reported by other similar studies conducted on conventionally ventilated operating theatres. However, it should be pointed out that these studies also differed considerably among themselves, again with regard to both sizes of particulates [9], [18].

It may reasonably be supposed that the utilization of surgical instruments that produce surgical smoke contributed to the high concentration of particulates. This supposition is supported by the fact that, with regard to particulates with a diameter of ≥0.5 μm, we found a significantly higher concentration ($p<0.001$) when the ultrasonic scalpel was being used than when it was not. Moreover, a statistically significant correlation emerged between the percentage use of this instrument and the mean concentration of ≥0.5 μm particles, and between procedure duration and the mean concentration of ≥0.5 μm particles. On the basis of these findings, it may be hypothesized that, as the duration of the procedure increases, so also does the use of the ultrasonic scalpel, i.e. the device responsible for the production of these particles.

For what concerns the heavier particles (≥5 μm), a correlation with the percentage use of the ultrasonic scalpel emerged only with regard to knee-replacement procedures. This could be explained by the fact that, as a proportion of the total particulates released by the ultrasonic scalpel, which is known to produce particulates in the 0.35–6.5 μm range, particulates with a diameter of ≥0.5 μm may prevail; by this token, the heavier particles could account for a smaller proportion of the total, becoming more detectable only after prolonged use of the device.

With regard to the correlation between ≥5 μm particles and the number of persons present in the room, the results obtained could be explained in terms of the fact that such particulates also includes the skin debris, the dimensions of which vary from 2.5 to 20 μm [18], and which are constantly being released by both theatre staff and patients. Moreover, the number of persons present influences the amount of movement taking place in the room, which, as already pointed out in other papers [18], tends to raise any dust that has already settled. Likewise, this can explain the correlation between microbial concentration and the number of persons present in the room.

In conclusion, this study showed that the use of surgical instruments that produce surgical smoke, such as the ultrasonic scalpel, can markedly contribute to the production of airborne particulates. However, neither fraction of these particulates (≥0.5 μm or ≥5 μm) displayed any correlation with the microbial load in either of the types of procedure considered.

However, one of the limitations of the present research is that only two particulate fractions were studied. We cannot therefore rule out the possibility that there may be a correlation between the number of particles/m^3 and CFU/m^3 if particulate fractions in narrower size-ranges are considered, as has been reported by Stocks et al. [9]. Moreover, further investigations should be carried out in operating theaters equipped with laminar-flow ventilation systems, an issue which has not yet been sufficiently addressed in studies of this kind.

Until these issues have been settled, microbiological monitoring remains the most suitable method of evaluating the quality of air in operating theatres.

Acknowledgments

The authors thank Dr. Bernard Patrick for translating the manuscript into English.

Author Contributions

Conceived and designed the experiments: MLC PO FP. Performed the experiments: GO DP. Analyzed the data: MS. Contributed reagents/materials/analysis tools: PO RG DP. Wrote the paper: AMS MLC.

References

1. Al-Waked R (2010) Effect of Ventilation Strategies on Infection Control inside Operating Theatres. Eng Appl Comp Fluid 4: 1–16.
2. Andersson AE, Bergh I, Karlsson J, Eriksson BI, Nilsson K (2012) Traffic flow in the operating room: An explorative and descriptive study on air quality during orthopedic trauma implant surgery. Am J Infect Control 40: 750–755.
3. Dharan S, Pittet D (2002) Environmental controls in operating theatres. J Hosp Infect 51: 79–84.
4. Weaving P, Cox F, Milton S (2008) Infection prevention and control in the operating theatre: reducing the risk of surgical site infections (SSIs). J Perioper Pract 18: 199–204.
5. Gould D (2001) Clean surgical wounds: prevention of infection. Nurs Stand 15: 45–52.
6. Landrin A, Bissery A, Kac G (2005) Monitoring air sampling in operating theatres: can particle counting replace microbiological sampling? J Hosp Infect 61: 27–29.
7. Wan GH, Chung FF, Tang CS (2011) Long-term surveillance of air quality in medical center operating rooms. Am J Infect Control 39: 302–308.
8. Seal DV, Clark RP (1990) Electronic particle counting for evaluating the quality of air in operating theatres: a potential basis for standards. J Appl Bacteriol 68: 225–230.
9. Stocks GW, Self SD, Thompson B, Adame XA, O'Connor DP (2010) Predicting bacterial populations based on airborne particulates: a study performed in nonlaminar flow operating rooms during joint arthroplasty surgery. Am J Infect Control 38: 199–204.
10. Sartini M, Ottria G, Dallera M, Spagnolo AM, Cristina ML (2006) Nitrous oxide pollution on operating theatres in relation to the type of leakage and the number of efficacious air exchanges per hour. J Prev Med Hyg 47: 155–159.
11. Diab-Elschahawi M, Berger J, Blacky A, Kimberger O, Oguz R, et al. (2011) Impact of different-sized laminar air flow versus no laminar air flow on bacterial counts in the operating room during orthopedic surgery. Am J Infect Control 39: e25–9.
12. Brüske-Hohlfeld I, Preissler G, Jauch KW, Pitz M, Nowak D, et al. (2008) Surgical smoke and ultrafine particles. J Occup Med Toxicol 3: 31.
13. EN ISO 14644-1 (ISO/TC 209) (1999) Cleanrooms and associated controlled environments, Part 1: Classification of air cleanliness International Organization for Standardization Technical Committee.
14. NF S 90–351 (2003) Norme - Etablissements de santé - Salles propres et environnements apparentés - Exigences relatives pour la maîtrise de la contamination aéroportée. Paris: Agence française de normalisation (AFNOR).
15. Istituto Superiore per la Prevenzione e Sicurezza sul Lavoro (ISPESL) (2010) Linee guida sugli standard di sicurezza e di igiene del lavoro nel reparto operatorio. Available: http://www.ispesl.it/linee_guida/Comparto_o_Settore/ISPESL-LG-SaleOperatorie.pdf. Accessed 2012 Jul 18.
16. Cristina ML, Spagnolo AM, Orlando P (2012) Prevention of Surgical Site Infections and Features of the Operating Theatre In: Nova Sciences Publishers, editors. Advances in Medicine and Biology vol. 34 63–92.
17. Orlando P, Cristina ML, Sartini M, Orlando M, Cordara R, et al. (1999) Risk of microbial contamination in operating room [Il rischio da contaminazione microbica in sala operatoria.] L'Igiene Moderna 112: 1253–1262.
18. Scaltriti S, Cencetti S, Rovesti S, Marchesi I, Bargellini A, et al. (2007) Risk factors for particulate and microbial contamination of air in operating theatres. J Hosp Infect 66: 320–326.

4

Socio-Economic Position Has No Effect on Improvement in Health-Related Quality of Life and Patient Satisfaction in Total Hip and Knee Replacement: A Cohort Study

J. Christiaan Keurentjes[1]*, David Blane[2], Melanie Bartley[3], Johan J. B. Keurentjes[4], Marta Fiocco[5], Rob G. Nelissen[1]

1 Department of Orthopaedic Surgery, Leiden University Medical Center, Leiden, The Netherlands, **2** Department of Primary Care and Public Health, Imperial College London, London, United Kingdom, **3** Department of Epidemiology and Public Health, University College London, London, United Kingdom, **4** Department of Information Management, Kadaster/Dutch Land Registry Office, Apeldoorn, The Netherlands, **5** Department of Medical Statistics and BioInformatics, Leiden University Medical Center, Leiden, The Netherlands

Abstract

Introduction: Considerable evidence suggests that patients with more advantaged Socio-Economic Positions undergo Total Hip and Knee Replacement (THR/TKR) more often, despite having a lower need. We questioned whether more disadvantaged Socio-Economic Position is associated with an lower improvement in Health-Related Quality of Life (HRQoL) and a lower patient satisfaction after THR/TKR.

Methods: Patients who underwent primary THR/TKR in one academic and three community hospitals between 2005 and 2009, were eligible for inclusion. The highest completed levels of schooling were aggregated to index social class. We compared the improvement in HRQoL and postoperative satisfaction with surgery (measured using the Short-Form 36 (SF36) and an 11-point numeric rating scale of satisfaction) between the aggregated groups of highest completed levels of schooling, using linear mixed model analysis, with center as a random effect and potential confounders (i.e. age, gender, Body Mass Index and Charnley's comorbidity classification) as fixed effects.

Results: 586 THR patients and 400 TKR patients (40% of all eligible patients) agreed to participate and completed all questionnaires sufficiently. We found no differences in HRQoL improvement in any dimension of the SF36 in THR patients. Patients with a higher completed level of schooling had a larger improvement in role-physical (9.38 points, 95%-CI:0.34–18.4), a larger improvement in general health (3.67 points, 95%-CI:0.56–6.79) and a smaller improvement in mental health (3.60 points, 95%-CI:0.82–6.38) after TKR. Postoperative patient satisfaction did not differ between different highest completed level of schooling groups.

Discussion: Completed level of schooling has no effect on the improvement in HRQoL and patient satisfaction in a Dutch THR population and a small effect in a similar TKR population. Undertreatment of patients with more disadvantaged Socio-Economic Position cannot be justified, given the similar improvement in HRQoL and postoperative level of satisfaction with surgery between the social groups examined.

Editor: Francois Rannou, Cochin Hospital (AP-HP), and the University Paris Descarte, France

Funding: Ongoing research grant of the Dutch Arthritis Association to Prof. Dr. Nelissen, Department of Orthopaedic Surgery, Leiden University Medical Center, grant number LLP-013 (http://www.reumafonds.nl/informatie-voor-doelgroepen/professionals/ongoing-research). The funders had no role in study design, data collection and analysis, decision to publish, or preparation of the manuscript.

Competing Interests: The authors have declared that no competing interests exist.

* E-mail: j.c.keurentjes@lumc.nl

Introduction

Total Hip Replacement (THR) and Total Knee Replacement (TKR) are effective surgical interventions, which alleviate pain and improve Health-Related Quality of Life (HRQoL) in patients with hip or knee joint degeneration.[1] Although on average patients improve markedly after THR or TKR, not all patients benefit from these surgeries. Persistent pain is reported in 9% of THR patients and 20% of TKR patients at long term follow-up.[2] Additionally, up to 30% of patients are dissatisfied after surgery, with higher reported dissatisfaction rates for TKR patients.[3–9] Therapeutic options are limited in patients with persistent pain or dissatisfaction after joint replacement: the outcome of revision surgery performed without a specific mechanical or physiological indication is highly unpredictable. Furthermore, revision THR or TKR surgery is associated with a higher probability of orthopaedic and medical complications. Given the projected increase of 137% and 601% in the annual number of THR and TKR performed in the United States in 2030, the absolute number of patients with unfavorable outcomes after joint replacement is expected to rise, potentially inducing large societal and medical problems.[10]

Predicting which patient groups are at increased risk of an unfavorable outcome after joint replacement may provide additional insights in the mechanisms involved and offer the possibility of intervention in order to optimise the outcome. At the very least, it allows patients to be well informed of their specific risks and expected gains before surgery.

People attain unequal societal positions according to their occupation, educational achievement, income level and status. The Socio-Economic Position (SEP) encompasses both resource-based measures and prestige-based measures in determining an individuals position in the socioeconomic hierarchy.[11] The patients SEP might be a good predictor of a favorable outcome after joint replacement: a more advantaged SEP is associated with better health,[12] which in turn is associated with better outcomes after joint replacement surgery.[13,14] As it does not require any invasive or expensive diagnostics, it would be easy to implement in clinical practice. We therefore questioned whether SEP was associated with the improvement in HRQoL and satisfaction after THR or TKR. We hypothesised that patients with more advantaged SEP would have a larger improvement in HRQoL after THR and TKR and a higher degree of satisfaction with their surgical results.

Methods

The presently reported study is an add-on to a multi-center follow-up study, conducted at the departments of orthopaedic surgery of the Leiden University Medical Center, the Slotervaart hospital in Amsterdam, the Albert Schweitzer hospital in Dordrecht and the Groene Hart hospital in Gouda, the Netherlands, from August 2010 until August 2011 (see Study Time-line in figure 1). The study was approved by the Medical Ethics Committee of the Leiden University Medical Center and the Medical Ethical Committees of all other participating centers; all patients gave written informed consent (CCMO-Nr: NL29018.058.09; MEC-Nr: P09.189). This study was registered in the Netherlands Trial Register (NTR2190). It concerned the clinical follow-up of a multi-center randomized controlled clinical trial, comparing different blood management modalities in THR and TKR surgery (Netherlands Trial Register: NTR303). In this trial, 2442 primary and revision hip or knee replacements in 2257 patients were included between 2004 and 2009 (see Study Time-line in figure 1).

All patients who participated in the randomized controlled trial and completed preoperative HRQoL questionnaires, who underwent primary THR of TKR and who were alive at the time of inclusion for the present follow-up study were eligible for inclusion. In contrast to the previous clinical trial, in which joint replacements were the subjects of interest, patients are the subject of interest in the current study. Patients who participated more than once in the previous trial, were only allowed to participate once in the current study; the first joint replacement performed in the previous trial was chosen as the index surgery.

Records of the financial administration of all participating centers were checked in order to ascertain that all eligible patients were still alive before being approached. All eligible patients were first sent an invitation letter signed by their treating orthopaedic surgeon, an information brochure and a reply card. Patients who did not respond within 4 weeks after the first invitation were sent another invitation letter. The remaining patients, who did not respond to this second invitation, were contacted by telephone.

The improvement in different dimensions of HRQoL and satisfaction with the surgical results were the outcome measures of interest. Important concepts in HRQoL are elements of health status that people usually value (e.g. stair climbing) and peoples rating of the value of their subjective experience of living.[15] In other words, both objective functioning and subjective well-being should be considered when measuring HRQoL.[16] We measured HRQoL preoperatively and in the present follow-up study using the Short-Form 36 (SF36),[17] a health status instrument which includes several sub-scales related to functioning as well as perceived well-being.[18,19] The SF36 is translated and validated in Dutch and allows studying small between-group differences in HRQoL.[20,21] The 36 items cover eight domains (physical function, role physical, bodily pain, general health, vitality, social function, role emotional, and mental health), for which a sub-scale score is calculated (100 indicating no symptoms and 0 indicating extreme symptoms). Additionally, these scales are incorporated into two summary measures: a Physical Component Summary (PCS) and Mental Component Summary (MCS). The HRQoL outcome measure was the mean improvement (i.e. the mean of each patients postoperative sub-scale score minus their preoperative sub-scale score).

At follow-up one question was asked about satisfaction with the result in general, namely: "How satisfied are you with your hip or knee replacement?". Such as a single item has been shown to provide additional insight into the impact of surgery, besides the measurement of HRQoL.[22] Patient satisfaction with the surgical result was measured using an 11-point Numeric Rating Scale of Satisfaction (NRSS; 0 indicating completely dissatisfied, 10 indicating completely satisfied). The satisfaction outcome measure was the mean NRSS score.

Exposure

The follow-up questionnaire contained the following question: "What is your highest completed level of schooling?". We have aggregated these levels of schooling into an approximation of the social classes, on the assumption that level of schooling indexes the type of qualifications obtained, which in turn indicates the type of occupations available to the subject and hence their own adult social class. Thus: University, Higher vocational education and Preparatory higher vocational & scientific education have been aggregated as indicating the professional and managerial social classes; Middle vocational education and Preparatory middle vocational education have been aggregated as indicating the skilled non-manual and manual social classes; and Lower vocational education, Elementary schooling and No formal education have been aggregated as indicating the semi- & unskilled manual social classes.

Potential confounders

Sociodemographic characteristics collected at baseline in the trial included: age at joint replacement and gender. Additionally, the following variables were collected in the questionnaire of the follow-up study: length and weight, in order to calculate the Body Mass Index (BMI) (<25, 25–30, 30–35, >35) and patient reported Charnley classification of co-morbidity (Class A: patients in which the index operated hip or knee are affected only; Class B: patients in which the other hip or knee is affected as well; Class C: patients with a hip or knee replacement and other affected joints and/or a medical condition which affects the patients' ability to ambulate).[23,24]

Statistical analysis

We performed descriptive analyses of patients baseline characteristics. In order to investigate the possible extent of self-selection bias, we compared the age at THR or TKR and gender of participants to non-participants.

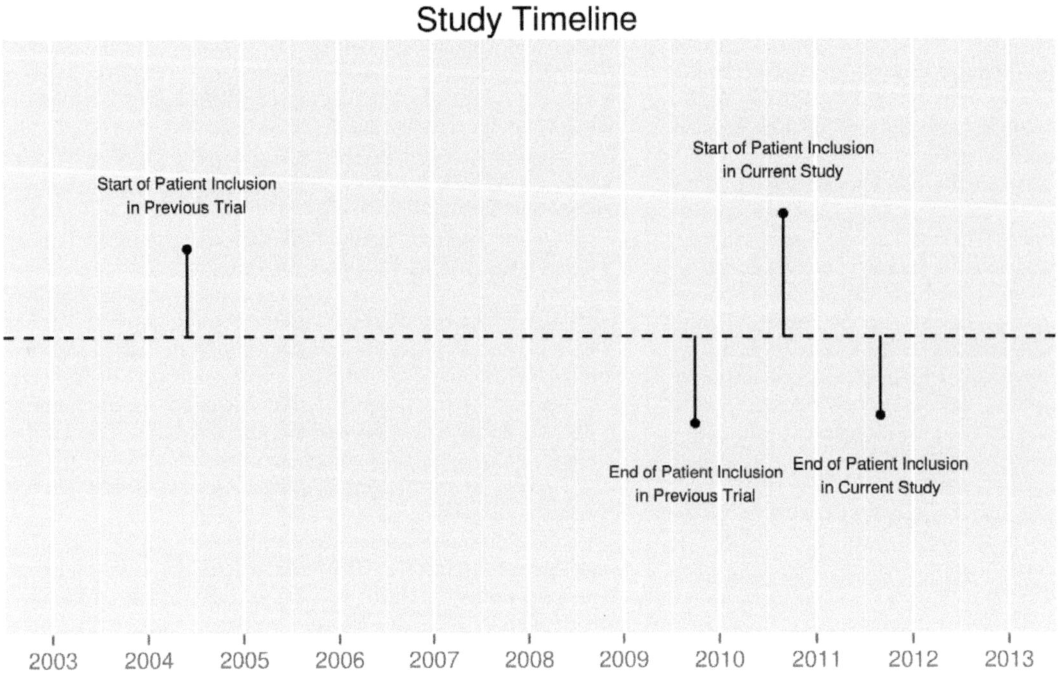

Figure 1. Study Timeline.

Patients with missing preoperative SF36 questionnaires, missing SF36 questionnaires at follow-up or missing highest level of schooling were excluded from analyses, as we could not exclude a Missing Not At Random (MNAR) mechanism. Missing values of the Charnley Co-morbidity Classification and BMI were deemed Missing At Random and imputed using Multiple Imputations (MI), in order to improve efficiency of the regression analyses and avert biased regression coefficients. We performed MI ($m = 10$) using an Expectation-Maximization algorithm,[25] which is implemented in the Amelia 2 package for R.[26,27]

We performed regression analyses in each imputed dataset in order to compare the mean improvement in HRQoL and the mean NRSS between patients from different social classes, whilst adjusting for confounders. As minimal clinically important differences (MCIDs) in HRQoL differ between THR patients and TKR patients,[28] we performed all analyses separately for THR and TKR. Possible confounders are age, gender, BMI and poly-articular morbidity in both THR and TKR patients. We used the Charnley classification as a proxy for poly-articular morbidity. As the length of follow-up varies considerably, we first stratified our data in quartiles of follow-up length for each imputed dataset. Within each stratum of follow-up length, we performed a multivariate mixed effect linear regression analysis, with the mean improvement in HRQoL and the mean NRSS as the dependent variable, the completed level of schooling and confounders as independent variables and center as a random effect. Stratum-specific mean differences in HRQoL between the KL grades were pooled using inverse variance weighting in order to produce an overall estimate of the mean difference in HRQoL for each imputed data-set. Finally, the $m = 10$ estimates of the mean differences in HRQoL were combined into one estimate, according to Rubin.[29]

All analyses were performed using R, version 2.14.0.[30]

Results

In the previous trial, 2579 THR and TKR were randomised in 2382 patients; 2442 joint replacements were evaluated. The first joint replacements of the 2382 patients consisted of 2206 primary THR and TKR and 176 revision THR and TKR. Of these 2206 patients who underwent primary joint replacement, 285 patients did not complete all preoperative questionnaires and 63 patients died, leaving 1858 patients with primary joint replacement eligible. 986 patients agreed to participate, of which 668 patients had returned all questionnaires sufficiently completed (response rate: 40%). Non-responding THR patients were on average 3.95 years older than participants (95%CI: 2.6–5.3 years); Non-responding TKR patients were on average 3.31 years older than participants (95%CI: 2.0–4.7 years). The proportion of males was similar in participants and non-responders. An overview of the patient characteristics is provided in table 1, an overview of preoperative HRQoL is presented in table 2 for THR patients and 3 for TKR patients.

Data on age, gender, highest completed level of schooling, pre- and postoperative SF36, satisfaction with surgery and length of follow-up was complete for all THR patients and all TKR patients. In 20 THR patients and 8 TKR patients, the Charnley classification was missing; in 12 THR patients and 13 TKR patients, the BMI was missing.

The mean improvement in HRQoL and mean NRSS per completed level of schooling is shown in table 4 for THR patients and table 5 for TKR patients. Adjusted differences in improvement in HRQoL and mean NRSS after joint replacement per increasing category of completed level of schooling are shown in table 6 for THR patients and table 7 for TKR patients. For each increasing completed level of schooling, THR patients improved 0.88 points more in physical functioning, 3.09 points less in role-physical, 0.60 points less in bodily pain, 0.66 points less in general health, 1.44 points less in vitality, 0.12 points more in social functioning, 0.34 points less in role-emotional, 1.35 points less in

Table 1. Patient Characteristics.

HIP	University, Higher Vocational Education and Preparatory Higher Vocational & Scientific Education: n = 100	Middle Vocational Education and Preparatory Middle Vocational Education n = 150	Lower Vocational Education, Elementary Schooling and No Formal Education n = 156	All Patients: n = 406
Age	62.5 (11.9)	63.8 (10.6)	66.3 (9.4)	64.4 (10.6)
Males	51.0%	34.7%	35.9%	39.2%
Follow-up period	3.13 (1.20)	3.19 (1.10)	3.17 (1.10)	3.16 (1.14)
Charnley:				
A	24.2%	20.0%	22.6%	22.0%
B	12.6%	17.9%	11.6%	14.2%
C	63.2%	62.1%	65.8%	63.7%
BMI:				
<25	50.0%	33.8%	27.0%	35.0%
25–30	35.1%	41.2%	48.0%	42.4%
30–35	12.8%	20.3%	19.1%	18.0%
>35	2.10%	4.70%	5.90%	4.60%
KNEE	**n = 42**	**n = 98**	**n = 122**	**n = 262**
Age	63.7 (12.7)	67.6 (9.0)	69.2 (9.3)	67.7 (10.0)
Males	40.5%	35.7%	29.5%	33.6%
Follow-up period	3.25 (1.2)	3.02 (1.0)	3.28 (1.2)	3.18 (1.13)
Charnley:				
A	14.6%	14.0%	11.7%	13.0%
B	14.6%	10.8%	10.0%	11.0%
C	70.6%	75.3%	78.3%	76.0%
BMI:				
<25	23.7%	13.7%	15.5%	16.1%
25–30	47.4%	56.8%	37.9%	46.6%
30–35	23.7%	21.1%	26.7%	24.1%
>35	5.30%	8.40%	19.8%	13.3%

Values are means (SD), unless stated otherwise.

Table 2. Quality of Life before Hip Replacement: A Comparison Between Patients with different Completed Levels of Schooling.

SF36 Sub-Scale	University, Higher Vocational Education and Preparatory Higher Vocational & Scientific Education: n = 100	Middle Vocational Education and Preparatory Middle Vocational Education n = 150	Lower Vocational Education, Elementary Schooling and No Formal Education n = 156	All Patients: n = 406
Physical Functioning	43.0 (20.2)	39.1 (21.7)	39.8 (22.5)	40.3 (21.6)
Role-Physical	38.4 (40.7)	31.7 (39.6)	28.6 (38.1)	32.2 (39.4)
Bodily Pain	44.3 (19.3)	41.7 (20.6)	38.4 (20.7)	41.1 (20.4)
General Health	70.0 (19.9)	69.1 (19.4)	67.6 (19.3)	68.7 (19.5)
Vitality	67.2 (20.7)	59.6 (20.6)	59.5 (22.8)	61.4 (21.7)
Social Functioning	69.0 (22.8)	66.2 (26.6)	63.8 (30.6)	66.0 (27.4)
Role Emotional	79.7 (36.4)	71.1 (41.7)	67.1 (41.7)	71.7 (40.6)
Mental Health	78.9 (15.8)	74.0 (18.1)	73.4 (19.6)	75.0 (18.3)
PCS	38.0 (11.1)	38.5 (9.10)	38.8 (9.40)	38.5 (9.70)
MCS	54.8 (9.30)	51.7 (10.9)	50.9 (11.1)	52.2 (10.7)

Values are means (SD).

mental health, 0.17 points less in the physical component summary and 0.80 points less in the mental component summary; however, none of these differences reached statistical significance (table 6). For each increasing completed level of schooling, TKR patients improved 3.64 points more in physical functioning, 9.38 points more in role-physical, 3.68 points more in bodily pain, 3.67 points more in general health, 1.78 points less in vitality, 0.62 points more in social functioning, 3.11 points less in role-emotional, 3.60 points less in mental health, 2.74 points more in the physical component summary and 2.08 points less in the mental component summary; however, only role-physical, general health, mental health, the physical component summary and the mental component summary reached statistical significance (table 7).

For each increasing completed level of schooling, the NRSS increased 0.1 points for THR patients and 0.0 points for TKR patients. None of these differences reached statistical significance (table 6 and 7).

Adjusted differences in improvement in HRQoL and mean NRSS after joint replacement between each completed level of schooling category are shown in table 8 for THR patients and table 9 for TKR patients. The larger improvement in role-physical functioning in patients with a higher level of completed schooling is mainly due to the large difference between patients with Middle Vocational Education or Preparatory Middle Vocational Education and patients with Lower Vocational Education, Elementary Schooling or No Formal Education. The larger improvement in general health is constant across all groups of level of completed schooling. The larger improvement in the Physical Component Summary Scale in patients with a higher level of completed schooling is mainly due to the large difference between patients with Middle Vocational Education or Preparatory Middle Vocational Education and patients with Lower Vocational Education, Elementary Schooling or No Formal Education.

The smaller improvement in mental health in patients with a higher level of completed schooling is mainly due to the large difference between patients with Middle Vocational Education or Preparatory Middle Vocational Education and patients with Lower Vocational Education, Elementary Schooling or No Formal Education.

Finally, the smaller improvement in the Mental Component Summary Scale in patients with a higher level of completed schooling is mainly due to the large difference between patients with Middle Vocational Education or Preparatory Middle Vocational Education and patients with Lower Vocational Education, Elementary Schooling or No Formal Education.

Discussion

Regardless of their completed level of schooling, patients improve in HRQoL and have a high satisfaction after THR. After TKR, we found that patients with higher completed levels of schooling had a larger improvement in role-physical functioning, general health and the Physical Component Summary scale and a smaller improvement in mental health and the Mental Component Summary scale, although the found differences in the SF36 subscales were smaller than recently published within-group MCIDs at two-years follow-up.[28] All other dimensions of HRQoL and patient satisfaction showed no differences between the completed levels of schooling, thereby failing to refute our hypothesis.

Strengths of our study include the rigorous efforts to minimise confounding and the generalisability of our study population, due to the multi-center setting and the similarity of the demographics of our study population to those of large-scaled national joint registries.[31]

Weaknesses of the study include the low participation rate and the variation in follow-up period after joint replacement. Although participation rates of 100% are feasible in small-scaled studies with hard endpoints,[32,33] participation rates in epidemiological studies have been steadily declining in the last 30 years.[34] Even sharper declines have been reported in the past few years.[35] Unfortunately, the participation rate of this study follows this general trend, and therefore we cannot exclude the presence of self-selection bias. In order to limit the extent of this bias, we have sent multiple reminders and have called all patients who did not answer our reminders and who did not return the questionnaire. As incentives, we have included an appealing information brochure in which the primary goals of the follow-up study were explained and a study pen as a small gift. Additionally, patients were urged to participate by their treating physician. However, the participation rate alone does not determine the extent of bias

Table 3. Quality of Life before Knee Replacement: A Comparison Between Patients with different Completed Levels of Schooling.

SF36 Sub-Scale	University, Higher Vocational Education and Preparatory Higher Vocational & Scientific Education: n = 42	Middle Vocational Education and Preparatory Middle Vocational Education n = 98	Lower Vocational Education, Elementary Schooling and No Formal Education n = 122	All Patients: n = 262
Physical Functioning	40.4 (19.4)	41.3 (19.1)	38.4 (22.1)	39.8 (20.6)
Role-Physical	41.7 (41.9)	40.4 (42.3)	38.1 (42.9)	39.5 (42.4)
Bodily Pain	45.5 (19.4)	45.4 (19.7)	42.2 (21.6)	43.9 (20.6)
General Health	62.5 (19.0)	65.2 (18.7)	59.0 (21.1)	61.9 (20.0)
Vitality	63.2 (18.0)	63.1 (21.2)	57.7 (22.3)	60.6 (21.4)
Social Functioning	72.6 (22.1)	72.2 (23.0)	67.3 (26.3)	70.0 (24.5)
Role Emotional	82.5 (33.1)	74.5 (39.4)	62.0 (44.8)	70.0 (41.8)
Mental Health	79.6 (10.4)	76.4 (15.7)	68.1 (20.3)	73.1 (18.0)
PCS	36.8 (11.8)	40.2 (9.20)	40.8 (9.70)	39.9 (10.0)
MCS	55.5 (7.40)	53.0 (9.50)	48.8 (11.2)	51.5 (10.4)

Table 4. Improvement in Health-Related Quality of Life and Satisfaction after Hip Replacement:: A Comparison Between Patients with different Completed Levels of Schooling.

SF36 Sub-Scale	University, Higher Vocational Education and Preparatory Higher Vocational & Scientific Education: n = 100	Middle Vocational Education and Preparatory Middle Vocational Education n = 150	Lower Vocational Education, Elementary Schooling and No Formal Education n = 156
Physical Functioning	27.8 (23.3–32.3)	26.6 (22.4–30.7)	24.9 (20.5–29.2)
Role-Physical	35.7 (26.6–44.7)	40.7 (32.9–48.6)	42.3 (35.0–49.5)
Bodily Pain	38.0 (33.1–42.9)	33.4 (29.3–37.6)	38.9 (34.9–42.9)
General Health	−1.20 (−4.80–2.50)	−0.70 (−3.70–2.30)	−0.20 (−3.50–3.10)
Vitality	3.40 (0.20–6.60)	8.50 (5.80–11.3)	6.70 (3.10–10.2)
Social Functioning	16.0 (11.3–20.7)	18.1 (13.5–22.7)	20.0 (15.4–24.5)
Role Emotional	5.70 (−2.60–13.9)	16.0 (8.80–23.2)	11.9 (4.70–19.0)
Mental Health	2.10 (−0.60–4.80)	6.40 (3.90–9.00)	5.90 (3.30–8.50)
PCS	12.8 (11.1–14.6)	10.8 (9.20–12.3)	11.4 (9.80–13.0)
MCS	−1.60 (−3.40–0.30)	1.50 (−0.10–3.00)	0.60 (−1.00–2.20)
NRS Satisfaction	8.9 (8.6–9.3)	8.7 (8.4–9.0)	8.6 (8.3–8.9)

present in any particular study.[35] The difference between participants and nonparticipants is far more important.[36] As the found differences in demographics were small, it is unlikely that the study results will be severely biased.

The follow-up period after joint replacement varies between 1.5 and 6 years in this study (Figure 1 and 2). Theoretically, this broad range could influence our findings. In order to exclude this variable, all patients should have been followed for the exact same amount of time. In our data, we found no clear evidence of a relationship between the improvement in HRQoL after joint replacement and the follow-up period (See Appendix S1 and S2 for scatter plots of the improvement in HRQoL as a function of the follow-up period length, stratified per completed levels of schooling and Appendix S3 and S4 for scatter plots of the NRSS after surgery as a function of the follow-up period length, stratified per completed levels of schooling). In order to account for this range, we stratified our analysis per quartile of follow-up period. Stratifying for an additional variable inevitably leads to a loss of power, thereby increasing the probability of a type 2-error. In our analysis, this loss of power was negligible, as unstratified analyses showed similar results, supporting our conclusions (data not shown).

Although a residual effect of follow-up length within each stratum cannot be excluded, we do not think this is very plausible, as recent evidence suggests that the improvement in HRQoL after completion of the initial rehabilitation-period is sustained up to 7 years after joint replacement surgery.[37,38] The minimum follow-up period is well beyond the length of the expected rehabilitation-period, suggested by a recently published systematic review.[39]

Two other studies have investigated the relation between SEP and patient-reported outcomes after THR or TKR.[40,41] Allen Butler et. al. have studied this relation in a randomised controlled trial, which compared two THR designs.[40] In this study, the

Table 5. Improvement in Health-Related Quality of Life and Satisfaction after Knee Replacement:: A Comparison Between Patients with different Completed Levels of Schooling.

SF36 Sub-Scale	University, Higher Vocational Education and Preparatory Higher Vocational & Scientific Education: n = 42	Middle Vocational Education and Preparatory Middle Vocational Education n = 98	Lower Vocational Education, Elementary Schooling and No Formal Education n = 122
Physical Functioning	20.4 (12.4–28.5)	14.0 (8.70–19.3)	10.3 (6.40–14.2)
Role-Physical	31.5 (15.6–47.5)	25.2 (14.4–35.9)	15.6 (7.40–23.7)
Bodily Pain	24.9 (17.6–32.2)	25.5 (19.7–31.2)	21.0 (16.5–25.5)
General Health	4.00 (−0.60–8.60)	−1.60 (−5.20–2.10)	−3.60 (−6.90–−0.30)
Vitality	1.30 (−3.60–6.30)	−1.00 (−4.70–2.80)	2.60 (−0.90–6.10)
Social Functioning	11.6 (2.80–20.4)	7.80 (1.80–13.8)	8.80 (4.40–13.2)
Role Emotional	9.50 (−1.50–20.5)	3.40 (−6.30–13.1)	10.9 (2.60–19.2)
Mental Health	3.30 (0.20–6.40)	1.30 (−2.30–4.90)	6.20 (3.40–9.10)
PCS	7.70 (4.20–11.3)	7.00 (4.90–9.00)	4.20 (2.70–5.70)
MCS	−0.40 (−3.00–2.20)	−1.70 (−3.7–0.30)	1.70 (0.00–3.40)
NRS Satisfaction	8.3 (7.6–9.1)	8.1 (7.6–8.6)	7.9 (7.4–8.4)

Table 6. Adjusted Difference in Improvement in Health-Related Quality of Life and Satisfaction after Hip Replacement: A Comparison Between Patients with different Completed Levels of Schooling.

SF36 Sub-Scale	Adjusted difference per increasing Completed Levels of Schooling (95% CI)	p-value
Physical Functioning	−0.88 (−4.14–2.38)	0.59
Role-Physical	3.09 (−2.89–9.07)	0.31
Bodily Pain	0.60 (−2.70–3.89)	0.72
General Health	0.66 (−1.81–3.13)	0.60
Vitality	1.44 (−1.04–3.92)	0.25
Social Functioning	−0.12 (−3.59–3.36)	0.94
Role Emotional	0.34 (−5.31–6.00)	0.90
Mental Health	1.35 (−0.61–3.30)	0.18
PCS	0.17 (−1.04–1.38)	0.79
MCS	0.80 (−0.42–2.03)	0.20
NRS Satisfaction	−0.1 (−0.4–0.1)	0.29

Negative values indicate a higher mean improvement in HRQoL after THR in patients with increasing Completed Levels of Schooling. The mean differences between education level are adjusted for age, sex, Body Mass Index and Charnley Classification of Comorbidity and stratified for quartiles of follow-up.

effect of SEP was studied on a multitude of outcome measures, including the WOMAC, Short Form-12 (SF12) and degree of patient satisfaction. An association was found between lower levels of education and a degree of satisfaction which was "less than very satisfied". Unfortunately, the authors have only reported their significant findings; differences in WOMAC or SF12 between social classes are not reported. Additionally, only p-values are reported instead of mean differences or relative risks, precluding any judgment on the clinical relevance of their findings. Finally, it is unclear for which factors any associations were adjusted, as the authors applied forward stepwise logistic regression modeling, without mentioning which variables were included in the final model. Davis et. al. have measured WOMAC scores before surgery and at 3, 12 and 24 months after TKR.[41] Whilst comparing WOMAC scores at each time point between patients of different income categories, patients with more disadvantaged SEP had worse preoperative WOMAC scores and similar postoperative WOMAC scores as patients with less disadvantaged SEP. These findings imply a larger improvement in disease-specific quality of life in patients with more disadvantaged SEP than in patients with less disadvantaged SEP. However, not all patients were measured at each time point. A cross-sectional comparison at each time point precludes judgment on the actual within-patient improvement in disease-specific quality of life. Due to methodological shortcomings of both other studies which investigated the relation between SEP and patient-reported outcomes after joint replacement, no meaningful comparison of results can be made.

Our findings have large implications for policymakers, as a more advantaged SEP is associated with greater use of health services in general.[12] A recent systematic review and numerous studies indicate that this also holds for THR[42–51] and TKR[42,46–48,50–52] in post-industrialised countries. Additionally, the need for

Table 7. Adjusted Difference in Improvement in Health-Related Quality of Life and Satisfaction after Knee Replacement: A Comparison Between Patients with different Completed Levels of Schooling.

SF36 Sub-Scale	Adjusted difference per increasing Completed Levels of Schooling (95% CI)	p-value
Physical Functioning	−3.64 (−8.03–0.74)	0.10
Role-Physical	−9.38 (−18.4–−0.34)	0.04
Bodily Pain	−3.68 (−8.39–1.03)	0.13
General Health	−3.67 (−6.79–−0.56)	0.02
Vitality	1.78 (−1.51–5.08)	0.29
Social Functioning	−0.62 (−5.37–4.14)	0.80
Role Emotional	3.11 (−5.07–11.3)	0.46
Mental Health	3.60 (0.82–6.38)	0.01
PCS	−2.74 (−4.41–−1.07)	0.001
MCS	2.08 (0.37–3.79)	0.02
NRS Satisfaction	0.0 (−0.5–0.4)	0.83

Negative values indicate a higher mean improvement in HRQoL after TKR in patients with increasing Completed Levels of Schooling. The mean differences between education level are adjusted for age, sex, Body Mass Index and Charnley Classification of Comorbidity and stratified for quartiles of follow-up.

Table 8. Adjusted Difference in Improvement in Health-Related Quality of Life and Satisfaction after Hip Replacement.: A Comparison Between Patients with different Completed Levels of Schooling.

SF36 Sub-Scale	Adjusted Difference Between U+HVE+PHVSE and MVE+PMVE* (95%CI)	Adjusted Difference Between MVE+PMVE and LVE+ES+NFE** (95%CI)	Adjusted Difference Between U+HVE+PHVSE and LVE+ES+NFE*** (95%CI)
Physical Functioning	−1.96 (−8.56–4.64)	0.91 (−5.16–6.97)	−1.94 (−8.53–4.66)
Role-Physical	6.21 (−5.85–18.3)	2.66 (−8.04–13.4)	6.21 (−5.91–18.3)
Bodily Pain	−6.27 (−12.9–0.33)	7.28 (1.69–12.7)	−0.33 (−6.94–6.29)
General Health	−0.70 (−5.72–4.31)	1.57 (−2.95–6.08)	1.16 (−3.85–6.17)
Vitality	5.11 (0.09–10.1)	−1.08 (−5.76–3.61)	3.18 (−1.83–8.19)
Social Functioning	−0.50 (−7.57–6.57)	0.85 (−5.72–7.42)	−0.34 (−7.37–6.70)
Role Emotional	5.63 (−5.81–17.1)	−2.95 (−13.3–7.42)	1.89 (−9.59–13.4)
Mental Health	3.43 (−0.59–7.44)	−0.19 (−3.86–3.48)	2.98 (−0.99–6.95)
PCS	−1.64 (−4.07–0.79)	1.85 (−0.29–3.99)	−0.05 (−2.49–2.38)
MCS	2.69 (0.20–5.19)	−0.70 (−2.95–1.55)	1.93 (−0.55–4.41)
NRS Satisfaction	−0.3 (−0.8–0.2)	0.1 (−0.3–0.6)	−0.3 (−0.9–0.2)

U+HVE+PHVSE: University, Higher Vocational Education and Preparatory Higher Vocational & Scientific Education; MVE+PMVE: Middle Vocational Education and Preparatory Middle Vocational Education; LVE+ES+NFE: Lower Vocational Education, Elementary Schooling and No Formal Education.
*Negative values indicate a higher mean improvement in HRQoL after THR in U+HVE+PHVSE patients, compared to MVE+PMVE patients.
**Negative values indicate a higher mean improvement in HRQoL after THR in MVE+PMVE patients, compared to LVE+ES+NFE patients.
***Negative values indicate a higher mean improvement in HRQoL after THR in U+HVE+PHVSE patients, compared to LVE+ES+NFE patients.
The mean differences between education level are adjusted for age, sex, Body Mass Index and Charnley Classification of Comorbidity and stratified for quartiles of follow-up.

joint replacement appears to be higher in patients with more disadvantaged SEP,[48,51,52] thereby increasing the inequity in access to joint replacement. Under-treatment of patients with more disadvantaged SEP cannot be justified, given the similar improvement in HRQoL and postoperative level of satisfaction with surgery between the examined groups of completed level of schooling.

A number of factors might explain the found differences in improvement in HRQoL after between THR and TKR patients per completed level of schooling groups. Biomechanical factors might play a role. The hip joint is a relatively simple ball and socket joint, which is adequately mimicked by a THR. The adequate mimicry of the biomechanics is reflected in a highly

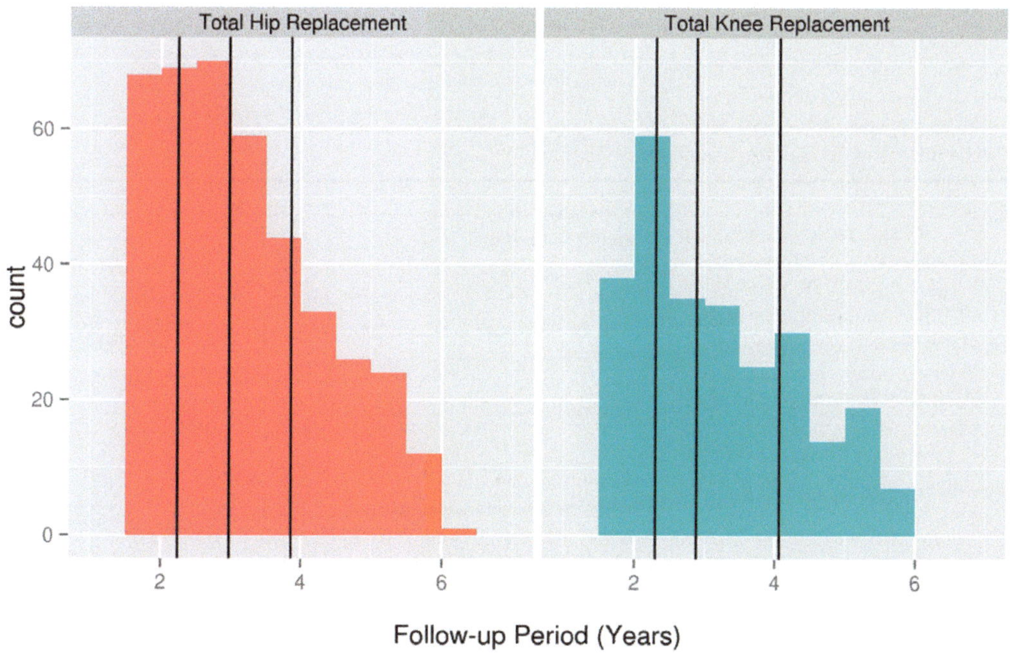

Figure 2. Follow-up Period in Years for THR and TKR patients. Vertical lines indicate quartiles of follow-up period length.

Table 9. Adjusted Difference in Improvement in Health-Related Quality of Life and Satisfaction after Knee Replacement::A Comparison Between Patients with different Completed Levels of Schooling.

SF36 Sub-Scale	Adjusted Difference Between U+HVE+PHVSE and MVE+PMVE* (95%CI)	Adjusted Difference Between MVE+PMVE and LVE+ES+NFE** (95%CI)	Adjusted Difference Between U+HVE+PHVSE and LVE+ES+NFE*** (95%CI)
Physical Functioning	−5.80 (−15.1–3.53)	−2.24 (−9.14–4.65)	−7.99 (−17.2–1.26)
Role-Physical	−3.37 (−22.5–15.7)	−12.2 (−26.5–2.18)	−16.5 (−35.4–2.53)
Bodily Pain	1.00 (−9.02–11.0)	−6.46 (−14.1–1.20)	−6.13 (−16.1–3.81)
General Health	−4.84 (−11.4–1.72)	−2.84 (−7.88–2.21)	−7.64 (−14.2–−1.10)
Vitality	−0.60 (−7.57–6.36)	3.57 (−1.70–8.83)	2.98 (−3.93–9.89)
Social Functioning	−3.22 (−13.4–6.94)	0.87 (−6.47–8.21)	−2.09 (−12.2–7.94)
Role Emotional	−1.26 (−18.8–16.2)	5.73 (−7.79–19.3)	4.49 (−12.8–21.8)
Mental Health	−0.80 (−6.69–5.08)	5.84 (1.11–10.6)	6.32 (0.53–12.1)
PCS	−1.36 (−4.90–2.18)	−3.42 (−6.04–−0.80)	−5.04 (−8.56–−1.52)
MCS	0.03 (−3.63–3.70)	3.04 (0.19–5.88)	3.58 (−0.03–7.19)
NRS Satisfaction	0.2 (−0.8–1.1)	−0.1 (−0.8–0.6)	−0.1 (−1.0–0.8)

U+HVE+PHVSE: University, Higher Vocational Education and Preparatory Higher Vocational & Scientific Education; MVE+PMVE: Middle Vocational Education and Preparatory Middle Vocational Education; LVE+ES+NFE: Lower Vocational Education, Elementary Schooling and No Formal Education.
*Negative values indicate a higher mean improvement in HRQoL after TKR in U+HVE+PHVSE patients, compared to MVE+PMVE patients.
**Negative values indicate a higher mean improvement in HRQoL after TKR in MVE+PMVE patients, compared to LVE+ES+NFE patients.
***Negative values indicate a higher mean improvement in HRQoL after TKR in U+HVE+PHVSE patients, compared to LVE+ES+NFE patients.
The mean differences between education level are adjusted for age, sex, Body Mass Index and Charnley Classification of Comorbidity and stratified for quartiles of follow-up.

consistent improvement in HRQoL, regardless of completed level of schooling. The biomechanical aspects of the knee joint are more difficult to imitate, as the knee is a pivotal hinge joint with 6 degrees of freedom. These degrees of freedom are generally not restored after TKR, which is substantiated in kinematic and kinetic studies.[53] However, more complex biomechanics might explain a less consistent improvement in HRQoL in TKR patients, but does not explain differences between patient groups with different completed levels of schooling.

Differences between THR and TKR patients might be part of the explanation. Better general health, physical, emotional and social function, motivation and self-efficacy and lower levels of pain before surgery and during the rehabilitation period are associated with improved short- and medium-term outcomes.[2] In our study population, differences in the preoperative health status between completed level of schooling groups are more pronounced in TKR patients than in THR patients (table 2 and table 3). Finally, differences in rehabilitational options could play an important role. TKR patients require more rehabilitation than THR patients in order to achieve optimal results.[54] TKR patients with higher completed Level of Schooling might have better access to physical therapy or other rehabilitational facilities, and therefore gain more in role-physical functioning and general health than less advantaged patients. This effect might be exacerbated by the higher prevalence of obesity and co-morbidity in TKR patients compared to THR patients. Unfortunately, we do not have any information on the rehabilitational regime of our THR and TKR patients, leaving this hypothesis to be addressed in future research.

Supporting Information

Appendix S1 Scatterplots of the improvement in HRQoL as a function of the follow-up period length, stratified per completed levels of schooling, for Total Hip Replacement Patients. U+HVE+PHVSE: University, Higher Vocational Education and Preparatory Higher Vocational & Scientific Education; MVE+PMVE: Middle Vocational Education and Preparatory Middle Vocational Education; LVE+ES+NFE: Lower Vocational Education, Elementary Schooling and No Formal Education.

Appendix S2 Scatterplots of the improvement in HRQoL as a function of the follow-up period length, stratified per completed levels of schooling, for Total Knee Replacement Patients. U+HVE+PHVSE: University, Higher Vocational Education and Preparatory Higher Vocational & Scientific Education; MVE+PMVE: Middle Vocational Education and Preparatory Middle Vocational Education; LVE+ES+NFE: Lower Vocational Education, Elementary Schooling and No Formal Education.

Appendix S3 Scatterplots of the NRSS after surgery as a function of the follow-up period length, stratified per completed levels of schooling, for Total Hip Replacement Patients. U+HVE+PHVSE: University, Higher Vocational Education and Preparatory Higher Vocational & Scientific Education; MVE+PMVE: Middle Vocational Education and Preparatory Middle Vocational Education; LVE+ES+NFE: Lower Vocational Education, Elementary Schooling and No Formal Education.

Appendix S4 Scatterplots of the NRSS after surgery as a function of the follow-up period length, stratified per completed levels of schooling, for Total Knee Replacement Patients. U+HVE+PHVSE: University, Higher Vocational Education and Preparatory Higher Vocational & Scientific Education; MVE+PMVE: Middle Vocational Education and Preparatory Middle Vocational Education; LVE+ES+NFE: Lower Vocational Education, Elementary Schooling and No Formal Education.

Author Contributions

Conceived and designed the experiments: JCK DB RGN. Performed the experiments: JCK. Analyzed the data: JCK DB MB JJK MF. Wrote the paper: JCK DB MB JJK MF RGN.

References

1. Ethgen O, Bruyère O, Richy F, Dardennes C, Reginster J-Y (2004) Health-related quality of life in total hip and total knee arthroplasty. A qualitative and systematic review of the literature. The Journal of bone and joint surgery American volume 86-A: 963–974.
2. Beswick AD, Wylde V, Gooberman-Hill R, Blom A, Dieppe P (2012) What proportion of patients report long-term pain after total hip or knee replacement for osteoarthritis? A systematic review of prospective studies in unselected patients. BMJ open 2: e000435.
3. Gandhi R, Davey JR, Mahomed NN (2008) Predicting patient dissatisfaction following joint replacement surgery. The Journal of rheumatology 35: 2415–2418. doi:10.3899/jrheum.080295
4. Noble PC, Conditt MA, Cook KF, Mathis KB (2006) The John Insall Award: Patient expectations affect satisfaction with total knee arthroplasty. Clinical orthopaedics and related research 452: 35–43. doi:10.1097/01.blo.0000238825.63648.1e
5. Brokelman RBG, Van Loon CJM, Rijnberg WJ (2003) Patient versus surgeon satisfaction after total hip arthroplasty. [Miscellaneous Article]. Journal of Bone & Joint Surgery - British Volume 85-B: 495–498.
6. Nilsdotter AK, Toksvig-Larsen S, Roos EM (2009) Knee arthroplasty: are patients' expectations fulfilled? A prospective study of pain and function in 102 patients with 5-year follow-up. Acta orthopaedica 80: 55–61. doi:10.1080/17453670902805007
7. Lingard EA, Sledge CB, Learmonth ID (2006) PATIENT EXPECTATIONS REGARDING TOTAL KNEE ARTHROPLASTY: DIFFERENCES AMONG THE UNITED STATES, UNITED KINGDOM, AND AUSTRALIA. Journal of Bone & Joint Surgery, American Volume 88: 1201–1207.
8. Garellick G, Malchau H, Herberts P (2000) Survival of hip replacements. A comparison of a randomized trial and a registry. ClinOrthopRelat Res: 157–167.
9. Baker PN, Van der Meulen JH, Lewsey J, Gregg PJ (2007) The role of pain and function in determining patient satisfaction after total knee replacement. Data from the National Joint Registry for England and Wales. The Journal of bone and joint surgery British volume 89: 893–900. doi:10.1302/0301-620X.89B7.19091
10. Kurtz S, Ong K, Lau E, Mowat F, Halpern M (2007) Projections of primary and revision hip and knee arthroplasty in the United States from 2005 to 2030. The Journal of Bone and Joint Surgery American Volume 89: 780–785.
11. Krieger N (2001) A glossary for social epidemiology. Journal of epidemiology and community health 55: 693–700.
12. Lostao L, Regidor E, Gimeno D, Netuveli G, Blane D (2011) Socioeconomic patterns in health services use in Great Britain and Spain before and after the health system reforms of the 1990s. Health & place 17: 830–835.
13. Quintana JM, Escobar A, Aguirre U, Lafuente I, Arenaza JC (2009) Predictors of health-related quality-of-life change after total hip arthroplasty. Clinical orthopaedics and related research 467: 2886–2894. doi:10.1007/s11999-009-0868-9
14. Escobar A, Quintana JM, Bilbao A, Azkárate J, Güenaga JI, et al. (2007) Effect of patient characteristics on reported outcomes after total knee replacement. Rheumatology (Oxford, England) 46: 112–119. doi:10.1093/rheumatology/kel184
15. Gill TMFeinstein AR(n.d.) A critical appraisal of the quality of quality-of-life measurements. JAMA: the journal of the American Medical Association 272: 619–626.
16. Muldoon MF, Barger SD, Flory JD, Manuck SB (1998) What are quality of life measurements measuring? BMJ (Clinical research ed) 316: 542–545.
17. Ware JE, Sherbourne CD (1992) The MOS 36-item short-form health survey (SF-36). I. Conceptual framework and item selection. Medical care 30: 473–483.
18. Stewart AL, Hays RD, Ware JE (1988) The MOS short-form general health survey. Reliability and validity in a patient population. Medical care 26: 724–735.
19. Jenkinson C, Coulter A, Wright L (1993) Short form 36 (SF36) health survey questionnaire: normative data for adults of working age. BMJ (Clinical research ed) 306: 1437–1440.
20. Aaronson NK, Muller M, Cohen PD, Essink-Bot ML, Fekkes M, et al. (1998) Translation, validation, and norming of the Dutch language version of the SF-36 Health Survey in community and chronic disease populations. Journal of clinical epidemiology 51: 1055–1068.
21. Ostendorf M, Van Stel HF, Buskens E, Schrijvers AJP, Marting LN, et al. (2004) Patient-reported outcome in total hip replacement. A comparison of five instruments of health status. The Journal of Bone and Joint Surgery British Volume 86: 801–808.
22. Grosse Frie K, Van der Meulen J, Black N (2012) Single item on patients' satisfaction with condition provided additional insight into impact of surgery. Journal of clinical epidemiology 65: 619–626.
23. Charnley J (1972) The long-term results of low-friction arthroplasty of the hip performed as a primary intervention. The Journal of bone and joint surgery British volume 54: 61–76.
24. Dunbar MJ, Robertsson O, Ryd L (2004) What's all that noise? The effect of co-morbidity on health outcome questionnaire results after knee arthroplasty. Acta orthopaedica Scandinavica 75: 119–126. doi:10.1080/00016470412331294355
25. Dempster AP, Laird NM, Rubin DB (1977) Maximum Likelihood Estimation from Incomplete Data Via the EM Algorithm. Journal of the Royal Statistical Association 39: 1–38.
26. Honaker J, King G, Blackwell M (2010) AMELIA II: A Program for Missing Data. Journal Of Statistical Software 45: 1–53. doi:10.1.1.149.9611
27. King G, Honaker J, Joseph A, Scheve K (2001) Analyzing Incomplete Political Science Data: An Alternative Algorithm for Multiple Imputation. American Political Science Review 95: 49–69. doi:10.2307/3117628
28. Keurentjes JC, Van Tol F, Fiocco M, Schoones J, Nelissen RG (2012) Minimal clinically important differences in health-related quality of life after total hip or knee replacement. Bone and Joint Research 1: 71–77. doi:10.1302/2046-3758.15.2000065
29. Rubin DB (1987) Multiple Imputation for Nonresponse in Surveys. Wiley. p.
30. Team RDC (2008) R: A Language and Environment for Statistical Computing. Vienna Austria R Foundation for Statistical Computing 1: ISBN 3–900051–07–0.
31. Malchau H, Garellick G, Eisler T, Kärrholm J, Herberts P (2005) Presidential guest address: the Swedish Hip Registry: increasing the sensitivity by patient outcome data. Clinical orthopaedics and related research 441: 19–29.
32. Schreurs BW, Keurentjes JC, Gardeniers JWM, Verdonschot N, Slooff TJJH, et al. (2009) Acetabular revision with impacted morsellised cancellous bone grafting and a cemented acetabular component: a 20- to 25-year follow-up. The Journal of bone and joint surgery British volume 91: 1148–1153. doi:10.1302/0301-620X.91B9.21750
33. Keurentjes JC, Fiocco M, Schreurs BW, Pijls BG, Nouta KA, et al. (2012) Revision surgery is overestimated in hip replacement. Bone and Joint Research 1: 258–262. doi:10.1302/2046-3758.110.2000104
34. Hartge P (2006) Participation in population studies. Epidemiology (Cambridge, Mass) 17: 252–254. doi:10.1097/01.ede.0000209441.24307.92
35. Galea S, Tracy M (2007) Participation rates in epidemiologic studies. Annals of epidemiology 17: 643–653. doi:10.1016/j.annepidem.2007.03.013
36. Jones J (1996) The effects of non-response on statistical inference. Journal of health & social policy 8: 49–62. doi:10.1300/J045v08n01_05
37. Bruyère O, Ethgen O, Neuprez A, Zégels B, Gillet P, et al. (2012) Health-related quality of life after total knee or hip replacement for osteoarthritis: a 7-year prospective study. Archives of orthopaedic and trauma surgery.
38. Ng CY, Ballantyne JA, Brenkel IJ (2007) Quality of life and functional outcome after primary total hip replacement. A five-year follow-up. The Journal of bone and joint surgery British volume 89: 868–873. doi:10.1302/0301-620X.89B7.18482
39. Vissers MM, Bussmann JB, Verhaar JAN, Arends LR, Furlan AD, et al. (2011) Recovery of physical functioning after total hip arthroplasty: systematic review and meta-analysis of the literature. Physical therapy 91: 615–629. doi:10.2522/ptj.20100201
40. Allen Butler R, Rosenzweig S, Myers L, Barrack RL (2011) The Frank Stinchfield Award: the impact of socioeconomic factors on outcome after THA: a prospective, randomized study. Clinical orthopaedics and related research 469: 339–347.
41. Davis ET, Lingard EA, Schemitsch EH, Waddell JP (2008) Effects of socioeconomic status on patients' outcome after total knee arthroplasty. International journal for quality in health care: journal of the International Society for Quality in Health Care/ISQua 20: 40–46.
42. Mujica-Mota RE, Tarricone R, Ciani O, Bridges JF, Drummond M (2012) Determinants of demand for total hip and knee arthroplasty: a systematic literature review. BMC health services research 12: 225.
43. Agabiti N, Picciotto S, Cesaroni G, Bisanti L, Forastiere F, et al. (2007) The influence of socioeconomic status on utilization and outcomes of elective total hip replacement: a multicity population-based longitudinal study. International journal for quality in health care: journal of the International Society for Quality in Health Care/ISQua 19: 37–44. doi:10.1093/intqhc/mzl065
44. Brennan SL, Stanford T, Wluka AE, Henry MJ, Page RS, et al. (2012) Cross-sectional analysis of association between socioeconomic status and utilization of primary total hip joint replacements 2006-7: Australian Orthopaedic Association National Joint Replacement Registry. BMC musculoskeletal disorders 13: 63. doi:10.1186/1471-2474-13-63
45. Dixon T, Shaw M, Ebrahim S, Dieppe P (2004) Trends in hip and knee joint replacement: socioeconomic inequalities and projections of need. Annals of the rheumatic diseases 63: 825–830. doi:10.1136/ard.2003.012724

46. Hawkins K, Escoto KH, Ozminkowski RJ, Bhattarai GR, Migliori RJ, et al. (2011) Disparities in major joint replacement surgery among adults with Medicare supplement insurance. Population health management 14: 231–238. doi:10.1089/pop.2010.0042
47. Judge A, Welton NJ, Sandhu J, Ben-Shlomo Y (2009) Geographical variation in the provision of elective primary hip and knee replacement: the role of socio-demographic, hospital and distance variables. Journal of public health (Oxford, England) 31: 413–422. doi:10.1093/pubmed/fdp061
48. Judge a., Welton NJ, Sandhu J, Ben-Shlomo Y (2010) Equity in access to total joint replacement of the hip and knee in England: cross sectional study. Bmj 341: c4092–c4092. doi:10.1136/bmj.c4092
49. Majeed A, Eliahoo J, Bardsley M, Morgan D, Bindman AB (2002) Variation in coronary artery bypass grafting, angioplasty, cataract surgery, and hip replacement rates among primary care groups in London: association with population and practice characteristics. Journal of public health medicine 24: 21–26.
50. Peterson MG, Hollenberg JP, Szatrowski TP, Johanson NA, Mancuso CA, et al. (1992) Geographic variations in the rates of elective total hip and knee arthroplasties among Medicare beneficiaries in the United States. The Journal of bone and joint surgery American volume 74: 1530–1539.
51. Steel N, Melzer D, Gardener E, McWilliams B (2006) Need for and receipt of hip and knee replacement–a national population survey. Rheumatology (Oxford, England) 45: 1437–1441. doi:10.1093/rheumatology/kel131
52. Yong PFK, Milner PC, Payne JN, Lewis Pa, Jennison C (2004) Inequalities in access to knee joint replacements for people in need. Annals of the rheumatic diseases 63: 1483–1489. doi:10.1136/ard.2003.013938
53. Wolterbeek N, Garling EH, Mertens BJ, Nelissen RGHH, Valstar ER (2011) Kinematics and early migration in single-radius mobile- and fixed-bearing total knee prostheses. Clinical biomechanics (Bristol, Avon). doi:10.1016/j.clinbiomech.2011.10.013
54. Roos EM (2003) Effectiveness and practice variation of rehabilitation after joint replacement. Current opinion in rheumatology 15: 160–162.

5

Patients with Severe Radiographic Osteoarthritis Have a Better Prognosis in Physical Functioning after Hip and Knee Replacement: A Cohort-Study

J. Christiaan Keurentjes[1]*, Marta Fiocco[2], Cynthia So-Osman[3], Ron Onstenk[4], Ankie W. M. M. Koopman-Van Gemert[5], Ruud G. Pöll[6], Herman M. Kroon[7], Thea P. M. Vliet Vlieland[1], Rob G. Nelissen[1]

1 Department of Orthopaedic Surgery, Leiden University Medical Center, Leiden, The Netherlands, **2** Department of Medical Statistics and BioInformatics, Leiden University Medical Center, Leiden, The Netherlands, **3** Department of Research and Development, Sanquin Blood Supply South West Region, Leiden, The Netherlands, **4** Department of Orthopaedic Surgery, Groene Hart Hospital, Gouda, The Netherlands, **5** Department of Anaesthesiology, Albert Schweitzer Hospital, Dordrecht, The Netherlands, **6** Department of Orthopaedic Surgery, Slotervaart Hospital, Amsterdam, The Netherlands, **7** Department of Radiology, Leiden University Medical Center, Leiden, The Netherlands

Abstract

Introduction: Although Total Hip and Knee Replacements (THR/TKR) improve Health-Related Quality of Life (HRQoL) at the group level, up to 30% of patients are dissatisfied after surgery due to unfulfilled expectations. We aimed to assess whether the pre-operative radiographic severity of osteoarthritis (OA) is related to the improvement in HRQoL after THR or TKR, both at the population and individual level.

Methods: In this multi-center observational cohort study, HRQoL of OA patients requiring THR or TKR was measured 2 weeks before surgery and at 2–5 years follow-up, using the Short-Form 36 (SF36). Additionally, we measured patient satisfaction on a 11-point Numeric Rating Scale (NRSS). The radiographic severity of OA was classified according to Kellgren and Lawrence (KL) by an independent experienced musculoskeletal radiologist, blinded for the outcome. We compared the mean improvement and probability of a relevant improvement (defined as a patients change score≥Minimal Clinically Important Difference) between patients with mild OA (KL Grade 0–2) and severe OA (KL Grade 3+4), whilst adjusting for confounders.

Results: Severe OA patients improved more and had a higher probability of a relevant improvement in physical functioning after both THR and TKR. For TKR patients with severe OA, larger improvements were found in General Health, Vitality and the Physical Component Summary Scale. The mean NRSS was also higher in severe OA TKR patients.

Discussion: Patients with severe OA have a better prognosis after THR and TKR than patients with mild OA. These findings might help to prevent dissatisfaction after THR and TKR by means of patient selection or expectation management.

Editor: Hamid Reza Baradaran, Tehran University of Medical Sciences, Islamic Republic of Iran

Funding: This study was funded by a grant from the Dutch Arthritis Association (Grant-number: LLP-13). Both the sponsors of the previous trial (ZON-MW, The Netherlands Organization for Health Research and Development; Roche Nederland BV; Sanquin Bloodbank Amsterdam; Haemonetics BV) and the sponsor of the current study (Dutch Arthritis Association) had no role in study design, data collection, data analysis, data interpretation, or writing of the report. The corresponding author had full access to all the data in the study. All authors had final responsibility for the decision to submit for publication.

Competing Interests: The authors have declared that no competing interests exist.

* E-mail: j.c.keurentjes@lumc.nl

Introduction

Total Hip Replacement (THR) and Total Knee Replacement (TKR) are effective surgical interventions, which alleviate pain and improve Health-Related Quality of Life (HRQoL) in patients with hip or knee joint degeneration at the population level. [1] Although on average patients improve markedly after THR or TKR, not all patients benefit from these surgeries. Persistent pain is reported in 9% of THR patients and 20% of TKR patients at long term follow-up. [2] Additionally, up to 30% of patients are dissatisfied after surgery, with higher reported dissatisfaction rates for TKR patients.[3–9] The relatively high dissatisfaction rate is especially worrying, as the therapeutic options are limited in dissatisfied patients after joint replacement. Moreover, given the projected increase in the annual number of THR and TKR performed in the United States, the absolute number of dissatisfied patients is expected to rise. [10].

Unattained expectations of surgery are thought to play an important role in dissatisfaction after joint replacement. [3,4,6,11] In order to successfully manage patient expectations, accurate prediction of the probability of a meaningful improvement for each individual patient is of paramount importance. This probability can be assessed at the individual level using the Minimal Clinically Important Difference (MCID), which is defined as the minimal difference in scores of an outcome measure that is perceived by patients as beneficial or harmful. [12,13]

MCIDs in HRQoL, measured using the Short-Form 36, have been established for THR and TKR.[14–16].

Reports of the effect of the preoperative radiographic severity of osteoarthritis (OA) on the outcome of THR are conflicting: at the population level, Nilsdotter et al showed no effect at one year follow-up, while Meding et al found less postoperative pain at one year follow-up in patients with more preoperative joint space narrowing. [17,18] At the individual level, patients with severe preoperative radiographic OA were more likely to improve in physical functioning. [19] We found no studies addressing the effect of the preoperative radiographic severity of osteoarthritis (OA) on the outcome of TKR.

From a clinical perspective, the preoperative radiographic severity of OA would be a helpful predictor of improvement in HRQoL, as it is both inexpensive and performed routinely for templating purposes. Moreover, the assessment of the severity of preoperative OA could be standardised, whereas this would be more difficult with subjective symptoms such as pain.

We questioned whether the radiographic severity of OA affects the improvement in HRQoL after THR and TKR, both at the population and individual level. Additionally, we questioned whether patient satisfaction with the surgical results differed between patients with mild or severe preoperative radiographical OA.

Methods

We conducted a multi-center follow-up study at the departments of orthopaedic surgery of the Leiden University Medical Center, the Slotervaart hospital in Amsterdam, the Albert Schweitzer hospital in Dordrecht and the Groene Hart hospital in Gouda, the Netherlands, from August 2010 until August 2011. [20] The study was approved by the Medical Ethics Committee of the Leiden University Medical Center and the Medical Ethical Committees of all other participating centers; all patients gave written informed consent (CCMO-Nr: NL29018.058.09; MEC-Nr: P09.189). This study was registered in the Netherlands Trial Register (NTR2190). It concerned the clinical follow-up of a multi-center randomized controlled clinical trial, comparing different blood management modalities in THR and TKR surgery (Netherlands Trial Register: NTR303). In this trial, 2442 primary and revision hip or knee replacements in 2257 patients were included between 2004 and 2009.

All patients who participated in the randomized controlled trial and completed preoperative HRQoL questionnaires, who underwent primary THR of TKR for primary OA and who were alive at the time of inclusion for the present follow-up study were eligible for inclusion. In this study, patients are the subject of interest. Patients who participated more than once in the previous trial, were only allowed to participate once in the current study; the first joint replacement performed in the previous trial was chosen as the index surgery.

Records of the financial administration of all participating centers were checked in order to ascertain that all eligible patients were still alive before being approached. All eligible patients were first sent an invitation letter signed by their treating orthopaedic surgeon, an information brochure and a reply card. Patients who did not respond within 4 weeks after the first invitation were sent another invitation letter. The remaining patients, who did not respond to this second invitation, were contacted by telephone.

Assessments

The assessments of the follow-up study consisted of patient-reported questionnaires, examination of patient records and preoperative radiographs.

Outcomes. HRQoL was measured preoperatively and in the present follow-up study using the SF36, which is translated and validated in the Dutch language. [21,22] The 36 items cover eight domains (physical function, role physical, bodily pain, general health, vitality, social function, role emotional, and mental health), for which a sub-scale score is calculated (100 indicating no symptoms and 0 indicating extreme symptoms). Additionally, these scales are incorporated into two summary measures: a Physical Component Summary (PCS) and Mental Component Summary (MCS).

At the population level, the HRQoL outcome measure was the mean change score, i.e. the mean of each patients postoperative sub-scale score minus their pre-operative sub-scale score). At the individual level, the change scores were used to categorise patients in responders and non-responders, using previously published MCIDs.[14–16] Patients with a change score equal to or larger than the MCID of that particular sub-scale were categorised as a responder; patients whose change score was less than the CID of that particular sub-scale were categorised as non-responders.

Patient satisfaction with the surgical result was measured using an 11-point Numeric Rating Scale of Satisfaction (NRSS; 0 indicating completely dissatisfied, 10 indicating completely satisfied). At the population level, the satisfaction outcome measure was the mean NRSS score. The proportion of patients who achieved a satisfactory outcome (defined as a NRSS>8, according to Brokelman et al [5]) was the satisfaction outcome measure at the individual level.

Exposure. Pre-operative radiographs of the hips (anterior–posterior) and knees (posterior–anterior) were collected from the participating patients' medical records and radiology department. These radiographs were routinely made in each participating center for pre-operative templating purposes. All radiographs were assessed by an experienced musculoskeletal radiologist (HMK), who was blinded for patient characteristics and HRQoL assessments. The method of scoring OA followed that described by Kellgren and Lawrence (KL) (0 indicating no OA, 1 doubtful OA, 2 minimal OA, 3 moderate OA and 4 indicating severe OA). [23] All radiographs were scored twice: both readings were used to establish intra-reader reliability (Intra-Class Correlation hip radiographs: 0.85 (95%CI: 0.82–0.88); Intra-Class Correlation knee radiographs: 0.87 (95%CI: 0.83–0.89)). The second reading was used for further statistical analyses.

As KL grade 0 to 2 and grade 3 and 4 are deemed similar from a clinical perspective, we grouped the severity of pre-operative OA in 2 categories: mild radiographic OA (KL grade 0, 1 or 2) and severe radiographic OA (KL grade 3 or 4).

Potential confounders. Socio-demographic characteristics collected at baseline in the trial included: age at joint replacement and gender. Additionally, the following socio-demographic variables were collected in the questionnaire of the follow-up study: length and weight, in order to calculate the Body Mass Index (BMI) (<25, 25–30, 30–35, >35) and patient reported Charnley classification of co-morbidity (Class A: patients in which the index operated hip or knee are affected only; Class B: patients in which the other hip or knee is affected as well; Class C: patients with a hip or knee replacement and other affected joints and/or a medical condition which affects the patients' ability to ambulate). [24,25].

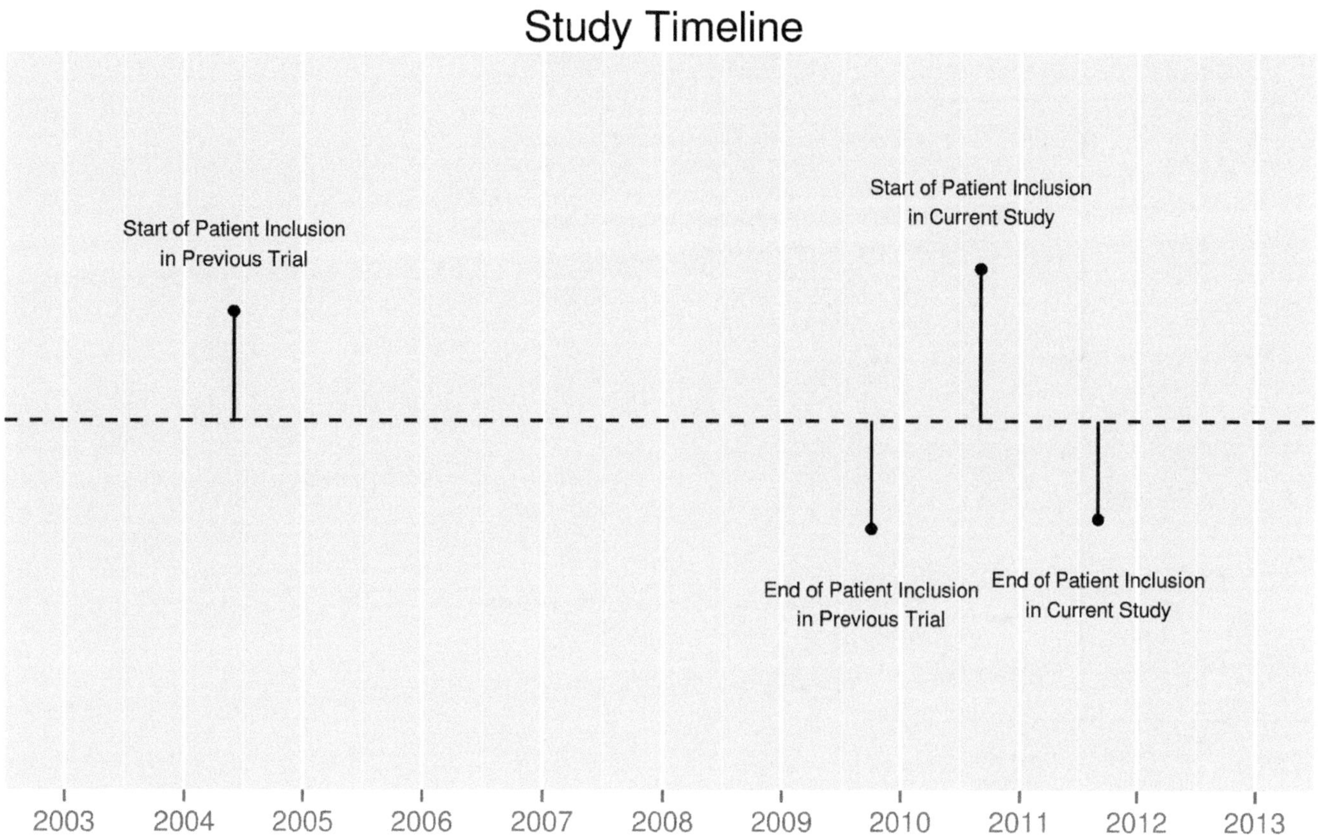

Figure 1. Study Timeline.

Statistical Analysis

We performed descriptive analyses of patients baseline characteristics. In order to investigate the possible extent of self-selection bias, we compared the age at THR or TKR and gender of participants to non-participants.

Patients with missing pre-operative SF36 questionnaires, missing SF36 questionnaires at follow-up or missing pre-operative radiographs were excluded from analyses, as we could not exclude a Missing Not At Random (MNAR) mechanism. Missing values of the Charnley Co-morbidity Classification and BMI were deemed Missing At Random and imputed using Multiple Imputations (MI), in order to improve efficiency of the regression analyses and avert biased regression coefficients. We performed MI ($m = 10$) using an Expectation-Maximization algorithm, [26] which is implemented in the Amelia 2 package for R. [27,28].

We performed regression analyses in each imputed dataset in order to compare the mean improvement in HRQoL and the probability of achieving a MCID in HRQoL after THR and TKR, between patients with KL grade 0, 1 or 2 and grade 3 or 4. As MCIDs in HRQoL differ between THR patients and TKR patients, we performed all analyses separately for THR and TKR. Possible confounders are age, gender, BMI and poly-articular OA in both THR and TKR patients. We used the Charnley classification as a proxy for poly-articular OA. As the length of follow-up varied considerably, we first stratified our data in quartiles of follow-up length for each imputed dataset. Within each stratum of follow-up length, we performed a multivariate mixed effect linear regression analysis, with the mean improvement in HRQoL and the mean NRSS as the dependent variable, the KL grade and confounders as independent variables and center as a random effect. Stratum-specific mean differences in HRQoL between the KL grades were pooled using inverse variance weighting in order to produce an overall estimate of the mean difference in HRQoL for each imputed data-set. Finally, the $m = 10$ estimates of the mean differences in HRQoL were combined into one estimate, according to Rubin. [29].

Within each stratum of follow-up length, we also performed a multivariate mixed effect logistic regression analysis, with the probability of attaining a MCID in HRQoL and a satisfactory NRSS as the dependent variable, the KL grade and confounders as independent variables and center as a random effect. Stratum-specific odds ratios of attaining a MCID in HRQoL between the KL grades were pooled using inverse variance weighting in order to produce an overall estimate of the odds ratio of attaining a MCID in HRQoL for each imputed data-set. Finally, the $m = 10$ estimates of the mean differences in HRQoL were combined into one estimate, according to Rubin. [29].

All analyses were performed using R, version 2.14.0. [30].

Results

At 2 to 5 years after joint replacement, 723 patients agreed to participate and returned the questionnaires sufficiently completed (participation rate: 46%, figure 1 and 2). Non-participating THR patients were on average 4.32 years older than participants (95%CI: 2.93–5.70 years); Non-participating TKR patients were on average 2.68 years older than participants (95%CI: 1.28–4.09 years). The proportion of males was similar in participants and non-responders. An overview of the patient characteristics is provided in table 1.

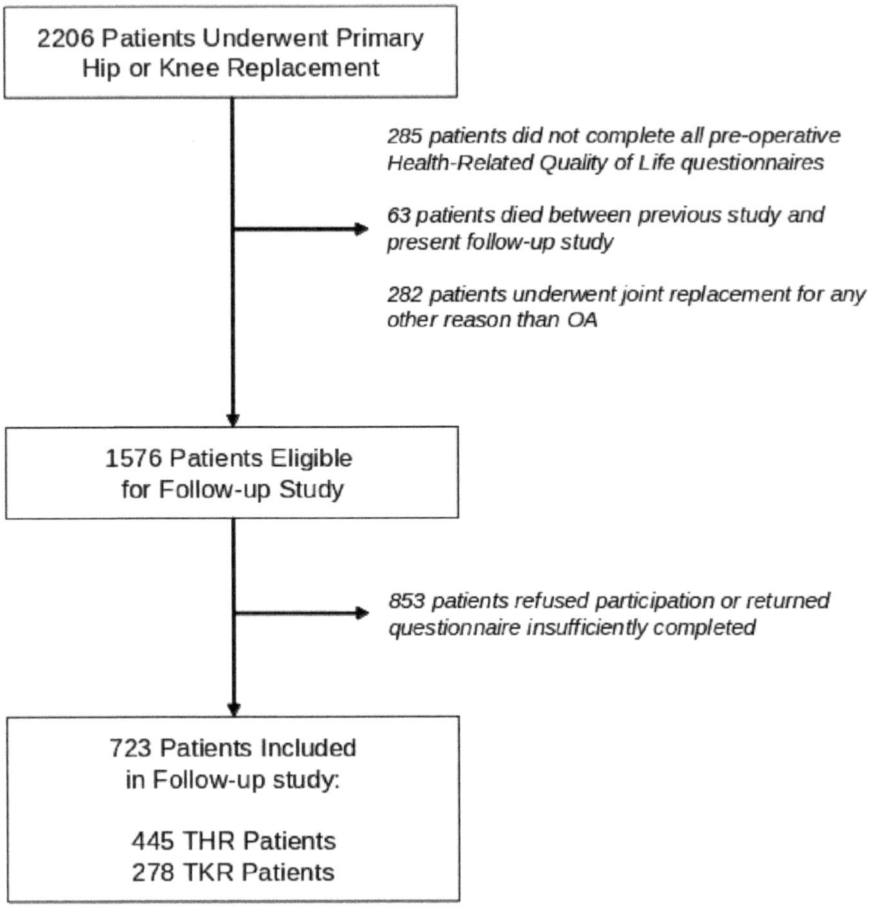

Figure 2. Patient Inclusion Flow-chart.

In 13 THR patients and 7 TKR patients, the Charnley classification was missing; in 9 THR patients and 11 TKR patients, the BMI was missing. These missing values were imputed using multiple imputation.

The mean improvement in HRQoL and mean NRSS per KL grade is shown in table 2 for THR patients and table 3 for TKR patients. In THR, patients with severe radiographic OA had a larger improvement in Physical Functioning than patients with mild radiographic OA. The improvement in other domains of HRQoL and the mean NRSS was similar for THR patients of all severities of radiographic OA. In TKR, patients with severe radiographic OA had a larger improvement in Physical functioning than patients with mild radiographic OA. Additionally, patients with severe radiographic OA had a larger improvement in General Health, a larger improvement in the Physical Component Summary Scale and a higher NRSS than patients with mild radiographic OA.

The crude probabilities of achieving a MCID in each dimension of HRQoL are presented in table 4 for THR patients and table 5 for TKR patients. In THR, the probability of achieving a relevant improvement in Physical Functioning was higher in patients with severe radiographic OA than in patients with mild radiographic OA. The probability of achieving a satisfactory outcome was also higher in patients with severe radiographic OA than in patients with mild radiographic OA. The probability of achieving a relevant improvement in other domains of HRQoL was similar for THR patients of all severities of radiographic OA. In TKR, the probability of achieving a relevant improvement in Physical Functioning was higher in patients with severe radiographic OA than in patients with mild radiographic OA. Additionally, the probability of achieving a relevant improvement in General Health and the probability of achieving a satisfactory outcome was also higher in patients with severe radiographic OA than in patients with mild radiographic OA.

Discussion

At the population level, patients with severe radiographic OA improve more in Physical Functioning than patients with mild radiographic OA, both for THR and TKR. At the individual level, THR and TKR patients with severe radiographic OA have a larger probability of a relevant improvement in Physical Functioning than patients with mild radiographic OA. The effects of the preoperative severity of radiographic OA on Physical Functioning are more pronounced in TKR patients than in THR patients. Other domains of HRQoL do not appear to be influenced by the preoperative severity of OA, except General Health and the Physical Component Summary Scale in TKR patients. Additionally, patient satisfaction appears to be better in patients with more severe preoperative radiographic OA.

Limitations of the study include the participation rate and range of follow-up period after joint replacement. Although participation rates of 100% are feasible in small-scaled studies with hard endpoints, [31,32] participation rates in epidemiological studies

Table 1. Patient Characteristics.

Primary THR	Kellgren Grade 0–2	Kellgren Grade 3+4	All Patients
Age at Joint Replacement	65.1 (7.8)	67.4 (8.7)	66.6 (8.5)
Males	23.9%	44.3%	37.5%
Follow-up (years)	2.83 (1.0)	2.79 (0.9)	2.8 (0.93)
Charnley:			
Class A:	25.8%	24.0%	24.6%
Class B:	14.6%	13.7%	14.0%
Class C:	59.6%	62.3%	61.4%
Body Mass Index:			
<25:	29.2%	34.1%	32.5%
25–30:	41.6%	46.4%	44.8%
30–35:	23.6%	16.2%	18.7%
>35:	5.60%	3.40%	4.10%
Primary TKR	**Kellgren Grade 0–2**	**Kellgren Grade 3+4**	**All Patients**
Age at Joint Replacement	65.1 (10.3)	69.5 (8.6)	69.1 (8.9)
Males	31.8%	30.9%	31.0%
Follow-up (years)	3.1 (1.1)	2.79 (0.9)	2.82 (0.93)
Charnley:			
Class A:	4.50%	19.0%	17.5%
Class B:	4.50%	11.4%	10.7%
Class C:	90.9%	69.6%	71.8%
Body Mass Index:			
<25:	33.3%	14.7%	16.3%
25–30:	27.8%	46.7%	45.0%
30–35:	33.3%	21.2%	22.3%
>35:	5.60%	17.4%	16.3%

All values are mean (SD), unless stated otherwise.

Table 2. Improvement in Health-Related Quality of Life and Satisfaction after Hip Replacement: A Comparison Between Patients with Mild to Moderate and Severe Radiographical Pre-Operative Osteoarthritis.

SF36 Sub-Scale	Kellgren Grade 0–2: Mean Improvement (95%CI)	Kellgren Grade 3+4: Mean Improvement (95%CI)	Kellgren Grade 0–2 VS Kellgren Grade 3+4: Mean Adjusted Difference (95%CI)	P-value
Physical Functioning	19.2 (14.2–24.1)	26.2 (22.4–30.0)	8.93 (2.14–15.7)	*0.01*
Role-Physical	36.3 (26.7–45.9)	42.2 (35.4–48.9)	6.39 (−5.89–18.7)	0.31
Bodily Pain	35.9 (30.4–41.3)	36.5 (32.8–40.2)	0.88 (−6.08–7.84)	0.80
General Health	0.60 (−3.50–4.60)	−1.50 (−4.50–1.50)	−0.66 (−5.66–4.34)	0.79
Vitality	9.30 (5.00–13.5)	3.70 (0.80–6.70)	−3.53 (−9.03–1.97)	0.21
Social Functioning	19.4 (13.6–25.2)	14.6 (10.7–18.4)	−4.11 (−11.2–2.97)	0.25
Role Emotional	6.90 (−1.10–14.9)	11.3 (4.70–17.8)	3.11 (−8.22–14.4)	0.59
Mental Health	7.20 (4.00–10.5)	4.60 (2.10–7.10)	−1.80 (−6.13–2.50)	0.41
PCS	10.7 (8.70–12.6)	11.2 (9.90–12.6)	1.94 (−0.57–4.44)	0.13
MCS	1.50 (−0.40–3.40)	−0.50 (−1.80–0.90)	−2.03 (−4.46–0.39)	0.10
NRS Satisfaction	8.5 (8.0–8.9)	8.9 (8.6–9.2)	0.3 (−0.2–0.9)	0.19

Positive values indicate a higher mean improvement in HRQoL after THR in patients with Kellgren Grade 3+4, compared to Grade 0–2.
The mean differences between radiographic severity are adjusted for age, sex, Charnley Comorbidity Classification and BMI and stratified for quartiles of follow-up.

Table 3. Improvement in Health-Related Quality of Life and Satisfaction after Knee Replacement: A Comparison Between Patients with Mild to Moderate and Severe Radiographical Pre-Operative Osteoarthritis.

SF36 Sub-Scale	Kellgren Grade 0–2: Mean Improvement (95%CI)	Kellgren Grade 3+4: Mean Improvement (95%CI)	Kellgren Grade 0–2 VS Kellgren Grade 3+4: Mean Adjusted Difference (95%CI)	P-value
Physical Functioning	−2.10 (−10.5–6.30)	15.1 (11.7–18.5)	19.1 (8.48–29.7)	*<0.001*
Role-Physical	9.10 (−11.9–30.1)	20.6 (−13.5–27.7)	17.4 (−6.32–41.1)	0.15
Bodily Pain	14.5 (3.50–25.5)	25.2 (21.5–29.0)	9.02 (−3.43–21.5)	0.15
General Health	−9.10 (−16.9– −1.30)	−1.50 (−3.80–0.80)	9.23 (1.31–17.2)	*0.02*
Vitality	−5.40 (−13.0–2.30)	1.20 (−1.40–3.80)	8.44 (−0.28–17.2)	0.06
Social Functioning	2.80 (−8.00–13.6)	8.90 (5.40–12.4)	7.44 (−4.18–19.1)	0.21
Role Emotional	4.50 (−17.5–26.6)	5.80 (−0.60–12.1)	8.87 (−11.8–29.6)	0.40
Mental Health	3.40 (−4.00–10.8)	3.00 (0.80–5.10)	0.29 (−6.93–7.50)	0.94
PCS	1.50 (−2.90–6.00)	6.40 (5.10–7.70)	5.64 (1.26–10.0)	*0.01*
MCS	0.10 (−4.30–4.40)	−0.30 (−1.60–1.00)	−0.18 (−4.45–4.10)	0.94
NRS Satisfaction	7.4 (6.1–8.6)	8.2 (7.9–8.6)	1.2 (0.1–2.4)	*0.04*

Positive values indicate a higher mean improvement in HRQoL after THR in patients with Kellgren Grade 3+4, compared to Grade 0–2. The mean differences between radiographic severity are adjusted for age, sex, Charnley Comorbidity Classification and BMI and stratified for quartiles of follow-up.

have been steadily declining in the last 30 years. [33] Even sharper declines have been reported in the past few years. [34] Unfortunately, the participation rate of this study follows this general trend, resulting in a participation rate of 46%. Therefore, we cannot exclude the presence of self-selection bias. In order to limit the extent of this bias, we have sent multiple reminders and have called all patients who did not answer our reminders and who did not return the questionnaire. As incentives, we have included an appealing information brochure in which the primary goals of the follow-up study were explained and a study pen as a small gift. Additionally, patients were urged to participate by their treating physician. However, the participation rate alone does not determine the extent of bias present in any particular study. [34] The difference between participants and non-participants is far more important. [35] As the found differences in demographics were of little clinical relevance, it is unlikely that the study results will be severely biased. Finally, the patient demographics of our study population were similar to those of large-scaled national joint registry studies, regarding age, gender, Charnley classification and BMI. [36,37].

The follow-up period after joint replacement varies between 2 and 5 years. Although a residual effect of follow-up length cannot be excluded, we do not think this is very plausible, as recent evidence suggests that the improvement in HRQoL is sustained up to 5 years after joint replacement surgery. [38,39].

Although joint replacements are highly effective in improving HRQoL at the group level, [1] this is not the case for each individual patient, judging from the relatively high dissatisfaction rates. [40,41] Studying HRQoL at the individual level, using the probability of achieving a clinically important difference as an outcome measure, enables a better prediction of a successful outcome. Moreover, it could provide a helpful way to fine-tune the indication for joint replacement, for which there are no clear cut-off points currently available. [42].

Table 4. Improvement in Health-Related Quality of Life and Satisfaction after Hip Replacement: A Comparison Between Patients with Mild to Moderate and Severe Radiographical Pre-Operative Osteoarthritis.

SF36 Sub-Scale	Kellgren Grade 0–2: Probability of Achieving a MCID (95%CI)	Kellgren Grade 3+4: Probability of Achieving a MCID (95%CI)	Kellgren Grade 0–2 VS Kellgren Grade 3+4: Adjusted Odds Ratio (95%CI)	P-value
Physical Functioning	64/92:69.6% (59.5–78.0)	146/185:78.9% (72.5–84.2)	1.87 (0.97–3.60)	0.06
Role-Physical	55/92:59.8% (49.6–69.2)	124/185:67.0% (60.0–73.4)	1.50 (0.82–2.72)	0.19
Bodily Pain	71/92:77.2% (67.6–84.6)	141/185:76.2% (69.6–81.8)	1.03 (0.52–2.05)	0.93
General Health	62/92:67.4% (57.3–76.1)	117/185:63.2% (56.1–69.9)	0.91 (0.47–1.77)	0.78
Vitality	34/92:37.0% (27.8–47.2)	54/185:29.2% (23.1–36.1)	0.84 (0.46–1.55)	0.58
Social Functioning	42/92:45.7% (35.9–55.8)	80/185:43.2% (36.3–50.4)	0.87 (0.49–1.55)	0.64
Role Emotional	21/92:22.8% (15.4–32.4)	51/185:27.6% (21.6–34.4)	1.01 (0.51–2.01)	0.98
Mental Health	17/92:18.5% (11.9–27.6)	40/185:21.6% (16.3–28.1)	1.26 (0.62–2.58)	0.53
NRS Satisfaction >8	53/92:57.6% (47.4–67.2)	136/185:73.5% (66.7–79.3)	1.95 (1.06–3.59)	*0.03*

Odds Ratios >1 indicate a higher probability of achieving a Minimal Clinically Important Difference in HRQoL after THR in patients with Kellgren Grade 3+4, compared to Grade 0–2.
The odds ratios adjusted for age, sex, Charnley Comorbidity Classification and BMI and stratified for quartiles of follow-up.

Table 5. Improvement in Health-Related Quality of Life and Satisfaction after Knee Replacement: A Comparison Between Patients with Mild to Moderate and Severe Radiographical Pre-Operative Osteoarthritis.

SF36 Sub-Scale	Kellgren Grade 0–2: Probability of Achieving a MCID (95%CI)	Kellgren Grade 3+4: Probability of Achieving a MCID (95%CI)	Kellgren Grade 0–2 VS Kellgren Grade 3+4: Adjusted Odds Ratio (95%CI)	P-value
Physical Functioning	5/22:22.7% (10.1–43.4)	105/191:55.0% (47.9–61.9)	5.44 (1.45–20.3)	*0.01*
Role-Physical	9/22:40.9% (23.3–61.3)	88/191:46.1% (39.2–53.2)	1.46 (0.49–4.32)	0.50
Bodily Pain	15/22:68.2% (47.3–83.6)	136/191:71.2% (64.4–77.2)	1.15 (0.32–4.16)	0.83
General Health	9/22:40.9% (23.3–61.3)	122/191:63.9% (56.9–70.4)	3.56 (1.23–10.4)	*0.02*
Vitality	8/22:36.4% (19.7–57)	86/191:45.0% (38.1–52.1)	1.09 (0.35–3.44)	0.88
Social Functioning	7/22:31.8% (16.4–52.7)	98/191:51.3% (44.3–58.3)	2.84 (0.87–9.32)	0.08
Role Emotional	6/22:27.3% (13.2–48.2)	41/191:21.5% (16.2–27.8)	0.85 (0.26–3.02)	0.85
Mental Health	8/22:36.4% (19.7–57)	79/191:41.4% (34.6–48.4)	2.79 (0.70–11.2)	0.15
NRS Satisfaction >8	9/22:40.9% (23.3–61.3)	116/191:60.7% (53.7–67.4)	2.25 (0.78–6.52)	0.14

Odds Ratios >1 indicate a higher probability of achieving a Minimal Clinically Important Difference in HRQoL after THR in patients with Kellgren Grade 3+4, compared to Grade 0–2.
The odds ratios adjusted for age, sex, Charnley Comorbidity Classification and BMI and stratified for quartiles of follow-up.

Regardless of age, gender, co-morbidity and BMI, we have shown that joint replacement patients with severe preoperative OA have a better prognosis in improvement in Physical Functioning and patient satisfaction with the surgical results. These effects are more pronounced in TKR patients than in THR patients, which might be explained in part by biomechanical factors. The hip joint is a relatively simple ball and socket joint, which is adequately mimicked by a THR. The biomechanical aspects of the knee joint are more difficult to imitate, as the knee is a pivotal hinge joint with 6 degrees of freedom. These degrees of freedom are generally not restored after TKR, which is substantiated in kinematic and kinetic studies. [43] This additional disadvantage of TKR patients who underwent joint replacement for mild radiographic OA is reflected in a smaller increase in Physical Functioning than THR patients who underwent joint replacement for mild radiographic OA. Additionally, the odds of achieving a MCID in Physical Functioning is smaller and the difference in satisfaction is larger.

Clinically, these are promising findings, as dissatisfaction rates are higher in TKR patients than in THR patients. [4,6] Patient satisfaction is thought to be closely related to unfulfilled expectations. Although patient expectations of THR and TKR are similar, recent evidence suggests that THR meets important patient expectations better than TKR. [6,11,44] Our findings could lead to a more fitting expectation management regarding the expected improvement in Physical Functioning, using a single predictor. This improvement in expectation management might lead to higher satisfaction rates.

Plain radiographs have a number of appealing aspects. In the first place, they are inexpensive and easily available, as they are currently a part of the clinical work-up to joint replacement. Secondly, due to the non-invasive character of the test, radiographs are a patient-friendly modality. Finally, they offer a more objective approach to joint complaints. These aspects would make it easy to implement the KL grade in clinical practice, in order to predict HRQoL and satisfaction after joint replacement.

Author Contributions

Conceived and designed the experiments: JCK MF CSO HMK TPMVV RGN. Performed the experiments: JCK RO AWMMKG RGP. Analyzed the data: JCK MF RGN. Contributed reagents/materials/analysis tools: JCK RO AWMMKG RGP RGN. Wrote the paper: JCK MF CSO RO AWMMKG RGP HMK TPMVV RGN.

References

1. Ethgen O, Bruyère O, Richy F, Dardennes C, Reginster J-Y (2004) Health-related quality of life in total hip and total knee arthroplasty. A qualitative and systematic review of the literature. The Journal of bone and joint surgery American volume 86-A: 963–974.
2. Beswick AD, Wylde V, Gooberman-Hill R, Blom A, Dieppe P (2012) What proportion of patients report long-term pain after total hip or knee replacement for osteoarthritis? A systematic review of prospective studies in unselected patients. BMJ open 2: e000435.
3. Gandhi R, Davey JR, Mahomed NN (2008) Predicting patient dissatisfaction following joint replacement surgery. The Journal of rheumatology 35: 2415–2418. doi:10.3899/jrheum.080295.
4. Noble PC, Conditt MA, Cook KF, Mathis KB (2006) The John Insall Award: Patient expectations affect satisfaction with total knee arthroplasty. Clinical orthopaedics and related research 452: 35–43. doi:10.1097/01.blo.0000238825.63648.1e.
5. Brokelman RBG, Van Loon CJM, Rijnberg WJ (2003) Patient versus surgeon satisfaction after total hip arthroplasty. [Miscellaneous Article]. Journal of Bone & Joint Surgery - British Volume 85-B: 495–498.
6. Nilsdotter AK, Toksvig-Larsen S, Roos EM (2009) Knee arthroplasty: are patients' expectations fulfilled? A prospective study of pain and function in 102 patients with 5-year follow-up. Acta orthopaedica 80: 55–61. doi:10.1080/17453670902805007.
7. Lingard EA, Sledge CB, Learmonth ID (2006) PATIENT EXPECTATIONS REGARDING TOTAL KNEE ARTHROPLASTY: DIFFERENCES AMONG THE UNITED STATES, UNITED KINGDOM, AND AUSTRALIA. Journal of Bone & Joint Surgery, American Volume 88: 1201–1207.
8. Garellick G, Malchau H, Herberts P (2000) Survival of hip replacements. A comparison of a randomized trial and a registry. Clinical orthopaedics and related research: 157–167.
9. Baker PN, Van der Meulen JH, Lewsey J, Gregg PJ (2007) The role of pain and function in determining patient satisfaction after total knee replacement. Data from the National Joint Registry for England and Wales. The Journal of bone and joint surgery British volume 89: 893–900. doi:10.1302/0301-620X.89B7.19091.
10. Bini SA, Sidney S, Sorel M (2011) Slowing demand for total joint arthroplasty in a population of 3.2 million. The Journal of arthroplasty 26: 124–128. doi:10.1016/j.arth.2011.03.043.
11. Scott CEH, Bugler KE, Clement ND, Macdonald D, Howie CR, et al. (2012) Patient expectations of arthroplasty of the hip and knee. The Journal of bone and joint surgery British volume 94: 974–981. doi:10.1302/0301-620X.94B7.28219.

12. Jaeschke R, Singer J, Guyatt GH (1989) Measurement of health status. Ascertaining the minimal clinically important difference. Controlled clinical trials 10: 407–415.
13. King MT (2011) A point of minimal important difference (MID): a critique of terminology and methods. Expert review of pharmacoeconomics & outcomes research 11: 171–184. doi:10.1586/erp.11.9.
14. Quintana JM, Escobar A, Bilbao A, Arostegui I, Lafuente I, et al. (2005) Responsiveness and clinically important differences for the WOMAC and SF-36 after hip joint replacement. Osteoarthritis and cartilage/OARS, Osteoarthritis Research Society 13: 1076–1083. doi:10.1016/j.joca.2005.06.012.
15. Escobar A, Quintana JM, Bilbao A, Aróstegui I, Lafuente I, et al. (2007) Responsiveness and clinically important differences for the WOMAC and SF-36 after total knee replacement. Osteoarthritis and cartilage/OARS, Osteoarthritis Research Society 15: 273–280. doi:10.1016/j.joca.2006.09.001.
16. Keurentjes JC, Van Tol F, Fiocco M, Schoones J, Nelissen R (2012) Minimal clinically important differences in health-related quality of life after total hip or knee replacement. Bone and Joint Research 1: 71–77. doi:10.1302/2046-3758.15.2000065.
17. Nilsdotter AK, Aurell Y, Siösteen AK, Lohmander LS, Roos HP (2001) Radiographic stage of osteoarthritis or sex of the patient does not predict one year outcome after total hip arthroplasty. Annals of the rheumatic diseases 60: 228–232.
18. Meding JB, Anderson AR, Faris PM, Keating EM, Ritter MA (2000) Is the preoperative radiograph useful in predicting the outcome of a total hip replacement? Clinical orthopaedics and related research: 156–160.
19. Judge A, Javaid MK, Arden NK, Cushnaghan J, Reading I, et al. (2012) Clinical tool to identify patients who are most likely to achieve long-term improvement in physical function after total hip arthroplasty. Arthritis care & research 64: 881–889. doi:10.1002/acr.21594.
20. Keurentjes JC, Blane D, Bartley M, Keurentjes JJB, Fiocco M, et al. (2013) Socio-Economic Position Has No Effect on Improvement in Health-Related Quality of Life and Patient Satisfaction in Total Hip and Knee Replacement: A Cohort Study. PLoS ONE 8: e56785. doi:10.1371/journal.pone.0056785.
21. Ware JE, Sherbourne CD (1992) The MOS 36-item short-form health survey (SF-36). I. Conceptual framework and item selection. Medical care 30: 473–483.
22. Aaronson NK, Muller M, Cohen PD, Essink-Bot ML, Fekkes M, et al. (1998) Translation, validation, and norming of the Dutch language version of the SF-36 Health Survey in community and chronic disease populations. Journal of clinical epidemiology 51: 1055–1068.
23. KELLGREN JH, LAWRENCE JS (1957) Radiological assessment of osteo-arthrosis. Annals of the rheumatic diseases 16: 494–502.
24. Dunbar MJ, Robertsson O, Ryd L (2004) What's all that noise? The effect of co-morbidity on health outcome questionnaire results after knee arthroplasty. Acta orthopaedica Scandinavica 75: 119–126. doi:10.1080/00016470412331294355.
25. Charnley J (1972) The long-term results of low-friction arthroplasty of the hip performed as a primary intervention. The Journal of bone and joint surgery British volume 54: 61–76.
26. Dempster AP, Laird NM, Rubin DB (1977) Maximum Likelihood Estimation from Incomplete Data Via the EM Algorithm. Journal of the Royal Statistical Association 39: 1–38.
27. Honaker J, King G, Blackwell M (2010) AMELIA II?: A Program for Missing Data. Journal Of Statistical Software 45: 1–53. doi:10.1.1.149.9611.
28. King G, Honaker J, Joseph A, Scheve K (2001) Analyzing Incomplete Political Science Data: An Alternative Algorithm for Multiple Imputation. American Political Science Review 95: 49–69. doi:10.2307/3117628.
29. Rubin DB (1987) Multiple Imputation for Nonresponse in Surveys. Wiley.
30. Team RC (2012) R: A language and environment for statistical computing. Vienna, Austria.: R Foundation for Statistical Computing.
31. Schreurs BW, Keurentjes JC, Gardeniers JWM, Verdonschot N, Slooff TJJH, et al. (2009) Acetabular revision with impacted morsellised cancellous bone grafting and a cemented acetabular component: a 20- to 25-year follow-up. The Journal of bone and joint surgery British volume 91: 1148–1153. doi:10.1302/0301-620X.91B9.21750.
32. Keurentjes JC, Fiocco M, Schreurs BW, Pijls BG, Nouta KA, et al. (2012) Revision surgery is overestimated in hip replacement. Bone and Joint Research 1 : 258–262. doi:10.1302/2046-3758.110.2000104.
33. Hartge P (2006) Participation in population studies. Epidemiology (Cambridge, Mass) 17: 252–254. doi:10.1097/01.ede.0000209441.24307.92.
34. Galea S, Tracy M (2007) Participation rates in epidemiologic studies. Annals of epidemiology 17: 643–653. doi:10.1016/j.annepidem.2007.03.013.
35. Jones J (1996) The effects of non-response on statistical inference. Journal of health & social policy 8: 49–62. doi:10.1300/J045v08n01_05.
36. Malchau HMD, GARELLICK GMD, Eisler TMD, Karrholm JMD, HERBERTS PMD (2005) Presidential guest address: The swedish hip registry: Increasing the sensitivity by patient outcome data. [Article]. Clinical Orthopaedics & Related Research 441: 19–29.
37. Hobbs T (n.d.) TWELVE YEAR REPORT.
38. Ng CY, Ballantyne JA, Brenkel IJ (2007) Quality of life and functional outcome after primary total hip replacement. A five-year follow-up. The Journal of bone and joint surgery British volume 89: 868–873. doi:10.1302/0301-620X.89B7.18482.
39. Bruyère O, Ethgen O, Neuprez A, Zégels B, Gillet P, et al. (2012) Health-related quality of life after total knee or hip replacement for osteoarthritis: a 7-year prospective study. Archives of orthopaedic and trauma surgery.
40. Mancuso CA, Salvati EA, Johanson NA, Peterson MG, Charlson ME (1997) Patients' expectations and satisfaction with total hip arthroplasty. The Journal of arthroplasty 12: 387–396.
41. Vissers MM, De Groot IB, Reijman M, Bussmann JB, Stam HJ, et al. (2010) Functional capacity and actual daily activity do not contribute to patient satisfaction after total knee arthroplasty. BMC musculoskeletal disorders 11: 121. doi:10.1186/1471-2474-11-121.
42. Gossec L, Paternotte S, Bingham CO, Clegg DO, Coste P, et al. (2011) OARSI/OMERACT initiative to define states of severity and indication for joint replacement in hip and knee osteoarthritis. An OMERACT 10 Special Interest Group. The Journal of rheumatology 38: 1765–1769. doi:10.3899/jrheum.110403.
43. Wolterbeek N, Garling EH, Mertens BJ, Nelissen RGHH, Valstar ER (2011) Kinematics and early migration in single-radius mobile- and fixed-bearing total knee prostheses. Clinical biomechanics (Bristol, Avon). doi:10.1016/j.clinbiomech.2011.10.013.
44. De Beer J, Petruccelli D, Adili A, Piccirillo L, Wismer D, et al. (2012) Patient perspective survey of total hip vs total knee arthroplasty surgery. The Journal of arthroplasty 27: 865–9. e1–5.

6

Deformation of the Durom Acetabular Component and Its Impact on Tribology in a Cadaveric Model—A Simulator Study

Feng Liu[a], **Zhefeng Chen**[a], **Yanqing Gu, Qing Wang, Weiding Cui, Weimin Fan***

Department of Orthopedics, the First Affiliated Hospital with Nanjing Medical University, Nanjing, China

Abstract

Background: Recent studies have shown that the acetabular component frequently becomes deformed during press-fit insertion. The aim of this study was to explore the deformation of the Durom cup after implantation and to clarify the impact of deformation on wear and ion release of the Durom large head metal-on-metal (MOM) total hips in simulators.

Methods: Six Durom cups impacted into reamed acetabula of fresh cadavers were used as the experimental group and another 6 size-paired intact Durom cups constituted the control group. All 12 Durom MOM total hips were put through a 3 million cycle (MC) wear test in simulators.

Results: The 6 cups in the experimental group were all deformed, with a mean deformation of 41.78 ± 8.86 μm. The average volumetric wear rate in the experimental group and in the control group in the first million cycle was 6.65 ± 0.29 mm^3/MC and 0.89 ± 0.04 mm^3/MC ($t = 48.43$, $p = 0.000$). The ion levels of Cr and Co in the experimental group were also higher than those in the control group before 2.0 MC. However there was no difference in the ion levels between 2.0 and 3.0 MC.

Conclusions: This finding implies that the non-modular acetabular component of Durom total hip prosthesis is likely to become deformed during press-fit insertion, and that the deformation will result in increased volumetric wear and increased ion release.

Clinical Relevance: This study was determined to explore the deformation of the Durom cup after implantation and to clarify the impact of deformation on wear and ion release of the prosthesis. Deformation of the cup after implantation increases the wear of MOM bearings and the resulting ion levels. The clinical use of the Durom large head prosthesis should be with great care.

Editor: Jie Zheng, University of Akron, United States of America

Funding: The authors have no support or funding to report.

Competing Interests: Zimmer International donated the cups used in this study. Zimmer International had no role in the study design, data collection and analysis, decision to publish, or preparation of the manuscript.

* E-mail: fanweimin@vip.sina.com

[a] These authors contributed equally to this work.

Introduction

Large-head metal-on-metal total hip prosthesis designs with non-modular acetabular components theoretically increase range of motion, reduce wear, and decrease dislocation rates [1,2]. Early and mid-term reports have produced encouraging results with some non-modular large-head MOM total hip acetabular designs [3]. The longest-term results of follow-up data with these designs to date are approximately 8 to 10 years and are available for only one design (Birmingham Hip Resurfacing, Smith and Nephew) [4]. Few or no long-term data are available for the majority of non-modular large-head MOM total hip devices currently in use.

Unacceptably high revision rates of the non-modular large head MOM hip replacements have been reported recently [5,6]. The biological effects of wear products generated by MOM components made of CoCrMo alloy also remain a major cause of concern. The term of ARMD (Adverse Reaction to Metal Debris) has been coined to describe the inflammatory reactions around joints, including large joint effusions, pseudotumour formation and aseptic soft tissue necrosis resulting from these reactions [7,8]. The systemic toxicity of cobalt and chromium ions on the vital organs and the immune system is also of significant concern [9]. Although the relationship between clinical performance and ion levels is still unclear [10], some researchers consider that malfunction and unexplainable groin pain may be correlated with high levels of metal ions [11,12]. Some surgeons have abandoned the use of large-head metal-on-metal total hip replacements for the above reasons [13].

Multiple variables influence serum metal ion levels after MOM total hip arthroplasty. Tribologic factors, such as increased sphericity, increased carbon content, decreased clearance and surface roughness, have been shown to decrease wear and therefore, presumably, serum metal ion levels [14,15]. Excessive

Table 1. Demographics of cadaver hip donors.

Specimen	Gender	Age(y)	Height(cm)	Weight(kg)	BMD(g/cm^2)	T-score
1R(right hip)	M	49	173	73	1.061	0.8
1L(left hip)					1.039	0.7
2R(right hip)	M	52	170	68	1.302	1.0
2L(left hip)					1.381	1.2
3R(right hip)	M	47	174	71	1.012	0.4
3L(left hip)					1.005	0.2

abduction and anteversion of the acetabular cups might also be a risk factor for elevated metal ion release [16].

In order to preserve more bone stock and to achieve fluid-film lubrication, non-modular MOM shells for resurfacing or total hip arthroplasty have been manufactured with thinner walls to maximize femoral head sizes. Initial stability of the acetabular components can be achieved with press-fit fixation. However, despite the potential benefits of this approach, deformation may occur around the peripheral rim of the cup. This deformation may damage the fluid-film lubrication between the cup and the femoral head, increasing the wear rate and releasing more metal ions [17,18,19]. The main objective of this study was to observe and detect deformation of the Durom total hip prosthesis's cups inserted into fresh cadaveric acetabula, thus to clarify the relationship between deformation, volumetric wear rate and ion levels using a simulator test.

Materials and Methods

1. Durom cup

The Durom large head total hip prosthesis cup (original design) is a non-modular acetabular component and uses a high-carbon, forged chromium-cobalt bearing surface with a titanium plasma spray surface for bone ingrowth. The implant is a 165° truncated hemisphere with an elliptical shape providing a 2-mm press fit circumferentially. Initial stability is achieved by the press-fit technique at the rim and the purchase of the peripheral rim fins in the acetabular bone.

2. Cadaver pelvis and preparation of the acetabulum

All procedures were reviewed and approved by Ethics Committee of the First Affiliated Hospital with Nanjing Medical University. Three fresh adult cadaver pelves (provided by Nanjing Medical University) were harvested and were cleaned of soft tissue, preserving the sacrospinous and sacrotuberous ligaments. The specimens were wrapped in saline-soaked gauze, covered with plastic, and stored at −20°C until the insertion of the Durom cups. On the day of testing, the specimens were thawed for 12 hours at room temperature. Detailed demographics of the donors are presented in Table 1. Bilateral acetabular replacements in all cadaver pelves were performed by a senior surgeon (Feng Liu) who inserted the Durom cups.

With the femoral heads removed from the specimens, the labrum and teres ligaments were excised. After all of the cartilage had been removed and the reamer neared the base of the notch, reaming was directed at an angle of 45° inclination and 15° to 20° anteversion. Larger reamers were used sequentially until the anterior and posterior walls were firmly engaged. Then Durom cups of the same size as the last reamer were fitted under 3D digital image correlation detection (3D DIC).

3. 3D Digital Image Correlation (3D DIC)

After impaction, the deformation of each cup was assessed by 3D digital image correlation (VIC-3D Correlation Solution, Inc. SC, USA, Precision: 1 μm). 3D DIC is a computer vision technique which is used to track the surface displacements of deforming materials. Before testing, proper preparation of the specimens is required. Black and white dots on the material surface are an absolute requirement for measuring the deformation. We initially sprayed a thin layer of white paint and then used a black spray to make black dots on the inner surface of all the 12 Durom cups (Figures 1a, 1b).

Before the 3D DIC measurement, hand-made support bases were made from plastic foam according to the size of the metal cups. After being put gently inside the foam support base, the foam supports with the cups were fixed on the base of the VIC-3D firmly. 6 Durom cups scheduled for implantation were then fixed for DIC detection, and the primary images were obtained. After that, the cups were removed from the support bases and impacted into the bone acetabula with 45°inclination and 15° to 20° anteversion. After the Durom cups were set in position, it was important to ensure that the cups were firmly engaged by the anterior and posterior walls, and that the rim fins of the cups had a firm purchase on the peripheral acetabular bone (Figure 1c). Then 6 specimens were inspected under 3D DIC again to detect any possible deformation. Twenty-four hours later, the specimens were

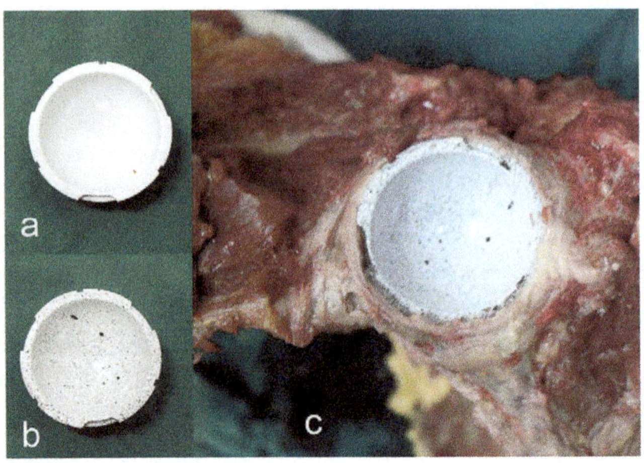

Figure 1. (a)Durom cup after white sprayed (b)Durom after black dots sprayed (c) Implantation of the Durom cup.

examined again, and then the cups were gently removed from the bone acetabula. On the 7th day, the third examination was conducted.

4. Simulator testing

After the deformation detection test, all the painted cups were ultrasonicated in 95% ethanol for 2 hours, and then the paint was removed by running water avoiding the damage to the inner surface of the cups. The six Durom cups which underwent deformation testing constituted the experimental group. The remaining 6 size-paired intact cups were the control group. They were tested in six station Prosim 2 hip simulators (Simsol, Stockport, UK) (Figure 2). The total of 12 cups were randomly divided into the two groups and housed randomly in different stations. The acetabular components were housed in stainless steel fixtures, supported by polymethyl methacrylate (PMMA) cement that was cast against the back ensuring full support. Flats were machined on the reverse of the cups to prevent rotation of the cups within the cement mantle and to ensure accurate repositioning of the components following each measurement.

The acetabular cups were mounted at 45° inclination and 15° anteversion and the rotational position were identical to their positions in acetabula. The femoral components were positioned vertically below the cups resulting in the contact region developing on the pole. The simulator had a flexion–extension range of −15° to 30° (on the head) and internal–external rotation of ±10° (on the cup). The motions were 90° out of phase to generate open elliptical and "figure of 8" wear paths to produce clinically relevant amounts of cross shear. Twin peak time-dependent loading was applied vertically to the femoral head. A peak load of 3 kN and a swing phase load of 280 N (ISO14242-1) were used. The test was conducted for 3.0 MC at a frequency of 1 Hz (Figure 3).

Testing was conducted in 25% (v/v) newborn bovine serum, containing 0.1% (w/v) sodium azide to retard bacterial growth. Each station was self-contained within a silicon bag containing 500 mL of lubricant to prevent evaporation. In the first 1.0 MC, the lubricant was changed after 0.33, 0.66, and 1.0 MC; between 1.0 and 3.0 MC, the lubricant was changed every 0.5 MC. At each change, the lubricant was collected and stored at −20°C for further quantification of wear debris and ion levels.

After 0.33, 0.66, 1.0, 1.5, 2.0, 2.5 and 3.0 MC, the hip simulator was stopped for measurements. The wear of the samples was

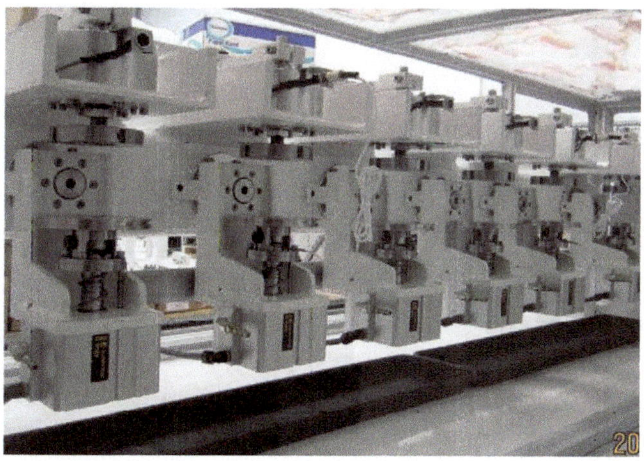

Figure 2. Six-Station Prosim 2 Hip Simulator (Simsol, Stockport, UK).

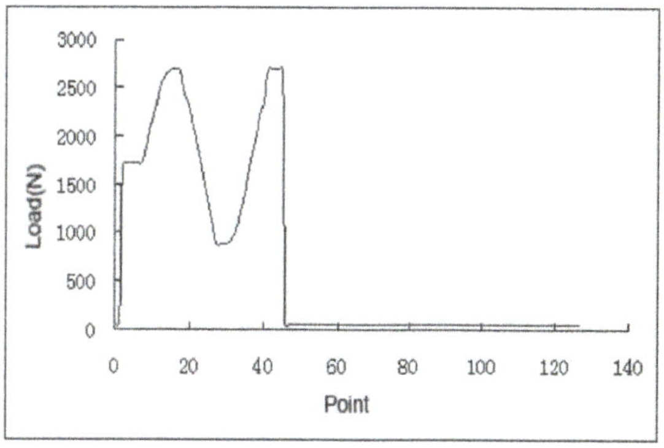

Figure 3. The loads used in hip simulator study.

quantified gravimetrically. After removal from the simulator, the test specimens were washed in detergent solution to remove all visible debris. Firstly, they were ultrasonicated in detergent solution for 10 min, then rinsed in water and soaked in Virkon to ensure all bacteria were killed. Then, specimens were rinsed with deionized water and ultrasonicated for 10 min in 70% isopropanol. Finally, after being allowed to air dry, they were put in a controlled environment for 24 h before weighing.

The components were weighed using a Mettler AT201 balance (accurate to 10 μg in a controlled environment) (Mettler-Toledo Ltd., Leicester, UK). Each component was weighed five times to determine average weight. Gravimetric data were converted into cumulative volumetric wear data (density of cobalt chromium [CoCr] 8.33 g/cm^3).

5. Measurement of ion levels

Inductively coupled plasma mass spectrometry was chosen to measure ion levels in the lubricant due to the great sensitivity of this method. The detection limits were 0.1 μg/L for Cr and 0.01 μg/L for Co. An aliquot of 10 mL serum lubricant was removed from each station after 0.33, 0.66, 1.0, 1.5, 2.0, 2.5 and 3 MC. The lubricant was centrifuged at 15,000× g for 15 minutes. The supernatant was digested with nitric acid, and the final sample was introduced into the instrument and compared with a background measurement of 25% (v/v) bovine serum with 0.1% (w/v) sodium azide to verify the results.

6. Bearing surface profile observation

The surface profile data of each bearing after 3.0 MC were acquired using an Ultrahigh Precision Surface 3D Profiler (MiaoXAM2.5X-50X, Westwood, Tucson, USA).

7. Wear debris analysis

Wear debris was isolated and analyzed according to the method developed by Brown *et al* [20]. Samples of serum lubricant (10 mL) were removed from each stations at every test point and centrifuged at 15,000× g for 20 min and the supernatant was removed. The pelleted samples were digested sequentially with papain, proteinase-k, lyticase and zymolyase. Following digestion, the particles were filtered onto 1.2 μm polycarbonate filters and dried for 4 hours. Filtered samples were analyzed using a scanning electron microscope (Hitachi, S-3000N, Hitachi, Ltd,Japan). Energy dispersive X-ray analysis (EDX, Finder-1000, KYKY Technology Development Ltd, Beijing, CHN) was used to confirm the elemental composition of the wear particles. The size of the particles was determined using a Zetasizer Nano-ZS90 (Malvern

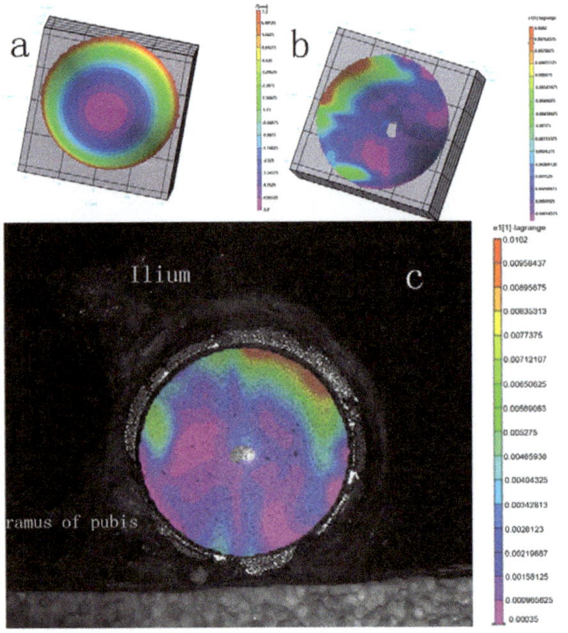

Figure 4. (a)The image of Durom cup before implantation (b)The image of Durom cup after implantation. (c) the image of the cup in the pelvis and location of deformation.

Instruments ZEN3590, Malvern, UK). Using Image Pro Plus (Media Cybernetics Inc., Bethesda, MD), maximum diameter measurements were taken of 150 particles per sample to generate size distributions as a function of size.

Statistical Analysis

Measurement data are expressed as Mean ± SD ($\bar{x} \pm s$). Differences between both groups were compared with Repeated Measurement Variance Analysis, Pillai's Trace and profile plots of the estimated marginal means. The p-value reported was two-sided and a value of less than 0.05 was considered statistically significant. All analyses were performed using SPSS software (Version 13.0, SPSS Inc., Chicago, IL)

Results

1. Durom cup deformation

After the final reaming, the sizes of the six cups were 2 of 50 mm, 2 of 52 mm and 2 of 54 mm. All cups were deformed following impaction into the surgically prepared pelves (Figure 4a,b). Most of the deformations were in the posterior-superior quadrant and the area of the ramus of ischium(Figure 4c). Small areas of deformation could also be seen in other areas. The average deformation value was 41.73±8.86 μm. Detailed demographics of the deformation of each cup along with the corresponding wear value for each bearing are presented in Table 2. The deformation of cups at 24 hours and 7 days were 41.72±7.97 μm and 41.63±7.93 μm. There was no significant difference (ANOVA, $F = 0.002$, $P = 0.998$) in deformation at three testing points.

2. Simulator testing

Detailed demographics of the cumulative volumetric wear of cups and heads are presented in Table 3. Two distinct phases of wear were observed for both the experimental and the control group; bedding in, which produced an elevated wear rate, and steady state, resulting in a reduced wear rate. The average volumetric wear rate in the experimental group and in the control group in the first million cycle was 6.65±0.29 mm^3/MC and 0.89±0.04 mm^3/MC ($t = 48.43$, $p = 0.000$). The bedding-in wear rate (0–1.0 MC) in the experimental group was almost 8 times greater than that in the control group. In the steady state (1.0–2.0 MC, 2.0–3.0 MC), the difference between the two groups became less significant. Overall, the wear rate of the experimental group was more than that in the control group over the entire testing cycle ($F = 2910.916$, $p < 0.001$ and $F = 1963.215$, $p < 0.001$) (Figures 5, 6).

The levels of Co in the lubricant of the experimental group were higher than in the control group at test-points of 0.33, 0.66, 1.0, 1.5, and 2.0 MC ($p = 0.000, 0.000, 0.000, 0.000, 0.011$). Although there was no significant difference in Co level between the two groups at the 2.5 and 3.0 MC test-points ($p = 0.102$, 0.359, respectively), the overall Co levels of experiment group were higher than those of control group ($F = 604.718$, $p < 0.001$).

The levels of Cr in the lubricant of the experimental group were higher than in the control group at the test-points of 0.33, 0.66, 1.0, 1.5 and 2.0 MC ($p = 0.000, 0.000, 0.000, 0.001, 0.046$). Although there was no significant difference in Cr levels between the two groups at the 2.5 and 3.0 MC test-points ($p = 0.094$, 0.157). As the lubricant was fully replaced regularly, care must be taken when interpreting these results. The ion levels at 0.33 MC were representative of the wear between 0 and 0.33 MC, the ion levels at 0.66 MC were representative of the wear between 0.33 and 0.66 MC, and so on (Figure 7). However, Repeated measurement variance analysis indicated that the overall levels of Cr in experimental group were higher than those in control group ($F = 851.469$, $p < 0.001$) (Figure 7).

Table 2. Demographics of the deformation of each cup along with the corresponding wear value for each bearing.

Cup Number	Diameter(mm)	Average Deformation (μm)	Cumulative Volumetric Wear of Cup(mm^3)	Cumulative Volumetric Wear of head (mm^3)
1	50	43.13	4.525	8.672
2	50	30.84	4.368	8.382
3	52	32.43	4.360	8.387
4	52	48.41	4.648	8.988
5	54	46.84	4.189	8.063
6	54	48.74	4.272	8.080

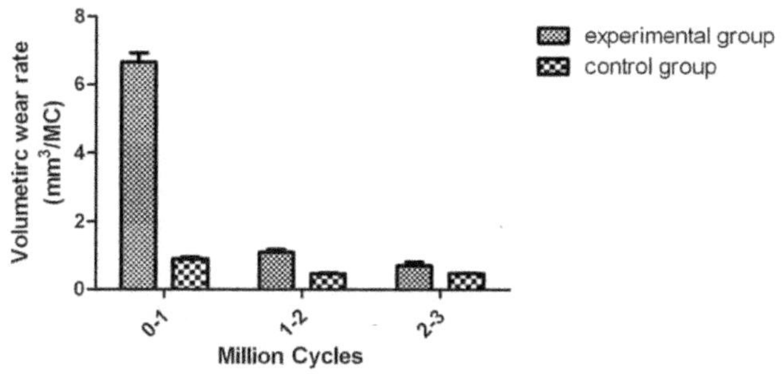

Figure 5. Volumetric wear rates during 0–1,1–2 and 2–3 MC.

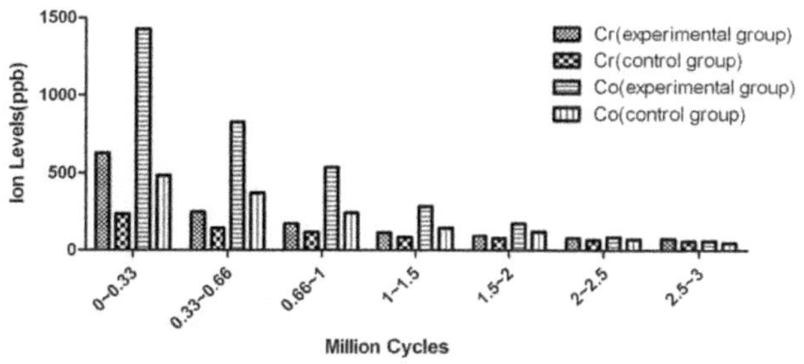

Figure 6. The ion levels(Levels of Co, Cr) in lubricant from 0.33, 0.66, 1.0, 1.5, 2.0. 2.5 and 3.0 MC test-points. Mean values displayed in parts per billion (ppb).

3. Bearing surface profile observation

We observed the evident wear zone on femoral heads in deformation group. The wear zones were at the weight loading area of the femoral heads (close to the pole). On the cup side, the wear patch corresponding to the wear zone of the head was also observed. But in the control group, only mild criss-cross scratching on the contact zone was observed. The surface profile data of each cup and femoral head components' wear zone after 3.0 MC were acquired using the Ultrahigh Precision Surface 3D Profiler. Grooves were widely seen on the surface of the in both groups. The non-uniform directions of the grooves suggested the complex regimen of the wear pattern. Less protein deposition was found on the components in the experimental group, and the grooves on the wear zone in the experimental group were deeper (Figure 7).

4. Wear Debris Analysis

No significant differences in mean particle sizes were seen between the two groups at 1.0 MC and 3.0 MC. Predominantly aggregated round or oval globular particles with a size range of 10–100 nm were observed (mean diameter≈50 nm). EDS analysis showed that the predominant chemical components of the wear particles were cobalt and chromium (cobalt≈61%, chromium≈35%) (Figure 8).

Discussion

Unacceptably high revision rates of the non-modular large head MOM hip replacements have been reported recently. An alternative explanation of the failure of large head metal on metal hips, both resurfacing and total hips, has been offered and is supported by evidence in the literature. With smaller and sub-optimally positioned cups, 'edge loading' or 'rim-wear' of the acetabular cup takes place. This rim-wear results in relatively large volumes of metallic wear debris which manifests itself as high ion levels in the blood of patients and a range of additional complications such as pain, swellings, pseudotumours etc. [6].

Moreover, the deformation of the acetabular component during insertion may damage the fluid-film lubrication between the cup and the femoral head, increasing the wear rate and releasing more metal ions. The Durom cup is a mono-block implant. The thickness of the cup wall is 3.7 mm and the interference of the press-fit is 2–3 mm. The Young's modulus of bone is much less than the modulus of cobalt-chrome alloy. During the implantation of the acetabular component, the bone acetabulum actually expands outwards. Kroeber M et al. [21] have confirmed this phenomenon. Theoretically, some degree of deformation would also occur on cup side during insertion more or less. In physics, $F = m \times a$. Although there are no exact data which can describe the actual strength applies on the acetabulum and metal cup during insertion, the high acceleration accompanies with every impact of the mallet. Therefore the strength applied to the bone acetabulum by the cup is imaginably huge. On the contrary, this huge strength will also act on the cup itself. By Hooke's law, the elastic deformation ends when the material reaches its yield strength. At this point plastic deformation occurs. Our study showed that the mean deformation of the Durom cups was 41.73±8.86 μm. Many literatures also have confirmed the deformation of a variety of metal acetabular components during the insertion [22,17,18]. In our study, the deformations of the cups were predominantly in the superior-posterior quadrant and in areas of the ramus of ischium. One possible reason is that the bone is harder in those areas. The bone acetabula were prepared and reamed manually with hemispheric reamers, but the Durom acetabular component is an elliptically shaped, truncated hemisphere (165°) with peripheral circumferential fins, and therefore there may be some mismatch between the bone cavity and the Durom cup. This may also explain why some of the deformations appeared in other areas.

We know that 150 μm clearance of Durom bearing is a critical distance to guarantee the fluid film lubrication. In the MOM prostheses with non-deformed cups, the fluid film lubrication will be intact. But uneven (localized) 40 micrometers reduction of the clearance may cause some problems; the fluid film lubrication

Table 3. Demographics of the cumulative volumetric wear of cups and heads.

number of cycles(million)		0.33	0.66	1.0	1.5	2.0	2.5	3.0
cup (mm^3)	control group	0.230±0.008	0.351±0.014	0.449±0.020	0.570±0.021	0.680±0.033	0.795±0.034	0.927±0.038
	experimental group	1.890±0.093	3.043±0.072	3.376±0.146	3.745±0.164	4.009±0.126	4.192±0.114	4.394±0.168
head (mm^3)	control group	0.222±0.009	0.341±0.016	0.443±0.023	0.566±0.024	0.665±0.036	0.782±0.040	0.892±0.038
	experimental group	1.865±0.090	3.079±0.117	3.271±0.147	3.501±0.173	3.723±0.153	3.910±0.153	4.035±0.192

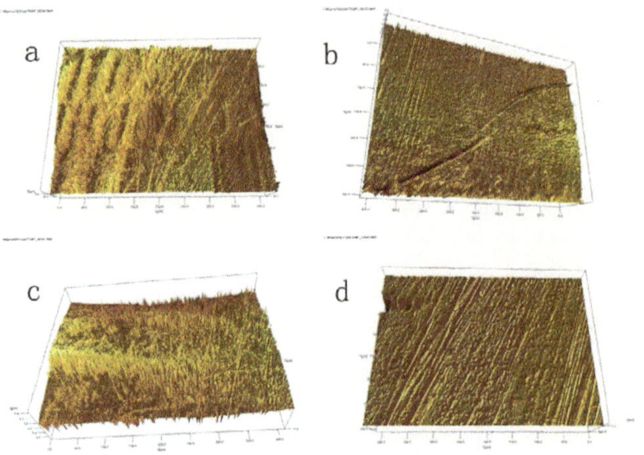

Figure 7. 3D profile micrographs from the center of the wear zone of the femoral head (a) and cup (c) in control group after 3MC wear test. More protein deposition, shallow grooves, less wear. 3D profile micrographs from the wear zone of the femoral head (b) and cup (d) in experimental group after 3MC wear test. Less protein deposition, deeper grooves, more wear.

would change to mixed lubrication or even the boundary lubrication. Since the Durom acetabular component is an elliptically shaped, truncated hemisphere (165°), the deformation at the cup rim would lead to articular contact closer to the rim of the cup, and this edge loading effect may increase the wear rate [23,24]. In this study, the surface of the cups and femoral heads was observed with a 3D profiler after a 3.0 MC test. Only mild criss-cross scratching on the contact zone in control group was observed which is in good agreement with Saikko's study [25] due to the similar experimental condition. On the contrary, the evident wear zone on bearing surface in deformation group was observed. These observations suggest that deformation may change the regimen of lubrication and adversely influence the wear mechanism. The decreased sphericity of bearing may result in equatorial bearing, leading to an increased frictional torque at the cup-bone interface, preventing bone in-growth, and culminating in acetabular loosening. According to our study, an average 41.78 μm deformation of the Durom cup occurred after insertion which would decrease the sphericity of the cup. The deformation of the Durom cup may possibly increase additional frictional torque at the interface.

The volumetric wear rate of the control group in the bedding-in stage was 0.8914±0.0429 mm^3/MC which is in agreement with the results of wear rate analysis of the 55 mm ASR resurfacing joint [26]. The cumulative volumetric wear in the experimental group is 8–9 times more than that in the control group, and ion levels increased significantly. The results of this study illustrate that the deformation of the Durom cup aggravates wear and ion release.

Predominantly aggregated round or oval globular particles were observed. The particle size ranged from 10–100 nm, with a mean size of around 50 nm, in which Co accounts for about 65% and Cr accounts for about 35%, quite similar to the results of other studies [26]. This large number of small particles has the potential to distribute throughout the body via the lymphatic system, with particles found in the lymph nodes, liver, spleen and bone marrow [27]. There are also concerns about the release of metal ions. Increased level of metal ions, such as cobalt and chromium ions, in the blood and urine of patients after metal-on-metal total hip arthroplasty has been reported. Significantly increased ion levels 2–3 years postoperatively are associated with the bedding-in state of the MOM prosthesis which agreed with the results of our study. Although the volumetric wear rate of the MOM prosthesis

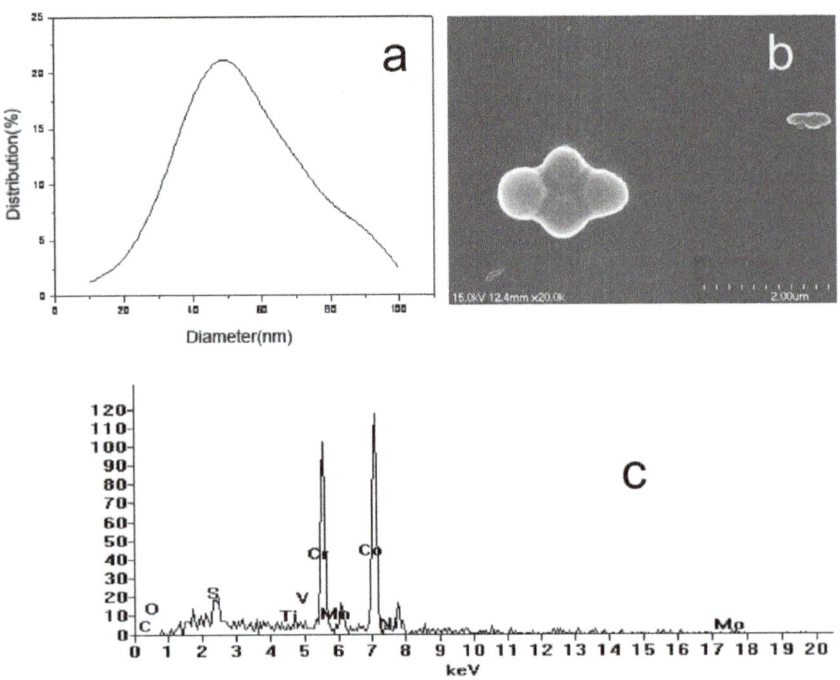

Figure 8. (a)Size distribution curve of wear particles (b)Image of aggregated CoCr wear particles (SEM, ×20,000) (c) The elemental composition in the wear particles by EDS analysis.

decreases markedly after 2–3 million cycles wear; the metal ions and metal particles released will be transported and accumulated causing potential adverse biological reactions. The patients are likely to be exposed to elevated metal levels throughout the life of the prosthesis. Maezawa K et al reported that the serum chromium level did not fall and was remained after 7 years from metal on metal total hip arthroplasty in most of their patients [28]. To date, there are no scientific or epidemiologic data suggesting an increased risk of carcinogenesis or teratogenesis related to increased ions levels after the use of a MOM bearings couple [29]. However, a large number of studies have demonstrated that ions have toxic effects on the liver, kidneys and the immune system [9,30].

To make the results more representative, this study selected specimens from medium build subjects with normal bone density as far as possible. The acetabula were reamed manually; all the procedures were carried out by one senior surgeon to minimize deviations and uncertainties. Since the deformation test is an *in vitro* test and the Durom cups may be restored to their original shape, we measured the deformation three times: the first was just after insertion; the second was 24 h later, then the cups were taken out of the specimens; and the third measurement was carried out 7 days after insertion. There was no statistical difference in deformation at three test points. Frozen cadaveric pelves were used in this study, freezing of allograft bone decreases its mechanical properties. Therefore, deformations seen in this study may be underestimated. In this study, 3D DIC was used to measure deformation, this method has obvious advantages in measuring small deformations, but there are some limitations to the use of this method. It is difficult to collect images at the very sharp edges of the Durom cups. As a result, the measured deformation data may be less than the actual deformation. We also used a digital caliper to measure deformation, but this method is too subjective to obtain accurate data. Only 6 cups were studied in this study, it is quite difficult to compare the deformation among the different size cups.

Conclusions

Deformation of the Durom cup after implantation increases the wear of MOM bearings and the resulting ion levels.

Acknowledgments

The authors are grateful to Zimmer International Ltd. for its assistance with the experimental studies.

Author Contributions

Conceived and designed the experiments: WF. Performed the experiments: FL ZC YG QW WC. Analyzed the data: FL ZC. Wrote the paper: FL ZC.

References

1. Kim RH, Dennis DA, Carothers JT (2008) Metal-on-metal total hip arthroplasty. J Arthroplasty 23:44–46.
2. Stuchin SA (2008) Anatomic diameter femoral heads in total hip arthroplasty: a preliminary report. J Bone Joint Surg [Am] 90(Suppl 3):52–56.
3. Saito S, Ryu J, Watanabe M, Ishii T, Saigo K (2006) Midterm results of Metasul metal-on-metal total hip arthroplasty. J Arthroplasty 21:1105–1110.
4. McMinn DJ, Daniel J, Ziaee H, Pradhan C (2008) Results of the Birmingham Hip Resurfacing dysplasia component in severe acetabular insufficiency: a six - to 9.6-year follow-up. J Bone Joint Surg [Br] 90:715–723.
5. Illgen RL 2nd, Heiner JP, Squire MW, Conrad DN (2010) Large-Head metal-on-metal total hip arthroplasty using the Durom acetabular component at minimum 1-year interval. J Arthroplasty 25(Suppl 6):26–30.
6. Langton DJ, Jameson SS, Joyce TJ, Hallab NJ, Natu S, et al. (2010) Early failure of metal-on-metal bearings in hip resurfacing and large-diameter total hip replacement. J Bone Joint Surg[Br] 92:38–46.
7. Pandit H, Glyn-Jones S, McLardy-Smith P, Gundle R, Whitwell D, et al. (2008) Pseudotumours associated with metal-on-metal hip resurfacings. J Bone Joint Surg [Br] 90:847–851.
8. Ollivere B, Darran C, Barker T, Nolan J, Porteous MJ (2009) Early clinical failure of the Birmingham metal-on-metal hip resurfacing is associated with metallosis and soft tissue necrosis. J Bone Joint Surg[Br] 91:1025–1030.
9. Whittingham-Jones PM, Dunstan E, Altaf H, Cannon SR, Revell PA, et al.(2008) Immune responses in patients with metal-on-metal hip articulations: a long-term follow-up. J Arthroplasty 23:1212–1218.
10. Imanishi T, Hasegawa M, Sudo A (2010) Serum metal ion levels after second-generation metal-on-metal total hip arthroplasty. Arch Orthop Trauma Surg 130:1447–1450.
11. De Smet K, De Haan R, Calistri A, Campbell PA, Ebramzadeh E, et al.(2008) Metal ion measurement as a diagnostic tool to identify problems with metal-on-metal hip resurfacing. J Bone Joint Surg[Am] 90(Suppl 4):202–208.
12. Hart AJ, Sabah S, Henckel J, Lewis A, Cobb J, et al.(2009) The painful metal-on-metal hip resurfacing. J Bone Joint Surg[Br] 91:738–744.
13. Berton C, Girard J, Krantz N, Migaud H (2010) The Durom large diameter head acetabular component: early results with a large-diameter metal-on-metal bearing. J Bone Joint Surg[Br] 92:202–208.
14. De Haan R, Pattyn C, Gill HS, Murray DW, Campbell PA, et al.(2008) Correlation between inclination of the acetabular component and metal ion levels in metal-on-metal hip resurfacing replacement. J Bone Joint Surg [Br] 90:1291–1297.
15. Langton DJ, Jameson SS, Joyce TJ, Webb J, Nargol AV (2008) The effect of component size and orientation on the concentrations of metal ions after resurfacing arthroplasty of the hip. J Bone Joint Surg[Br] 90:1143–1151.
16. Brodner W, Grübl A, Jankovsky R, Meisinger V, Lehr S, et al. (2004) Cup inclination and serum concentration of cobalt and chromium after metal-on-metal total hip arthroplasty. J Arthroplasty 19(Suppl 3):66–70.
17. Squire M, Griffin WL, Mason JB, Peindl RD, Odum S (2006) Acetabular component deformation with press-fit fixation. J Arthroplasty 21(Suppl 2):72–77.
18. Jin ZM, Meakins S, Morlock MM, Parsons P, Hardaker C, et al. (2006) Deformation of press-fitted metallic resurfacing cups. Part 1: Experimental simulation. Proc Inst Mech Eng H 220:299–309.
19. Yew A, Jin ZM, Donn A, Morlock MM, Isaac G (2006) Deformation of press-fitted metallic resurfacing cups. Part 2: Finite element simulation. Proc Inst Mech Eng H 220:311–319.
20. Brown C, Williams S, Tipper JL, Fisher J, Ingham E (2007) Characterisation of wear particles produced by metal on metal and ceramic on metal hip prostheses under standard and microseparation simulation. J Mater Sci Mater Med 18:819–827.
21. Kroeber M, Ries MD, Suzuki Y, Renowitzky G, Ashford F, et al. (2002) Impact biomechanics and pelvic deformation during insertion of press-fit acetabular cups. J Arthroplasty 17:349–354.
22. Markel D, Day J, Siskey R, Liepins I, Kurtz S, et al. (2011) Deformation of metal-backed acetabular components and the impact of liner thickness in a cadaveric model. Int Orthop 35:1131–1137.
23. Morlock MM, Bishop N, Zustin J, Hahn M, Rüther W, et al. (2008) Modes of implant failure after hip resurfacing: morphological and wear analysis of 267 retrieval specimens. J Bone Joint Surg[Am] 90(suppl 3):89–95.
24. De Haan R, Campbell PA, Su EP, De Smet KA (2008) Revision of metal-on-metal resurfacing arthroplasty of the hip: the influence of malpositioning of the components. J Bone Joint Surg[Br] 90:1158–1163..
25. Saikko V (2005) A 12-station anatomic hip joint simulator. Proc Inst Mech Eng H 219:437–448.
26. Leslie I, Williams S, Brown C, Isaac G, Jin Z, et al.(2008) Effect of bearing size on the long-term wear, wear debris, and ion levels of large diameter metal-on-metal hip replacements-An in vitro study. J Biomed Mater Res B Appl Biomater 87:163–172.
27. Case CP, Langkamer VG, James C, Palmer MR, Kemp AJ, et al.(1994) Widespread dissemination of metal debris from implant. J Bone Joint Surg [Br] 76:701–712.
28. Maezawa K, Nozawa M, Yuasa T, Aritomi K, Matsuda K, et al.(2010) Seven years of chronological changes of serum chromium levels after Metasul metal-on-metal total hip arthroplasty. J Arthroplasty 25(8):1196–1200.
29. MacDonald SJ (2004) Metal-on-metal total hip arthroplasty: the concerns. Clin Orthop Relat Res 429:86–93.
30. Goodman SB (2007) Wear particles, periprosthetic osteolysis and the immune system. Biomaterials 28:5044–5048.

7

Genome Wide Analysis Indicates Genes for Basement Membrane and Cartilage Matrix Proteins as Candidates for Hip Dysplasia in Labrador Retrievers

Ineke C. M. Lavrijsen[1], Peter A. J. Leegwater[1]*, Alan J. Martin[2], Stephen J. Harris[2], Marianna A. Tryfonidou[1], Henri C. M. Heuven[1], Herman A. W. Hazewinkel[1]

1 Department of Clinical Sciences of Companion Animal, Faculty of Veterinary Medicine, Utrecht University, Utrecht, The Netherlands, **2** Waltham Centre for Pet Nutrition, Leicestershire, United Kingdom

Abstract

Hip dysplasia, an abnormal laxity of the hip joint, is seen in humans as well as dogs and is one of the most common skeletal disorders in dogs. Canine hip dysplasia is considered multifactorial and polygenic, and a variety of chromosomal regions have been associated with the disorder. We performed a genome-wide association study in Dutch Labrador Retrievers, comparing data of nearly 18,000 single nucleotide polymorphisms (SNPs) in 48 cases and 30 controls using two different statistical methods. An individual SNP analysis based on comparison of allele frequencies with a χ^2 statistic was used, as well as a simultaneous SNP analysis based on Bayesian variable selection. Significant association with canine hip dysplasia was observed on chromosome 8, as well as suggestive association on chromosomes 1, 5, 15, 20, 25 and 32. Next-generation DNA sequencing of the exons of genes of seven regions identified multiple associated alleles on chromosome 1, 5, 8, 20, 25 and 32 ($p<0.001$). Candidate genes located in the associated regions on chromosomes 1, 8 and 25 included *LAMA2*, *LRR1* and *COL6A3*, respectively. The associated region on CFA20 contained candidate genes *GDF15*, *COMP* and *CILP2*. In conclusion, our study identified candidate genes that might affect susceptibility to canine hip dysplasia. These genes are involved in hypertrophic differentiation of chondrocytes and extracellular matrix integrity of basement membrane and cartilage. The functions of the genes are in agreement with the notion that disruptions in endochondral bone formation in combination with soft tissue defects are involved in the etiology of hip dysplasia.

Editor: Yi-Hsiang Hsu, Harvard Medical School, United States of America

Funding: This study was funded by the Waltham Centre for Pet Nutrition, a division of Mars Petcare UK (http://www.mars.com/global/brands/petcare.aspx). The co-authors Alan J Martin and Stephen J Harris were employed by Mars Petcare UK. They took part in the study design, data collection and analysis, decision to publish and preparation of the manuscript.

Competing Interests: It should be noted that the co-authors AJ Martin and SJ Harris are employed by Waltham Centre for Pet Nutrition, a division of Mars Petcare, which also funded this study. This company has applied for patents based on the results of this work: Application 1310552.3; Name: Composition for Canine Animals and Application 1310558.0; Name: Genetic Test.

* E-mail: P.A.J.Leegwater@uu.nl

Introduction

Hip dysplasia is characterised by an abnormal formation of the hip joint, causing incongruity and/or laxity of the joint, which can lead to osteoarthritis. It has been observed in several mammals, including humans, where it is referred to as developmental dysplasia of the hip (DDH), and in dogs where the term canine hip dysplasia (CHD) is used. In both species delayed femoral capital ossification, hip joint laxity and subluxation are observed in dysplastic hips [1] [2].

The reported incidence of DDH varies widely, depending on screening methods and DDH definition employed at medical centres. Between 0.5% and 4.2% of screened neonates and infants receive treatment [2] [3]. Risk factors include a family history of DDH, female sex, other skeletal abnormalities and hormonal and environmental factors. CHD is one of the most common developmental skeletal disorders in dogs and affects predominantly breeds of medium and large sized dogs [4]. In Bulldogs up to 72% of the screened animals are affected (www.offa.org/stats_hip.html). For some breeds a sex predisposition has been described [5]. Hereditary and environmental factors are thought to play a role in the manifestation of this disorder. The involvement of one gene with a major effect in combination with genes with small contributions is considered likely in a number of breeds [6] [7].

In recent years, several attempts have been made to gain understanding of the molecular genetic basis of hip dysplasia in man and dog. Occurrence of hip dysplasia in humans has been associated with variations in asporin (an extracellular matrix protein belonging to the small leucine-rich repeat protein family), interleukin-6 and transforming growth factor β1 [8] (both involved in bone remodelling [9] [10]), growth differentiation factor 5 [11], T-box 4 (involved in hind limb development) [12], the vitamin D receptor and estrogen receptor 1 [13] and pregnancy-associated plasma protein A2 [14]. In canines, genome-wide studies have been performed in Portuguese Water Dogs, German Shepherd Dogs, Labrador Retrievers and Greyhound/Labrador Retriever crossbreeds. Different definitions of CHD were used, including hip joint laxity measured as Norberg Angle or distraction index and hip scores according to the Fédération Cynologique Internationale (FCI) for CHD grading. These studies found quantitative trait loci (QTLs) on multiple chromosomal regions and a variant of the fibrillin 2 gene (*FBN2*) to be associated with CHD [15–21]. None of the loci could account for more than 18% of the genetic variance, confirming the polygenic nature of the disorder. Additional genes play an essential role in the correct formation of the hip joint, and identification of these genes would provide insight into the molecular processes that lead to CHD.

We describe a SNP-based genome-wide association study for CHD in Labrador Retrievers from The Netherlands, and subsequent fine mapping of the identified regions by case-control comparison of DNA sequences of gene exons included in the regions.

Methods

Ethics Statement

The dogs were privately owned and included with informed consent of the owners. They were handled by licensed veterinarians only. Thus we complied to the conditions set forth in the Dutch 'Wet op de Uitoefening van de Diergeneeskunde' (Law on the Practice of Veterinary Medicine) of March 21, 1990 and approval of an ethics committee for the use of samples of the animals was not necessary.

Animals

Hip radiographs and DNA from blood samples of 122 unrelated purebred Labrador retrievers born between 1980 and 2005 were assessed. All dogs were registered by the Dutch Kennel Club or descendants of registered dogs only. DNA was isolated from blood

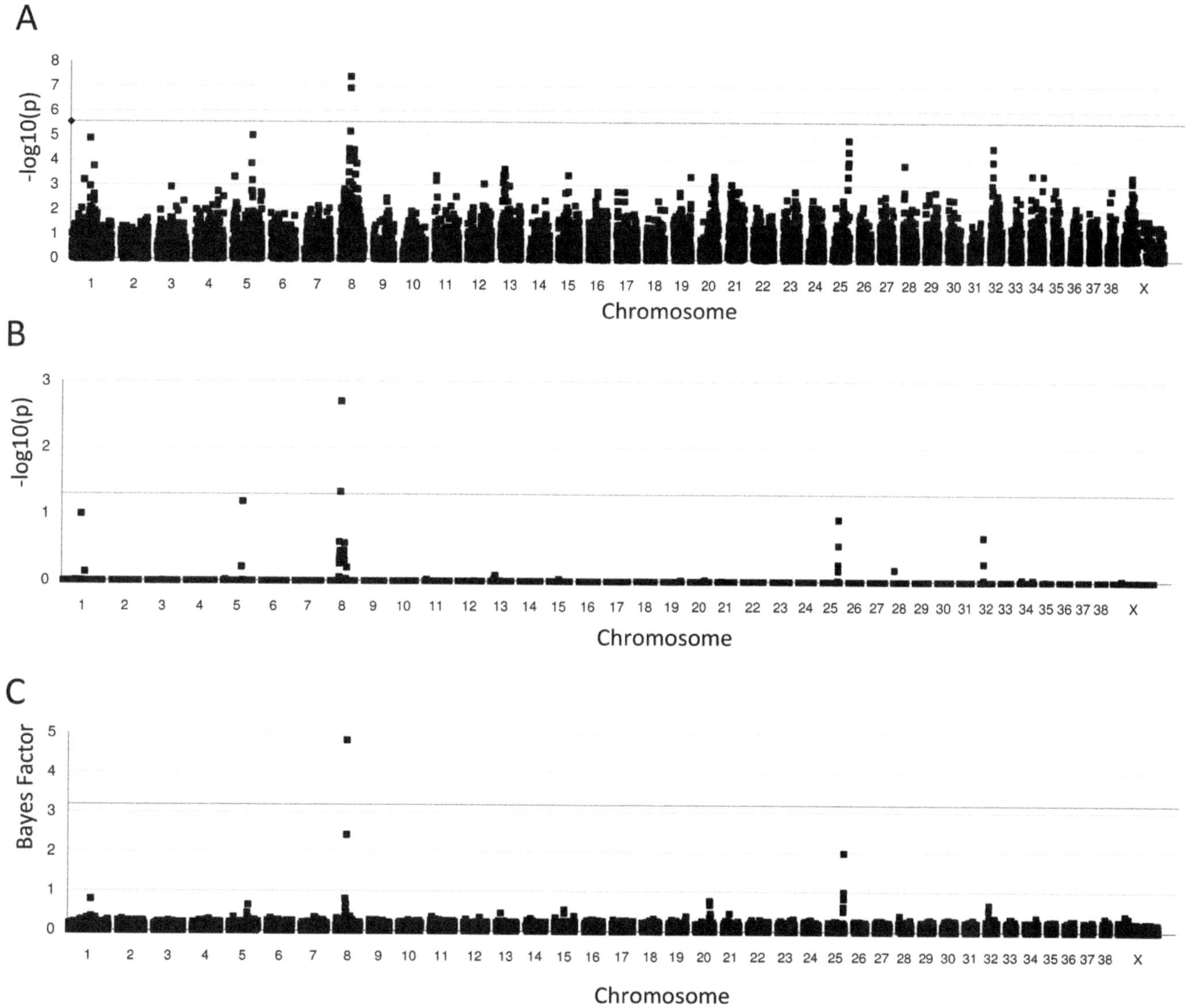

Figure 1. Genome wide association analysis of hip dysplasia in Labrador retrievers. Genotypes of 17,859 SNPs were compared between 48 cases and 30 controls. A. Allele frequency based χ^2 statistics. The dotted line indicates the significance threshold after Bonferroni correction. B. Multiple testing correction of the χ^2 statistics by 1,000 permutations of the phenotypes to determine empirical p-values. The dotted line indicates the significance threshold ($\alpha = 0.05$). C. Genome wide association analysis using Bayesian variable selection to detect SNPs with a high probability to have an effect on the CHD phenotype. The dotted line indicates the significance level.

Table 1. Array SNPs associated with hip dysplasia in Labrador Retrievers [a].

			MAF[b]		score	
CFA	location	SNP	cases	controls	PLINK[c]	iBay[d]
1	70962581	BICF2P1446667	0.24	0.02	3.76	0.79
5	62363747	BICF2S23057444	0.22	0.57	5.02	0.66
8	29868871	BICF2P950415	0.28	0.62	4.47	0.81
8	31218201	BICF2S23118415	0.46	0.15	4.12	0.57
8	32367889	BICF2S2305197	0.56	0.23	4.26	0.68
8	33707642	BICF2S23913508	0.20	0.63	7.41	2.43
8	33990753	BICF2P601580	0.64	0.20	6.94	4.82
15	32865368	BICF2G630433123	0.28	0.57	3.42	0.54
20	46604376	BICF2P1445357	0.40	0.68	3.32	0.77
20	47759323	BICF2S22943564	0.40	0.67	3.00	0.68
20	47926376	BICF2P878084	0.34	0.63	3.39	0.75
25	50228063	BICF2G630160005	0.54	0.23	3.83	0.63
25	50458146	BICF2S23326254	0.28	0.03	3.97	0.52
25	50637313	BICF2G630159246	0.55	0.20	4.85	1.98
25	51127510	BICF2P909436	0.53	0.20	4.39	1.00
25	51155516	BICF2P770517	0.53	0.20	4.39	0.84
32	11802242	BICF2S23211582	0.07	0.33	4.54	0.54
32	12336449	rs8795055	0.20	0.47	3.43	0.68

[a]SNPs with a Bayes Factor >0.5 were included.
[b]MAF = minor allele frequency.
[c]$-^{10}$log p-values.
[d]Bayes Factor.

samples using a standard salt-extraction method [22]. Blood samples were not available from 26 dogs and the DNA was isolated from buccal swabs from these dogs using the QIAamp DNA Blood Mini Kit (QIAgen, Hilden, Germany).

Phenotypes

A ventrodorsal hip radiograph of the dog in dorsal recumbency with extended hind limbs was made, examined by the CHD-panel of the Dutch Kennel Club and graded according to FCI guidelines, distinguishing CHD-A (normal), CHD-B (subnormal/borderline), CHD-C (mild), CHD-D (moderate) and CHD-E (severe). Most dogs were graded at age between 12 and 20 months. The six exceptions were one CHD-C graded dog of 50 months; three CHD-D dogs of 26, 27 and 40 months; and two CHD-D/E graded dogs of 33 and 63 months of age. We chose to analyze canine hip dysplasia as a binomial trait with affected (CHD-C/D/E) versus unaffected (CHD-A) dogs excluding CHD-B dogs from the study.

Generation of Genotypes and Quality Control

The Illumina Infinium CanineSNP20 BeadChip was used to genotype more than 22,000 SNPs in our sample set. Of these, the 17,859 SNPs that had a minor allele frequency higher than 0.01 and that were successfully genotyped in more than 90% of the samples were included in the data analysis. PLINK software was used to generate an "identical by state" similarity matrix [44]. The first two principal components of this multidimensional similarity matrix were used to depict each individual in a 2-dimensional plot.

Association Analysis

A χ^2 statistic for the comparison of allele frequencies of 17,859 SNPs in 48 cases (21 males and 27 females) and 30 unaffecteds (12 males and 18 females) was generated using PLINK software [23]. Of the cases, 17 were graded CHD-C, 25 CHD-D and 6 CHD-D/E. The unaffecteds were all graded CHD-A.

A Bonferroni correction was used as multiple-testing correction, but because this is a rather stringent correction method, a series of 1,000 permutations were also run on our data set and compared against the best result from all SNPs to estimate the significance of the peaks (EMP2 in PLINK).

Simultaneous analysis of multiple randomly selected SNPs was performed using a Bayesian procedure with the program iBay [24] [25] assuming a mixture model to identify associated SNPs. The model assumed that SNPs belong to one of two normal distributions; the first distribution contained SNPs that had very little effect on the phenotype and the second distribution comprised SNPs that had an effect on the phenotype. Bayesian analysis required values for the hyper parameters of the priors. It was assumed that less than 5% of our SNPs belonged to the second distribution explaining 99.5% of the genetic variance.

The genetic variance was obtained from the phenotypic variance assuming a heritability of 20%. This value was an average of the heritability derived for four dog breeds (unpublished results). The prior variances of the two distributions were calculated using these assumptions. The Bayesian procedure is based on Gibbs sampling and three million Bayesian iterations were run to calculate the posterior variances as well as the posterior probabilities that SNPs belong to either of the two distributions. Odds ratios were calculated for each SNP by dividing the posterior probability by the a priori probability, which was inherent to the assumptions made. A Bayes factor BF was calculated by dividing the posterior by the prior odds ratio for each SNP. BF larger than 3.2 indicate 'substantial' evidence for association while a BF larger than 10 indicates 'strong' evidence and a value larger than 100 as 'decisive' [26]. We considered SNPs with a BF>3 as regions for follow up.

Next-Generation Sequencing and Analysis

Five regions were selected for targeted exon enrichment and sequencing on a SOLiD4 at the University of Liverpool, UK. For each annotated gene in these regions, exons, intron/exon boundaries (30 bp) and the intergenic regions flanking both sides of each gene (2×500 bp), were targeted for enrichment. When the gene was smaller than 3 kb, the 5′ (upstream) flanking region was increased until this criterion was met, to facilitate haplotype analysis. To minimize the chance of missing genes or exons due to a faulty annotation of the dog genome build, the synthenic regions in the human genome were compared and human cDNA of genes in these regions were compared with the reference dog genome using BLAST software. When the orientation of the alignments was corresponding to the homologous gene in the dog and located within 100 kb of the gene, this alignment was considered a putative non-annotated exon. These exons, as well as alignments of canine expressed sequence tags (ESTs) compared with the dog genome were targeted for enrichment. Microarray-based enrichment of all targeted loci was performed using a custom Comparative Genomic Hybridization Array by Roche NimbleGen.

A subset of "interesting" genes, based on their known function and position within the association peak regions, was selected and the exons were sequenced in 48 cases and 30 controls (priority genes), while the exons of remainder of the genes were sequenced in 15 cases and 15 controls (non priority genes).

Table 2. Variant DNA sequences associated with hip dysplasia in Labrador Retrievers.

			number		MAF [a]				
CFA	location	alleles	cases	controls	cases	controls	score [b]	gene	position in gene [c]
1	70938018	(T/A)	36	30	0.28	0.02	4.35	*LAMA2*	intron
1	70997779	(A/T)	33	30	0.26	0.02	3.94	*LAMA2*	exon, synonymous
5	59194609	(G/−)	15	15	0.33	0.77	3.13	*KLHL17*	3′-UTR
5	62929475	(C/T)	14	8	0.04	0.63	4.85	*NPHP4*	5′-UTR
8	29247021	(C/T)	33	30	0.73	0.35	4.67	*LRR1*	3′-UTR
8	31496895	(C/T)	33	30	0.55	0.23	3.46	*PTGDR*	downstream
8	31496910	(C/T)	32	30	0.53	0.22	3.51	*PTGDR*	downstream
20	45260332	(A/G)	32	30	0.30	0.07	3.01	*LTF*	exon, non-synonymous
20	46671813	(C/G)	15	15	0.53	0.10	3.51	*PBX4*	inton
20	46706734	(A/G)	27	28	0.63	0.27	3.87	*CILP2*	3′-UTR
20	47636184	(G/A)	29	30	0.55	0.23	3.41	*GDF15*	3′-UTR
20	47714388	(G/A)	29	29	0.24	0.66	5.13	*LSM4*	5′-UTR
20	48071192	(G/A)	34	30	0.26	0.63	4.56	*INSL3*	upstream
20	48243399	(G/−)	12	13	0.17	0.65	3.31	*UNC13A*	3′-UTR
20	48804130	(G/A)	13	14	0.19	0.71	3.92	*NWD1*	exon, synonymous
20	49019261	(T/C)	29	30	0.57	0.25	3.38	*CHERP*	intron
20	49318725	(C/T)	7	12	0.64	0.04	4.31	*CIB3*	exon, synonymous
25	47629272	(C/T)	26	29	0.06	0.36	3.94	*INPP5D*	upstream
25	47666842	(G/A)	28	30	0.02	0.28	4.10	*INPP5D*	exon, synonymous
25	47685188	(C/T)	31	30	0.68	0.37	3.23	*INPP5D*	intron
25	48075297	(C/G)	15	15	0.37	0.00	3.62	*LOC100688622*	exon, non-synonymous
25	48076278	(G/A)	15	15	0.37	0.00	3.62	*LOC100688622*	downstream
25	48396330	(C/T)	25	30	0.54	0.23	3.03	*SPP2*	inron
25	50050076	(G/A)	9	6	0.78	0.08	3.71	*ASB18*	downstream
25	50228063	(C/G)	13	15	0.27	0.73	3.28	*IQCA1*	intron
25	51029326	(G/A)	28	30	0.57	0.27	3.06	*COL6A3*	intron
25	51031100	(A/G)	32	30	0.39	0.10	3.73	*COL6A3*	exon, synonymous
25	51040259	(A/G)	33	30	0.52	0.20	3.61	*COL6A3*	exon, synonymous
25	51046607	(G/A)	31	30	0.53	0.22	3.49	*COL6A3*	exon, synonymous
25	51736576	(T/C)	27	30	0.56	0.23	3.38	*HES6*	upstream
32	11265116	(−/T)	15	15	0.03	0.40	3.25	*LOC487839*	downstream

[a]minor allele frequency.
[b]$-^{10}$log p-value.
[c]UTR lengths based on human cDNA data.

Minor allele read frequencies for each sequenced location were calculated by dividing the number of observed reads for the less prevalent allele by the number of the reads that covered the position of the SNP. Genotypes were estimated using thresholds for minor allele read frequencies of more than 0.2 and less than 0.8 for heterozygotes. Individuals with a minor allele read frequency of less than 0.2 at a certain location were considered homozygous for the major allele, and over 0.8 were considered homozygous for the minor allele. These inferred genotypes were used to calculate allelic association with a standard $\chi 2$ statistic as well as with iBay. All raw SNP data and DNA sequencing data are available upon request.

Results

Population stratification analysis revealed genetic divergence within the group of Labrador Retrievers. The Dutch Labrador Retrievers were identified as the main group, and samples that deviated from this group were dogs imported from the USA or their first generation descendants ($n = 44$). There were no cases in this subpopulation and we excluded this group, leaving 48 cases (mild, moderate or severe CHD) and 30 controls (no signs of CHD) for further analysis.

Individual and Multiple SNP Association Analysis

Individual SNP association to CHD was tested using a χ^2-based statistic for the comparison of allele frequencies using PLINK software, and revealed association to multiple chromosomal regions, including chromosome 1, 3, 5, 8, 11, 12, 13, 15, 19, 20,

25, 28, 32, 34 and the X chromosome (P-value <0.001, Figure 1). A Bonferroni correction of $\alpha = 0.05$ over 17,859 tests was performed to correct for multiple testing and only the region on chromosome 8 was significantly associated to CHD, with BICF2S23913508 located at position 33707642 bp of the reference genome CanFam2 as the most strongly associated SNP in this region (corrected P-value = 0.0007, Figure 1A). Permutations were performed as a less stringent correction for multiple testing, but it also resulted in significant association of the region on chromosome 8 only (corrected *P*-value = 0.002, Figure 1B).

A Bayesian variable selection method was used to study the combined effect of all SNPs simultaneously to distinguish between chromosomal regions likely to have an effect on the phenotype and false positives. The effect of a SNP is corrected for all other SNPs in the model. The underlying assumption in this simultaneous SNP association analysis is that SNPs belong to either of two distributions; one that contains SNPs that contribute to the phenotype, and one that contains SNPs that do not. The program iBay was used to generate posterior probabilities, expressed as Bayesian factors (BF), for each SNP to belong to the distribution of SNPs that had an effect on the phenotype. Bayesian factors larger than three were considered significant. Analysis of the SNP data of the 48 cases and 30 controls identified one genomic region located on chromosome 8 to have an effect on the phenotype with BF greater than 3. Additional regions were identified that have a minor contribution (BF>0.5) to the phenotype on chromosomes 1, 5, 15, 20, 25 and 32 (Figure 1C). In Table 1 the results of the 18 SNPs with a BF larger than 0.5 are summarized. At least one SNP in each of the seven regions passed this threshold. The strongest association with the highest number of SNPs and the highest BFs were observed on chromosome 8 and on chromosome 25 and only eight SNPs were identified in the other five regions together. Regions nominated for follow-up analysis were selected based on the individual and multiple SNP analyses, and included regions on CFA01 (70.7–71.9 Mb), CFA05 (58.6–63.5 Mb), CFA08 (28.0–34.5 Mb), CFA15 (32.2–33.6 Mb), CFA20 (46.3–51.2 Mb), CFA25 (47.1–51.9 Mb), CFA32 (11.2–13.0 Mb).

Targeted Fragment Enrichment and Next-Generation Sequencing

The seven regions that displayed association were selected for microarray-based enrichment and DNA sequencing. The total size of these 7 regions was ~25 Mb. An exon sequencing approach was chosen to increase the coverage per analyzed position, resulting in 2.3 Mb of target DNA. Priority genes in the regions were selected based on the function of the encoded proteins. The processes involved were cartilage or bone development and synthesis or maintenance of extracellur matrix. The priority gene exons totaled 300 kb and these were analyzed in 69 DNA samples from the Dutch Labrador Retriever population. The exons of the remaining non-priority genes, 2 Mb in total size, were enriched and sequenced in 15 cases and 15 controls. For both sets, approximately 30% of the generated reads could be mapped to the targeted regions.

In the priority samples, approximately 81% of the targeted regions were sequenced at least once, but only 65% of the targeted regions were covered 10 times or more. For the non-priority samples, these percentages were slightly lower (80% and 60%, respectively) per sample. Overall, 74.4% of the priority regions and 58.0% of the non-priority regions were sequenced at least 10 times in 10 cases and 10 controls. We identified 5388 variations that were covered at least 10 times in both cases and controls and that had a minor allele frequency higher than 0.01 (Table S1). Genotypes were inferred from the number of reads per allele and used to calculate χ^2-based allelic association. The SNPs that were most strongly associated with CHD are listed in Table 2 together with the genes at the position or in the vicinity of these SNPs.

Discussion

CHD is considered a complex trait and multiple chromosomal regions have been associated with the disease in various dog breeds [15–20]. Around the world different protocols are in use to classify the severity of the disease based on radiographs. In this study, the severity grade was not taken into account due to the limited number of samples and CHD was analysed as a binomial trait. Given that HD is a complex disease two statistical analyses were applied. In contrast to the single SNP-analysis with PLINK software, the multiple-SNP analysis of iBay takes this complexity into account and therefore more weight was given to the results obtained with the latter program.

As could be expected for a complex disorder, our genome-wide analysis revealed multiple regions associated with CHD. Several of these regions had been implicated in CHD before. The region on CFA08 at position 28–34.5 Mb that was strongly associated in our study overlaps largely with the region of 29–34 Mb found by Marshall and Distl [16] in the German Shepherd Dog. The less strongly associated region on CFA01 at 70.7–71.9 Mb overlaps with a region around position70 Mb identified by Phavaphutanon et al. [18] in Labrador Retrievers and the region on chromosome 20 at 46.3–51.2 Mb overlaps with the region of 40–47 Mb described by Todhunter et al. [20] in the offspring of affected Labrador Retrievers and unaffected Greyhounds. The minor associated region on CFA32 at 11.2–13.0 Mb is flanked by regions identified in Labrador Retrievers around 5 Mb [18] and German Shepherd Dogs (16–20 Mb) [16].

We found no evidence for association of other regions on chromosomes 1, 2, 10, 20 (two regions around 30 Mb and 60 Mb) and CFA22 previously reported to be associated in Labrador Retrievers [18]. We also did not observe association to the region of CFA11 that contains *FBN2* coding for fibrillin 2. A deletion in an intron of this gene was found to be associated with suppression of the gene and with hip dysplasia in Labrador Retrievers from the USA [21]. The discrepant results might be due to population differences. Indeed, the population stratification analysis indicated that the Dutch and American populations of Labrador Retrievers have diverged.

CHD is a common disorder occurring in many breeds, and alternate genetic factors may be involved in different breeds or even populations. The etiology of CHD is not understood, although two broad etiological categories have been proposed i.e., laxity of the peri-articular soft tissues (ligaments, muscles, joint capsule) [27–30], and an abnormal progression of the endochondral ossification in the hip joint, or a combination of both processes [31] [32]. A majority of 88% of the affected dogs in our sample was graded before the age of 20 months. We were not concerned with the possibility of including phenocopies by adding dogs that were diagnosed at a later age, because their number was small and these could not have led to falsely positive results.

One of the identified SNPs associated with CHD is located near the *LRR1* gene on CFA08. the encoded protein has been described as down regulating the 4-1BB-mediated signal transduction pathways JNK1 and NfkappaB [33]. JNK1 and NFkappaB play a role in proteoglycan synthesis by chondrocytes [34] [35] making a role for *LRR1* in cartilage development and physiology plausible. Functional studies are needed to corroborate the possible role of *LRR1* in CHD.

Additional analysis of the data resulted in the selection of other SNPs of interest that were associated with CHD status together with *LRR1*. These SNPs were located in the top regions of the multiple SNP association analysis in or near the genes *COL6A3* on CFA25, and *LAMA2* on CFA01 (Table 2). The specific function of these genes in cartilage and muscle as described below facilitates their implication in CHD. First, *COL6A3* codes for the alpha 3 chain of collagen VI that forms a fine fibrillar network in many connective tissues [36] and is a specific component of the pericellular matrix of chondrocytes with a protective role for these cells [37]. Furthermore, one of the characterising features of myopathies related to mutations in the *COL6A3* gene is joint hyper laxity [38]. Second, laminins with a *LAMA2* encoded chain are found in the basal lamina of basement membranes [39]; the chain is also related to cartilage development [40] and has been implicated in congenital muscular dystrophy [41]. Third, the region of interest on CFA20 contains three genes involved in connective tissue integrity. This region displays strong linkage disequilibrium and it is not possible to discriminate between the genes based on the association data. Good candidate genes for involvement in CHD in this region are *GDF15* encoding growth-differentiating factor 15, *COMP* for cartilage oligomeric matrix protein and the gene encoding cartilage intermediate layer protein 2 (*CILP2*). *GDF15* is a gene with a role not only in bone remodelling [42], but has also been related to osteoarthritis in humans [43]. Mutations in *COMP* are associated with pseudoachondroplasia (OMIM177170) and multiple epiphyseal dysplasia (OMIM132400). *CILP-2* is expressed in cartilaginous tissues and muscles; specifically there are indications that it is associated with collagen VI microfibrils mediating interactions between matrix components in cartilage [44]. It should be noted that our DNA sequencing strategy aimed at identification of mutations in exons and in intron/exon junctions. Intron mutations at positions not close to exons can affect RNA splicing and these were not captured by our strategy.

The associated regions support the view that cartilage, as a specified connective tissue, plays an important role in the pathophysiology of CHD. A delay in endochondral ossification of the femoral head has been demonstrated in dysplastic Labrador dogs [45–47], in correspondence with earlier findings in German Shepherd dogs [28]. Furthermore, CHD in American Labrador Retrievers is associated with a deletion in *FBN2* that codes for fibrillin2, a component of the extracellular matrix in fibrous joint capsule and articular cartilage [21]. Another study observed a difference in muscle composition of two months old German Shepherd Dogs that developed CHD later in life compared to controls [28]. In addition, structural alterations were found in collagen fibers of the joint capsule of the hip joint and of the round ligament of dysplastic Labrador Retrievers when compared to these structures in tight-hipped Labradors [1].

Conclusions

This study identified several SNPs associated with CHD in or near genes that are involved in extracellular matrix development. The combination of the candidate genes implicates bone and soft tissue development in CHD. First, disturbances during the process of endochondral bone formation attributing to the abnormal formation of the hip joint may well be related to disturbances in the hypertrophic differentiation of the chondrocytes. Second, there are indications for soft tissue involvement (cartilage, muscles, and ligaments). The association results described here need to be confirmed by analysis of an independent replication cohort. Additional mechanistic studies are essential for the understanding of the molecular processes that lead to hip dysplasia.

Supporting Information

Table S1 Observed DNA sequence variations in genome regions associated with canine hip dysplasia.

Acknowledgments

The Royal Dutch Guide Dog Foundation (KNGF = Koninklijk Nederlands Geleidehonden Fonds) are acknowledged for consent to include DNA samples and phenotypes of their dogs and for supplying pedigree data.

Author Contributions

Conceived and designed the experiments: ICL PAL AJM SJH HCH HAH. Performed the experiments: ICL PAL AJM SJH HCH. Analyzed the data: ICL PAL AJM SJH MAT HCH. Contributed reagents/materials/analysis tools: AJM SJH MAT HCH HAH. Wrote the paper: ICL PAL AJM SJH HCH HAH.

References

1. Todhunter RJ, Lust G (2003) Canine hip dysplasia pathogenesis. In: Slatter D, editor. Textbook of small animal surgery. Philadelphia: WB Saunders Co. 2009–2019.
2. Boere-Boonekamp MM, Verkerk PH (1998) Screening for developmental dysplasia of the hip. Seminars in Neonatology 3: 49–59.
3. Peled E, Eidelman M, Katzman A, Bialik V (2008) Neonatal incidence of hip dysplasia: Ten years of experience. Clin Orthop Relat Res 466: 771–775.
4. Priester WA, Mulvihill JJ (1972) Canine hip dysplasia: Relative risk by sex, size, and breed, and comparative aspects. J Am Vet Med Assoc 160: 735–739.
5. Malm S, Strandberg E, Danell B, Audell L, Swenson L, et al (2007) Impact of sedation method on the diagnosis of hip and elbow dysplasia in swedish dogs. Prev Vet Med 78: 196–209.
6. Mäki K, Janss LL, Groen AF, Liinamo AE, Ojala M (2004) An indication of major genes affecting hip and elbow dysplasia in four finnish dog populations. Heredity 92: 402–408.
7. Janutta V, Hamann H, Distl O (2006) Complex segregation analysis of canine hip dysplasia in german shepherd dogs. J Hered 97: 13–20.
8. Kolundzic R, Trkulja V, Mikolaucic M, Kolundzic MJ, Pavelic SK, et al (2011) Association of interleukin-6 and transforming growth factor-beta1 gene polymorphisms with developmental hip dysplasia and severe adult hip osteoarthritis: A preliminary study. Cytokine 54: 125–128.
9. Hinke V, Seck T, Clanget C, Scheidt-Nave C, Ziegler R, et al (2001) Association of transforming growth factor-beta1 (TGFbeta1) T29–> C gene polymorphism with bone mineral density (BMD), changes in BMD, and serum concentrations of TGF-beta1 in a population-based sample of postmenopausal german women. Calcif Tissue Int 69: 315–320.
10. Kwan Tat S, Padrines M, Theoleyre S, Heymann D, Fortun Y (2004) IL-6, RANKL, TNF-alpha/IL-1: Interrelations in bone resorption pathophysiology. Cytokine Growth Factor Rev 15: 49–60.
11. Dai J, Shi D, Zhu P, Qin J, Ni H, et al (2008) Association of a single nucleotide polymorphism in growth differentiate factor 5 with congenital dysplasia of the hip: A case-control study. Arthritis Res Ther 10: R126.
12. Wang K, Shi D, Zhu P, Dai J, Zhu L, et al (2010) Association of a single nucleotide polymorphism in Tbx4 with developmental dysplasia of the hip: A case-control study. Osteoarthritis Cartilage 18: 1592–1595.
13. Kapoor B, Dunlop C, Wynn-Jones C, Fryer AA, Strange RC, et al (2007) Vitamin D and oestrogen receptor polymorphisms in developmental dysplasia of the hip and primary protrusio acetabuli–a preliminary study. J Negat Results Biomed 6: 7. 10.1186/1477-5751-6-7.
14. Jia J, Li L, Zhao Q, Zhang L, Ru J, et al (2012) Association of a single nucleotide polymorphism in pregnancy-associated plasma protein-A2 with developmental dysplasia of the hip: A case-control study. Osteoarthritis Cartilage 20: 60–63.
15. Chase K, Lawler DF, Adler FR, Ostrander EA, Lark KG (2004) Bilaterally asymmetric effects of quantitative trait loci (QTLs): QTLs that affect laxity in the right versus left coxofemoral (hip) joints of the dog (canis familiaris). Am J Med Genet A 124: 239–247.
16. Marschall Y, Distl O (2007) Mapping quantitative trait loci for canine hip dysplasia in german shepherd dogs. Mamm Genome 18: 861–870.
17. Zhu L, Zhang Z, Feng F, Schweitzer P, Phavaphutanon J, et al (2008) Single nucleotide polymorphisms refine QTL intervals for hip joint laxity in dogs. Anim Genet 39: 141–146.

18. Phavaphutanon J, Mateescu RG, Tsai KL, Schweitzer PA, Corey EE, et al (2009) Evaluation of quantitative trait loci for hip dysplasia in labrador retrievers. Am J Vet Res 70: 1094–101.
19. Zhou Z, Sheng X, Zhang Z, Zhao K, Zhu L, et al (2010) Differential genetic regulation of canine hip dysplasia and osteoarthritis. PLoS One 5: e13219. 10.1371/journal.pone.0013219.
20. Todhunter RJ, Mateescu R, Lust G, Burton-Wurster NI, Dykes NL, et al (2005) Quantitative trait loci for hip dysplasia in a cross-breed canine pedigree. Mamm Genome 16: 720–730.
21. Friedenberg SG, Zhu L, Zhang Z, Foels WS, Schweitzer PA, et al (2011) Evaluation of a fibrillin 2 gene haplotype associated with hip dysplasia and incipient osteoarthritis in dogs. Am J Vet Res 72: 530–540.
22. Miller SA, Dykes DD, Polesky HF (1988) A simple salting out procedure for extracting DNA from human nucleated cells. Nucleic Acids Res 16: 1215.
23. Purcell S, Neale B, Todd-Brown K, Thomas L, Ferreira MA, et al (2007) PLINK: A tool set for whole-genome association and population-based linkage analyses. Am J Hum Genet 81: 559–575.
24. George EI, McCulloch RE (1993) Variable selection via gibbs sampling. Journal of the American Statistical Association 88: 881–889.
25. Heuven HC, Janss LL (2010) Bayesian multi-QTL mapping for growth curve parameters BMC Proc 4 Suppl 1: S12.
26. Kass RE, Raftery AE (1995) Bayes Factors. Journal of the American Statistical Association 90: 773–795.
27. Paatsama S (2000) Fédération cynologique internationale (FCI). In: Morgan JP, Wind A, Davidson AP, editors. Hereditary Bone and Joint Diseases in the Dog - Osteochondroses, hip dysplasia, elbow dysplasia -. Hannover: Schlütersche. 263–266.
28. Ihemelandu EC, Cardinet GH 3rd, Guffy MM, Wallace LJ (1983) Canine hip dysplasia: Differences in pectineal muscles of healthy and dysplastic german shepherd dogs when two months old. Am J Vet Res 44: 411–416.
29. Lust G, Craig PH, Geary JC, Ross GE,Jr (1972) Changes in pelvic muscle tissues associated with hip dysplasia in dogs. Am J Vet Res 33: 1097–1108.
30. Cardinet GH 3rd, Guffy MM, Wallace LJ, Laben RC (1983) Canine hip dysplasia in german shepherd dog-greyhound crossbreeds. J Am Vet Med Assoc 182: 393–395.
31. Riser WH (1975) Growth and development of the normal canine pelvis, hip joints, and femur from birth to maturity. Veterinary Pathology 12: 264–278.
32. Riser WH (1975) The dysplastic hip joint: Radiologic and histologic development. Vet Pathol 12: 279–305.
33. Jang LK, Lee ZH, Kim HH, Hill JM, Kim JD, et al (2001) A novel leucine-rich repeat protein (LRR-1): Potential involvement in 4–1BB-mediated signal transduction. Mol Cells 12: 304–312.
34. Zhou Y, Millward-Sadler SJ, Lin H, Robinson H, Goldring M, et al (2007) Evidence for JNK-dependent up-regulation of proteoglycan synthesis and for activation of JNK1 following cyclical mechanical stimulation in a human chondrocyte culture model. Osteoarthritis Cartilage 15: 884–893.
35. Chowdhury TT, Salter DM, Bader DL, Lee DA (2008) Signal transduction pathways involving p38 MAPK, JNK, NFkappaB and AP-1 influences the response of chondrocytes cultured in agarose constructs to IL-1beta and dynamic compression. Inflamm Res 57: 306–313.
36. Groulx JF, Gagné D, Benoit YD, Martel D, Basora N, et al (2011) Collagen VI is a basement membrane component that regulates epithelial cell-fibronectin interactions. Matrix Biol 30: 195–206.
37. Peters HC, Otto TJ, Enders JT, Jin W, Moed BR, et al (2011) The protective role of the pericellular matrix in chondrocyte apoptosis. Tissue Eng Part A 17: 2017–2024.
38. Demir E, Sabatelli P, Allamand V, Ferreiro A, Moghadaszadeh B, et al (2002) Mutations in COL6A3 cause severe and mild phenotypes of ullrich congenital muscular dystrophy. Am J Hum Genet 70: 1446–1458.
39. Shibuya S, Wakayama Y, Inoue M, Kojima H, Oniki H (2003) Merosin (laminin-2) localization in basal lamina of normal skeletal muscle fibers and changes in plasma membrane of merosin-deficient skeletal muscle fibers. Med Electron Microsc 36: 213–220.
40. Durr J, Lammi P, Goodman SL, Aigner T, von der Mark K (1996) Identification and immunolocalization of laminin in cartilage. Exp Cell Res 222: 225–233.
41. Helbling-Leclerc A, Zhang X, Topaloglu H, Cruaud C, Tesson F, et al (1995) Mutations in the laminin alpha 2-chain gene (LAMA2) cause merosin-deficient congenital muscular dystrophy. Nat Genet 11: 216–218.
42. Hinoi E, Ochi H, Takarada T, Nakatani E, Iezaki T, et al (2011) Positive regulation of osteoclastic differentiation by growth differentiation factor-15 up-regulated in osteocytic cells under hypoxia. J Bone Miner Res 27: 938–949.
43. Iliopoulos D, Malizos KN, Oikonomou P, Tsezou A (2008) Integrative microRNA and proteomic approaches identify novel osteoarthritis genes and their collaborative metabolic and inflammatory networks. PLoS One 3: e3740.
44. Bernardo BC, Belluoccio D, Rowley L, Little CB, Hansen U, et al (2011) Cartilage intermediate layer protein 2 (CILP-2) is expressed in articular and meniscal cartilage and down-regulated in experimental osteoarthritis. J Biol Chem 286: 37758–37767.
45. Todhunter RJ, Zachos TA, Gilbert RO, Erb HN, Williams AJ, et al (1997) Onset of epiphyseal mineralization and growth plate closure in radiographically normal and dysplastic labrador retrievers. J Am Vet Med Assoc 210: 1458–1462.
46. Foels WS (2000) Secondary center of ossification differs in developmental dysplasia of the hip (abstract). Proceedings of the 46th Annual Meeting, Orthopaedic Research Society.
47. Madsen JS, Reiman NI, Svalastoga E (1991) Delayed ossification of the femoral head in dogs with hip dysplasia. Journal of Small Animal Practice 32: 351–354.

8

Serum Metalloproteinases 2 and 9 as Predictors of Gait Status, Pressure Ulcer and Mortality after Hip Fracture

David N. Gumieiro[1], Bruna P. M. Rafacho[2], Andrea F. Gonçalves[2], Priscila P. Santos[2], Paula S. Azevedo[2], Leonardo A. M. Zornoff[2], Gilberto J. C. Pereira[1], Luiz S. Matsubara[2], Sergio A. R. Paiva[2], Marcos F. Minicucci[2]*

1 Surgery and Orthopedic Department, Botucatu Medical School, UNESP - Univ Estadual Paulista, Botucatu, Brazil, 2 Internal Medicine Department, Botucatu Medical School, UNESP – Univ Estadual Paulista, Botucatu, Brazil

Abstract

Introduction: The aim of this study is to evaluate the serum activity of metalloproteinases (MMPs) -2 and -9 as predictors of pressure ulcer (PU), gait status and mortality 6 months after hip fracture.

Methods: Eighty-seven patients over the age of 65 admitted to the orthopedic unit from January to December 2010 with hip fracture were prospectively evaluated. Upon admission, patient demographic information, including age, gender and concomitant diseases, was recorded. Blood samples were taken for analysis of MMP -2 and -9 activity by gel zymography and for biochemical examination within the first 72 hours of the patient's admission, after clinical stabilization. The fracture pattern (neck, trochanteric or subtrochanteric), time from admission to surgery, surgery duration and length of hospital stay were also recorded.

Results: Two patients were excluded due to the presence of pathological fractures (related to cancer), and three patients were excluded due to the presence of PU before admission. Eighty-two patients, with a mean age of 80.4 ± 7.3 years, were included in the analysis. Among these patients, 75.6% were female, 59.8% had PU, and 13.4% died 6 months after hip fracture. All patients underwent hip fracture repair. In a univariate analysis, there were no differences in serum MMP activity between hip fracture patients with or without PU. In addition, the multiple logistic regression analysis models, which were adjusted by age, gender, length of hospital stay and C-reactive protein, showed that the pro-MMP-9 complexed with neutrophil gelatinase-associated lipocalin form (130 kDa) was associated with gait status recovery 6 months after hip fracture.

Conclusions: In conclusion, serum pro-MMP-9 is a predictor of gait status recovery 6 months after hip fracture.

Editor: Ulrich Thiem, University of Bochum, Germany

Funding: This work was supported by Botucatu Medical School. The funders had no role in study design, data collection and analysis, decision to publish, or preparation of the manuscript.

Competing Interests: The authors have declared that no competing interests exist.

* E-mail: minicucci@fmb.unesp.br

Introduction

The incidence of hip fractures has been rising in recent years, and it will most likely continue to increase due to an aging population [1–3]. According to Hu et al., 1.5 million hip fractures occur annually worldwide, and this number may reach 4.5 million in 2050 [4].

Pressure ulcer (PU) is a frequent complication of hip fracture, with an incidence of 8.8% to 55%. It has a major impact on the cost of hospital care, quality of life, and mortality [5]. However, the adoption of a care recommendation standard for PUs did not reduce their incidence[6]. Healing of PUs normally occurs in a predictable sequence of phases that ends with scar formation. These processes are regulated by numerous molecules, including growth factors, cytokines, proteinases, and the inhibitors of these molecules [7]. Some studies that analyze wound fluids and biopsies collected from PUs showed that the presence of excessive concentrations of activated forms of matrix metalloproteinases (MMP) -2 and MMP-9 might impede the healing process. These data suggest that these proteinases could destroy growth factors, receptors and extracellular proteins essential for PUs healing [7–8].

The MMPs are a family of more than 25 species of zinc-dependent proteases that are essential for normal tissue remodeling and are involved in a number of pathological conditions such as cancer, inflammatory and cardiovascular diseases[9]. These enzymes are synthesized as inactive zymogens and are secreted in the extracellular matrix as proenzymes of pro-MMPs, which remain quiescent until the propeptide domain is cleaved. The activity of MMPs is controlled by the action of specific MMPs inhibitors or TIMPs[9].

These proteinases also participate in bone remodeling and in fracture healing[10]. Delays in bone healing or even nonunion of the bones could be related to the concentrations of MMPs or the

Table 1. Demographic and clinical data of 82 patients with hip fracture.

Variables	Pressure Ulcer		P value
	No (n = 33)	Yes (n = 49)	
Age (yrs)	79.0 (71.0–84.0)	83.0 (77.0–85.3)	0.06
Female, % (n°)	75.8 (25)	75.8 (37)	0.81
Hypertension, % (n°)	60.6 (20)	55.1 (27)	0.79
Diabetes, % (n°)	24.2 (8)	24.5 (12)	0.80
Cardiovascular disease, % (n°)	30.3 (10)	36.7 (18)	0.72
Statins, % (n°)	15.1 (5)	4.1 (2)	0.11
Fracture type, % (n°)			
Femoral neck	36.4 (12)	40.8 (20)	0.84
Trochanteric	54.5 (18)	53.1 (26)	
Subtrochanteric	9.1 (3)	6.1 (3)	
LOS, (days)	7.0 (4.8–9.0)	8.0 (6.0–11.3)	0.06
A-S time, (days)	5.0 (3.8–7.0)	6.0 (4.0–8.3)	0.10
Mortality, % (n°)	6.1 (2)	18.4 (9)	0.19

LOS: length of hospital stay; A-S time: admission to surgery time. Data are expressed as median (including the lower and upper quartiles).

behavior of these enzymes over time. Henle et al. studied serum concentrations of MMPs and TIMPs during normal and delayed fracture healing[11]. They showed that systemic MMP and TIMP concentrations could be a reflection of local enzyme regulatory mechanisms during fracture healing. In addition, an increased MMP/TIMP ratio was associated with the pathophysiological processes leading to fracture nonunion [11]. However, the association between the serum activity of MPPs -2 and -9, PU development, gait status and the mortality in hip fracture patients has not yet been established.

Thus, the aim of this study is to evaluate the serum activity of MMPs -2 and -9 as predictors of PU, gait status and mortality 6 months after hip fracture.

Table 3. Demographic and clinical data of 82 patients with hip fracture.

Variables	Mortality in 6 months		P value
	No (n = 71)	Yes (n = 11)	
Age (yrs)	80.0 ± 7.39	82.5 ± 6.8	0.29
Female, % (n°)	76.1 (54)	72.7 (8)	1.00
Hypertension, % (n°)	57.7 (41)	54.5 (6)	1.00
Diabetes, % (n°)	23.9 (17)	27.3 (3)	1.00
Cardiovascular disease, % (n°)	35.2 (25)	27.2 (3)	0.74
Statins, % (n°)	9.9 (7)	0 (0)	0.59
Fracture type, % (n°)			
Femoral neck	38.0 (27)	45.5 (5)	0.59
Trochanteric	53.5 (38)	54.5 (6)	
Subtrochanteric	8.5 (6)	0 (0)	
LOS, (days)	8.0 (6.0–10.8)	6.0 (4.0–7.0)	0.07
A-S time, (days)	6.0 (4.0–8.0)	4.0 (3.0–6.0)	0.05

LOS: length of hospital stay; A-S time: admission to surgery time. Data are expressed as the mean ± standard deviation or median (including the lower and upper quartiles).

Materials and Methods

This study was approved by the Ethics Committee of the Botucatu Medical School of Medicine. Written informed consent was obtained from all patients. Eighty-seven consecutive patients over the age of 65 admitted to the orthopedic unit with hip fractures from January to December 2010 were prospectively evaluated. The presence of a pathological hip fracture and a PU before hospital admission was the exclusion criterion. All patients were treated according to specific protocols depending on the type of fracture.

The number of the patients needed using t test to achieve 80% power was 84. The sample size was calculated based on the MMP-9 values in hypertension patients. It is import to note that we could not found any MMP results in hip fracture patients [12].

Upon admission, patient demographic information, including age, gender and concomitant diseases, was recorded. Blood

Table 2. Baseline biochemical and zymography results of 82 patients with hip fracture.

Variables	Pressure Ulcer		P value
	No (n = 33)	Yes (n = 49)	
CRP, (mg/dL)	4.8 (3.3–6.9)	5.4 (3.6–12.4)	0.32
Creatinine, (mg/dL)	0.8 (0.7–1.1)	0.8 (0.7–1.1)	0.46
Urea, (mg/dL)	58.0 (36.8–75.5)	55.7 (38.8–72.4)	0.88
Glucose, (mg/dL)	111.5 (95.5–136.5)	122.5 (93.0–149.5)	0.35
Albumin, (g/L)	3.2 ± 0.6	3.2 ± 0.5	0.97
225 kDa (homodimer pro-MMP 9), (%)	21.3 (19.8–26.0)	24.9 (19.8–26.4)	0.26
130 kDa (pro-MMP 9 +NGAL), (%)	8.5 ± 3.3	8.8 ± 3.9	0.67
92 kDa (pro-MMP 9), (%)	51.1 ± 8.2	52.4 ± 7.1	0.44
72 kDa (pro-MMP 2), (%)	15.8 (11.3–21.3)	11.7 (9.6–8.3)	0.07

CRP: C-reactive protein, MMP: matrix metalloproteinase; NGAL: neutrophil gelatinase-associated lipocalin. Data are expressed as the mean ± standard deviation or median (including the lower and upper quartiles).

Table 4. Baseline biochemical and zymography results of 82 patients with hip fracture.

Variables	Mortality in 6 months		P value
	No (n = 71)	Yes (n = 11)	
CRP, (mg/dL)	5.2 (3.5–8.0)	4.6 (3.5–15.8)	0.78
Creatinine, (mg/dL)	0.8 (0.7–1.0)	1.2 (0.8–1.8)	0.04
Urea, (mg/dL)	53.0 (36.3–69.8)	73.6 (52.0–107.3)	0.03
Glucose, (mg/dL)	121.0 (96.0–141.8)	101.0 (88.5–172.3)	0.68
Albumin, (g/L)	3.2 ± 0.5	3.1 ± 0.5	0.65
225 kDa (homodimer pro-MMP 9), (%)	23.8 (19.9–26.5)	24.0 (19.7–26.1)	0.95
130 kDa (pro-MMP 9 +NGAL), (%)	8.9 ± 3.8	7.5 ± 2.4	0.23
92 kDa (pro-MMP 9), (%)	51.7 ± 7.7	53.0 ± 6.7	0.61
72 kDa (pro-MMP 2), (%)	13.6 (10.3–18.5)	12.7 (10.6–20.9)	0.73

CRP: C-reactive protein, MMP: matrix metalloproteinase; NGAL: neutrophil gelatinase-associated lipocalin. Data are expressed as the mean ± standard deviation or median (including the lower and upper quartiles).

samples were taken for analysis of MMP -2 and -9 activity and biochemical examination within the first 72 hours of the patient's admission, after clinical stabilization. The fracture pattern (neck, trochanteric or subtrochanteric), time from admission to surgery, surgery duration and length of hospital stay were also recorded.

All patients were followed for 6 months after the fracture. The presence of PU, gait status, and mortality were recorded. These outcomes were evaluated by two examiners (orthopedists) with expertise in this issue on the first day after surgery, at hospital discharge and at 15, 45, 90 and 180 days after hospital discharge. For the patients who died before 6 months after discharge, we considered PU and gait status evaluation at the last report. Patients were classified according to gait status as ambulators (patients who walk with or without help = 0) or non-ambulators (patients who could not walk = 1).

A PU was defined as an injury to the skin or underlying tissue over a bony prominence in any of the four stages defined by the National Pressure Ulcer Advisory Panel [13]. Patients were considered to have diabetes or hypertension if they were using medication chronically for these diseases. Cardiovascular diseases were considered when patients had stroke, coronary heart disease, peripheral artery disease or heart failure.

Laboratory Analysis

Total serum levels of C-reactive protein (CRP), albumin, glucose, creatinine and urea were measured using the dry chemistry method (Ortho-Clinical Diagnostics VITROS 950®, Johnson & Johnson).

Zymography

Serum MMP activity was determined as reported by Tyagi et al [14]. In brief, 2 µg of serum were diluted in application sample buffer consisting of 0.5 M Tris, pH 6.8, 100% glycerol, and 0.05% bromophenol blue. The samples were loaded into the wells of 8% SDS-polyacrylamide containing 1% gelatin. Electrophoresis was carried out in a Bio-Rad apparatus at 80 V for 2 hours, until the bromophenol blue reaches the bottom of the gel. The gel was removed and washed 2 times with 2.5% Triton-X-100 and then washed with 50 mM Tris pH 8.4. The gel was then incubated at 37°C overnight in activation solution consisting of 50 mMTris pH 8.4, 5 mM $CaCl_2$ and Zn Cl_2. The staining was performed for 2 hours with 0.5% coomassie blue, and destaining was performed in 30% methanol and 10% acetic acid until clear bands over a dark background were observed. Staining and destaining were performed at room temperature on a rotatory shaker. The gels were photographed, and the intensity of gelatinolytic action (clear

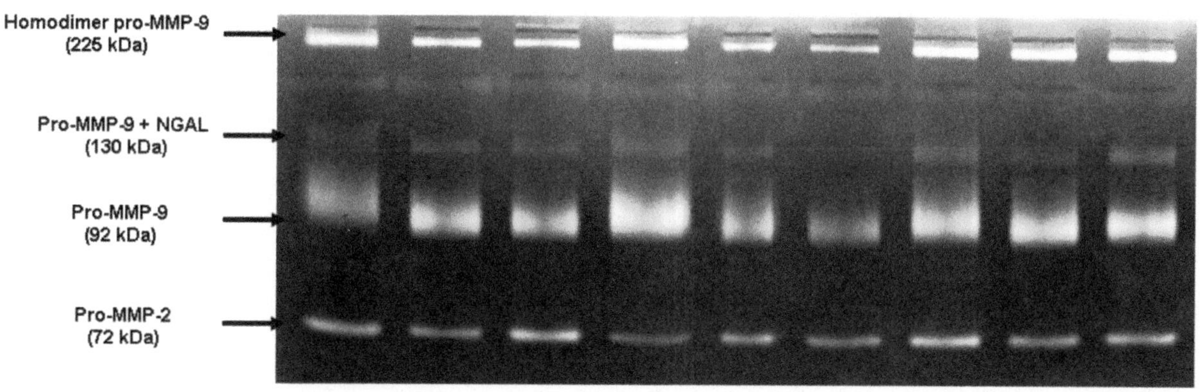

Figure 1. Gelatin zymograms of serum samples with all forms of MMPs usually found in human: the homodimer of the pro-MMP-9 form (225 kDa), the pro-MMP-9 complexed with neutrophil gelatinase-associated lipocalin form (130 kDa), the pro-MMP-9 form (92 kDa) and the pro-MMP-2 (72 kDa) form.

Table 5. Logistic regression for prediction of pressure ulcer 6 months after hip fracture.

	Odds Ratio	95% Confidence Interval	P value
225 kDa (homodimer pro-MMP 9)	1.02	0.94 - 1.10	0.63
130 kDa (pro-MMP 9 +NGAL)	1.03	0.91 - 1.16	0.66
92 kDa (pro-MMP 9)	1.02	0.96 - 1.09	0.44
72 kDa (pro-MMP 2)	0.96	0.91 - 1.02	0.15
225 kDa (homodimer pro-MMP 9)*	1.02	0.94 - 1.11	0.59
130 kDa (pro-MMP 9 +NGAL)*	1.05	0.91 - 1.21	0.51
92 kDa (pro-MMP 9)*	1.02	0.96 - 1.09	0.46
72 kDa (pro-MMP 2)*	0.95	0.89 - 1.02	0.14

MMP: matrix metalloproteinase; NGAL: neutrophil gelatinase-associated lipocalin
*Adjusted by age, gender, length of hospital stay and C-reactive protein.

bands) was analyzed in UVP, UV, and a White Darkhon image analyzer.

Statistical Methods

Data are expressed as the mean ± SD or the median (including the lower and upper quartiles). Comparisons between groups for continuous variables were performed using Student's t-test (normal distribution) or Mann-Whitney U-test (non-normal distribution). Fisher's test or the χ^2 test was used for all categorical data. Logistic regression was used to predict the presence of PU and gait status, and Cox regression model was used to predict mortality 6 months after hip fracture. The MMPs were tested as independent variables and adjusted by age, gender, CRP and length of hospital stay (LOS). Except for age, all independent variables in the regression models were included as continuous variables. These variables were chosen considering their clinically important significance for pressure ulcer, gait status and mortality [15–19].

Data analysis was performed using SigmaPlot software for Windows v12.0 (Systat Software Inc., San Jose, CA, USA). The significance level was considered to be 5%.

Results

Eighty-seven patients were evaluated. Two patients were excluded due to the presence of pathological fractures (related to cancer), and three patients were excluded due to the presence of PU before admission. Eighty-two patients, with a mean age of 80.4 ± 7.3 years, were included in the analysis. Among these patients, 75.6% were female, 59.8% had PU, and 13.4% died 6 months after hip fracture. All patients underwent hip fracture repair.

Considering PU development as the outcome, the demographic and clinical data are presented in Tableô 1. The majority of patients had trochanteric fractures (53.7%), and the fracture type did not influence PU development. The clinical features did not influence PU development. Laboratory data and MMP activity are presented in Tableô 2. There were no differences between hip fracture patients with or without PU.

Considering mortality as the outcome, creatinine and urea, accessed at baseline, were higher in patients who died 6 months after hip fracture (Tablesô 3 and 4).

A representative zymogram of serum samples is shown in Figureô 1. Gelatin zymograms of serum samples showed all forms of MMPs usually found in human, including the homodimer of the pro-MMP-9 form (225 kDa), the pro-MMP-9 complexed with neutrophil gelatinase-associated lipocalin form (130 kDa), the pro-MMP-9 form (92 kDa) and the pro-MMP-2 (72 kDa) form.

In the logistic regression and Cox regression analysis, serum MMP-2 and MMP-9 activity were not associated with PU and mortality 6 months after hip fracture (Tableô 5 and 6), even when they were adjusted for age, gender, LOS and CRP. On the other hand, the pro-MMP-9 complexed with neutrophil gelatinase-associated lipocalin form (130 kDa) was a predictor of gait status recovery 6 months after hip fracture. Each 1 unit increase of pro-MMP-9 increased the chance of gait recovery by 21%. (Tableô 7)

Table 6. Cox regression models for prediction of mortality 6 months after hip fracture.

	Hazard Ratio	95% Confidence Interval	P value
225 kDa (homodimer pro-MMP 9)	0.99	0.89 - 1.10	0.10
130 kDa (pro-MMP 9 +NGAL)	0.90	0.76 - 1.07	0.23
92 kDa (pro-MMP 9)	1.02	0.94 - 1.11	0.61
72 kDa (pro-MMP 2)	1.01	0.93 - 1.08	0.85
225 kDa (homodimer pro-MMP 9)*	0.98	0.87 - 1.09	0.66
130 kDa (pro-MMP 9 +NGAL)*	0.85	0.71 - 1.03	0.10
92 kDa (pro-MMP 9)*	1.03	0.93 - 1.14	0.14
72 kDa (pro-MMP 2)*	1.04	0.94 - 1.14	0.44

MMP: matrix metalloproteinase; NGAL: neutrophil gelatinase-associated lipocalin
*Adjusted by age, gender, length of hospital stay and C-reactive protein.

Table 7. Logistic regression for prediction of gait status recovery 6 months after hip fracture.

	Odds Ratio	95% Confidence Interval	P value
225 kDa (homodimer pro-MMP 9)	1.03	0.94 - 1.12	0.53
130 kDa (pro-MMP 9 +NGAL)	1.14	0.99 - 1.31	0.07
92 kDa (pro-MMP 9)	0.98	0.92 - 1.04	0.55
72 kDa (pro-MMP 2)	0.98	0.92 - 1.04	0.45
225 kDa (homodimer pro-MMP 9)*	1.03	0.94 - 1.12	0.55
130 kDa (pro-MMP 9 +NGAL)*	1.21	1.03 - 1.43	0.02
92 kDa (pro-MMP 9)*	0.97	0.90 - 1.04	0.34
72 kDa (pro-MMP 2)*	0.98	0.92 - 1.05	0.52

MMP: matrix metalloproteinase; NGAL: neutrophil gelatinase-associated lipocalin
*Adjusted by age, gender, length of hospital stay and C-reactive protein.

Discussion

The aim of this study was to evaluate the serum activity of MMPs -2 and -9 as predictors of pressure ulcer, gait status and mortality 6 months after hip fracture. Our data showed that the pro-MMP-9 was associated with gait status recovery 6 months after hip fracture. On the other hand, serum MMP-2 and MMP-9 were not associated with PU and mortality in hip fracture patients.

It is important to recognize that PU is a frequent complication after hip fracture, despite efforts employed to reduce its incidence. In our study, up to 60% of the patients had this complication within 6 months after hip fracture. The healing of PUs depends on a sequence of four phases, which are hemostasis, inflammation, proliferation, and remodeling. For a wound to heal successfully, these phases and their biophysiological functions must occur in the proper sequence and at a specific time [20].

There are local and systemic factors that influence PU healing. Among the local factors, the most important are tissue oxygenation, infection and excess production of proteinases [20]. Some studies have shown that MMPs were elevated in acute wound fluids and that MMP concentrations decreased 2 weeks after the ulcers began to heal [21–22]. A separate study that analyzed wound fluids and biopsies collected from PUs showed that elevated concentrations of MMP -2 and MMP-9 may influence the healing process [7]. Thus, local increases in the concentrations of MMPs could predict PU healing times. Serum concentrations of MMPs were also studied in the wound healing process. Utz et al. showed that elevated serum concentrations of MMP-2 and -7 were associated with delayed traumatic wound healing [23].

These data suggest that local MMP concentration and serum MMP concentration influence wound healing, although there is no data regarding the activity of these proteinases in ulcer development. This issue is extremely important after bone fractures because the concentrations of local and serum MMPs also increase in these situations. Henle et al. showed that serum MMPs were increased following fractures and that an increased serum MMP/TIMP ratio was associated with alterations in fracture healing [11]. Other studies also showed that high levels of serum MMPs were related with loosening of total hip replacement implants [24–25]. In addition, a recent study suggests that urinary levels of MMP-9 and MMP-13 may have potential as metabolic markers to monitor the progression of fracture healing [26].

Therefore, considering that the concentrations of MMPs might influence wound healing, we hypothesized that serum MMP concentrations might be associated with gait status. In accordance with this concept, our data showed that higher pro-MMP-9 concentration was a predictor of gait status recovery. This phenomenon can be explained by the decreased transformation from the inactive form to the active form of MMP-9.

Taking into account the relationship between MMP and wound healing, we also hypothesized that serum MMP concentrations would be associated with PU. Importantly, the identification of predictors of PU creates an opportunity to prevent its development. However, in our study, serum concentrations of MMP -2 and -9 were not predictors of PU development. This result could be due to the lack of the effect of these proteinases on previously intact skin.

Serum MMP levels were also associated with mortality in patients with cancer, sepsis and cardiovascular diseases [27–29]. The positive correlation between MMP activity and the inflammatory response is one of the explanations for the increased mortality observed in patients with high serum concentrations of MMPs. However, the role of these proteinases in mortality prediction had not yet been studied in patients with hip fractures. Our study did not show any influence of MMP-2 and MMP-9 activity on mortality prediction 6 months after hip fracture.

Finally, we should considerer the major limitations of this study. The concentration of TIMP was not measured in the serum samples of our patients, so we could not determine a ratio between collagen degradation and deposition. In addition, our study included a small sample size and patients from a unique medical center.

In conclusion, our data suggested that serum pro-MMP-9 is a predictor of gait status recovery 6 months after hip fracture.

Author Contributions

Conceived and designed the experiments: LAMZ SARP GJCP MFM. Performed the experiments: DNG BPMR AFG PPS PSA. Analyzed the data: MFM DNG LSM. Wrote the paper: DNG MFM.

References

1. Lefaivre KA, Macadam SA, Davidson DJ, Gandhi R, Chan H, et al. (2009) Length of stay, mortality, morbidity and delay to surgery in hip fractures. J Bone Joint Surg(br)91: 922–927.
2. Dunbar MJ, Howard A, Bogosh ER, Parvizi J, Kreder HJ, et al. (2009) An AOA-COA symposium. Orthopaedics in 2020: Predictors of musculoskeletal needs. J Bone Joint Surg Am 91: 2278–2286.

3. El Maghraoui A, Ngbanda AR, Bensaoud N, Bensaoud M, Rezqi A, et al. (2012) Age-adjusted incidence rates of hip fractures between 2006 and 2009 in Rabat, Morocco. Osteoporos Int. doi: 0.1007/s00198-012-2061-3.
4. Hu F, Jiang C, Shen J, Tang P, Wang Y (2012) Preoperative predictors for mortality following hip fractures surgery a systematic review and meta analysis. Injury 43: 676–685.
5. Lindholm C, Sterner E, Romanelli M, Pina E, Torra y Bou J, et al. (2008) Hip fracture and pressure ulcers the Pan-European Pressure Ulcer Study intrinsic and extrinsic risk factors. Int Wound J 5:315–328
6. Baumgarten M, Margolis D, Berlin JA, Strom BL, Garino J, et al. (2003) Risk factors for pressure ulcers among elderly hip fracture patients. Wound Repair Regen11:96–103.
7. Ladwig GP, Robson MC, Liu R, Kuhn MA, Muir DF, et al. (2002) Ratios of activated matrix metalloproteinase-9 to tissue inhibitor of matrix metalloproteinase-1 in wound fluids are inversely correlated with healing of pressure ulcers. Wound Repair Regen 10:26–37.
8. Yager DR, Zhang LY, Liang HX, Diegelmann RF, Cohen IK (1996) Wound fluids from human pressure ulcers contain elevated matrix metalloproteinase levels and activity compared to surgical wound fluids. J Invest Dermatol 107:743–748.
9. Brew K, Dinakarpandian D, Nagase H (2000) Tissue inhibitors of metalloproteinases: evolution, structure and function. BiochimBiophysActa1477: 267–283.
10. Ortega N, Behonick D, Stickens D, Werb Z (2003) How proteases regulate bone morphogenesis. Ann N Y AcadSci 995:109–116.
11. Henle P, Zimmermann G, Weiss S (2005) Matrix metalloproteinases and failed fracture healing. Bone 37:791–798.
12. Ahmed SH, Clark LL, Pennington WR, Webb CS, Bonnema DD, et al. (2006) Matrix metalloproteinases/tissue inhibitors of metalloproteinases: relationship between changes in proteolytic determinants of matrix composition and structural, functional, and clinical manifestations of hypertensive heart disease. Circulation 113: 2089–2096.
13. EPUAP (European Pressure Ulcer Advisory Panel) (1999) Guidelines on treatment of pressure ulcers. EPUAP Rev 1:31–33.
14. Tyagi SC, Matsubara L, Weber KT (1993) Direct extraction and estimation of collagenase(s) activity by zymography in microquantities of rat myocardium and uterus. Clin Biochem 26:191–198.
15. Beloosesky Y, Grinblat J, Pirotsky A, Weiss A, Hendel D (2004) Different C-reactive protein kinetics in post-operative hip-fractured geriatric patients with and without complications. Gerontology 50: 216–222.
16. Gumieiro DN, Rafacho BPM, Gradella LM, Azevedo PS, Gaspardo D, et al. (2012) Handgrip strength predicts pressure ulcers in patients with hip fracture. Nutrition 28: 438–442.
17. Kurtinaitis J, Dadonienė J, Kvederas G, Porvaneckas N, Butenas T (2012) Mortality after femoral neck fractures: a two-year follow-up. Medicina (Kaunas) 48: 145–149.
18. Shoda N, Yasunaga H, Horiguchi H, Matsuda S, Ohe K, et al. (2012) Risk factors affecting inhospital mortality after hip fracture: retrospective analysis using the Japanese Diagnosis Procedure Combination Database. BMJ Open 2, e000416, doi: 10.1136/bmjopen-2011-000416.
19. Vidal EI, Moreira-Filho DC, Pinheiro RS, Souza RC, Almeida LM, et al. (2012) Delay from fracture to hospital admission: a new risk factor for hip fracture mortality? Osteoporos Int 23: 2847–2859.
20. Guo S, DiPietro LA (2010) Factors affecting wound healing. J Dent Res 89:219–229.
21. Trengove NJ, StaceyMC, Macauley S, Bennett N, Gibson J, et al. (1999) Analysis of the acute and chronic wound environments: the role of proteases and their inhibitors. Wound Rep Reg7:442–452.
22. Wysocki AB, Staiano-Coico L, Grinnell F (1993) Wound fluid from chronic leg ulcers contains elevated levels of metalloproteinases MMP-2 and MMP-9. J Invest Dermatol101:64–68.
23. Utz ER, Elster EA, Tadaki DK, Gage F, Perdue PW, et al. (2010) Metalloproteinase expression is associated with traumatic wound failure. J Surg Res 159:633–639.
24. Ma GF, Ali A, Verzijl N, Hanemaaijer R, TeKoppele J, et al. (2006) Increased collagen degradation around loosened total hip replacement implants. Arthritis Rheum54:2928–2933.
25. Yokohama Y, Matsumoto T, Hirakawa M, Kuroki Y, Fujimoto N, et al. (1995) Production of matrix metalloproteinases at the bone-implant interface in loose total hip replacements. Lab Invest 73:899–911.
26. Wigner NA, Kulkarni N, Yakavonis M, Young M, Tinsley B, et al. (2012) Urine matrix metalloproteinases (MMPs) as biomarkers for the progression of fracture healing. Injury 43:274–278.
27. Lauhio A, Hästbacka J, Pettilä V, Tervahartiala T, Karlsson S, et al. (2011)Serum MMP-8, -9 and TIMP-1 in sepsis: high serum levels of MMP-8 and TIMP-1 are associated with fatal outcome in a multicenter, prospective cohort study. Hypothetical impact of tetracyclines. Pharmacol Res 64:590–594
28. Szarvas T, Jäger T, Becker M, Tschirdewahn S, Niedworok C, et al. (2011)Validation of circulating MMP-7 level as an independent prognostic marker of poor survival in urinary bladder cancer. Pathol Oncol Res 17:325–332.
29. Hansson J, Vasan RS, Ärnlöv J, Ingelsson E, Lind L, et al. (2011) Biomarkers of extracellular matrix metabolism (MMP-9 and TIMP-1) and risk of stroke, myocardial infarction, and cause-specific mortality: cohort study. PLoS One 6:e16185.

9

Comparison of Genome-Wide Association Methods in Analyses of Admixed Populations with Complex Familial Relationships

Naveen K. Kadri*, Bernt Guldbrandtsen, Peter Sørensen, Goutam Sahana

Centre for Quantitative genetics and Genomics, Department of Molecular Biology and Genetics, Aarhus University, Aarhus, Denmark

Abstract

Population structure is known to cause false-positive detection in association studies. We compared the power, precision, and type-I error rates of various association models in analyses of a simulated dataset with structure at the population (admixture from two populations; *P*) and family (*K*) levels. We also compared type-I error rates among models in analyses of publicly available human and dog datasets. The models corrected for none, one, or both structure levels. Correction for *K* was performed with linear mixed models incorporating familial relationships estimated from pedigrees or genetic markers. Linear models that ignored *K* were also tested. Correction for *P* was performed using principal component or structured association analysis. In analyses of simulated and real data, linear mixed models that corrected for *K* were able to control for type-I error, regardless of whether they also corrected for *P*. In contrast, correction for *P* alone in linear models was insufficient. The power and precision of linear mixed models with and without correction for *P* were similar. Furthermore, power, precision, and type-I error rate were comparable in linear mixed models incorporating pedigree and genomic relationships. In summary, in association studies using samples with both *P* and *K*, ancestries estimated using principal components or structured assignment were not sufficient to correct type-I errors. In such cases type-I errors may be controlled by use of linear mixed models with relationships derived from either pedigree or from genetic markers.

Editor: Yun Li, University of North Carolina, United States of America

Funding: This work was supported by a grant (No. 3405-10-0137) funded jointly by the Green Development and Demonstration Programme of the Danish Ministry of Food, Agriculture and Fisheries, The Milk Levy Fund, Viking Genetics, and Nordic Cattle Genetic Evaluation. The funders had no role in study design, data collection and analysis, decision to publish, or preparation of the manuscript.

Competing Interests: The authors have the following interests to declare: They received funding from commercial companies Viking Genetics, and Nordic Cattle Genetic Evaluation.

* E-mail: NaveenK.Kadri@agrsci.dk

Introduction

The power of an association study depends on the phenotypic variance explained by the causal variant, the extent of linkage disequilibrium (LD) between the causal variant and the markers, and, not least, the size of the study sample. Several recent association studies have thus focused on collecting large samples to obtain higher powers of detection [1,2] but this practice is often associated with population stratification problems. Among the factors thought to cause lack of reproducibility in association studies reviewed [3], population stratification has probably been the most cited reason [4].

Population stratification refers to the inclusion of individuals from isolated subpopulations in the population of interest. In such a population, individuals from a subpopulation are, on average, more closely related to each other than to other individuals in the population as a whole. Population structure is common in nature. It manifests in the form of herds, colonies, and ethnic groups, and as a consequence of geographic isolation and natural or artificial selection [5]. A subtle form of stratification can also occur at the family level, especially in livestock when animals are bred in full-sib or half-sib families [6].

Genetic association studies aim to correlate differences in trait level with differences in genotypes at a tested marker. This correlation is assumed to arise from the co-occurrence of the marker with the quantitative trait locus (QTL), i.e., LD. The presence of LD is usually equated with physical linkage. However, in a stratified population with differences at the trait level, markers with different frequencies across populations will also correlate with trait levels. Thus the use of a structured population in an association study may yield false associations due to differences in allele frequencies among subpopulations [7].

Examination of an unstratified sample is thus optimal in an association study [5]. However, combining samples from multiple populations is often necessary to increase the power of detection. In some cases, study of a structured population may be advantageous. Markers tightly linked to causal variants achieve similar significance in tests of association, making it difficult to distinguish them from the causal variant. In such cases, the use of a structured sample may enable precise localization of the causal variant, as a marker in strong LD with the causal variant in one population may not be in strong LD in the other [8]. Thus, the use of statistical methods that correct for stratification at the population and family level, especially in livestock are important for the present and future association studies that aim to genotype large samples.

Several methods, such as structured analysis (SA) [9], principal component analysis (PCA) [10] and the use of linear mixed models (LMM) [5], have been reported to be useful in correcting for stratification in genome-wide association (GWA) samples. It has been noted that correcting for stratification is more challenging when family structure is present along with population stratification [11]. In this study, we simulated an admixed population (variable ancestry from two populations) with familial relatedness as generally observed in commercial cattle populations and compared the power, precision and false-positive detection rates of analyses using the SA, PCA, and LMM approaches. We also applied these methods to two publicly available real datasets and compared the incidence of false-positive associations.

Materials and Methods

The study uses a simulated dataset and 2 publicly available datasets, so no ethical approval was required.

Simulation Study

An admixed population (Fig. 1) was simulated using the QMSim software package [12]. First, an historic population (HP) was simulated to generate the initial linkage disequilibrium (LD) and to allow for mutation (2.5×10^{-3}/locus/generation) and drift. The HP consisted of 5,000 individuals that were randomly mated for 1,000 generations. The genome was assumed to have 20 chromosomes of 100 cM each with 40,000 evenly distributed bi-allelic SNP markers with equal frequencies (0.5) for the two alleles in the base population. Only two QTLs with two equally frequent alleles were simulated, both located on chromosome 1 at 20 cM and 80 cM. The QTL mutation rate was 2.5×10^{-5}/generation. The number of recombination per Morgan (per chromosome) was sampled from a Poisson distribution of mean = 1 and the cross-overs were randomly placed on the chromosomes. QTL effects were introduced in the last generation of the HP for a trait (mean = 0, variance = 1) with a heritability of 0.3. The allelic effects were sampled from a gamma distribution with a shape parameter of 0.4 as implemented in QMSim [12], so that the two QTLs together explained 10% of phenotypic variance. The remaining genetic variance was simulated as a polygenic effect. After 1,000 generations, the population size was reduced to 2,500 individuals (2,000 females, 500 males).

Next, two populations were generated from the HP by mating two separate parent groups in isolation. The parent groups (1,000 females, 50 males each) were randomly selected from the last generation of the HP. Each sire was mated to 20 dams, with each mating producing one offspring. This procedure yielded a total of 1,000 offspring with an equal sex ratio (500 males, 500 females) from each parent group. Fifty randomly selected male offspring from each group were used as sires for the next generation, whereas all female offspring along with 500 randomly selected dams from the previous generation were used as dams for the next generation. This mating scheme was continued for 30 generations.

After 30 generations, the average genetic distance between populations in 100 replicates, estimated as mean F_{st} from all 40,000 SNP markers, was 0.025 [standard deviation (SD) = 0.0006]. The allele frequencies of the markers (Fig. 2) and mean phenotype levels (Fig. 3) differed between populations.

In the next step of the simulation, individuals from two isolated populations were mated to yield an admixed population. Twenty-five males and 500 females were selected from each population to serve as parents. These individuals were randomly mated for four generations to yield an admixed population of 1,000 individuals (500 males, 500 females), following the mating scheme described above. After admixture, QTLs in the last generation explained 0–13% of the total phenotypic variance. The individuals' ancestries, calculated as average genetic contributions from one parent population to individuals in the admixed population over four generations, are presented in Figure 4. Data on phenotypes for

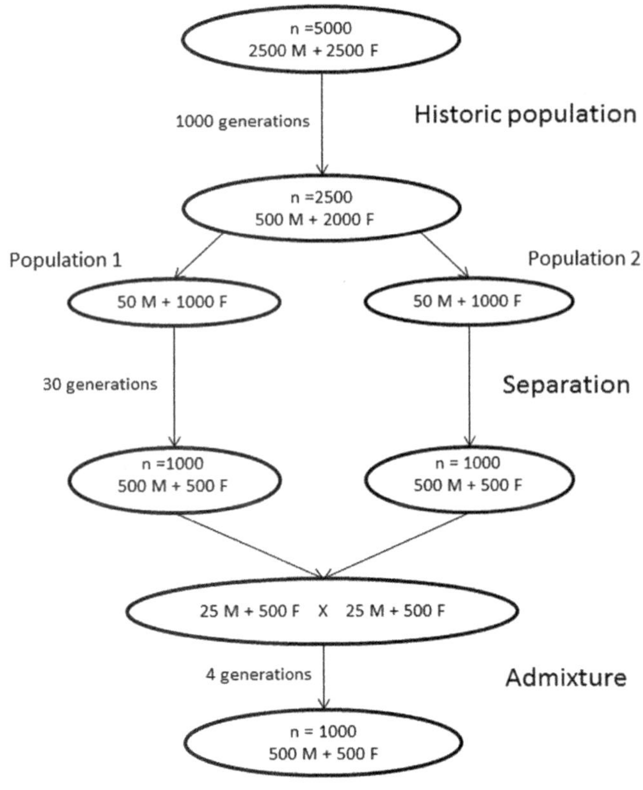

Figure 1. Schematic representation of the simulation.

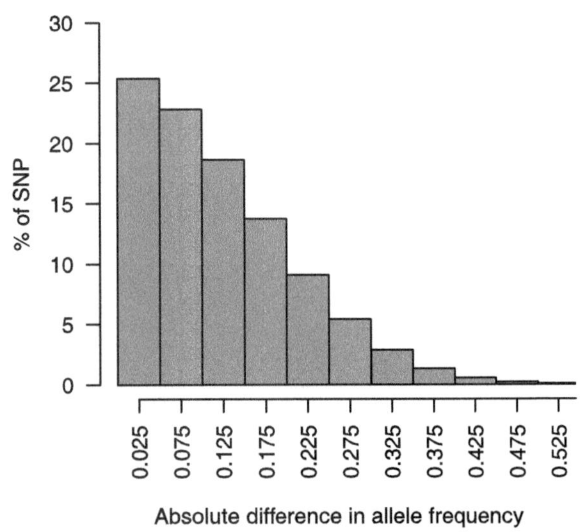

Figure 2. Absolute differences in allele frequencies of single-nucleotide polymorphism (SNP) markers between populations (100 replicates).

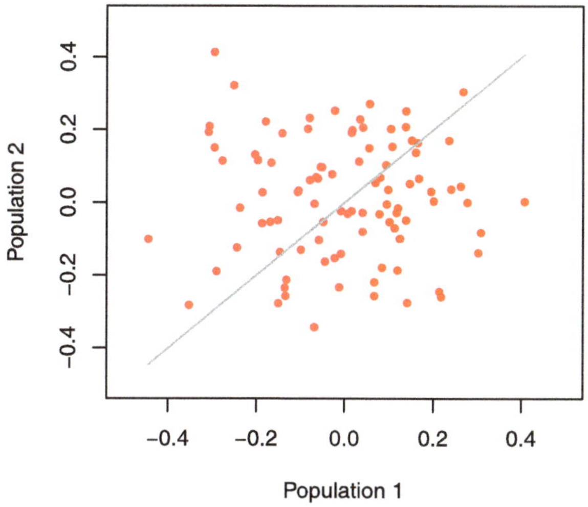

Figure 3. Differences in mean phenotypes of two populations after separation for 30 generations (100 replicates).

these 1,000 samples, along with their genotypes for 40,000 SNP markers, were used in our association analyses.

Chromosome 1, which contained two simulated QTLs, was used to assess the power and precision of the models and five chromosomes (chromosomes 2–6) without simulated QTLs (null chromosomes) were used to assess the false-positive rate (type-I error). A total of 100 replications were used to compare the models.

Publicly Available Real Data

In addition to the simulated datasets, the models for GWA studies were applied to the following two publicly available datasets to assess their ability to control type-I error.

Human GOLDN Dataset. This human stature dataset was collected from 1,315 European American individuals genotyped for 637 genetic markers as part of the Genetics of Lipid Lowering Drugs and Diet Network (GOLDN) study [13,14]. Individuals' height, sex, and age were recorded. Previous studies have found no significant population structure in this sample and no significant association between height and any of these genotyped markers.

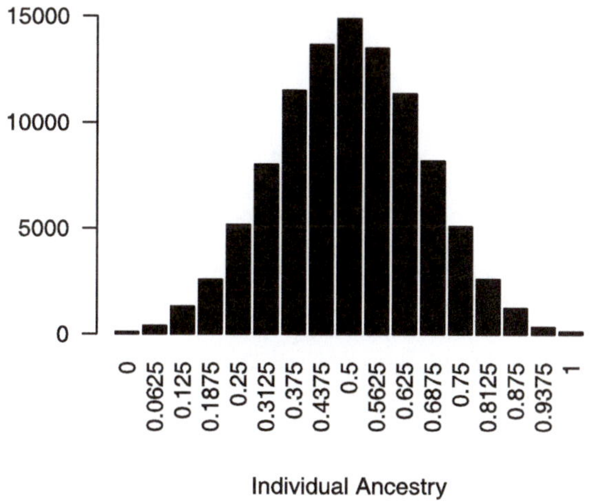

Figure 4. Distribution of individuals' ancestries after admixture (100 replicates).

Dog Data on Hip Dysplasia. This dataset contains hip dysplasia data from 292 dogs of two breeds (Labrador retriever and greyhound) and their crosses (F_1, F_2, and backcrosses). The samples were genotyped for 23,500 SNPs and hip dysplasia was measured using the Norberg angle [15]. The relationship matrix was estimated from pedigree. The ancestors of each dog were traced back as far as possible. We used 1,000 randomly chosen markers assumed to be unlinked to the variants controlling hip dysplasia [14].

Association Models

The allele substitution effect (b) of an SNP was estimated by successively fitting the marker in the following models. The simulated data contained two confounding factors: admixture (P) and familial relatedness (K). The models compared corrected for none, one, or both factors.

The significance of estimated b was then tested against the null hypothesis ($b = 0$) using a t-test with Bonferroni correction for multiple testing, at a significance level of $\alpha = 0.05$. All analyses were carried out with the DMU software package [16].

1) **Linear Model (LM).** A linear model (LM) ignoring K and P was used to estimate the allele substitution effect:

$$y = \mu\mathbf{1} + b\mathbf{g} + \mathbf{e}$$

where **y** was a vector of phenotypes, μ was an overall mean, $\mathbf{1}$ was a vector of ones, b was the allele substitution effect of the SNP, **g** was a vector of additively coded (0, 1 and 2) SNP genotypes and **e** was a vector of random residuals with normal distribution $N(0, \mathbf{I}\sigma_e^2)$, where σ_e^2 is the error variance and $\mathbf{I}$ is the identity matrix.

2) **Linear Mixed Model Including Pedigree-Based Relationship (LMMped).** An LMM accounting only for K was used to test the associations of single SNPs with the phenotype:

$$y = \mu\mathbf{1} + b\mathbf{g} + \mathbf{u} + \mathbf{e}$$

The terms in the model are similar to those in the LM, with the addition of random polygenic effects ($\mathbf{u}$). K was included in the model as the variance-covariance structure ($\mathbf{A}$) of $\mathbf{u}$, estimated from the pedigree relationships. $\mathbf{u}$ was assumed to be multivariate normally distributed $\mathbf{u} \sim N(0, \sigma_g^2\mathbf{A})$, where σ_g^2 is the genetic variance and $\mathbf{A}$ is the additive genetic relationship matrix derived from pedigree records for the last three generations.

3) **Linear Mixed Model Including Genomic Relationship (LMMgmat).** This LMM was similar to the LMMped accounting for K, differing only in the estimation of the variance-covariance matrix of $\mathbf{u}$. Instead of a pedigree-based relationship matrix ($\mathbf{A}$), genome-wide SNP markers were used to estimate the genomic relationship matrix ($\mathbf{G}$) [17]. $\mathbf{u}$ was assumed to be multivariate normally distributed $\mathbf{u} \sim N(0, \sigma_g^2\mathbf{G})$.

4) **Structured Association.** A model based on the clustering method of the STRUCTURE software package [9] was used to correct for P. One thousand markers evenly distributed over the genome were selected and individuals were assigned to two clusters ($k = 2$) in a structure linkage model [18].

Admixture was assumed and partial membership to a cluster was allowed. The membership of an individual in a cluster ($\boldsymbol{s}$, varying continuously between 0 and 1) was used as a covariate in the following models to correct for *P*.

1) **4a) Linear Model with STRUCTURE (LMstr).** This model was similar to the LM, with additional fixed regression (c) of the phenotype on $\boldsymbol{s}$ to account only for P while ignoring K:

$$y = \mu \boldsymbol{1} + b\boldsymbol{g} + c\boldsymbol{s} + \boldsymbol{e}$$

2) **4b) Linear Mixed Model with STRUCTURE (LMMstr).** This model was similar to LMMped, with the addition of fixed regression of the phenotype on $\boldsymbol{s}$ to correct for K and P:

$$y = \mu \boldsymbol{1} + b\boldsymbol{g} + \boldsymbol{u} + c\boldsymbol{s} + \boldsymbol{e}$$

5) **Principal Component Analysis (PCA).** PCA was performed to correct for *P* in the sample. Principal components (PCs) for the covariance matrix, estimated from all 40,000 SNP markers, were calculated. SNP genotypes and phenotypes were corrected for the first two PCs, as described elsewhere [10].

5) In the simulated datasets on an average the top two PCs explained 2.23% of the total variance in the range of 2.05 to 2.62. Although the fraction of the total variance explained was low, in most cases one of the first two PCs for the simulated datasets (Fig. S1) or the first PC for the dog dataset (Fig. S2) showed the strongest correlations with known ancestries and separated samples on ancestries. We also found that in most of the cases the correlation between PCs and known ancestries decayed rapidly beyond the first two PCs (Fig. S3). Thus, the first two PCs were used to correct for *P*. Although PCs did not separate the human samples, two PCs were used to correct the genotypes and phenotypes for comparison. The corrected genotypes ($\boldsymbol{g}^*$) and phenotypes ($\boldsymbol{y}^*$) were fitted in the following models to correct for *P*.

1) **5a) Principal Component Analysis in a Linear Model (LMpca).** Here, $\boldsymbol{y}^*$ and $\boldsymbol{g}^*$ were fitted in the LM to account only for *P* while ignoring *K*:

$$y^* = \mu \boldsymbol{1} + b\boldsymbol{g} + \mathbf{e}$$

2) **5b) Principal Component Analysis in a Linear Mixed Model (LMMpca).** Here, $\boldsymbol{y}^*$ and $\boldsymbol{g}^*$ were fitted in LMMped to correct for *K* and *P*:

$$y^* = \mu \boldsymbol{1} + b\boldsymbol{g} + \boldsymbol{u} + \boldsymbol{e}$$

Comparison of the Models

Type-I Error. *Simulated Data.* SNPs on five null chromosomes (with no simulated QTL) were used to assess the type-I error rates of all described models. A total of 1,000,000 SNPs over 100 replicates were fitted into the models to estimate b. The distribution of $-\log_{10}$ p-values of the t-test was plotted against the null (uniform) distribution in a quantile-quantile (QQ) plot. Deviation from the null distribution was used to assess the type-I error rate. In addition, the number of observed significant SNPs on null chromosomes was compared with the expected number at different significance levels.

Real Data. The human data were analyzed with LM, LMMped, LMMpca (first two PCs), and LMMstr ($k = 2$), with the inclusion of sex, age, and squared age as covariates [14]. Previous studies have reported no significant association between the SNPs and height. The deviation of $-\log_{10}$ p-values of the t-test from the expected uniform distribution in a QQ plot was used to assess the type-I error rate.

The data on hip dysplasia in dogs were fitted to the LM, LMMped, LMMpca (first two PCs), LMMstr ($k = 2$), and LMMpedB, a model similar to LMMped but with the addition of breed (as proportion of Labrador retriever) as a fixed regression. The 1,000 randomly chosen markers were assumed to be unassociated with the causal variants for hip dysplasia. The distribution of $-\log_{10}p$-values of the test of association was compared with the expected distribution under the assumption of no association in a QQ plot. Deviation from the expected distribution was used to assess the type-I error rate.

Power and Precision. The power of the models to detect the QTL was assessed from chromosome 1, with 2 simulated QTL, i.e., for 199 QTLs over 100 replicates (one QTL fixed for an allele was left out of the analysis). A QTL was considered detected when an SNP within 1 cM of the simulated QTL showed significance after Bonferroni correction (for 12,000 SNPs tested on six chromosomes) at $\alpha = 0.05$. The absolute distance between the detected and simulated QTL positions was calculated to ascertain the precision of the methods in locating the QTL. Power and precision were estimated separately for small effect (explaining $<5\%$ of σ_p^2) and large effect QTL (explaining $>5\%$ of σ_p^2).

Results

Results from the simulation study

Type-I Error. The distributions of $-\log_{10}$ p-valuesfor the SNPs on the five null chromosomes were compared with expected uniform distributions (Fig. 5). In general, type-I error rates were lower in LMMs, where familial relationship (K) was used to model the covariance structure of the random individual effect than in LMs (which did not account for *K*). Among LMMs, LMMpca closely followed the expected type-I error rate, whereas LMMgmat was the most conservative, showing a lower than expected type-I error rate.

The average number of significant SNPs on the null chromosomes is compared with expected numbers under the null hypothesis at different significance levels in Table 1. At a Bonferroni-corrected significance level, $\alpha = 0.05$ (corrected for 10,000 SNPs tested on five chromosomes) LMs that did not account for *K* (LM, LMstr, and LMpca) showed significantly higher false-positive results than expected ($p<0.01$), whereas LMMs that corrected for *K* (LMMped, LMMstr, LMMpca, and LMMgmat) showed better control of false-positive results.

Power. The power of the models to detect two simulated QTLs on chromosome 1 using 100 replicates with 199 QTLs is summarized in Figure 6. Power was compared only among LMMs

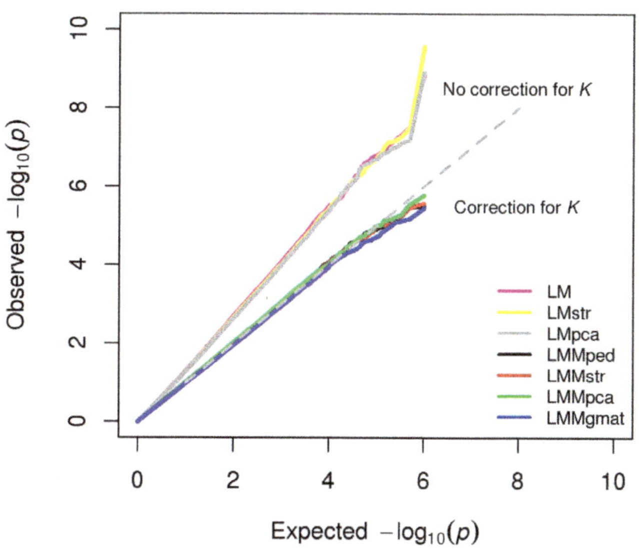

Figure 5. Quantile-quantile plot of $-\log_{10}p$-values for association tests using different models in the simulated dataset.

because the LMs had very high false-positive detection rates (Fig. 5). No LMM had the power to detect small-effect (<5% of σ_p^2) QTLs. The power was ~5%, at the level expected with $\alpha = 0.05$. In contrast, all models tested showed 53–60% power to detect large-effect (explaining >5% of σ_p^2) QTLs. LMMped and LMMstr had the highest powers (59.6%), followed by LMMpca (57.6%) and LMMgmat (53.5%), although this difference was not significant [$\chi 2$ (3, $n = 99$) = 0.9925; $p = 0.8031$]. Overall, LMMped had the highest power, detecting 32% of simulated QTLs, followed by LMMstr (31.7%), LMMpca (30.7%), and LMMgmat (28.1%); however, this difference was also not significant [χ^2 (3, $n = 199$) = 0.8983; $p = 0.8258$].

Out of the total 199 simulated QTLs, 53 were detected by all the four models, the majority (50) of which being large effect QTL (mean genetic variance = 0.087, SD = 0.02). On the other hand 133 QTLs were not detected by any of the models, majority (95) of them being small effect QTL (mean genetic variance = 0.031, SD = 0.032).

Precision. The precision of the models, measured as the absolute distance (cM) between the positions of simulated and detected QTLs, is described in Figure 6 and Table 2. All four methods compared showed greater precision for the localization of large-effect compared with small-effect QTLs. On average, large-effect QTLs were localized within 0.36–0.39 cM of the simulated QTL positions, whereas small-effect QTLs were localized within 0.62–0.66 cM. LMMped was most precise (±0.62 cM) for small-effect QTLs, and LMMgmat was most precise (±0.36 cM) for large-effect QTLs.

Results from the Published Data

Human GOLDN Dataset. For the Human GOLDN dataset, type-I error was compared among the LM, LMMped, LMMstr, and LMMpca. The distribution of test statistic is given in a QQ plot (Figure 7). The LM without correction for K and P showed the highest false-positive rate. The three LMMs (LMMped, LMMstr, and LMMpca), showed similar distributions of −log10 p-values, which were slightly higher than expected.

Dog Data on Hip Dysplasia. The dog data were analyzed using the LM, LMMped, LMMpedB, LMMstr, and LMMpca. The type-I error rates for these methods are compared in a QQ plot in Figure 8. The LM showed the highest rate of type-I errors, and this rate was comparable among LMMs, with LMMpedB and LMMstr showing the lowest type-I error rates.

Discussion

We compared the power, precision and false-positive association rates of several GWA models in analyses of simulated admixed data with familial relationships. LMs that did not model K (LM, LMstr, and LMpca) showed higher rates of false-positive associations than did LMMs accounting for K (Fig. 5, Table 1). Regardless of whether they corrected for population stratification, LMMs controlled for false-positive results at the nominal level. This is probably due to the capture of the ancestry of individuals by the variance-covariance structure modeled into the random

Table 1. Average number of significant single-nucleotide polymorphisms (SNPs; 100 replicates) in five chromosomes (10,000 SNPs) without simulated quantitative trait loci.

Model		Significance level			
	Correction for	0.05	0.005	0.0005	0.000005
LMMped	K	514.73* (7.83)	53* (1.7)	5.5 (0.4)	0.02 (0.014)
LMMstr	$P+K$	511.88 (7.9)	51.97 (1.6)	5.64* (0.4)	0.02 (0.014)
LMMpca	$P+K$	520.89** (7.6)	53.92** (1.6)	5.88** (0.4)	0.02 (0.014)
LMMgmat	K	472.15 (5.7)	44.92 (1.2)	4.45 (0.3)	0.01 (0.01)
LM	-	1014.51** (18.9)	190.2** (6.8)	36.93** (2.0)	1.43** (0.17)
LMstr	P	998.22** (17.8)	184.33** (6.4)	34.78** (1.8)	1.34** (0.16)
LMpca	P	968.01** (18.7)	175.27** (6.5)	32.01** (1.7)	1.17** (0.16)
Expected false-positive associations		500	50	5	0.05

Standard errors are given in parentheses. The average number of significant SNPs (S_{obs}) in 100 replicates was compared with the expected number (S_{exp}) at different significance levels using t-tests. (H_0: $S_{obs} = S_{exp}$; H_1: $S_{obs} > S_{exp}$; *$p<0.05$, **$p<0.01$). Significance level of 0.000005 corresponds to a nominal significance level of 0.05 after Bonferroni correction for 10000 tests.

LMMped = Linear Mixed Model Including Pedigree-Based Relationship, LMMstr = Linear Mixed Model with STRUCTURE, LMMpca = Principal Component Analysis in a Linear Mixed Model, LMMgmat = Linear Mixed Model Including Genomic Relationship, LM = Linear Model, LMstr = Linear Model with STRUCTURE, LMpca = Principal Component Analysis in a Linear Model, P = admixture, K = Familial relationships.

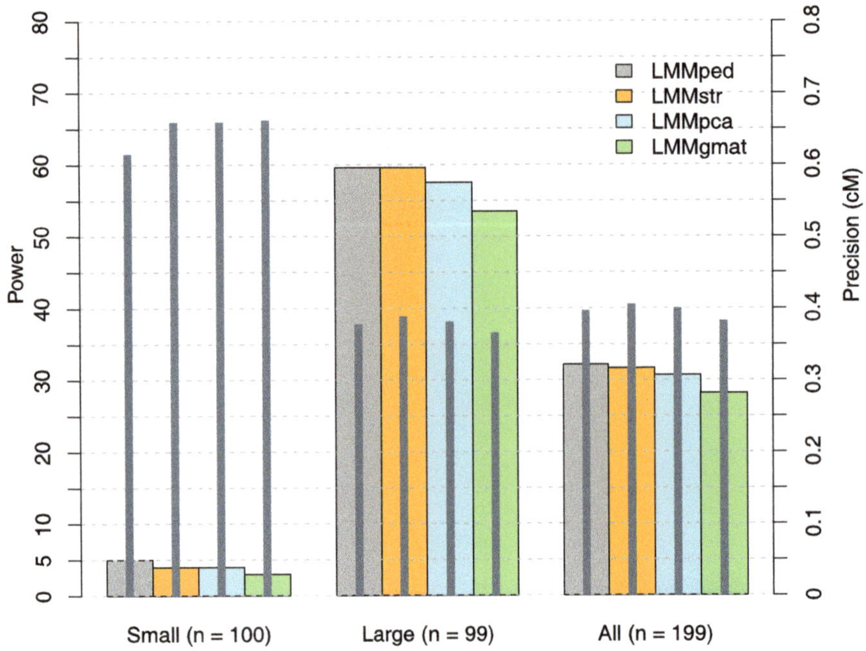

Figure 6. The power [% of quantitative trait loci (QTLs) detected] and precision (absolute distance between simulated and detected QTL; gray bars) of the models in QTL localization.

polygenic effect, as previously shown [5]. The results of analyses of publicly available human and dog data also show that LMMped was comparable to LMMstr and LMMpca in controlling for type-I errors (Figs. 7 and 8). Thus, in a sample with structure at the family and population levels, correction for *K* alone might be sufficient to control for false-positive associations arising from population structure.

In contrast, correction for *P* alone in the LMpca and LMstr was insufficient to control for false-positive associations. This is probably because STRUCTURE [9] and PCA [10] corrected for *P*, but subtle admixture at the family level was not captured by STRUCTURE ($k=2$) and LMpca (two PCs). Thus our findings indicate that correction for structure at the population level alone is not sufficient in samples with structure at the population and family levels. In such samples, LMMs can be effectively used to control for false-positive results.

Among LMMs, LMMgmat was the most conservative and consequently suffered a slight loss of power. In this model, the relationship matrix (G) was estimated from the whole genome, including markers linked to the simulated QTL. This probably led to correction of part of the QTL effects in the data, thereby reducing the model's power to detect QTLs.

The compared models had powers of ~60% in detecting large-effect QTLs. In our simulation, the same set of QTLs were segregating in the two ancestral populations, which might not accurately reflect the situation in real populations, where subpopulations may have different causal variants affecting the same trait, thereby reducing the power to detect such QTLs. Thus, our power results likely reflect the upper boundary of detection power in structured populations for QTLs with similar effects using the same sample size. In our study, none of the tested methods had the power to detect small-effect QTLs in the simulated dataset. This finding might be explained by a lower average LD ($r^2=0.07$) between adjacent markers and a similar LD between markers and the QTL. Increasing the marker density and sample size might increase the power to detect small-effect QTLs in such a dataset.

It should also be noted that the LD levels in the dataset is defined by the specific parameters (mutation rate, recombination rate and type of mating) used in the simulation. The mutation rate for markers assumed in this study was higher than what is observed in real life (e.g. 10^{-8} per base per generation in human, The 1000 Genomes Project Consortium. 2010 [21]). However, we had only 2000 marker per chromosome (100 cM≈100 MB). Therefore, the mutation rate considered in the study reflects the chance of having a mutation for a genomic region the SNP represents. Altering the genetic parameters may change the LD structure; however we do not expect a change in the relative ranking of the methods in the power of QTL detection; the same is true for the type-I error rate. Moreover, we use chromosomes devoid of the simulated QTL to assess the type-I error rate; hence the false associations arise only due to stratification and not because of the LD between markers and the QTL. Our study focuses on quantitative trait, but the findings can be generalized to case-control data as reported by

Table 2. Absolute error (cM) in quantitative trait loci localization.

	Small effect	Large effect	All
LMMped	0.62	0.38	0.40
LMMstr	0.66	0.39	0.41
LMMpca	0.66	0.38	0.40
LMMgmat	0.66	0.37	0.38

Precision is given as the absolute genetic distance between simulated and detected quantitative trait loci (±1 cM).
LMMped = Linear Mixed Model Including Pedigree-Based Relationship, LMMpca = Principal Component Analysis in a Linear Mixed Model, LMMstr = Linear Mixed Model with STRUCTURE, LMMgmat = Linear Mixed Model Including Genomic Relationship.

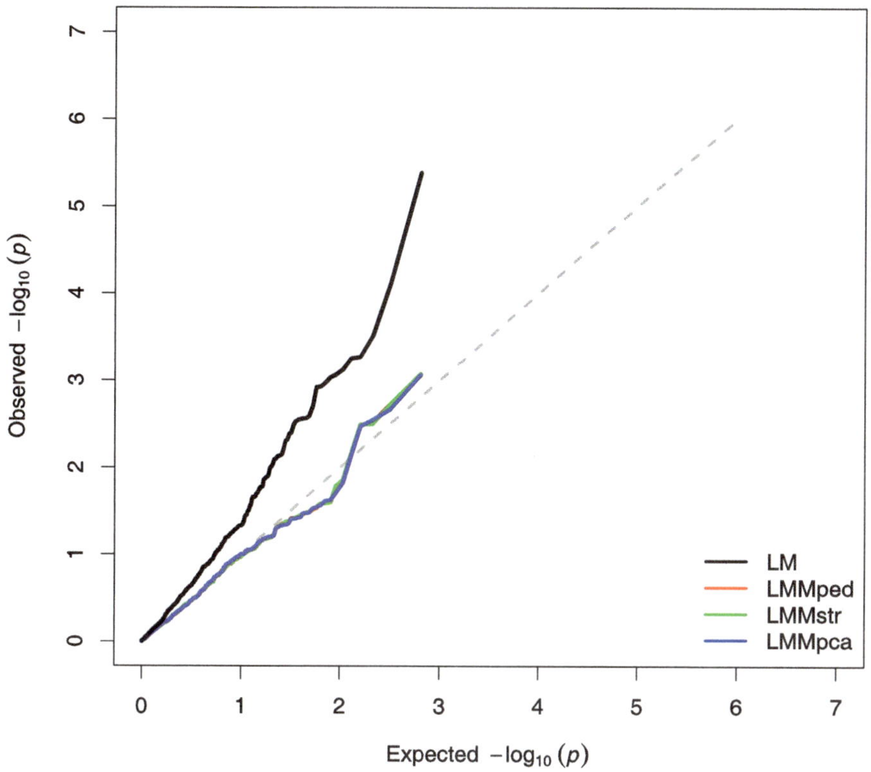

Figure 7. Quantile-quantile plot of $-\log_{10}p$-values for association tests of the human GOLDN dataset using different models.

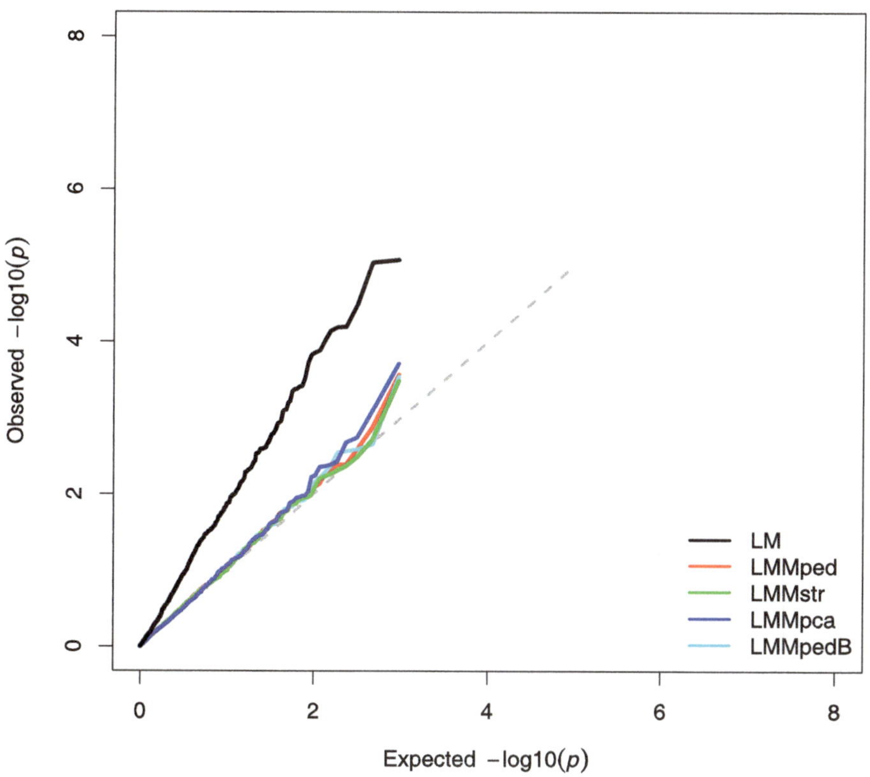

Figure 8. Quantile-quantile plot of $-\log_{10}p$-values for association tests of the dog hip dysplasia dataset using different models.

Kang et al., 2010 [19]; who found variance components based method to be effective in correcting for stratification.

The models showed comparable precision in QTL localization. Large-effect QTLs were localized with higher precision than were small-effect QTLs. This result contrasts with that of MacLeod et al. [20], who found that small-effect QTLs were mapped more precisely than large-effect QTLs. This difference is probably due to sampling bias, as the models in our study had no/very low power to detect small-effect QTLs, but ~60% power for large-effect QTLs; this situation allowed comparison of only a few observations.

In our simulation, we found that in most cases (86) the first principal component captures the genetic variation due to population stratification (correlation of 0.77 with ancestry; see Fig. S1). However, in nine cases the second PC, in three cases the third PC and in two cases the fourth PC had showed the highest correlation with the ancestries (0.67, 0.58, and 0.52, respectively). These observations suggest that in a dataset with structure at both population and family level, the latter may account for more genetic variation than the former. Therefore correction for only the first two PCs might not always be sufficient to correct for population stratification. It may thus be important to find out which PCs explain the cryptic relationship better in each dataset and include those to correct population stratification.

Our findings show that LMM approaches accounting for K are able to correct for structure at the family and population levels. We also found that the power and type-I error rate of LMMgmat with G were comparable to those of LMMped with A. Thus, LMMs may be used to correct for structure at the family and population levels by including K estimated from pedigree or genetic markers.

Supporting Information

Figure S1 Top two axes of variation in the simulated datashowsseparation of samples along the top two axes of variation in 4 replicates of simulated data. The samples are color coded with the individual ancestry (IA).Replicates i and iii show separation along the first axis whereas replicates ii and iv show separation along the second axis. Over 100 replicates, in 86 cases the first PC had the highest correlation (mean of 0.77) with the ancestries, in 9 cases with the second PC (0.67), in 3 cases with third PC (0.58) and in 2 cases with the fourth PC (0.52).

Figure S2 Top two axes of variation in the Dog hip dysplasia datashows separation of Dog breeds, Labrador (L), Greyhound (G), and crosses along the top 2 PCs. The first PC had a correlation of 0.91 with the breed proportions.

Figure S3 Correlation between the top 20 PCs and the known ancestries in the simulated dataset (100 replicates).

Author Contributions

Conceived and designed the experiments: NKK GS BG PS. Performed the experiments: NKK. Analyzed the data: NKK GS BG PS. Wrote the paper: NKK.

References

1. Cho YS, Go MJ, Kim YJ, Heo JY, Oh JH, et al. (2009) A large-scale genome-wide association study of Asian populations uncovers genetic factors influencing eight quantitative traits. Nature Genetics 41: 527–534.
2. Sanna S, Jackson AU, Nagaraja R, Willer CJ, Chen WM, et al. (2008) Common variants in the GDF5-UQCC region are associated with variation in human height. Nature Genetics 40: 198–203.
3. Hirschhorn JN, Lohmueller K, Byrne E, Hirschhorn K (2002) A comprehensive review of genetic association studies. Genetics in Medicine 4: 45–61.
4. Cardon LR, Palmer LJ (2003) Population stratification and spurious allelic association. The Lancet 361: 598–604.
5. Yu J, Pressoir G, Briggs WH, Bi IV, Yamasaki M, et al. (2005) A unified mixed-model method for association mapping that accounts for multiple levels of relatedness. Nature Genetics 38: 203–208.
6. Goddard ME, Hayes BJ (2009) Mapping genes for complex traits in domestic animals and their use in breeding programmes. Nature Reviews Genetics 10: 381–391.
7. Li C (1969) Population subdivision with respect to multiple alleles. Annals of human genetics 33: 23–29.
8. Zaitlen N, Paşaniuc B, Gur T, Ziv E, Halperin E (2010) Leveraging genetic variability across populations for the identification of causal variants. The American Journal of Human Genetics 86: 23–33.
9. Pritchard JK, Stephens M, Donnelly P (2000) Inference of population structure using multilocus genotype data. Genetics 155: 945–959.
10. Price AL, Patterson NJ, Plenge RM, Weinblatt ME, Shadick NA, et al. (2006) Principal components analysis corrects for stratification in genome-wide association studies. Nature Genetics 38: 904–909.
11. Price AL, Zaitlen NA, Reich D, Patterson N (2010) New approaches to population stratification in genome-wide association studies. Nature Reviews Genetics 11: 459–463.
12. Sargolzaei M, Schenkel FS (2009) QMSim: a large-scale genome simulator for livestock. Bioinformatics 25: 680–681.
13. Lai CQ, Arnett DK, Corella D, Straka RJ, Tsai MY, et al. (2007) Fenofibrate effect on triglyceride and postprandial response of apolipoprotein A5 variants. Arteriosclerosis, thrombosis, and vascular biology 27: 1417–1425.
14. Zhang Z, Ersoz E, Lai CQ, Todhunter RJ, Tiwari HK, et al. (2010) Mixed linear model approach adapted for genome-wide association studies. Nature Genetics 42: 355–360.
15. Zhang Z, Zhu L, Sandler J, Friedenberg SS, Egelhoff J, et al. (2009) Estimation of heritabilities, genetic correlations, and breeding values of four traits that collectively define hip dysplasia in dogs. American journal of veterinary research 70: 483–492.
16. Madsen P, Jensen J (2010) DMU, A package for analysing Multivariate Mixed Models. http://dmuagrscidk/dmuv6_guide50pdf Version 6, release 5.0.
17. VanRaden P (2008) Efficient methods to compute genomic predictions. Journal of dairy science 91: 4414–4423.
18. Falush D, Stephens M, Pritchard JK (2003) Inference of population structure using multilocus genotype data: linked loci and correlated allele frequencies. Genetics 164: 1567–1587.
19. Kang HM, Sul JH, Zaitlen NA, Kong S, Freimer NB, et al. (2010) Variance component model to account for sample structure in genome-wide association studies. Nature Genetics 42: 348–354.
20. MacLeod I, Hayes B, Savin K, Chamberlain A, McPartlan H, et al. (2010) Power of a genome scan to detect and locate quantitative trait loci in cattle using dense single nucleotide polymorphisms. Journal of Animal Breeding and Genetics 127: 133–142.
21. Abecasis GR, Altshuler D, Auton A, Brooks LD, Durbin RM, et al. (2010) A map of human genome variation from population-scale sequencing. Nature 467: 1061–1073.

Structural Brain Changes in Chronic Pain Reflect Probably Neither Damage Nor Atrophy

Rea Rodriguez-Raecke[1], Andreas Niemeier[2], Kristin Ihle[1], Wolfgang Ruether[2], Arne May[1]*

1 Department of Systems Neuroscience, University Medical Center Hamburg Eppendorf, Hamburg, Germany, 2 Department of Orthopaedics, University Medical Center Hamburg Eppendorf, Hamburg, Germany

Abstract

Chronic pain appears to be associated with brain gray matter reduction in areas ascribable to the transmission of pain. The morphological processes underlying these structural changes, probably following functional reorganisation and central plasticity in the brain, remain unclear. The pain in hip osteoarthritis is one of the few chronic pain syndromes which are principally curable. We investigated 20 patients with chronic pain due to unilateral coxarthrosis (mean age 63.25±9.46 (SD) years, 10 female) before hip joint endoprosthetic surgery (pain state) and monitored brain structural changes up to 1 year after surgery: 6–8 weeks, 12–18 weeks and 10–14 month when completely pain free. Patients with chronic pain due to unilateral coxarthrosis had significantly less gray matter compared to controls in the anterior cingulate cortex (ACC), insular cortex and operculum, dorsolateral prefrontal cortex (DLPFC) and orbitofrontal cortex. These regions function as multi-integrative structures during the experience and the anticipation of pain. When the patients were pain free after recovery from endoprosthetic surgery, a gray matter increase in nearly the same areas was found. We also found a progressive increase of brain gray matter in the premotor cortex and the supplementary motor area (SMA). We conclude that gray matter abnormalities in chronic pain are not the cause, but secondary to the disease and are at least in part due to changes in motor function and bodily integration.

Editor: Berthold Langguth, University of Regensburg, Germany

Funding: This work was supported by grants from the DFG (German Research Foundation) (MA 1862/2-3) and BMBF (The Federal Ministry of Education and Research) (371 57 01 and NeuroImage Nord). The funders had no role in study design, data collection and analysis, decision to publish, or preparation of the manuscript.

Competing Interests: The authors have declared that no competing interests exist.

* E-mail: a.may@uke.uni-hamburg.de

Introduction

Evidence of functional and structural reorganization in chronic pain patients support the idea that chronic pain should not only be conceptualized as an altered functional state, but also as a consequence of functional and structural brain plasticity [1,2,3,4,5,6]. In the last six years, more than 20 studies were published demonstrating structural brain changes in 14 chronic pain syndromes. A striking feature of all of these studies is the fact that the gray matter changes were not randomly distributed, but occur in defined and functionally highly specific brain areas – namely, involvement in supraspinal nociceptive processing. The most prominent findings were different for each pain syndrome, but overlapped in the cingulate cortex, the orbitofrontal cortex, the insula and dorsal pons [4]. Further structures comprise the thalamus, dorsolateral prefrontal cortex, basal ganglia and hippocampal area. These findings are often discussed as cellular atrophy, reinforcing the idea of damage or loss of brain gray matter [7,8,9]. In fact, researchers found a correlation between brain gray matter decreases and duration of pain [6,10]. But the duration of pain is also linked to the patient's age, and the age dependent global, but also regionally specific decline of gray matter is well documented [11]. On the other hand, these structural changes could also be a decrease in cell size, extracellular fluids, synaptogenesis, angiogenesis or even due to blood volume changes [4,12,13]. Whatever the source is, for our interpretation of such findings it is important to see these morphometric findings in the light of a wealth of morphometric studies in exercise dependant plasticity, given that regionally specific structural brain changes have been repeatedly shown following cognitive and physical exercise [14].

It is not understood why only a relatively small proportion of humans develop a chronic pain syndrome, considering that pain is a universal experience. The question arises whether in some humans a structural difference in central pain transmitting systems may act as a diathesis for chronic pain. Gray matter changes in phantom pain due to amputation [15] and spinal cord injury [3] indicate that the morphological changes of the brain are, at least in part, a consequence of chronic pain. However, the pain in hip osteoarthritis (OA) is one of the few chronic pain syndrome which is principally curable, as 88% of these patients are regularly free of pain following total hip replacement (THR) surgery [16]. In a pilot study we have analysed ten patients with hip OA before and shortly after surgery. We found decreases of gray matter in the anterior cingulated cortex (ACC) and insula during chronic pain before THR surgery and found increases of gray matter in the corresponding brain areas in the pain free condition after surgery [17]. Focussing on this result, we now expanded our studies investigating more patients (n = 20) after successful THR and monitored structural brain changes in four time intervals, up to one year following surgery. To control for gray matter changes due to motor improvement or depression we also administered questionnaires targeting improvement of motor function and mental health.

Materials and Methods

Volunteers

The patients reported here are a subgroup of 20 patients out of 32 patients published recently who were compared to an age- and gender-matched healthy control group [17] but participated in an additional one year follow-up investigation. After surgery 12 patients dropped out because of a second endoprosthetic surgery ($n = 2$), severe illness ($n = 2$) and withdrawal of consent ($n = 8$). This left a group of twenty patients with unilateral primary hip OA (mean age 63.25±9.46 (SD) years, 10 female) who were investigated four times: before surgery (pain state) and again 6–8 and 12–18 weeks and 10–14 months after endoprosthetic surgery, when completely pain free. All patients with primary hip OA had a pain history longer than 12 months, ranging from 1 to 33 years (mean 7.35 years) and a mean pain score of 65.5 (ranging from 40 to 90) on a visual analogue scale (VAS) ranging from 0 (no pain) to 100 (worst imaginable pain). We assessed any occurrence of minor pain events, including tooth-, ear- and headache up to 4 weeks prior to the study. We also randomly selected the data from 20 sex- and age matched healthy controls (mean age 60,95±8,52 (SD) years, 10 female) of the 32 of the above mentioned pilot study [17]. None of the 20 patients or of the 20 sex- and age matched healthy volunteers had any neurological or internal medical history. The study was given ethical approval by the local Ethics committee and written informed consent was obtained from all study participants prior to examination.

Behavioural Data

We collected data on depression, somatization, anxiety, pain and physical and mental health in all patients and all four time points using the following standardized questionnaires: Beck Depression Inventory (BDI) [18], Brief Symptom Inventory (BSI) [19], Schmerzempfindungs-Skala (SES = pain unpleasantness scale) [20] and Health Survey 36-Item Short Form (SF-36) [21] and the Nottingham Health Profile (NHP). We conducted repeated measures ANOVA and paired two-tailed t-Tests to analyse the longitudinal behavioural data using SPSS 13.0 for Windows (SPSS Inc., Chicago, IL), and used Greenhouse Geisser correction if the assumption for sphericity was violated. The significance level was set at $p<0.05$.

VBM - Data Acquisition

Image acquisition. High-resolution MR scanning was performed on a 3T MRI system (Siemens Trio) with a standard 12-channel head coil. For each of the four time points, scan I (between 1 day and 3 month before endoprosthetic surgery), scan II (6 to 8 weeks after surgery), scan III (12 to 18 weeks after surgery) and scan IV (10–14 months after surgery), a T1 weighted structural MRI was acquired for each patient using a 3D-FLASH sequence (TR 15 ms, TE 4.9 ms, flip angle 25°, 1 mm slices, FOV 256×256, *voxel size 1×1×1 mm*).

Image Processing and Statistical Analysis

Data pre-processing and analysis were performed with SPM2 (Wellcome Department of Cognitive Neurology, London, UK) running under Matlab (Mathworks, Sherborn, MA, USA) and containing a voxel-based morphometry (VBM)-toolbox for longitudinal data, that is based on high resolution structural 3D MR images and allows for applying voxel-wise statistics to detect regional differences in gray matter density or volumes [22,23]. In summary, pre-processing involved spatial normalization, gray matter segmentation and 10 mm spatial smoothing with a Gaussian kernel. For the pre-processing steps, we used an optimized protocol [22,23] and a scanner- and study-specific gray matter template [17]. We used SPM2 rather than SPM5 or SPM8 to make this analysis comparable to our pilot study [17]. as it allows an excellent normalisation and segmentation of longitudinal data. However, as a more recent update of VBM (VBM8) became available recently (http://dbm.neuro.uni-jena.de/vbm/), we also used VBM8.

Cross-sectional Analysis

We used a two-sample t-test in order to detect regional differences in brain gray matter between groups (patients at time point scan I (chronic pain) and healthy controls). We applied a threshold of $p<0.001$ (uncorrected) across the whole brain because of our strong *a priory* hypothesis, which is based on 9 independent studies and cohorts showing decreases in gray matter in chronic pain patients [7,8,9,15,24,25,26,27,28], that gray matter increases will appear in the same (for pain processing relevant) regions as in our pilot study (17). The groups were matched for age and sex with no significant differences between the groups. To investigate whether the differences between groups changed after one year, we also compared patients at time point scan IV (pain free, one year follow-up) to our healthy control group.

Longitudinal Analysis

To detect differences between time points (Scan I–IV) we compared the scans before surgery (pain state) and again 6–8 and 12–18 weeks and 10–14 months after endoprosthetic surgery (pain free) as repeated measure ANOVA. Because any brain changes due to chronic pain may need some time to recede following operation and cessation of pain and because of the post surgery pain the patients reported, we compared in the longitudinal analysis scan I and II with scan III and IV. For detecting changes that are not closely linked to pain, we also looked for progressive changes over all time intervals. We flipped the brains of patients with OA of the left hip ($n = 7$) in order to normalize for the side of the pain for both, the group comparison and the longitudinal analysis, but primarily analysed the unflipped data. We used the BDI score as a covariate in the model.

Results

Behavioral Data

All patients reported chronic hip pain before surgery and were pain free (regarding this chronic pain) immediately after surgery, but reported rather acute post-surgery pain on scan II which was different from the pain due to osteoarthritis. The mental health score of the SF-36 ($F(1.925/17.322) = 0.352$, $p = 0.7$) and the BSI global score GSI ($F(1.706/27.302) = 3.189$, $p = 0.064$) showed no changes over the time course and no mental co-morbidity. None of the controls reported any acute or chronic pain and none showed any symptoms of depression or physical/mental disability.

Before surgery, some patients showed mild to moderate depressive symptoms in BDI scores that significantly decreased on scan III ($t(17) = 2.317$, $p = 0.033$) and IV ($t(16) = 2.132$, $p = 0.049$). Additionally, the SES scores (pain unpleasantness) of all patients improved significantly from scan I (before the surgery) to scan II ($t(16) = 4.676$, $p<0.001$), scan III ($t(14) = 4.760$, $p<0.001$) and scan IV ($t(14) = 4.981$, $p<0.001$, 1 year after surgery) as pain unpleasantness decreased with pain intensity. The pain rating on scan 1 and 2 were positive, the same rating on day 3 and 4 negative. The SES only describes the quality of perceived pain. It was therefore positive on day 1 and 2 (mean 19.6 on day 1 and 13.5 on day 2) and negative (n.a.) on day 3 & 4. However, some patients did not understand this procedure and used the SES as a global "quality of life" measure. This is why all patients were asked on the same day individually and by the same person regarding pain occurrence.

In the short form health survey (SF-36), which consists of the summary measures of a *Physical Health Score* and a *Mental Health Score* [29], the patients improved significantly in *the Physical Health score* from scan I to scan II ($t(17) = -4.266$, $p = 0.001$), scan III ($t(16) = -8.584$, $p<0.001$) and IV ($t(12) = -7.148$, $p<0.001$), but not in the *Mental Health Score.* The results of the NHP were similar, in the subscale "pain" (reversed polarity) we observed a significant change from scan I to scan II ($t(14) = -5.674$, $p<0.001$, scan III ($t(12) = -7.040$, $p<0.001$ and scan IV ($t(10) = -3.258$, $p = 0.009$). We also found a significant increase in the subscale "physical mobility" from scan I to scan III ($t(12) = -3.974$, $p = 0.002$) and scan IV ($t(10) = -2.511$, $p = 0.031$). There was no significant change between scan I and scan II (six weeks after surgery).

Structural Data

Cross-sectional analysis. We included age as a covariate in the general linear model and found no age confounds. Compared to sex and age matched controls, patients with primary hip OA ($n = 20$) showed pre-operatively (Scan I) reduced gray matter in the anterior cingulate cortex (ACC), the insular cortex, operculum, dorsolateral prefrontal cortex (DLPFC), right temporal pole and cerebellum (Table 1 and Figure 1). Except for the right putamen ($x = 31$, $y = -14$, $z = -1$; $p<0.001$, $t = 3.32$) no significant increase in gray matter density was found in patients with OA compared to healthy controls. Comparing patients at time point scan IV with matched controls, the same results were found as in the cross-sectional analysis using scan I compared to controls.

Flipping the data of patients with left hip OA ($n = 7$) and comparing them with healthy controls did not change the results significantly, but for a decrease in the thalamus ($x = 10$, $y = -20$, $z = 3$, $p<0.001$, $t = 3.44$) and an increase in the right cerebellum ($x = 25$, $y = -37$, $z = -50$, $p<0.001$, $t = 5.12$) that did not reach significance in the unflipped data of the patients compared to controls.

Longitudinal analysis. In the longitudinal analysis, a significant increase ($p<.001$ uncorrected) of gray matter was detected by comparing the first and second scan (chronic pain/post-surgery pain) with the third and fourth scan (pain free) in the ACC, insular cortex, cerebellum and pars orbitalis in the patients with OA (Table 2 and Figure 1). Gray matter decreased over time ($p<.001$ whole brain analysis uncorrected) in the secondary somatosensory cortex, hippocampus, midcingulate cortex, thalamus and caudate nucleus in patients with OA (Figure 2).

Flipping the data of patients with left hip OA ($n = 7$) did not change the results significantly, but for a decrease of brain gray matter in the Heschl's Gyrus ($x = -41$, $y = -21$, $z = 10$, $p<0.001$, $t = 3.69$) and Precuneus ($x = 15$, $y = -36$, $z = 3$, $p<0.001$, $t = 4.60$).

By contrasting the first scan (presurgery) with scans 3+4 (postsurgery), we found an increase of gray matter in the frontal cortex and motor cortex ($p<0.001$ uncorrected). We note that this contrast is less stringent as we have now less scans per condition (pain vs. non-pain). When we lower the threshold we repeat what we have found using contrast of 1+2 vs. 3+4.

By looking for areas that increase over all time intervals, we found changes of brain gray matter in motor areas (area 6) in patients with coxarthrosis following total hip replacement (scan I<scan II<scan III<scan IV)). Adding the BDI scores as a covariate did not change the results. Using the recently available software tool VBM8 including DARTEL normalisation (http://dbm.neuro.uni-jena.de/vbm/) we could replicate this finding in the anterior and mid-cingulate cortex and both anterior insulae.

We calculated the effect sizes and the cross-sectional analysis (patients vs. controls) yielded a Cohen's d of 1.78751 in the peak voxel of the ACC ($x = -12$, $y = 25$, $z = -16$). We also calculated Cohen's d for the longitudinal analysis (contrasting scan 1+2 vs. scan 3+4). This resulted in a Cohen's d of 1.1158 in the ACC ($x = -3$, $y = 50$, $z = 2$). Regarding the insula ($x = -33$, $y = 21$, $z = 13$) and related to the same contrast, Cohen's d is 1.0949. Additionally, we calculated the mean of the non-zero voxel values of the Cohen's d map within the ROI (comprised of the anterior

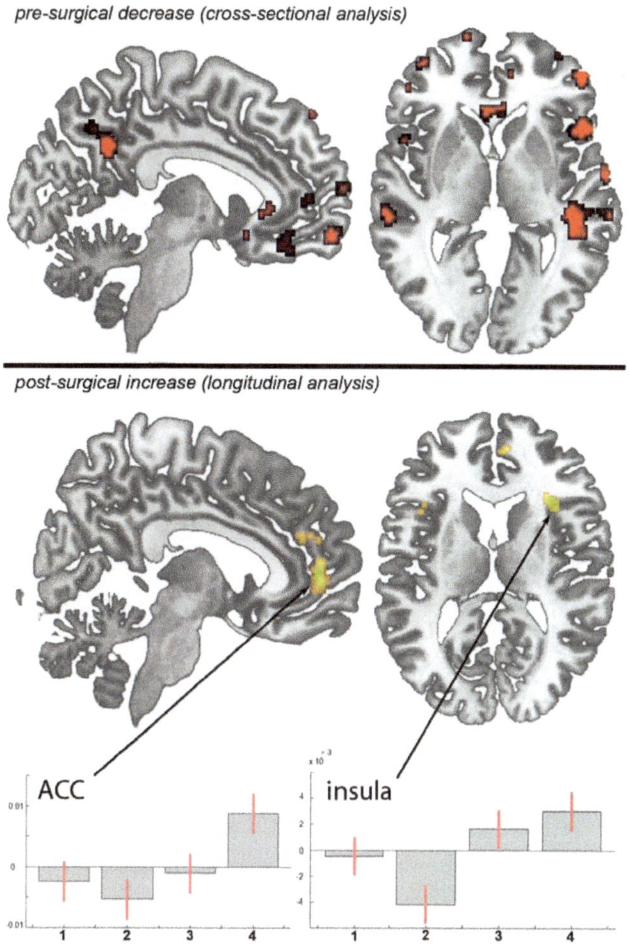

Figure 1. Statistical parametric maps demonstrating the structural differences in gray matter in patients with chronic pain due to primary hip OA compared to controls and longitudinally compared to themselves over time. Significant gray matter changes are shown superimposed in color, cross-sectional data is depicted in red and longitudinal data in yellow. Axial plane: the left side of the picture is the left side of the brain. top: Areas of significant decrease of gray matter between patients with chronic pain due to primary hip OA and unaffected control subjects. $p<0.001$ uncorrected bottom: Gray matter increase in 20 pain free patients at the third and fourth scanning period after total hip replacement surgery, as compared to the first (preoperative) and second (6–8 weeks post surgery) scan. $p<0.001$ uncorrected Plots: Contrast estimates and 90% Confidence interval, effects of interest, arbitrary units. x-axis: contrasts for the 4 timepoints, y-axis: contrast estimate at −3, 50, 2 for ACC and contrast estimate at 36, 39, 3 for insula.

Table 1. Cross-sectional data (not flipped, patients with OA<healthy controls), gray matter decrease in OA (p<0.001 uncorrected).

	MNI				
Anatomical locations	**x**	**y**	**z**	**Peak t-scores**	**number of voxels**
anterior cingulate cortex	−12	25	−16	5.51	2678
insular cortex/operculum	54	22	5	5.00	1527
Cerebellum	26	−42	−27	4.16	1913
pars orbitalis/orbital gyrus	48	47	−9	3.77	1080
superior frontal gyrus	−14	68	2	3.97	96
mid temporal gyrus	−63	−29	−7	4.15	1961
superior medial gyrus	10	67	13	4.35	222
pars opercularis	48	18	0	4.25	1527
DLPFC	45	35	29	4.69	1332
superior temporal gyrus/S2	64	−5	4	4.37	324

division of the cingulate gyrus and the subcallosal cortex, derived from the Harvard-Oxford Cortical Structural Atlas): 1.251223.

Discussion

Monitoring whole brain structure over time, we confirm and expand our pilot data published recently [17]. We found changes in brain gray matter in patients with primary hip osteoarthritis in the chronic pain state, which reverse partly when these patients are pain free, following hip joint endoprosthetic surgery. The partial increase in gray matter after surgery is nearly in the same areas where a decrease of gray matter has been seen before surgery. Flipping the data of patients with left hip OA (and therefore normalizing for the side of the pain) had only little impact on the results but additionally showed a decrease of gray matter in the Heschl's gyrus and Precuneus that we cannot easily explain and, as no a priori hypothesis exists, regard with great caution. However, the difference seen between patients and healthy controls at scan I was still observable in the cross-sectional analysis at scan IV. The relative increase of gray matter over time is therefore subtle, i.e. not sufficiently distinct to have an effect on the cross sectional analysis, a finding that has already been shown in studies investigating experience dependant plasticity [30,31]. We note that the fact that we show some parts of brain-changes due to chronic pain to be reversible does not exclude that some other parts of these changes are irreversible.

Interestingly, we observed that the gray matter decrease in the ACC in chronic pain patients before surgery seems to continue 6 weeks after surgery (scan II) and only increases towards scan III and IV, possibly due to post-surgery pain, or decrease in motor

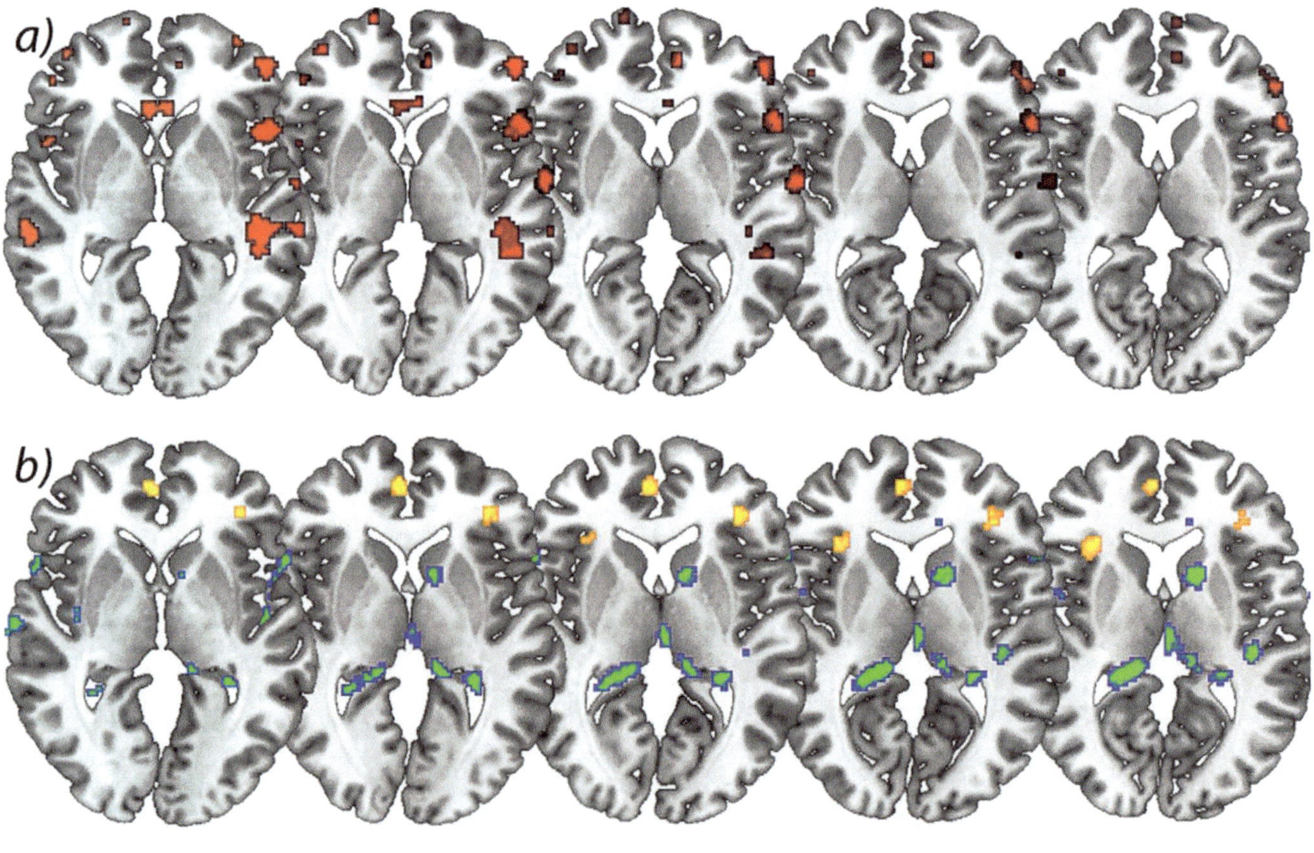

Figure 2. Significant increases in brain gray matter following successful operation. a) Axial view of significant decrease of gray matter in patients with chronic pain due to primary hip OA compared to control subjects. p<0.001 uncorrected (cross-sectional analysis), **b)** Longitudinal increase of gray matter over time in yellow comparing scan I&II<scan III<scan IV) and longitudinal decrease of gray matter over time in blue/green comparing scan I&II>scan III>scan IV) in patients with OA. p<0.001 uncorrected (longitudinal analysis). The left side of the picture is the left side of the brain.

Table 2. Longitudinal data, significant changes in gray matter in patients with chronic pain due to primary hip osteoarthritis.

	MNI					
Anatomical locations	**x**	**y**	**z**	**Peak t-scores**	**number of voxels**	**Increase/decrease**
anterior cingulate cortex	−3	50	2	4.21	674	increase
insular cortex	−33	21	13	4.13	420	increase
pars orbitalis	4	39	10	3.77	77	increase
Cerebellum	47	−71	−22	5.00	5139	increase
mid cingulate cortex	11	−26	43	5.04	1713	decrease
caudate nucleus	11	9	8	4.14	791	decrease
pars opercularis	−58	16	2	4.53	445	decrease
Area 44	64	9	8	4.59	1155	decrease
Thalamus	3	−17	6	4.17	1540	decrease
operculum/S2	−66	−26	17	5.66	2935	decrease
Operculum	41	−26	11	4.41	283	decrease
Hippocampus	−18	−37	7	4.50	1662	decrease

The changes are tabulated in terms of the brain region and the corresponding Brodmann's area (BA). The x, y, z co-ordinates are according to the MNI atlas. Each location is the peak within a cluster (defined as the voxel with the highest T-score). (Patients with OA, not flipped) Increase = increase in gray matter scan I/scan II>scan III>scan IV. Decrease = decrease in gray matter scan I/scan II<scan III<scan IV; $p<0.001$ uncorrected).

function. This is in line with the behavioural data of the physical mobility score included in the NHP, which post-operatively did not show any significant change at time point II but significantly increased towards scan III and IV. Of note, our patients reported no pain in the hip after surgery, but experienced post-surgery pain in surrounding muscles and skin which was perceived very differently by patients. However, as patients still reported some pain at scan II, we also contrasted the first scan (pre-surgery) with scans III+IV (post-surgery), revealing an increase of gray matter in the frontal cortex and motor cortex. We note that this contrast is less stringent because of less scans per condition (pain vs. non-pain). When we lowered the threshold we repeat what we have found using contrast of I+II vs. III+IV.

Our data strongly suggest that gray matter alterations in chronic pain patients, which are usually found in areas involved in supraspinal nociceptive processing [4] are neither due to neuronal atrophy nor brain damage. The fact that these changes seen in the chronic pain state do not reverse completely could be explained with the relatively short period of observation (one year after operation versus a mean of seven years of chronic pain before the operation). Neuroplastic brain changes that may have developed over several years (as a consequence of constant nociceptive input) need probably more time to reverse completely. Another possibility why the increase of gray matter can only be detected in the longitudinal data but not in the cross-sectional data (i.e. between cohorts at time point IV) is that the number of patients (n = 20) is too small. It needs to be pointed out that the variance between brains of several individuals is quite large and that longitudinal data have the advantage that the variance is relatively small as the same brains are scanned several times. Consequently, subtle changes will only be detectable in longitudinal data [30,31,32]. Of course we cannot exclude that these changes are at least partly irreversible although that is unlikely, given the findings of exercise specific structural plasticity and reorganisation [4,12,30,33,34]. To answer this question, future studies need to investigate patients repeatedly over longer time frames, possibly years.

We note that we can only make limited conclusions regarding the dynamics of morphological brain changes over time. The reason is that when we designed this study in 2007 and scanned in 2008 and 2009, it was not known whether structural changes would occur at all and for reasons of feasibility we chose the scan dates and time frames as described here. One could argue that the gray matter changes in time, which we describe for the patient group, might have happened in the control group as well (time effect). However, any changes due to aging, if at all, would be expected to be a decrease in volume. Given our a priori hypothesis, based on 9 independent studies and cohorts showing decreases in gray matter in chronic pain patients [7,8,9,15,24,25,26,27,28], we focussed on regional increases over time and therefore believe our finding not to be a simple time effect. Of note, we cannot rule out that the gray matter decrease over time that we found in our patient group could be due to a time effect, as we have not scanned our control group in the same time frame. Given the findings, future studies should aim at more and shorter time intervals, given that exercise dependant morphometric brain changes may occur as fast as after 1 week [32,33].

In addition to the impact of the nociceptive aspect of pain on brain gray matter [17,34] we observed that changes in motor function probably also contribute to the structural changes. We found motor and premotor areas (area 6) to increase over all time intervals (Figure 3). Intuitively this may be due to improvement of motor function over time as the patients were no more restricted in living a normal life. Notably we did not focus on motor function but an improvement in pain experience, given our original quest to investigate whether the well-known reduction in brain gray matter in chronic pain patients is in principle reversible. Consequently, we did not use specific instruments to investigate motor function. Nevertheless, (functional) motor cortex reorganization in patients with pain syndromes is well documented [35,36,37,38]. Moreover, the motor cortex is one target in therapeutic approaches in medically intractable chronic pain patients using direct brain stimulation [39,40], transcranial direct current stimulation [41], and repetitive transcranial magnetic stimulation [42,43]. The exact mechanisms of such modulation (facilitation vs. inhibition, or simply interference in the pain-related networks) are not yet elucidated [40]. A recent study demonstrated that a specific motor experience can alter the structure of the brain [13]. Synaptogenesis, reorganisation of movement representations and angiogenesis in motor cortex may occur with special demands of a motor task. Tsao et al. showed reorganisation in the motor cortex of patients with chronic low back pain that seem to be back pain-specific [44] and Puri et al. observed a reduction in left supplemental motor area gray matter in fibromyalgia sufferers [45]. Our study was not designed to disentangle the different factors that may change the brain in chronic pain but we interpret our data concerning the gray matter changes that they do not exclusively mirror the consequences of constant nociceptive input. In fact, a recent study in neuropathic pain patients pointed out abnormalities in brain regions that encompass emotional, autonomic, and pain perception, implying that they play a critical role in the global clinical picture of chronic pain [28].

Two recent pilot studies focussed on hip replacement therapy in osteoarthritis patients, the only chronic pain syndrome which is principally curable with total hip replacement [17,46] and these data are flanked by a very recent study in chronic low back pain patients [47]. These studies need to be seen in the light of several longitudinal studies investigating experience-dependent neuronal plasticity in humans on a structural level [30,31] and a recent study on structural brain changes in healthy volunteers experiencing repeated painful stimulation [34]. The key message of all these studies is that the main difference in the brain structure between pain patients and controls may recede when the pain is cured. However, it must be taken into account that it is simply not clear whether the changes in chronic pain patients are solely due to nociceptive input or due to the consequences of pain or both. It is more than likely that behavioural changes, such as deprivation or enhancement of social contacts, agility, physical training and life style changes are sufficient to shape the brain [6,12,28,48]. Particularly depression as a co-morbidity or consequence of pain is a key candidate to explain the differences between patients and controls. A small group of our patients with OA showed mild to moderate depressive symptoms that changed with time. We did not find the structural alterations to covary significantly with the BDI-score but the question arises how many other behavioural changes due to the absence of pain and motor improvement may contribute to the results and to what extent they do. These behavioural changes can possibly influence a gray matter decrease in chronic pain as well as a gray matter increase when pain is gone.

Another important factor which may bias our interpretation of the results is the fact that nearly all patients with chronic pain took medications against pain, which they stopped when they were pain free. One could argue that NSAIDs such as diclofenac or ibuprofen have some effects on neural systems and the same holds true for opioids, antiepileptics and antidepressants, medications which are frequently used in chronic pain therapy. The impact of pain killers and other medications on morphometric findings may well be important (48). No study so far has shown effects of pain medication on brain morphology but several papers found that changes in brain structure in chronic pain patients are neither solely explained by pain related inactivity [15], nor by pain medication [7,9,49]. However, specific studies are lacking. Further research should focus the experience-dependent changes in cortical plasticity, which may have vast clinical implications for the treatment of chronic pain.

We also found decreases of gray matter in the longitudinal analysis, possibly due to reorganisation processes that accompany changes in motor function and pain perception. There is little information available about longitudinal changes in brain gray matter in pain conditions, for this reason we have no hypothesis for a gray matter decrease in these areas after the operation. Teutsch et al. [25] found an increase of brain gray matter in the somatosensory and midcingulate cortex in healthy volunteers that experienced painful stimulation in a daily protocol for eight consecutive days. The finding of gray matter increase following experimental nociceptive input overlapped anatomically to some degree with the decrease of brain gray matter in this study in patients that were cured of long-lasting chronic pain. This implies that nociceptive input in healthy volunteers leads to exercise dependant structural changes, as it possibly does in patients with chronic pain, and that these changes reverse in healthy volunteers when nociceptive input stops. Consequently, the decrease of gray matter in these areas seen in patients with OA could be interpreted to follow the same fundamental process: exercise dependant changes brain changes [50]. As a non-invasive procedure, MR Morphometry is the ideal tool for the quest to find the morphological substrates of diseases, deepening our understanding of the relationship between brain structure and function, and even to monitor therapeutic interventions. One of the great challenges in the future is to adapt this powerful tool for multicentre and therapeutic trials of chronic pain.

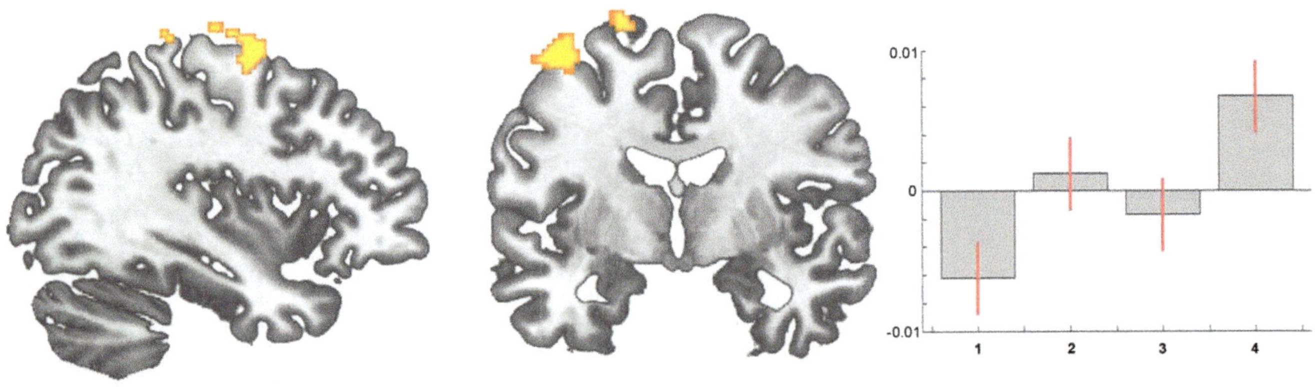

Figure 3. Statistical parametric maps demonstrating a significant increase of brain gray matter in motor areas (area 6) in patients with coxarthrosis before compared to after THR (longitudinal analysis, scan I<scan II<scan III<scan IV). Contrast estimates at x = 19, y = −12, z = 70.

Table 3. Longitudinal data, significant increase in gray matter comparing scan 1 with scan 3 and 4 (excluding scan 2) in patients with chronic pain due to primary hip osteoarthritis.

		MNI			
Anatomical locations	**x**	**y**	**z**	**Peak t-scores**	**number of voxels**
Right precentral gyrus	48	−6	62	3.61	419
Right precentral gyrus	24	−17	80	3.50	200
Right superior frontal gyrus, Area 6	17	0	74	4.00	98
Left superior medial gyrus	−9	46	24	3.93	65
Right postcentral gyrus	40	−32	71	3.59	3
Left cerebellum	−10	−63	−22	3.51	17
Left middle frontal gyrus	−34	9	64	3.42	8
Right precentral gyrus	26	−17	78	3.36	2

The changes are tabulated in terms of the brain region and the corresponding Brodmann's area (BA). The x, y, z co-ordinates are according to the MNI atlas. Significance level $p<0.001$, uncorrected.

Limitations of this Study

Although this study is an extension of our previous study expanding the follow-up data to 12 months and investigating more patients, our principle finding that morphometric brain changes in chronic pain are reversible is rather subtle. The effect sizes are small (see above) and the effects are partly driven by a further reduction of regional brain gray matter volume at the time-point of scan 2. When we exclude the data from scan 2 (directly after the operation) only significant increases in brain gray matter for motor cortex and frontal cortex survive a threshold of $p<0.001$ uncorrected (Table 3).

Conclusion

It is not possible to distinguish to what extent the structural alterations we observed are due to changes in nociceptive input, changes in motor function or medication consumption or changes in well-being as such. Masking the group contrasts of the first and last scan with each other revealed much less differences than expected. Presumably, brain alterations due to chronic pain with all consequences are developing over quite a long time course and may also need some time to revert. Nevertheless, these results reveal processes of reorganisation, strongly suggesting that chronic nociceptive input and motor impairment in these patients leads to altered processing in cortical regions and consequently structural brain changes which are in principle reversible.

Acknowledgments

We thank all volunteers for the participation in this study and the Physics and Methods group at NeuroImage Nord in Hamburg. The study was given ethical approval by the local Ethics committee and written informed consent was obtained from all study participants prior to examination.

Author Contributions

Conceived and designed the experiments: RR AM. Performed the experiments: AN KI WR. Analyzed the data: RR AM. Contributed reagents/materials/analysis tools: AM WR. Wrote the paper: RR AM.

References

1. Woolf CJ, Salter MW (2000) Neuronal plasticity: increasing the gain in pain. Science 288: 1765–1769.
2. Flor H, Nikolajsen L, Staehelin Jensen T (2006) Phantom limb pain: a case of maladaptive CNS plasticity? Nat Rev Neurosci 7: 873–881.
3. Wrigley PJ, Gustin SM, Macey PM, Nash PG, Gandevia SC, et al. (2009) Anatomical changes in human motor cortex and motor pathways following complete thoracic spinal cord injury. Cereb Cortex 19: 224–232.
4. May A (2008) Chronic pain may change the structure of the brain. Pain 137: 7–15.
5. May A (2009) Morphing voxels: the hype around structural imaging of headache patients. Brain.
6. Apkarian AV, Baliki MN, Geha PY (2009) Towards a theory of chronic pain. Prog Neurobiol 87: 81–97.
7. Apkarian AV, Sosa Y, Sonty S, Levy RM, Harden RN, et al. (2004) Chronic back pain is associated with decreased prefrontal and thalamic gray matter density. J Neurosci 24: 10410–10415.
8. Rocca MA, Ceccarelli A, Falini A, Colombo B, Tortorella P, et al. (2006) Brain gray matter changes in migraine patients with T2-visible lesions: a 3-T MRI study. Stroke 37: 1765–1770.
9. Kuchinad A, Schweinhardt P, Seminowicz DA, Wood PB, Chizh BA, et al. (2007) Accelerated brain gray matter loss in fibromyalgia patients: premature aging of the brain? J Neurosci 27: 4004–4007.
10. Tracey I, Bushnell MC (2009) How neuroimaging studies have challenged us to rethink: is chronic pain a disease? J Pain 10: 1113–1120.
11. Franke K, Ziegler G, Kloppel S, Gaser C (2010) Estimating the age of healthy subjects from T1-weighted MRI scans using kernel methods: exploring the influence of various parameters. Neuroimage 50: 883–892.
12. Draganski B, May A (2008) Training-induced structural changes in the adult human brain. Behav Brain Res 192: 137–142.
13. Adkins DL, Boychuk J, Remple MS, Kleim JA (2006) Motor training induces experience-specific patterns of plasticity across motor cortex and spinal cord. J Appl Physiol 101: 1776–1782.
14. Duerden EG, Laverdure-Dupont D (2008) Practice makes cortex. J Neurosci 28: 8655–8657.
15. Draganski B, Moser T, Lummel N, Ganssbauer S, Bogdahn U, et al. (2006) Decrease of thalamic gray matter following limb amputation. Neuroimage 31: 951–957.
16. Nikolajsen L, Brandsborg B, Lucht U, Jensen TS, Kehlet H (2006) Chronic pain following total hip arthroplasty: a nationwide questionnaire study. Acta Anaesthesiol Scand 50: 495–500.
17. Rodriguez-Raecke R, Niemeier A, Ihle K, Ruether W, May A (2009) Brain gray matter decrease in chronic pain is the consequence and not the cause of pain. J Neurosci 29: 13746–13750.
18. Beck AT, Ward CH, Mendelson M, Mock J, Erbaugh J (1961) An inventory for measuring depression. Arch Gen Psychiatry 4: 561–571.
19. Franke G (2002) Die Symptom-Checkliste nach L.R. Derogatis - Manual. Göttingen Beltz Test Verlag.
20. Geissner E (1995) The Pain Perception Scale–a differentiated and change-sensitive scale for assessing chronic and acute pain. Rehabilitation (Stuttg) 34: XXXV–XLIII.
21. Bullinger M, Kirchberger I (1998) SF-36 - Fragebogen zum Gesundheitszustand. Hand-anweisung. Göttingen: Hogrefe.
22. Ashburner J, Friston KJ (2000) Voxel-based morphometry–the methods. Neuroimage 11: 805–821.

23. Good CD, Johnsrude IS, Ashburner J, Henson RN, Friston KJ, et al. (2001) A voxel-based morphometric study of ageing in 465 normal adult human brains. Neuroimage 14: 21–36.
24. Baliki MN, Chialvo DR, Geha PY, Levy RM, Harden RN, et al. (2006) Chronic pain and the emotional brain: specific brain activity associated with spontaneous fluctuations of intensity of chronic back pain. J Neurosci 26: 12165–12173.
25. Lutz J, Jager L, de Quervain D, Krauseneck T, Padberg F, et al. (2008) White and gray matter abnormalities in the brain of patients with fibromyalgia: a diffusion-tensor and volumetric imaging study. Arthritis Rheum 58: 3960–3969.
26. Wrigley PJ, Gustin SM, Macey PM, Nash PG, Gandevia SC, et al. (2008) Anatomical Changes in Human Motor Cortex and Motor Pathways following Complete Thoracic Spinal Cord Injury. Cereb Cortex 19: 224–232.
27. Schmidt-Wilcke T, Hierlmeier S, Leinisch E (2010) Altered Regional Brain Morphology in Patients With Chronic Facial Pain. Headache.
28. Geha PY, Baliki MN, Harden RN, Bauer WR, Parrish TB, et al. (2008) The brain in chronic CRPS pain: abnormal gray-white matter interactions in emotional and autonomic regions. Neuron 60: 570–581.
29. Brazier J, Roberts J, Deverill M (2002) The estimation of a preference-based measure of health from the SF-36. J Health Econ 21: 271–292.
30. Draganski B, Gaser C, Busch V, Schuierer G, Bogdahn U, et al. (2004) Neuroplasticity: changes in grey matter induced by training. Nature 427: 311–312.
31. Boyke J, Driemeyer J, Gaser C, Buchel C, May A (2008) Training-induced brain structure changes in the elderly. J Neurosci 28: 7031–7035.
32. Driemeyer J, Boyke J, Gaser C, Buchel C, May A (2008) Changes in gray matter induced by learning–revisited. PLoS ONE 3: e2669.
33. May A, Hajak G, Ganssbauer S, Steffens T, Langguth B, et al. (2007) Structural brain alterations following 5 days of intervention: dynamic aspects of neuroplasticity. Cereb Cortex 17: 205–210.
34. Teutsch S, Herken W, Bingel U, Schoell E, May A (2008) Changes in brain gray matter due to repetitive painful stimulation. Neuroimage 42: 845–849.
35. Flor H, Braun C, Elbert T, Birbaumer N (1997) Extensive reorganization of primary somatosensory cortex in chronic back pain patients. Neurosci Lett 224: 5–8.
36. Flor H, Denke C, Schaefer M, Grusser S (2001) Effect of sensory discrimination training on cortical reorganisation and phantom limb pain. Lancet 357: 1763–1764.
37. Swart CM, Stins JF, Beek PJ (2009) Cortical changes in complex regional pain syndrome (CRPS). Eur J Pain 13: 902–907.
38. Maihofner C, Baron R, DeCol R, Binder A, Birklein F, et al. (2007) The motor system shows adaptive changes in complex regional pain syndrome. Brain 130: 2671–2687.
39. Fontaine D, Hamani C, Lozano A (2009) Efficacy and safety of motor cortex stimulation for chronic neuropathic pain: critical review of the literature. J Neurosurg 110: 251–256.
40. Levy R, Deer TR, Henderson J (2010) Intracranial neurostimulation for pain control: a review. Pain Physician 13: 157–165.
41. Antal A, Brepohl N, Poreisz C, Boros K, Csifcsak G, et al. (2008) Transcranial direct current stimulation over somatosensory cortex decreases experimentally induced acute pain perception. Clin J Pain 24: 56–63.
42. Teepker M, Hotzel J, Timmesfeld N, Reis J, Mylius V, et al. (2010) Low-frequency rTMS of the vertex in the prophylactic treatment of migraine. Cephalalgia 30: 137–144.
43. O'Connell N, Wand B, Marston L, Spencer S, Desouza L (2010) Non-invasive brain stimulation techniques for chronic pain. A report of a Cochrane systematic review and meta-analysis. Eur J Phys Rehabil Med 47: 309–326.
44. Tsao H, Galea MP, Hodges PW (2008) Reorganization of the motor cortex is associated with postural control deficits in recurrent low back pain. Brain 131: 2161–2171.
45. Puri BK, Agour M, Gunatilake KD, Fernando KA, Gurusinghe AI, et al. (2010) Reduction in left supplementary motor area grey matter in adult female fibromyalgia sufferers with marked fatigue and without affective disorder: a pilot controlled 3-T magnetic resonance imaging voxel-based morphometry study. J Int Med Res 38: 1468–1472.
46. Gwilym SE, Fillipini N, Douaud G, Carr AJ, Tracey I (2010) Thalamic atrophy associated with painful osteoarthritis of the hip is reversible after arthroplasty; a longitudinal voxel-based-morphometric study. Arthritis Rheum.
47. Seminowicz DA, Wideman TH, Naso L, Hatami-Khoroushahi Z, Fallatah S, et al. (2011) Effective treatment of chronic low back pain in humans reverses abnormal brain anatomy and function. J Neurosci 31: 7540–7550.
48. May A, Gaser C (2006) Magnetic resonance-based morphometry: a window into structural plasticity of the brain. Curr Opin Neurol 19: 407–411.
49. Schmidt-Wilcke T, Leinisch E, Straube A, Kampfe N, Draganski B, et al. (2005) Gray matter decrease in patients with chronic tension type headache. Neurology 65: 1483–1486.
50. May A (2009) Morphing voxels: the hype around structural imaging of headache patients. Brain 132(Pt 6): 1419–1425.

11

Cortical Thickness Mapping to Identify Focal Osteoporosis in Patients with Hip Fracture

Kenneth E. S. Poole[1]*, Graham M. Treece[2], Paul M. Mayhew[1], Jan Vaculík[3], Pavel Dungl[3], Martin Horák[4], Jan J. Štěpán[5], Andrew H. Gee[2]

1 Department of Medicine, University of Cambridge, Cambridge, Cambridgeshire, United Kingdom, 2 Department of Engineering, University of Cambridge, Cambridge, Cambridgeshire, United Kingdom, 3 Department of Orthopaedics, Faculty of Medicine, Charles University Prague and Bulovka Hospital, Prague, Czech Republic, 4 Department of Radiology, Homolka Hospital, Prague, Czech Republic, 5 Department of Rheumatology, Faculty of Medicine 1, Charles University Prague and Institute of Rheumatology, Prague, Czech Republic

Abstract

Background: Individuals with osteoporosis are predisposed to hip fracture during trips, stumbles or falls, but half of all hip fractures occur in those without generalised osteoporosis. By analysing ordinary clinical CT scans using a novel cortical thickness mapping technique, we discovered patches of markedly thinner bone at fracture-prone regions in the femurs of women with acute hip fracture compared with controls.

Methods: We analysed CT scans from 75 female volunteers with acute fracture and 75 age- and sex-matched controls. We classified the fracture location as femoral neck or trochanteric before creating bone thickness maps of the outer 'cortical' shell of the intact contra-lateral hip. After registration of each bone to an average femur shape and statistical parametric mapping, we were able to visualise and quantify statistically significant foci of thinner cortical bone associated with each fracture type, assuming good symmetry of bone structure between the intact and fractured hip. The technique allowed us to pinpoint systematic differences and display the results on a 3D average femur shape model.

Findings: The cortex was generally thinner in femoral neck fracture cases than controls. More striking were several discrete patches of statistically significant thinner bone of up to 30%, which coincided with common sites of fracture initiation (femoral neck or trochanteric).

Interpretation: Femoral neck fracture patients had a thumbnail-sized patch of focal osteoporosis at the upper head-neck junction. This region coincided with a weak part of the femur, prone to both spontaneous 'tensile' fractures of the femoral neck, and as a site of crack initiation when falling sideways. Current hip fracture prevention strategies are based on case finding: they involve clinical risk factor estimation to determine the need for single-plane bone density measurement within a standard region of interest (ROI) of the femoral neck. The precise sites of focal osteoporosis that we have identified are overlooked by current 2D bone densitometry methods.

Editor: Xing-Ming Shi, Georgia Health Sciences University, United States of America

Funding: This analysis was funded by Arthritis Research UK via a Clinician Scientist Fellowship award to KESP. Cambridge National Institute for Health Research Biomedical Research Centre funded PMM. The Evelyn Trust funded GMT. The funders had no role in study design, data collection and analysis, decision to publish, or preparation of the manuscript.

Competing Interests: GMT and KESP are co-inventors on a related GB patent application A method of determining the cortical thickness of a patients bone (GB0917524.1 Accurate cortical thickness measurement from clinical CT data, A method of determining the cortical thickness of a patients bone. International (PCT) Patent Application No PCT/GB2010/051671, CU ref: TRE-2326-09-01, International search ref: PC925159WO. Title: Image data processing systems, Inventors: G.M. Treece & K.E.S Poole). The other authors have declared that no competing interests exist.

* E-mail: kp254@nhs.net

Introduction

The annual incidence of hip fractures is projected to rise fourfold to 6.3 million worldwide by 2050, because of the exponentially increasing risk of fracture as people live longer. Studying femoral neck and trochanteric fractures is therefore a health priority [1]. In older people, the proximal femur breaks when the loads placed on it overcome its strength, with common loading scenarios being sideways falls, stumbles or sudden unusual movements [2]. However, a spontaneous or 'impact-free' mechanism accounts for up to 6% of hip fractures (fig. 1) [3,4]. We know that women with osteoporosis (who have generally thinner and more porous bones) are more likely to suffer hip fracture, but most people who will sustain hip fracture do not have generalised osteoporosis [5]. We also know that the outer 'cortical' bone of the femur where fractures initiate [6] thins rapidly with age [7,8], is a key determinant of bone strength and fracture risk [9–13] and responds well to certain osteoporosis drugs [14,15]. Here we ask; Is there a pattern of femoral bone thinning common to hip fracture patients and, if so, is it generalised or focal? Could focal osteoporosis of the femur be a cause of hip fracture in the elderly? The answer to these questions might illuminate why hip fractures tend to initiate in particular zones (fig. 1).

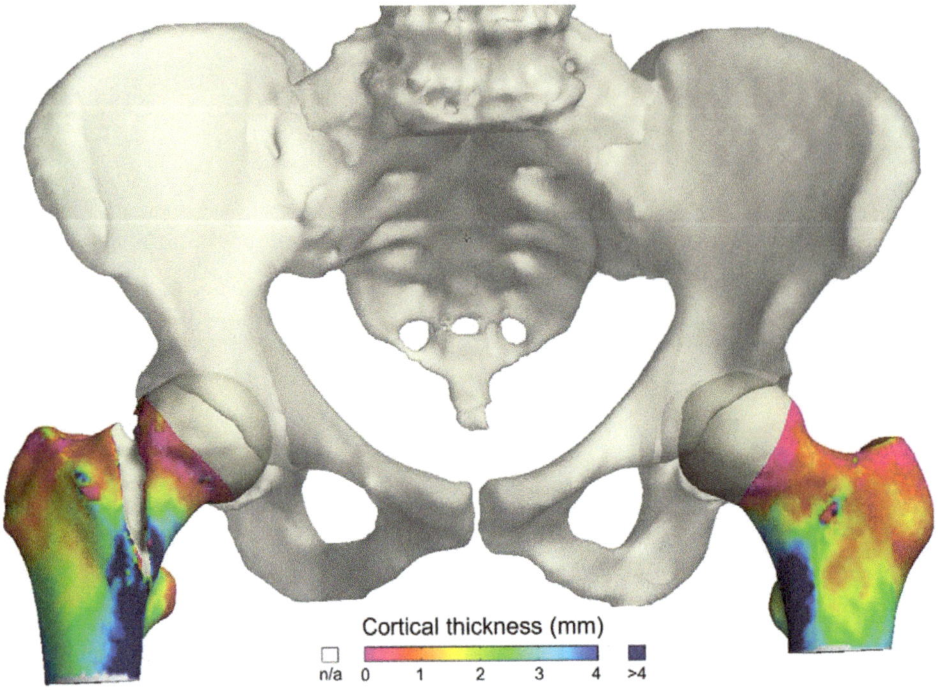

Figure 1. Cortical Thickness Colour Mapping using ordinary clinical CT data. Femora and pelvis from an 84-year-old osteoporotic female who sustained a fracture without falling. She felt her right hip break as she placed her right foot on a low step. Femoral neck BMD was 0.46 g/cm2, T score −3.3. From the Arthritis Research UK FEMCO study (07/H0305/61).

A new CT image processing technique [16] allows us to display cortical thickness as a colour map over the bone surface, with several thousand independent measurements across each proximal femur and sufficient sensitivity to detect even small differences (~30 microns) when expressed systematically by a suitably sized cohort. We use it here to pinpoint differences in bone thickness between women with and without hip fracture. We examined the contra-lateral side as a surrogate for the broken hip in these female fracture patients, having previously identified symmetry in femoral neck cortical thickness [8].

Methods

From 2006 to 2009, women admitted to Bulovka University Hospital, Prague with an acute hip fracture were consented to the pragmatic 'Surgical treatment of the hip joint in trauma' study (PI Professor P Dungl), part of which involved a clinical CT scan of both hips before surgical fixation [17]. Participants were positioned on the Siemens two-compartment Osteo phantom and a single CT scan (either Siemens Sensation 40 or 16 detector, B10/20 kernel, ≤1 mm reconstructed slice thickness) was performed including both hips from above the acetabulum to just below the lesser trochanter. Women were aged over 50, were awaiting surgical repair of a cervical or trochanteric fracture and had sustained a low energy injury. Women were excluded if they had metalwork in either hip, high trauma injury, metastatic cancer, unilateral bone disease, subtrochanteric fracture or terminal illness. Using the same criteria, a convenience control sample of older women without fracture was recruited by invitation at rheumatology clinics and two residential care centres in the same districts of Prague. From 204 invitations, 108 fracture-free women responded of whom 81 were eligible for CT scanning at Homolka hospital, Prague (Siemens Sensation 16 detector B20 kernel, ≤1mm reconstructed slice thickness). At the image quality control step, 6 scans were excluded (due to insufficient scan length or undisclosed metalwork) leaving 75 female controls. One age-matched case was selected for each of the 75 eligible control participants, from the total sample of 242 women with hip fracture. Where precise birth year age matching was not possible, the next nearest matching case was selected up to a maximum 5-year age difference. The final sample taken forward for cortical thickness mapping comprised 150 femurs from 75 women in each group (mean ages of femoral neck fracture cases 78.1+/−7.1 years, trochanteric fracture cases 75.2+/−7.9, controls 76.6+/−7.3 years). There were 36 femoral neck fractures and 39 trochanteric fractures.

The analysis method is illustrated in figure 2. Anonymised axial dicom images were received in Cambridge via the secure DICOM internet connection ePACS (ICZ, Brno, Czech Rep.) where they were reconstructed to classify fracture side and site according to AO criteria. Standard clinical hip bone density (2D areal DXA-equivalent) was measured in the 'total hip' region of interest (ROI) of each femur using QCTpro software (v4.2.3 Mindways, Austin, Texas, USA). The unfractured contralateral hip (or matching side in controls) was segmented semi-automatically in Stradwin v4.2 software (Treece, Gee, Cambridge) before mapping cortical thickness at approximately 6000 surface points per femur. Cortical thickness was estimated from the CT data using the method described by Treece et al. [16]. By making reasonable assumptions about both the anatomy and the imaging blur, thickness can be measured to super-resolution accuracy across the entire proximal femur, apart from at the femoral head where the proximity of the acetabulum is problematic. The methodology has been validated against thickness measurements obtained from high resolution micro-CT scans of cadaveric femurs [16]. Analysis of the 150 thickness maps followed established practice within the neuroimaging community, who have pioneered techniques for statistical inference from dense, spatially correlated data. To account for variations in inter-subject morphology, each map was spatially realigned with a canonical femur surface using a B-spline free-form deformation calculated by the iterative closest point registration algorithm [18]. The spatially normalized maps were then smoothed with a 10 mm full-width-half-maximum filter. We investigated differences in cortical thickness between i) femoral neck fractures (n36) and all controls or ii) trochanteric fractures (n39) and all controls. Formal inference was accomplished by statistical parametric mapping (SPM) [19], as implemented in the SurfStat package [20]. Model effects were group (case*control), age, height and weight. Missing height and weight values (2 fracture cases) were replaced with group mean values. T-statistics were calculated to test the significance of the group term. Random field theory then furnished p-values, corrected for multiple comparisons to control the overall image-wise chance of false positives. Figure 3 shows corrected p maps based on the magnitude of peaks (sensitive to focal effects) and on the extent of connected clusters exceeding an uncorrected p-value threshold of 0.001 (sensitive to distributed effects). All participants with fracture gave written informed consent. Control participants gave verbal consent which was documented in the medical notes as agreed with the Ethics Committee. Ethics committees approved the study in the Czech Republic (Ethical Committee of the Institute of Rheumatology and Ethical Committee of Bulovka Hospital, ref IRB0002384101) and in the UK (Cambridgeshire 4, ref 07/H0305/61).

Results

Percentage differences in cortical thickness between each hip fracture group and the control group were displayed on an average right femur surface map using a colour scale. Views from several anatomical planes were chosen to illustrate the differences (femoral neck fractures vs. controls; fig. 3 *left upper panel* and trochanteric fractures vs controls; fig. 3 *right upper panel*). Similar maps were created to visualise the statistical significance of differences (fig 3. *lower panels*). Several distinct patches of up to 30% thinner cortical bone were identified in fracture cases which coincided with typical sites of hip fracture. No regions of statistically significant thicker bone were seen in fracture cases. WHO-defined osteoporosis (a total hip DXA-equivalent bone mineral density T score <-2.5) was present in less than half of hip fracture patients (31/75, 41.3%) and 9/75 (12%) controls. The age, height and weight adjusted values for the clusters of thinner bone associated with each fracture type are shown in table 1. The mean, unadjusted value of whole proximal femur cortical thickness among femoral neck fracture patients was 1.20 mm±0.17 mm, compared with a value of 1.25 mm±0.20 mm among trochanteric fracture patients and 1.30 mm±0.21 mm among controls (ANOVA $p = 0.0388$). Whole femur cortical thickness was statistically significantly lower in femoral neck fracture compared with control (Dunnett's values* were 0.012 for neck fracture, $p = 0.024$, and -0.04 for trochanteric fracture, $p = 0.34$; *[absolute difference in sample means] - [least significant difference]). The age and weight terms were significant within the 150 femurs (age range 55–98 and weight range 40–89 kg). Significant thinning of approximately 0.02 mm per year from age 55–98 was apparent in the infero-medial region. Significant thickening of approximately 0.02 mm per kilogram was evident in a similar infero-medial region.

Discussion

We used cortical thickness mapping to explore differences between women with and without recent hip fracture and identified generalised thinning of the femoral cortex in fracture patients. We also discovered focal differences manifest as several well-defined patches of markedly thinner femoral cortex in hip fracture patients compared to controls. Since osteoporosis is defined as microarchitectural deterioration of bone tissue, we consider that these areas of focally thinner bone are best described as patches of focal osteoporosis (fig. 4, right panel). The patches were evident at common sites involved in fracture, the most severe being a thumbnail-sized patch of up to 30% thinner bone at the head-neck junction in patients with femoral neck fracture (figs. 3, 4 and 5). Focal osteoporosis at the head-neck junction may play an important role in fractures associated with falls, and might even be involved in 'spontaneous' hip fracture on rare occasions. While the locations of the patches of focal osteoporosis appear to be critical in determining fracture type, we cannot judge whether they are involved in causing hip fracture, which requires prospective research. However it is noteworthy that among all the bone structural parameters measured in the largest prospective study of hip CT in older men and women conducted to date, cortical thickness estimates from a supero-anterior part of the femoral neck were the best predictor of subsequent hip fracture [9].

We assume that a fall onto or near the hip was the principal fracture mechanism in these women, but we did not routinely collect information on how these women fell, a priority for future work. The largest patch of thinner femoral cortex that we identified (fig 3c) appears to correspond to a key site of fracture initiation in a simulation of femoral neck fracture during a sideways fall to the ground [21]. Although the women we studied with trochanteric fracture also had patches of thinner bone in

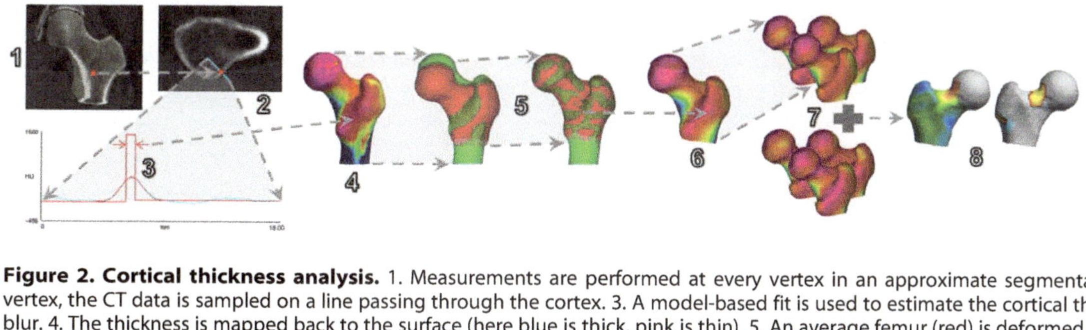

Figure 2. Cortical thickness analysis. 1. Measurements are performed at every vertex in an approximate segmentation of the hip. 2. At each vertex, the CT data is sampled on a line passing through the cortex. 3. A model-based fit is used to estimate the cortical thickness, allowing for image blur. 4. The thickness is mapped back to the surface (here blue is thick, pink is thin). 5. An average femur (red) is deformed to match the current femur (green). 6. Thickness estimates are then transferred to the average femoral surface and smoothed. 7. This process is repeated for all subjects, producing subject-specific thickness estimates all mapped to the same, average surface. 8. The data is analysed using statistical parametric mapping, to obtain mean thickness differences between groups and also the significance of these differences.

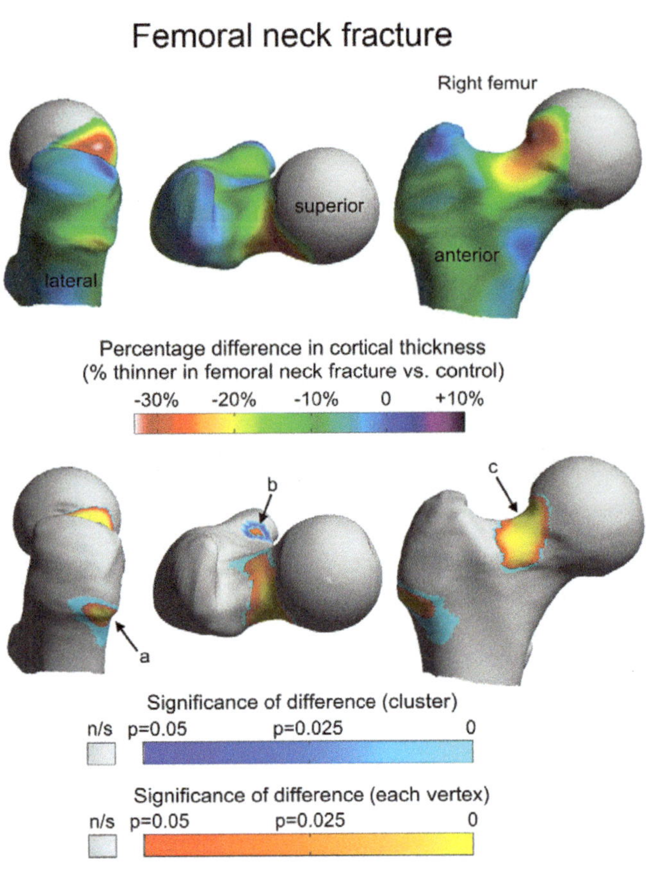

Figure 3. Results for femoral neck fracture (left) and trochanteric fracture (right). Upper colour maps show the average percentage difference in cortical thickness for each fracture type versus control (displayed on an average right femur model). The lower colour maps are the significance of the differences adjusted for age, height and weight, either point by point (vertex) or as a whole patch (blue clusters). Note that all the blue clusters extend uninterrupted beneath their respective orange/yellow vertices. Table 1 gives adjusted thickness values and significance of the clusters a–e.

fracture-relevant zones (fig. 3d and 3e), it is not clear whether they correspond to trochanteric fracture initiation sites in the relevant simulations [21]. Nevertheless, it is interesting to note that the focally thin bone in the lateral facet of the greater trochanter (fig. 3d) in the trochanteric fracture patients coincided with one of the insertion sites of gluteus medius, which receives considerable force during locomotion.

While most hip fractures in the elderly are a result of injurious falls, spontaneous fractures of the femoral neck prior to falls have been implicated in up to 6% of cases, translating to more than

Table 1. Details of thinner patches of femoral cortex in hip fracture.

Hip fracture type	**Location of 'cluster' Patch where bone cortex was thinner in hip fracture cases**	**Mean adjusted cortical thickness in cluster (Cases)**		**Mean adjusted cortical thickness in cluster (Cluster)**		**p value for difference**
		Millimetres	**±SD**	**Millimetres**	**±SD**	
Femoral neck fractures						
Patch a (fig.3a)	Greater trochanter	1.14	0.15	1.34	0.26	0.00407
Patch b (fig.3b)	Lesser trochanter	0.85	0.16	0.98	0.19	0.0319
Patch c (fig.3c)	Head-neck junction	0.62	0.10	0.77	0.14	0.00000350
Trochanteric fractures						
Patch d (fig.3d)	Greater trochanter	1.05	0.25	1.21	0.27	0.0237
Patch e (fig.3e)	Lesser trochanter	0.78	0.15	0.88	0.17	0.0108

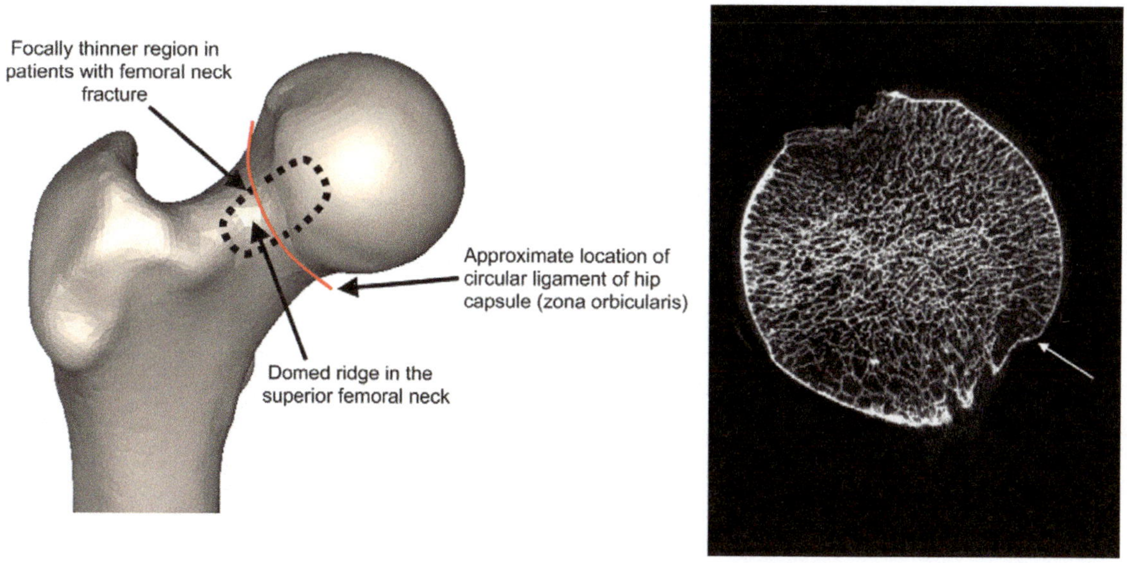

Figure 4. Anatomical context of focal thinning in women with femoral neck fracture. The left pane is a right proximal femur model seen from the front. The thin patch of cortex (fig 3c) in femoral neck fracture patients occurs on the domed ridge called the femoral neck eminence [25]. The right pane is a high resolution CT image through the femoral head of a 90 year old female (aBMD total hip T-score −1.9) which suggests that the patch is osteoporotic with microarchitectural thinning (white arrow). Femur courtesy of the Melbourne Femur Collection, Chairman Professor John Clement (Melbourne Dental School).

4000 hip fractures annually in the UK [22]. Previously, several research groups have reproduced these impact-free hip fractures in cadaveric femurs by simulating either the effects of increasing loads in stance or sudden large hip flexor muscle contractions. In Cristofolini's specimens, increasing the load by simulating one-legged stance (as in fig. 5b), led to crack initiation at the junction between the femoral head and neck, with the subsequent catastrophic failure of the femur closely resembling that observed in our patient with impact-free fracture (fig. 1) [3]. Likewise simulating sudden psoas muscle contraction (as happens when a person attempts to stabilise their trunk on a fixed leg during a slip or stumble) led to subcapital fracture in a similar location [23]. The conserved patch of focal osteoporosis we identified among our femoral neck fracture patients (fig. 3c) appears to correspond with the sites of high tensile stress induced in those simulations. In the light of our findings we wonder what effect osteoporosis medicines might have on the thin patches of bone and in particular if strengthening the thin areas could prevent stumbling-induced or spontaneous hip fractures. Analysis of large clinical trials with serial CT is needed to address this question.

We are currently unable to answer a key question generated by these results; namely how did the focal patches of thin cortex arise? Several intriguing ideas come from histological and macroscopic studies of the head-neck junction in patients with fracture and from cadavers. Freeman et al. discovered that in fracture specimens, the underlying bone from the head-neck junction frequently contains microcallus, considered to be evidence of tensile fatigue damage [24]. Modelling the behaviour of the head-neck junction during habitual locomotion and falls is therefore a priority for biomechanics research. Although there were marked age and weight effects within the women we studied, the decreasing cortical thickness associated with age and increasing thickness associated with weight affected the inferior femur; i.e. on the opposite side of the femoral neck to the patch of focally thin bone. Thus we assume that neither younger nor heavier women were necessarily protected from having a thin cortex at the head-neck junction. The patch of focal osteoporosis in femoral neck fracture patients corresponds macroscopically with the junction between femoral head cartilage and bone, and tracks along the domed ridge running along the top of the femoral neck (called the femoral neck eminentia, or eminence [25], fig. 4). Since the thin cortical bone is so well circumscribed at this site, we concur with Panzer et al. in describing the differences as 'focal osteoporosis', but acknowledge that higher resolution and histological studies would be useful to further characterise the cortical and sub-cortical bone [26]. The circular fibres of the hip capsule (the zona orbicularis) also encircle the femoral neck at the focally thin patch. Pitt and others described a mechanical, abrasive action of the overlying hip capsule, ligaments and psoas muscle at this patch that commonly results in a 'reaction area' with occasional underlying radiolucency. This lucency can be appreciated on plain x-rays and is known to radiologists as 'Pitt's Pit' [27]. Studies of the underlying histology of this zone in femoral neck fracture cases are clearly warranted [28,29], and Pitt suggested that the zone could be involved in hip fracture pathogenesis.

This work has several weaknesses, namely pragmatic case selection, the use of a convenience sample of controls and reliance on the intact hip as a surrogate for the fractured hip. The results need replication in a better-characterised population sample, with particular attention to recalled injury mechanism. Statistical Parametric Mapping does not indicate causality; for instance it is possible (but unlikely) that controls could have substantial thickening of bone at various sites through unknown mechanisms. Finally, although studying the cortex is important in determining bone strength, alternative methods such as finite element (FE) models use whole bone biomechanics, and can therefore be informative in determining how and why individuals fracture their hips (as reviewed recently by Cristofolini et al [30]). In this regard, it is interesting to note that our cortical thickness maps have the potential to be converted into inner and outer surfaces for optimal delineation of cortical and trabecular compartments, which may

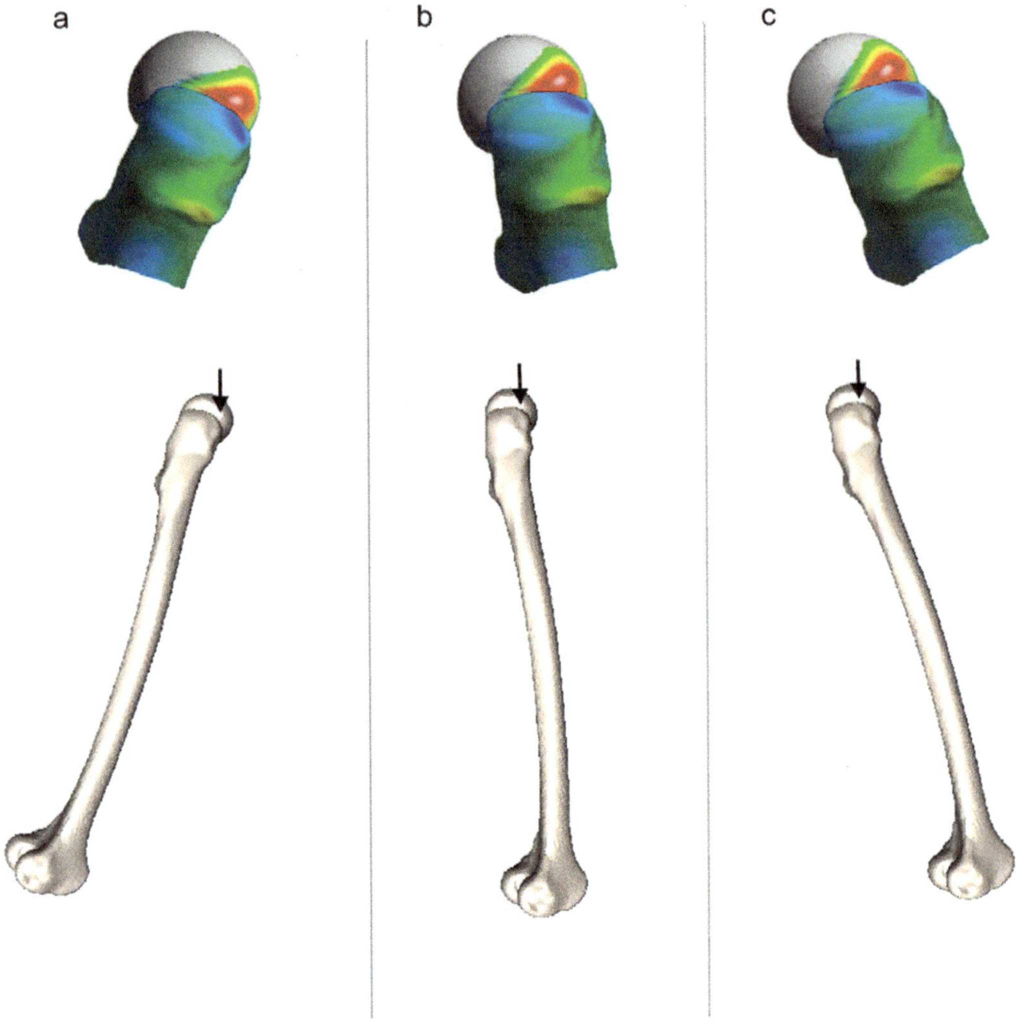

Figure 5. Approximate orientation of the focally thin (red) zone during the different phases of gait. Right femur (a) toe-off, (b) single leg stance and (c) heel strike. A slightly modified stance position (b) conferred the greatest risk of spontaneous femoral neck fracture in the laboratory simulations of Cristofolini et al [3]. The focally thin patch we identified coincides with a region of high tensile stress during simulations of spontaneous fracture.

help to improve the FE methods that currently assume a constant cortical thickness throughout the bone.

In related work, Li et al applied SPM to 3D density maps of femurs and discovered focal regions where clustered voxels of bone density differed significantly between hip fracture cases and controls [31]. In their analysis, several fracture-relevant density ROI's showed promise in defining a hip fracture phenotype. The fact that Li's head-neck junction femoral ROI based on volumetric density appears to coincide with the focally thinner femoral cortex we find at the head-neck junction suggests that having poor quality bone here is particularly concerning for future fracture risk. Previous prospective studies indicated that combining measures (e.g one measure of density, one of cortical thickness and one of bone shape) resulted in the optimum prediction of incident hip fracture [11,32]. However, large prospective studies are necessary to determine what thresholds of cortical thickness or density in these newly discovered zones are predictive of hip fracture and might be a trigger for intervention in an individual. Our work is useful in defining ROI's for cortical bone analysis that can then be taken forward for testing in prospective studies. Current hip fracture prevention strategies are based on case finding: they involve clinical risk factor estimation to determine the need for single plane bone density measurement within a standard femoral neck ROI. The precise sites of focal osteoporosis that we have now identified are overlooked by current 2D bone densitometry methods.

Acknowledgments

We thank Dr Jonathan Reeve, Department of Medicine, University of Cambridge, UK for his help with the Prague-Cambridge collaboration and for guidance on the selection of appropriate control participants.

Author Contributions

Conceived and designed the experiments: KESP PMM JS MH JV PD GMT AHG. Performed the experiments: KESP PMM GMT AHG. Analyzed the data: KESP AHG GMT. Contributed reagents/materials/analysis tools: JS MH JV PD PMM. Wrote the paper: KESP GMT AHG PMM JS MH JV PD. Designed the study to recruit patients with hip fracture in Prague: JV PD. Methods section critical review: JV PD.

References

1. Pulkkinen P, Gluer CC, Jamsa T (2011) Investigation of differences between hip fracture types: a worthy strategy for improved risk assessment and fracture prevention. Bone 49: 600–604.
2. Sievanen H, Kannus P, Jarvinen TL (2007) Bone quality: an empty term. PLoS Med 4: e27.
3. Cristofolini L, Juszczyk M, Martelli S, Taddei F, Viceconti M (2007) In vitro replication of spontaneous fractures of the proximal human femur. J Biomech 40: 2837–2845.
4. Yli-Kyyny T, Tamminen I, Syri J, Venesmaa P, Kröger H (2011) Bilateral hip pain. The Lancet 377: 2248.
5. Wainwright SA, Marshall LM, Ensrud KE, Cauley JA, Black DM, et al. (2005) Hip fracture in women without osteoporosis. J Clin Endocrinol Metab 90: 2787–2793.
6. de Bakker PM, Manske SL, Ebacher V, Oxland TR, Cripton PA, et al. (2009) During sideways falls proximal femur fractures initiate in the superolateral cortex: evidence from high-speed video of simulated fractures. J Biomech 42: 1917–1925.
7. Feik SA, Thomas CD, Clement JG (1997) Age-related changes in cortical porosity of the midshaft of the human femur. J Anat 191 (Pt 3): 407–416.
8. Poole KE, Mayhew PM, Rose CM, Brown JK, Bearcroft PJ, et al. (2010) Changing structure of the femoral neck across the adult female lifespan. J Bone Miner Res 25: 482–491.
9. Johannesdottir F, Poole KE, Reeve J, Siggeirsdottir K, Aspelund T, et al. (2011) Distribution of cortical bone in the femoral neck and hip fracture: a prospective case-control analysis of 143 incident hip fractures; the AGES-REYKJAVIK Study. Bone 48: 1268–1276.
10. Mayhew PM, Thomas CD, Clement JG, Loveridge N, Beck TJ, et al. (2005) Relation between age, femoral neck cortical stability, and hip fracture risk. Lancet 366: 129–135.
11. Gluer CC, Cummings SR, Pressman A, Li J, Gluer K, et al. (1994) Prediction of hip fractures from pelvic radiographs: the study of osteoporotic fractures. The Study of Osteoporotic Fractures Research Group. J Bone Miner Res 9: 671–677.
12. Hansen S, Jensen JE, Ahrberg F, Hauge EM, Brixen K (2011) The combination of structural parameters and areal bone mineral density improves relation to proximal femur strength: an in vitro study with high-resolution peripheral quantitative computed tomography. Calcif Tissue Int 89: 335–346.
13. Holzer G, von Skrbensky G, Holzer LA, Pichl W (2009) Hip fractures and the contribution of cortical versus trabecular bone to femoral neck strength. J Bone Miner Res 24: 468–474.
14. Borggrefe J, Graeff C, Nickelsen TN, Marin F, Gluer CC (2009) Quantitative Computed Tomography Assessment of the Effects of 24 months of Teriparatide Treatment on 3-D Femoral Neck Bone Distribution, Geometry and Bone Strength: Results from the EUROFORS Study. J Bone Miner Res 25: 472–481.
15. Poole KE, Treece GM, Ridgway GR, Mayhew PM, Borggrefe J, et al. (2011) Targeted regeneration of bone in the osteoporotic human femur. PLoS One 6: e16190.
16. Treece GM, Gee AH, Mayhew PM, Poole KE (2010) High resolution cortical bone thickness measurement from clinical CT data. Med Image Anal 14: 276–290.
17. Vaculík J, Malkus T, Majerníček M, Podškubka A, Dungl P (2007) Incidence of proximal femoral fractures. Ortopedie 1: 62–68.
18. Rueckert D, Frangi AF, Schnabel JA (2003) Automatic construction of 3-D statistical deformation models of the brain using nonrigid registration. IEEE Trans Med Imaging 22: 1014–1025.
19. Friston KJ, Holmes AP, Worsley KJ, Poline J-P, Frith CD, et al. (1994) Statistical parametric maps in functional imaging: A general linear approach. Human Brain Mapping 2: 189–210.
20. Worsley K, Taylor J, Carbonell F, Chung M, Duerden E, et al. (2009) SurfStat: A Matlab toolbox for the statistical analysis of univariate and multivariate surface and volumetric data using linear mixed effects models and random field theory. NeuroImage Organization for Human Brain Mapping 2009 Annual Meeting 47: S102.
21. Bessho M, Ohnishi I, Matsumoto T, Ohashi S, Matsuyama J, et al. (2009) Prediction of proximal femur strength using a CT-based nonlinear finite element method: differences in predicted fracture load and site with changing load and boundary conditions. Bone 45: 226–231.
22. Parker MJ, Twemlow TR (1997) Spontaneous hip fractures, 44/872 in a prospective study. Acta Orthop Scand 68: 325–326.
23. Yang KH, Shen KL, Demetropoulos CK, King AI, Kolodziej P, et al. (1996) The relationship between loading conditions and fracture patterns of the proximal femur. Journal of Biomechanical Engineering-Transactions of the Asme 118: 575–578.
24. Freeman MA, Todd RC, Pirie CJ (1974) The role of fatigue in the pathogenesis of senile femoral neck fractures. J Bone Joint Surg Br 56-B: 698–702.
25. Odgers PNB (1931) Two details about the neck of the femur: (1) The eminentia. (2) The empreinte. Journal of Anatomy 65: 352–U321.
26. Panzer S, Esch U, Abdulazim AN, Augat P (2010) Herniation pits and cystic-appearing lesions at the anterior femoral neck: an anatomical study by MSCT and microCT. Skeletal Radiol 39: 645–654.
27. Pitt M, Graham A, Shipman J, Birkby W (1982) Herniation pit of the femoral neck American Journal of Roentgenology 138 1115–1121.
28. Zebaze RM, Ghasem-Zadeh A, Bohte A, Iuliano-Burns S, Mirams M, et al. (2010) Intracortical remodelling and porosity in the distal radius and post-mortem femurs of women: a cross-sectional study. Lancet 375: 1729–1736.
29. Bell KL, Loveridge N, Power J, Garrahan N, Meggitt BF, et al. (1999) Regional differences in cortical porosity in the fractured femoral neck. Bone 24: 57–64.
30. Cristofolini L, Schileo E, Juszczyk M, Taddei F, Martelli S, et al. (2010) Mechanical testing of bones: the positive synergy of finite-element models and in vitro experiments. Philos Transact A Math Phys Eng Sci 368: 2725–2763.
31. Li W, Kornak J, Harris T, Keyak J, Li C, et al. (2009) Identify fracture-critical regions inside the proximal femur using statistical parametric mapping. Bone 44: 596–602.
32. Kaptoge S, Beck TJ, Reeve J, Stone KL, Hillier TA, et al. (2008) Prediction of incident hip fracture risk by femur geometry variables measured by hip structural analysis in the study of osteoporotic fractures. J Bone Miner Res 23: 1892–1904.

Increased Risk of Major Depression in the Three Years following a Femoral Neck Fracture–A National Population-Based Follow-Up Study

Chih-Yu Chang[1,2,3]⁹, Wen-Liang Chen[2]⁹, Yi-Fan Liou[3], Chih-Chi Ke[4], Hua-Chin Lee[2], Hui-Ling Huang[2,3], Li-Ping Ciou[3], Chu-Chung Chou[1,5,6], Mei-Chueh Yang[1], Shinn-Ying Ho[2,3]*, Yan-Ren Lin[1,2,5]*

1 Department of Emergency Medicine, Changhua Christian Hospital, Changhua, Taiwan, **2** Department of Biological Science and Technology, National Chiao Tung University, Hsinchu, Taiwan, **3** Institute of Bioinformatics and Systems Biology, National Chiao Tung University, Hsinchu, Taiwan, **4** Institute of Multimedia Engineering, National Chiao Tung University, Hsinchu, Taiwan, **5** School of Medicine, Chung Shan Medical University, Taichung, Taiwan, **6** School of Medicine, Taipei Medical University, Taipei, Taiwan

Abstract

Femoral neck fracture is common in the elderly, and its impact has increased in aging societies. Comorbidities, poor levels of activity and pain may contribute to the development of depression, but these factors have not been well addressed. This study aims to investigate the frequency and risk of major depression after a femoral neck fracture using a nationwide population-based study. The Taiwan Longitudinal Health Insurance Database was used in this study. A total of 4,547 patients who were hospitalized for femoral neck fracture within 2003 to 2007 were recruited as a study group; 13,641 matched non-fracture participants were enrolled as a comparison group. Each patient was prospectively followed for 3 years to monitor the occurrence of major depression. Cox proportional-hazards models were used to compute the risk of major depression between members of the study and comparison group after adjusting for residence and socio-demographic characteristics. The most common physical comorbidities that were present after the fracture were also analyzed. The incidences of major depression were 1.2% (n = 55) and 0.7% (n = 95) in the study and comparison groups, respectively. The stratified Cox proportional analysis showed a covariate-adjusted hazard ratio of major depression among patients with femoral neck fracture that was 1.82 times greater (95% CI, 1.30–2.53) than that of the comparison group. Most major depressive episodes (34.5%) presented within the first 200 days following the fracture. In conclusion, patients with a femoral neck fracture are at an increased risk of subsequent major depression. Most importantly, major depressive episodes mainly occurred within the first 200 days following the fracture.

Editor: Nick Harvey, University of Southampton, United Kingdom

Funding: The authors thank the National Chiao Tung University, Changhua Christian Hospital and National Science Council (NSC 102-2314-B-371-010) for financially supporting this research. The funders had no role in study design, data collection and analysis, decision to publish, or preparation of the manuscript.

Competing Interests: The authors have declared that no competing interests exist.

* E-mail: syho@mail.nctu.edu.tw (SYH); h6213.lac@gmail.com (YRL)

⁹ These authors contributed equally to this work.

Introduction

Femoral neck fracture is a common medical problem in patients over 60 years old. The incidence of this type of fracture is generally reported to be as high as 10%. [1–3] As the average life expectancy of the population increases, the number of femoral neck fractures increases each year; [4,5] one previous study further predicted that the incidence of hip fracture will double by the year 2050. [6] Globally, the impact of femoral neck fracture has increased in a number of developed (or developing) countries, especially in those with large populations of aged individuals. [6] Physical complications after femoral neck fracture, including increased comorbidities (infections and cardiovascular diseases; 50%), poor self-care in functional and routine activities (40%) and acute or chronic pain (60%), have been reported. [7–10] Overall, high mortality rates are associated with hip fracture; recent studies have reported that the one-year mortality rate ranged from 14.7% (Korea) to 41.7% (Spain). [11–14] Acute stress and poorer quality of life are usually present in most femoral neck fracture patients. Indeed, one study reported that 50 to 75% of patients with femoral neck fracture never reach their previous functional levels [8].

A depressive episode is characterized by disturbances in major life areas, including mood, psychomotor activity, cognition, and vegetative function. Furthermore, specific risk factors for depression have been reported: female gender, social isolation, low socioeconomic status, comorbid medical conditions, uncontrolled pain and functional impairment. [15] Therefore, we suspect that femoral neck fracture patients may experience major depression after injury related to several risk factors during the post-fracture period. Some previous studies have reported that hip fracture could increase the chance of suffering depressive symptoms (including anxiety and insomnia) in patients with older age or poorer quality of life; [16,17] however, no published study has focused on major depression. Unlike anxiety or insomnia, major depression presents with more severe psychosis symptoms, and the principles of diagnosis must establish, through rigorous criteria,

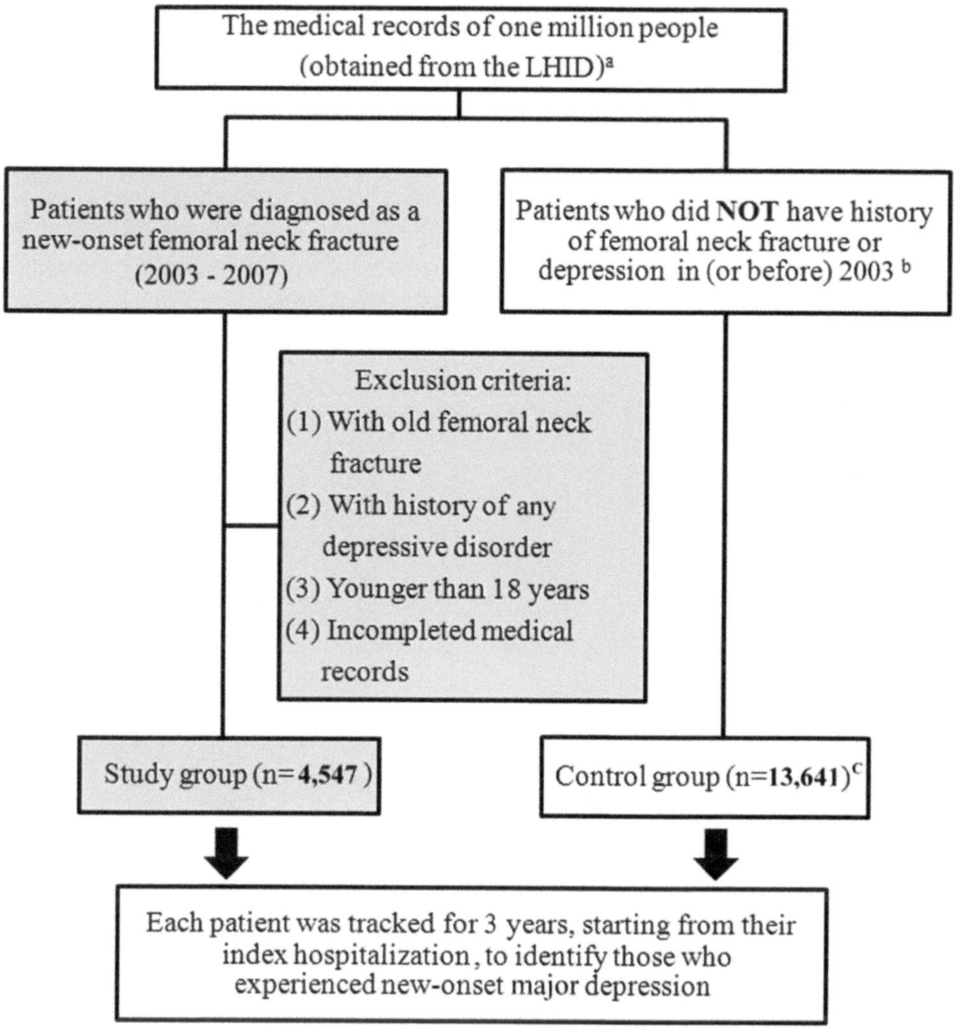

Figure 1. Flowchart of the selection methods in study and comparison patients. [a] The LHID contained medical records of one million people, which was randomly selected from the Taiwan National Health Insurance (NHI) program (supported by Taiwan government and over 98% of the Taiwanese population was enrolled in this program). [b] All personal medical records (diagnosis, treatments, medications), which had been recorded by different hospitals, were finally input into the NHI for requiring payments. Because almost all hospitals in Taiwan have joined the NHI; therefore, we could use it to screen patients' past histories. [C] Three comparison patients for each femoral neck fracture patient (matched with study group patients in terms of sex, age and years of healthcare use).

clinical distress and psychosocial impairment. In this study, we used a nationwide Taiwanese population database to prospectively examine the relationship between femoral neck fracture and the risk of major depression in a 3-year follow-up period in an Asian society. In our study, a diagnosis of femoral neck fracture was a warning sign to screen for increased risk of an impending major depressive episode.

Methods

2.1 Database

The Longitudinal Health Insurance Database (LHID) was used for this study; the LHID enables researchers to examine the use of medical services in Taiwan starting from the year 1995. The LHID is maintained by the Bureau of National Health Insurance and provided to scientists in Taiwan for research purposes. The Taiwanese government launched its National Health Insurance (NHI) program in 1995 to provide affordable health care for all people residing in Taiwan. As of 2007, over 98% of the Taiwanese population was enrolled in this program. The LHID contains original data collected from approximately one million people. The data used in this study were randomly sampled from data collected within 2003 to 2007. No significant differences were found in the gender and age distributions or average payroll-related insurance premiums between people in the LHID and all people served by the NHI program. The details of the generation of the LHID are published online by the Taiwan National Health Research Institutes.

2.2 Study Setting and Population

This is a prospective cohort study. During the period from January 1, 2003, to December 31, 2007, two patient groups were classified using the LHID, which included the study group (i.e., patients with femoral neck fracture) and the comparison group (i.e., patients without femoral neck fracture). The first hospitalization for treatment of femoral neck fracture during this period was coded as the index hospitalization. The comparison group's index

Table 1. Characteristics and personal histories between patients with femoral neck fracture and comparison patients.

	Patients with femoral neck fracture (n = 4,547)		Comparison patients (n = 13,641)		
	No.	%	No.	%	*p*-value
Gender					1.000
Male	2029	44.6	6087	44.6	
Female	2518	55.4	7554	55.4	
Mean age (y/o) (Mean±SD)	71.4±16.6		70.4±16.2		1.000
Age group (y/o)					1.000
18–39	324	7.1	972	7.1	
40–49	234	5.2	702	5.2	
50–59	324	7.1	972	7.1	
60–69	617	13.6	1851	13.6	
70–79	1506	33.1	4518	33.1	
>=80	1542	33.9	4626	33.9	
Economic level (monthly income) (USD$)*					<0.001
<600	2744	60.4	7783	57.1	
601~1000	1682	37.0	5167	37.9	
>1000	121	2.7	691	5.1	
Urbanization					<0.001
1 (most)	921	20.3	3207	23.5	
2	339	7.5	959	7.0	
3	1021	22.5	3003	22.0	
4	2266	49.9	6472	47.5	
Geographic regions of Taiwan*					0.004
Northern	2019	44.4	6380	46.8	
Central	900	19.8	2492	18.3	
Southern	1472	32.4	4389	32.2	
Eastern	156	3.4	380	2.8	
Personal history					
Diabetes Mellitus*	959	21.1	2619	19.2	0.006
Hypertension	1349	29.7	4038	29.6	0.941
Renal failure*	832	18.3	1491	11.0	<0.001
Liver cirrhosis*	223	4.9	418	3.1	<0.001
Stroke*	943	20.7	1809	13.3	<0.001
Osteoporosis*	1660	36.5	2237	16.4	<0.001

*Significant differences.

hospitalizations were set to be in the same month as those of the study patients. For control patients, the date that they were extracted was their index hospitalization. In this study, all patients were prospectively followed for 3 years after their index hospitalization. The probability of experiencing new-onset depression during the 3-year follow-up period was analyzed between the two groups.

2.3 Inclusion Criteria

Definition of patients with femoral neck fracture. We defined our group of femoral neck fracture patients as patients who were hospitalized with a principal diagnosis of femoral neck fracture according to criteria in the International Classification of Diseases, 9th Revision, Clinical Modification (ICD-9-CM; code 820).

Definition of patients with major depression. Major depression was defined as a principal diagnosis using ICD-9-CM criteria listed under codes 296.2, 296.3. The diagnosis of major depression adhered to the Diagnostic and Statistical Manual of Mental Disorders (DMS) - IV published by the American Psychiatric Association. The ICD-9-CM diagnosis of major depression was made by psychiatrists in this study.

2.4 Exclusion Criteria

All patients aged <18 years (n = 82) were excluded from this study. All patients who were previously diagnosed with femoral neck fracture or major depression prior to their index hospitalization were excluded from this study. Bipolar depression, substance-caused depression, dysthymic disorder and postpartum depression were not included. Moreover, affective disorder and depressive disorder were also not included because the principles

Table 2. Crude HR for the presence of new-onset major depression among patients with femoral neck fracture and the comparison patients.

Presence of depression	Total sample (n = 18,188)		Patients with femoral neck fracture (n = 4,547)		Comparison patients (n = 13,641)	
3-year follow-up	No.	%	No.	%	No.	%
Yes	150	0.8	55	1.2	95	0.7
No	18,038	99.2	4,492	98.8	13,546	99.3
Crude HR (95% CI)	–		1.82* (1.30–2.53)		1.00	

*p- value = 0.001.
HR, hazard ratio.

of their diagnosis and their clinical presentations are different from those of major depression. Affective disorder may include manic attacks, and depressive disorder has only some of the same symptoms as major depression.

2.5 Quality Control for Potential ICD-9 over Coding and Treatments

To make sure the medical resource (budget) that provided by NHI program (government supported) would not be over used by the treating hospitals or patients; therefore, the diagnosis, treatments, medications of each patient was randomly and routinely inspected by specialists. Over treatment or over ICD-9 coding was not permitted and might result in fines.

2.6 Study Protocol

Our study group included 4,547 patients with femoral neck fractures. The comparison group was selected from the remaining NHI beneficiaries registered in the LHID. We randomly selected 13,641 comparison patients (three comparison patients for each femoral neck fracture patient) who were matched with study group patients in terms of sex, age (<40, 40 to 49, 50 to 59, 60 to 69, 70 to 79, and >80 years) and years of healthcare use. As a result, a total of 18,118, patients were included in this study. The selection methods of study and comparison patients were summarized in Figure 1.

2.7 Data Analysis

The statistical package SAS was used for the analyses in this study. SAS was used to select the study and comparison groups (SAS Institute Inc., Cary, NC, USA). Descriptive analyses of the independent variables (patient characteristics, demographics, personal history at baseline, surgical interventions, the amount of time between fracture and the onset of depression and other comorbidities) are reported as percentages or the mean ± standard deviation (SD). The X^2 test was used to make between-groups comparisons of patient demographics, including economic status (monthly income: USD$>1000, USD$601~1000, USD$< 600), urbanization of their home city (level 1 to 4), the geographic location of patients' residence (northern, central, southern, and eastern Taiwan), personal history at baseline (diabetes mellitus, hypertension, renal failure, liver cirrhosis, stroke and osteoporosis) and mortality rate between patients with fracture and non-fracture. The urbanization of patients' home city was defined by population and certain indicators of the city's level of development. Level 1 urbanization was defined as having a population greater than 1,250,000 people and a specific status of political, economic, cultural and metropolitan development. Level 2 urbanization was defined as having a population between 500,000 and 1,250,000 and an important role in the Taiwanese political system, economy and culture. Urbanization levels 3 and 4 were defined as having a population between 150,000 and 500,000 and less than 150,000, respectively. Furthermore, a crude hazard ratio (HR) was calculated using Cox's stratified proportional hazards model (stratified with age, sex and the number of years since index hospitalization) to analyze the risk of new-onset major depression between the study and comparison groups. The covariate-adjusted HR was analyzed after adjusting for diabetes mellitus, hypertension, renal failure, liver cirrhosis, stroke, osteoporosis, geographic regions, post-fracture co-morbidities, monthly income and urbanization of patients' home cities. In addition, we used SAS to analyze the eight most common post-fracture comorbidities during the study period. The relationship between post-fracture comorbidities and major depression was also analyzed. We used the Kaplan-Meier method and Log-rank test to estimate survival curves and compare the 3-year major depression-free survival rate between patients with femoral neck fracture and those without. Among the femoral neck fracture patients, the amount of time before the onset of major depression was recorded and divided into 6 periods (<200, 201–400, 401–600, 601–800, 801–1000 and >1000 days). Additionally, the relationship between surgical interventions (including hip replacement and open reduction of internal fixation of the hip) and the chance of suffering new-onset major depression was analyzed for this group (X^2 test). Hip replacement included hip arthroplasty in this study. A p-value <0.05 was considered to be statistically significant.

2.8 Ethics Statement

This study was exempt from a full review by the Institutional Review Board (permission code: 121007) because the data set consists of de-identified secondary data, which was released without restrictions for research purposes.

Results

3.1 Demographic and Medical Treatment Data Collected from Patients with Femoral Neck Fracture

The characteristics and personal histories between patients with femoral neck fracture (n = 4,547) and those in the comparison group (without fracture; n = 13,641) are presented in Table 1. Females were the majority in both groups. Most femoral neck fractures occurred in the age groups of 70 to 79 (33.12%) and >80 years (33.91%). Compared with the control patients, femoral neck fracture patients had generally lower economic and urbanization levels. Fracture patients also had a higher prevalence of diseases in their personal medical histories at baseline compared with the non-fracture patients. These diseases included diabetes mellitus,

Table 3. Covariate-adjusted HR for major depression during the 3-year follow-up period for major depression among the total patient sample (n = 18,118).

	Occurrence of new-onset depression		
Variables	**HR**	**95% CI**	***p*-value**
Groups			
Patients with femoral neck fracture	3.54	1.21–10.35	0.021
Comparison*	1.00	1.00	1.000
Personal history			
Diabetes Mellitus**	1.90	1.02–3.53	0.044
Hypertension	0.78	0.40–1.51	0.459
Renal failure**	2.94	1.54–5.61	0.001
Liver cirrhosis	0.34	0.05–2.56	0.297
Stroke	0.49	0.19–1.25	0.135
Osteoporosis	1.16	0.63–2.15	0.638
Cormobidity (post-fracture)			
Cellulitis	0.99	0.52–1.87	0.970
Pneumonia	1.13	0.57–2.24	0.731
Chronic obstructive pulmonary disease	1.45	0.76–2.78	0.262
Arrhythmia	0.96	0.47–1.95	0.906
Heart failure	0.70	0.33–1.49	0.358
Deep vein thrombosis	1.64	0.74–3.63	0.222
Peptic ulcer	1.45	0.79–2.68	0.232
Stroke**	3.49	1.45–8.45	0.003
Geographic regions of Taiwan			
Northern*	1.00	1.00	1.000
Central	1.15	0.51–2.60	0.729
Southern	1.29	0.65–2.56	0.464
Eastern	0.88	0.31–2.46	0.803
Economic level (monthly income) (USD$)			
>1000*	1.00	1.00	1.000
601~1000	0.51	0.11–2.47	0.406
<600	0.80	0.17–3.70	0.774
Urbanization			
1 (most)*	1.00	1.00	1.000
2	0.85	0.37–1.93	0.694
3	1.14	0.48–2.71	0.776
4	0.94	0.29–3.05	0.918

*Reference group.
** Higher risk of major depression.
HR, hazard ratio.
CI, confidence interval.

renal failure, liver cirrhosis, stroke, and osteoporosis (for all of the above findings, $p<0.05$). The overall mortality rate during the study period was higher in patients with fractures (12.8%, n = 525) than in those without fractures (6.9%, n = 857) ($p<0.001$). Peptic ulcer (n = 1,644), chronic obstructive pulmonary disease (n = 1,547), pneumonia (n = 1,376), cellulitis (n = 1,041), heart failure (n = 896), arrhythmia (n = 832), stroke (n = 801) and deep vein thrombosis (n = 356) were the most common post-fracture comorbidities.

3.2 Depression Likelihood based on the Crude HR

During the 3-year follow-up period, we found that the risk of presenting with new-onset major depression was significantly higher in patients with femoral neck fracture than in comparison patients. In this study, 1.2% (n = 55) of patients experienced new-onset major depression after a femoral neck fracture, while the percentage of new-onset depression was only 0.7% (n = 95) in the comparison group. The stratified Cox proportional hazard analysis showed that the femoral neck fracture group had a crude HR 1.82 times greater than that of the comparison group (95% CI, 1.30–2.53; $p = 0.001$) (Table 2). After adjusting for patients'

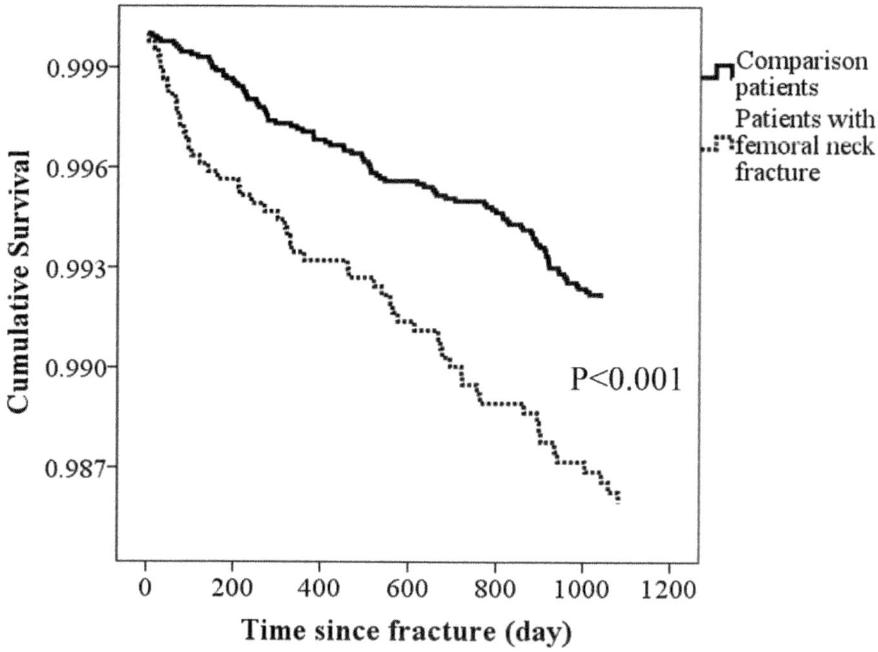

Figure 2. Time-related factor associated with the major depression occurrence. (A) Major depression-free survival curves for patients with femoral neck fracture and the comparison patients during the 3-year follow-up period ($p = <0.001$).

geographic regions, monthly incomes, and personal histories at baseline, patients with femoral neck fracture were more likely to experience new-onset depression than were the comparison group patients (HR: 1.46, 95% CI: 1.03–2.08) (data not shown). Furthermore, the HR obviously increased to 3.54 (95% CI: 1.21–10.35) after considering the eight most common post-fracture comorbidities (Table 3). Among the 4,547 patients with femoral neck fracture, most of them received surgical interventions (n = 3,600, 78.2%). Open reduction of internal fixation was the most common surgical method (n = 2,392, 52.6%). Comparing with the non-operation patients (n = 947), the prevalence of depression did not significantly decrease in those who had received operation ($p = 0.505$).

3.3 Major Depression-Free Survival Curves for Patients

The major depression-free survival curves generated for the study period pertaining to femoral neck fracture patients and the comparison patients appear in Figure 2. We noted that patients with femoral neck fracture had significantly lower rates of 3-year

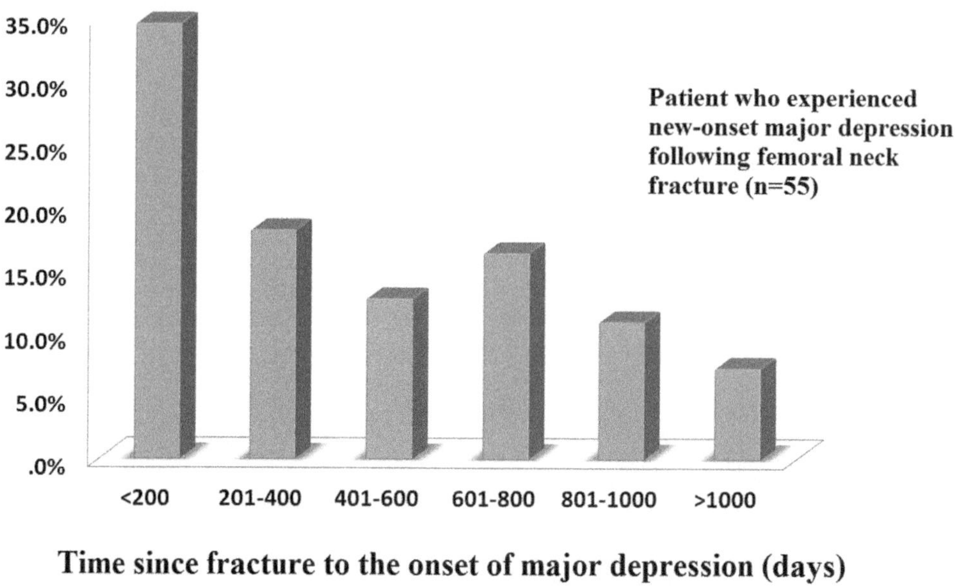

Figure 3. Most major depressive episodes (34.5%) occurred within the first 200 days following femoral neck fracture. The percentage of major depression patients also gradually decreased as the observation period prolonged.

major depression-free survival than the comparison patients did ($p<0.001$).

3.4 The Time between Fracture and the Onset of Depression

The amount of time between fracture and the presentation of new-onset major depression during the study period is shown in Figure 3. Most major depressive episodes occurred within the first 200 days following fracture.

Discussion

In this 3-year follow-up study, we found that femoral neck fracture was significantly related to the occurrence of new-onset major depression (1.82 times the rate among the control subjects without femoral neck fracture). After adjusting for patients' demographic data, including personal histories at baseline, economic status and geographic regions, femoral neck fracture was associated with a statistically significant increased risk of major depression (HR:1.46). After the fracture, the condition of recovery might also influence patients' emotions. Phillips AC et al. reported that poorer long-term recovery post-injury increased the chance of suffering depressive disorder; [16] however, post-fracture comorbidities were not well addressed. In this study, we noted that the HR of major depression obviously increased (1.46 to 3.54) after considering the comorbidities after femoral neck fracture. Among these, the adjusting analysis revealed that having a history of diabetes, renal failure or post-fracture stroke was the most powerful risk factor for major depression. The development of major depression is typically complex (including endocrine, gene, and immune activation), [18–20] and might not only relate to the risk factors that we have shown in this study.

Reduced quality of life and stress are usually present in femoral neck fracture patients. [15] It is well-known that life stress may be associated with depressive disorders. Some previous studies attempted to analyze elderly patients with hip fracture regarding cognitive impairment and mood disorder. These studies showed that 13 to 37.6% of the elderly had depressive mood or anxiety after hip fracture by self-report or score evaluation. [21–23] Compared with these studies, the incidence in this study was relatively low (1.2%) for three possible reasons. First, major depression has more serious diagnosis criteria than do depressive disorder or anxiety (in this study, bipolar depression, substance-caused depression, dysthymic disorder and postpartum depression were all excluded). Second, the diagnoses in this study were confirmed by a psychiatrist (not by self-report). Finally, our population not only focused on the elderly, and patients who had a history of depression were excluded before the study began.

Gambatesa M et al. analyzed 40 hip fracture patients for 30 days and found that their fracture-related anxiety scores did not obviously decrease, particularly among those who did not receive proper post-fracture education. [17] In this study, we further extended the observation period. Most major depressive episodes (34.5%) occurred within the first 200 days following a femoral neck fracture. The percentage of patients with major depression also gradually decreased as the observation period continued (<200 days: 34.5%; 201–400 days: 18.2%; 401–600 days: 12.7%; 601–800 days: 16.4%; 801–1000 days: 10.9%; >1000 days: 7.3%). Therefore, emotional support and depression prevention should be emphasized with primary physicians during the early stage of femoral neck fracture (early psychological intervention may be necessary).

Some studies have reported that surgical intervention for femoral neck fracture may improve quality of life. [8,24,25] In this study, 3,600 patients with femoral neck fracture underwent early surgical intervention (hip replacement and ORIF); only a small number, 46 (1.3%), of these patients experienced major depression. The percentage of surgical patients who experienced major depression was similar to that among the patients (n = 9; 1.0%) who did not undergo surgery. We suspect that life stress may persist after an operation because of increased medical costs (to pay for the operation) or the stress of wound care.

In conclusion, femoral neck fracture patients are at a high risk of experiencing subsequent major depression. More importantly, 34.5% of major depressive episodes occurred within the first 200 days following fracture. Early mental support or psychological intervention may be useful.

4.1 Limitation

The nature limitation of database study was the ICD-9 coding (which depending on the treating physicians). However, as the statements that we mentioned in the method section (quality control), the diagnosis and treatments of each patient were randomly and routinely inspected by specialists for controlling the government budget. For example, the payments for treating femoral neck fracture would be retrospectively inspected with patient's medical records and image reports. In addition, a new-onset major depressive disorder was favor to be diagnosed with a detailed history taking, social worker's records and psychiatrist's consultations. Therefore, we suspected this nature limitation has been obviously decreased in this study. Because the LHID started in 1995, diagnoses made before 1995 were not included. This is a natural limitation for researchers who analyze data using the LHID database. [26,27,28] Therefore, we suspected that some patients had diagnoses of femoral neck fracture or depression before 1995, but they could not be clearly excluded. To decrease this limitation, patients who had any medical record of femoral neck fracture or major depression from 1995 to 2003 were excluded. Finally, because of some specific medications, psychological treatment and counseling are only provided by psychiatrists with the Taiwanese government's permission. Therefore, nearly all patients who are suspected of initial major depression are referred to psychiatrists for complete evaluation. Therefore, we only included the psychiatrists' diagnoses.

Author Contributions

Conceived and designed the experiments: SYH HLH WLC HCL YRL. Performed the experiments: CYC WLC. Analyzed the data: SYH YFL CCK MCY HCL. Contributed reagents/materials/analysis tools: CYC HCL CCK WLC HLH CCC LPC YFL. Wrote the paper: CYC WLC.

References

1. Cannada LK, Viehe T, Cates CA, Norris RJ, Zura RD, et al. (2009) A retrospective review of high-energy femoral neck-shaft fractures. J Orthop Trauma 23: 254–260.
2. Wolinsky PR, Johnson KD (1995) Ipsilateral femoral neck and shaft fractures. Clin Orthop Relat Res (318): 81–90.
3. Alho A (1997) Concurrent ipsilateral fractures of the hip and shaft of the femur. A systematic review of 722 cases. Ann Chir Gynaecol 86: 326–336.
4. Hartholt KA, Oudshoorn C, Zielinski SM, Burgers PT, Panneman MJ, et al. (2011) The epidemic of hip fractures: Are we on the right track? PLoS One 6: e22227.
5. Miyanishi K, Jingushi S, Torisu T (2010) Mortality after hip fracture in japan: The role of nutritional status. J Orthop Surg (Hong Kong) 18: 265–270.
6. Browne JA, Pietrobon R, Olson SA (2009) Hip fracture outcomes: Does surgeon or hospital volume really matter? J Trauma 66: 809–814.

7. Roche JJ, Wenn RT, Sahota O, Moran CG (2005) Effect of comorbidities and postoperative complications on mortality after hip fracture in elderly people: Prospective observational cohort study. BMJ 331: 1374.
8. Valaviciene R, Macijauskiene J, Tarasevicius S, Smailys A, Dobozinskas P, et al. (2012) Femoral neck fractures in lithuania and sweden. the differences in care and outcome. Int Orthop 36: 1681–1686.
9. Enocson A, Pettersson H, Ponzer S, Tornkvist H, Dalen N, et al. (2009) Quality of life after dislocation of hip arthroplasty: A prospective cohort study on 319 patients with femoral neck fractures with a one-year follow-up. Qual Life Res 18: 1177–1184.
10. Shyu YI, Chen MC, Liang J, Lu JF, Wu CC, et al. (2004) Changes in quality of life among elderly patients with hip fracture in taiwan. Osteoporos Int 15: 95–102.
11. Kim SM, Moon YW, Lim SJ, Yoon BK, Min YK, et al. (2012) Prediction of survival, second fracture, and functional recovery following the first hip fracture surgery in elderly patients. Bone 50: 1343–1350.
12. Gordon J, Pham CT, Karnon J, Crotty M (2012) Monitoring progress in the management of hip fractures in south australia, australia. Arch Osteoporos 7: 267–273.
13. Holvik K, Ranhoff AH, Martinsen MI, Solheim LF (2010) Predictors of mortality in older hip fracture inpatients admitted to an orthogeriatric unit in oslo, norway. J Aging Health 22: 1114–1131.
14. Gonzalez-Rozas M, Perez-Castrillon JL, Gonzalez-Sagrado M, Ruiz-Mambrilla M, Garcia-Alonso M (2012) Risk of mortality and predisposing factors after osteoporotic hip fracture: A one-year follow-up study. Aging Clin Exp Res 24: 181–187.
15. Cole MG, Dendukuri N (2003) Risk factors for depression among elderly community subjects: A systematic review and meta-analysis. Am J Psychiatry 160: 1147–1156.
16. Phillips AC, Upton J, Duggal NA, Carroll D, Lord JM (2013) Depression following hip fracture is associated with increased physical frailty in older adults: The role of the cortisol: Dehydroepiandrosterone sulphate ratio. BMC Geriatr 13: 60-2318-13-60.
17. Gambatesa M, D'Ambrosio A, D'Antini D, Mirabella L, De Capraris A, et al. (2013) Counseling, quality of life, and acute postoperative pain in elderly patients with hip fracture. J Multidiscip Healthc 6: 335–346.
18. Ancelin ML, Carriere I, Scali J, Ritchie K, Chaudieu I, et al. (2013) Angiotensin-converting enzyme gene variants are associated with both cortisol secretion and late-life depression. Transl Psychiatry 3: e322.
19. Fenn AM, Gensel JC, Huang Y, Popovich PG, Lifshitz J, et al. (2013) Immune activation promotes depression 1 month after diffuse brain injury: A role for primed microglia. Biol Psychiatry.
20. Shen HP, Chen YS, Hsieh JC, Su TP, Chen LF (2012) Abnormal neural responses to facial expression images in major depressive patients. J. Neurosci. Neuroeng. 1, 90–96.
21. Holmes J, House A (2000) Psychiatric illness predicts poor outcome after surgery for hip fracture: A prospective cohort study. Psychol Med 30: 921–929.
22. Duggal NA, Upton J, Phillips AC, Hampson P, Lord JM (2013) Depressive symptoms are associated with reduced neutrophil function in hip fracture patients. Brain Behav Immun 33: 173–182.
23. Piscitelli P, Metozzi A, Benvenuti E, Bonamassa L, Brandi G, et al. (2012) Connections between the outcomes of osteoporotic hip fractures and depression, delirium or dementia in elderly patients: Rationale and preliminary data from the CODE study. Clin Cases Miner Bone Metab 9: 40–44.
24. Sendtner E, Renkawitz T, Kramny P, Wenzl M, Grifka J (2010) Fractured neck of femur–internal fixation versus arthroplasty. Dtsch Arztebl Int 107: 401–407.
25. Shyu YI, Liang J, Wu CC, Cheng HS, Chen MC (2010) An interdisciplinary intervention for older taiwanese patients after surgery for hip fracture improves health-related quality of life. BMC Musculoskelet Disord 11: 225-2474-11-225.
26. Hsu CS, Huang CJ, Kao JH, Lin HH, Chao YC, et al. (2013) Interferon-based therapy decreases risks of hepatocellular carcinoma and complications of cirrhosis in chronic hepatitis C patients. PLoS One 8: e70458.
27. Chen YH, Kang JH, Lin HC (2011) Patients with traumatic brain injury: Population-based study suggests increased risk of stroke. Stroke 42: 2733–2739.
28. Lai SC, Chang YY, Chang CY, Yang MC, Hsu HY, et al. (2013) Urticaria increases the risk of depression in adult patients: a national database study. J. Neurosci. Neuroeng. 2, 465–469.

13

Post-Operative Auto-Transfusion in Total Hip or Knee Arthroplasty: A Meta-Analysis of Randomized Controlled Trials

Zhao Haien[1], Jiang Yong[2], Ma Baoan[1]*, Guo Mingjun[1], Fan Qingyu[1]*

1 Department of Orthopaedic Surgery, Tangdu Hospital, The Fourth Military Medical University, Xi'an, China, 2 Department of Orthopaedic Surgery, Hong Hui Hospital, Xi'an Jiaotong University College of Medicine, Xi'an, China

Abstract

Background: Total hip or knee arthroplasty is an elective procedure that is usually accompanied by substantial blood loss, which may lead to acute anemia. As a result, almost half of total joint arthroplasty patients receive allogeneic blood transfusions (ABT). Many studies have shown that post-operative auto-transfusion (PAT) significantly reduces the need for ABT, but other studies have questioned the efficacy of this method.

Methods: The protocol for this trial and supporting CONSORT checklist are available as supporting information; see Checklist S1. To evaluate the efficacy of PAT, we conducted a Cochrane systematic review that combined all available data from randomized controlled trials. Data from the six included trials were pooled for analysis. We then calculated relative risks with 95% confidence intervals (CIs) for dichotomous outcomes and mean differences with 95% CIs for continuous outcomes.

Findings and Conclusion: To our knowledge, this is the first meta-analysis to compare the clinical results between PAT and a control in joint replacement patients. This meta-analysis has proven that the use of a PAT reinfusion system reduced significantly the demand for ABT, the number of patients who require ABT and the cost of hospitalization after total knee and hip arthroplasty. This study, together with other previously published data, suggests that PAT drains are beneficial. Larger, sufficiently powered studies are necessary to evaluate the presumed reduction in the incidence of infection as well as DVT after joint arthroplasty with the use of PAT.

Editor: Robert K. Hills, Cardiff University, United Kingdom

Funding: The authors have no support or funding to report.

Competing Interests: The authors have declared that no competing interests exist.

* E-mail: 53383365@qq.com (FQ); zhe992000@eyou.com (MB)

Introduction

Total hip or knee arthroplasty is an elective procedure that is usually accompanied by substantial blood loss, which may lead to acute anemia. As a result, almost half of total joint arthroplasty patients receive allogeneic blood transfusions (ABT) to prevent postoperative anemia [1–4]. However, ABT is an increasingly expensive and scarce resource, and ABT itself is not a risk-free therapeutic method. ABT can lead to the transmission of infectious diseases such as HIV, hepatitis, cytomegalovirus, Epstein-Barr virus, syphilis, and malaria as well as transfusion-related acute lung injury, hemolytic reactions, fluid overload, and an increased rate of postoperative infection [5,6].

An increased awareness of the greater incidence of postoperative complications and other potential hazards of ABT has prompted a review of transfusion practices and a search for blood conservation measures, such as the correction of peri-operative anemia (e.g., intravenous iron, recombinant human erythropoietin), the use of pharmacological agents to reduce peri-operative blood loss (eg, aprotinin, tranexamic acid), and the use of different measures of autologous blood transfusion [5–7]. Autologous blood transfusion includes pre-operative donation, intra-operative auto-transfusion (IAT), and post-operative auto-transfusion (PAT) [8]. In PAT, the post-operative blood drainage collected in drains is salvaged and returned. Many studies have shown that PAT significantly reduced the need for ABT [9–11], but other studies have questioned the efficacy of this method [12,13] or found that PAT after arthroplasty had a limited effect in terms of blood conservation [3,4].

The main objective of this study was to compare the clinical results of post-operative auto-transfusion (PAT) with the results of a control group that received standardized drainage (if necessary, patients were given allogeneic blood transfusion) following total hip or knee arthroplasty. To evaluate the clinical efficacy of PAT, we conducted a meta-analysis that combined all of the available data from randomized controlled trials (RCTs).

Materials and Methods

Literature Search

We searched for the published results of relevant trials in the Cochrane Library (Issue 2, 2011), PubMed (January 1995 to

February 2011), Ovid (January 1995 to February 2011), ScienceDirect Online (January 1995 to February 2011), ISI Web of Knowledge (January 1995 to February 2011), several orthopedic journals, transfusion journals, and conference proceedings. When necessary, the authors of the articles were contacted for original information. The search terms used included "total hip replacement", "total hip arthroplasty", "total knee replacement", "total knee arthroplasty", "total joint arthroplasty", "autotransfusion", "autologous transfusion", "post-operative blood salvage", "post-operative transfusion" and "randomized controlled trials".

Inclusion and Exclusion Criteria

We retrieved all randomized controlled trials (RCTs) that compared the PAT system group with the control group in patients undergoing total knee or hip arthroplasty. Properly randomized trials were eligible for inclusion if (i) the results included at least one of the outcome measures; (ii) at least one of the data points was presented as the mean ± SD; (iii) all data were shown as the medians and/or ranges, and we obtained the original information by contacting the corresponding author; (iv) there was no consideration of primary replacement or revision replacement of the joint.

Patients were excluded from the trials if (i) they had received any other blood-saving strategy including preoperative autologous blood donation, erythropoietin treatment, iron supplementation; (ii) all data were shown as the medians and/or ranges, and it was not possible to obtain the original information by contacting the author.

The data were extracted by 2 reviewers independently to ensure accuracy. In cases of disagreement, a consensus was reached by discussion. Study quality was evaluated according to the method for RCTs described in the Cochrane Reviewer's Handbook 5.0 [14].

Outcome Measures

The primary outcome measures assessed in this analysis include the number of patients requiring at least one unit of allogeneic RBCs (patients requiring homologous blood transfusions).

The secondary outcome measures include the ABT index (units of RBC transfused per patient), the total volume of blood loss following surgery, postoperative hemoglobin (Hb) level, transfusion reactions, infections, deep vein thrombosis (DVT), and the length of the hospital stay (LOHS).

Statistical Analysis

The data were pooled using REVMAN 5.0 software (The Nordic Cochrane Centre, Copenhagen, Denmark). For each study, we calculated relative risks (RRs) with 95% confidence intervals (CIs) for dichotomous data and mean differences (MDs) with 95% CIs for continuous data. Where appropriate, we pooled the results of comparable groups of trials using the fixed-effect (Mantel-Haenszel test) and random-effect (DerSimonian-Laird method) models. A random-effect model was used when significant heterogeneity was detected between studies ($P<0.10$; $I^2>50\%$). Otherwise, a fixed-effect model was used.

Results

Literature Search

The preliminary literature search yielded 729 potentially relevant articles. Most of these studies, however, were non-randomized cohort studies, retrospective studies, biomechanical studies, case reports, or other forms of investigation that did not fit our inclusion criteria. Finally, six studies were identified as eligible for data extraction and meta-analysis [3,12,13,15,18,19]. These six studies were adequately randomized studies of RCTs in which consensus was reached by discussion (Figure 1). The allocation concealments of all six eligible studies were unclear. None of the studies included adequate blinding procedures. In total, 829 patients from these six trials were included in our analysis; 469 of these patients received post-operative auto-transfusion (PAT) and 360 patients served as the control group. The quality of the trials included in this meta-analysis is presented in Table 1.

Outcome Measures

All of the six RCTs reported the number of patients requiring at least one unit of allogeneic RBCs following the arthroplasty surgery. So we included the six RCTs as the data of the meta-analysis in figure 2. In one of the studies (Soosman 2006), patients were randomized to three groups: group A as a control group, and group B and group C as two different re-infusion system groups. In our analysis, as a results, Soosman's study was divided into two studies, as Soosman 2006b and Soosman 2006c. Because significant heterogeneity was detected between the studies ($P=0.0009$; $I^2=74\%$), a random-effect model was used. The pooled result indicated a significant difference between treatment groups in the numbers of patients requiring at least one unit of allogeneic RBCs (RRs, 0.65; 95% CIs, 0.42 to 1.00; $P=0.05$) (Figure 2).

Two RCTs (Soosman 2006 and Konstantino 2010) was included in the meta-analysis of ABT index. In these two studies, patients were randomized to three groups: group A as a control group, and group B and group C as two different re-infusion system groups. As a results, Soosman's study and Konstantino's study was divided into two studies, as Soosman 2006b and Soosman 2006c, Konstantino 2010b and Konstantino 2010c, respectively. It demonstrated that there was no heterogeneity between subtotal ($P=0.99$; $I^2=0\%$) and we could pooled the two autotransfusion techniques in a meta-analysis. A random-effect model was used because significant heterogeneity was detected among the two studies of autotransfusion devices ($P<0.00001$; $I^2=94\%$). The pooled result of RCTs indicated that the ABT index differences between the PAT group and the control group were not statistically significant (MDs, −0.23; 95% CIs, −0.95 to 0.48; $P=0.52$) (Figure 3).

Among six of the trials, three studies reported the volume of the blood loss following surgery compared the total amount of blood loss in the PAT group with a control group, including both the intra-operative and post-operative blood loss. One of the five studies (Soosman 2006) provided the volume as a median and range rather than as the mean ± SD. Although we tried to contact the corresponding author, we could not obtain the original information. Thus, two studies were included in our comparison of the volume of blood loss. We pooled the two RCTs data in Figure 4. Because no significant heterogeneity was observed among these studies ($P=0.15$), a fixed-effect model was used. The pooled results indicated less volume of blood loss in the autotransfusion group than in the control group (MDs, −131.10; 95% CIs, −257.13 to −5.07; $P=0.04$) (Figure 4). The result showed differences between the groups were statistically significant.

The post-operation Hb level data were divided into 5 subgroups (1, 2, 3, 5, and 7 days post-operation) based on the post-operative time at which the Hb level data were acquired. Because no significant heterogeneity was observed among the subgroups ($P=0.46$; $I^2=0\%$) in this comparison, a fixed-effect model was employed. The pooled results of RCTs revealed a significant difference in the post-operative Hb level between the PAT group

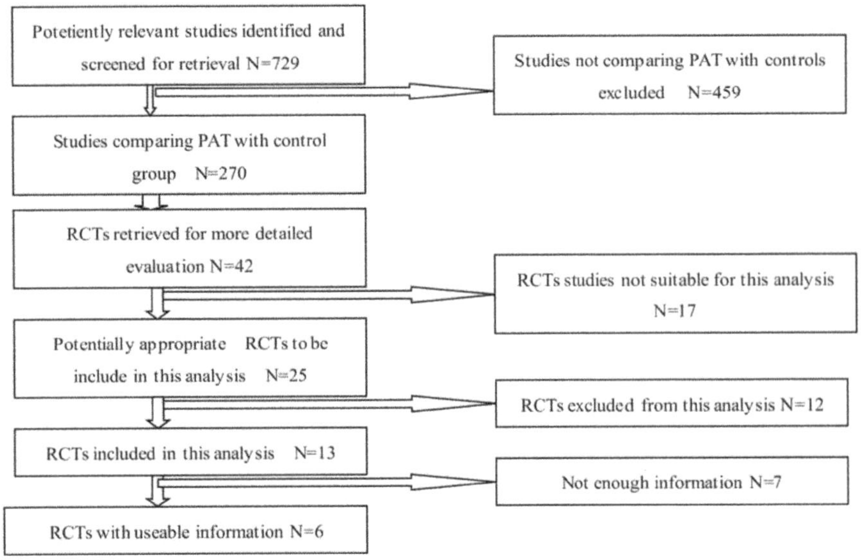

Figure 1. The QUOROM diagram for review. RCT, randomized controlled trial.

and the control group. The results demonstrated a higher level of post-operative Hb in the auto-transfusion group than in the control group (MDs, 0.25; 95% CIs, 0.12 to 0.37; P = 0.0001) (Figure 5).

Four RCTs trials reported febrile reactions among patients who received PAT versus ABT. Heterogeneity between the two treatment groups was not statistically significant (P = 0.29; $I^2 = 19\%$), so we employed a fixed-effect model to study the febrile reaction. The pooled results revealed a significant difference in the febrile reaction rate between the transfusion treatment groups (RRs, 0.65; 95% CIs, 0.46 to 0.93; P = 0.02) (Figure 6).

Four RCTs was included in the study of the infection rate. We pooled the results of the RCTs in Figure 7. Figure 7 shows the difference in the infection rate between PAT patients and ABT patients after total joint arthroplasty surgery. We found no significant heterogeneity between studies (P = 0.62; $I^2 = 0\%$) and thus compared the data with a fixed-effect model. The pooled result revealed no significant difference between the treatment groups (RRs, 1.09; 95% CIs, 0.54 to 2.21; P = 0.80).

Three RCTs were included in the study of LOHS and we pooled these RCTs in the study of LOHS in Figure 8. With no significant heterogeneity among the data compared in LOHS (P = 0.23; $I^2 = 30\%$; fixed-effect analysis), the pooled result revealed a significant difference in LOHS between the treatment groups (MDs, −0.79; 95% CIs, −1.54 to −0.05; P = 0.04) (Figure 8). It demonstrated LOHS in the PAT patients was shorter than patients in the control group after surgery. Two RCTs studies reported the incidence of DVT and revealed a lack of significant differences between the PAT group and the control group (RRs, 0.38; 95% CIs, 0.06 to 2.51; P = 0.31) (figure not shown).

Discussion

Total knee or hip arthroplasty is usually accompanied by substantial blood loss and regularly results in a postoperative requirement for blood transfusion. Because of the disadvantages of allogeneic blood transfusion (ABT) such as the risk of transfusion-associated infections, incompatibility-related transfusion fatalities or immuno-modulatory effects, a continuing effort to reduce ABT is important. Thus, the reinfusion of drained blood via a postoperative wound drainage and reinfusion system and the need for ABT was evaluated.

As mentioned above, autologous blood transfusion includes pre-operative blood donation, intra-operative auto-transfusion (IAT), and PAT. In pre-operative blood donation, the patient's own blood is collected a few weeks before the operation and transfused

Table 1. Quality evaluation of included RCTs.

Inclusion study	Design	Number		Random	Concealment	Blinding	Follow-up	Grade
		PAT	CG					
A.Amin 2008	RCT	92	86	Y	Y	UC	Y	B
Adrianus 2007	RCT	80	80	Y	Y	UC	Y	B
C.soosman 2006	RCT	47	22	Y	Y	UC	Y	B
Konstantino2010	RCT	163	85	Y	UC	UC	Y	C
Newman 1997	RCT	35	35	Y	UC	UC	Y	B
T.abuzakuk 2007	RCT	52	52	Y	UC	UC	Y	B

RCTs: Randomized controlled trials; PAT: Post-operative autotransfusion group; CG: Control group; Y: Yes; UC: Unclear.

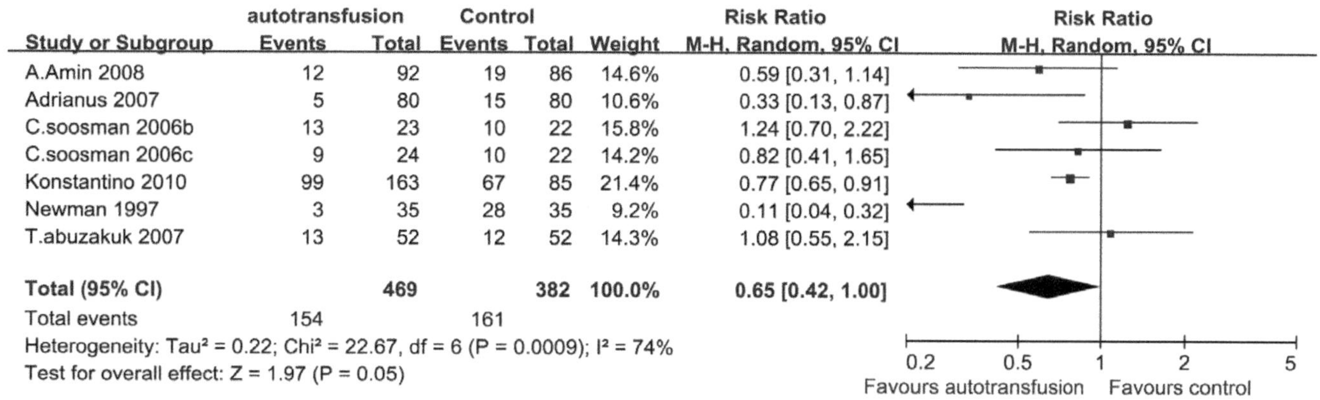

Figure 2. The RRs and 95% CIs for the number of patients requiring at least one unit of ABT among patients treated with vs. without PAT. It indicated that RRs of patients requiring ABT in the PAT group was significantly lower than that in the control group.

post-operatively as needed. In IAT, the patient's blood is collected from the operating field and reinfused. In PAT, the post-operative blood drainage collected in drains is salvaged and returned [20].

Recent techniques have facilitated autologous blood transfusion, and the concept of reinfusing blood collected in the drain following total joint arthroplasty is becoming increasingly attractive to many surgeons. However, PAT following surgery continues to be a controversial topic in the orthopedic literature, and many studies have reported considerable doubt with respect to its benefits [21,22].

In orthopedic surgery, the auto-transfusion of washed (RRs, 0.33; 95% CIs, 0.23 to 0.47) or unwashed cells (RRs, 0.30; 95% CIs, 0.21 to 0.43) decreased the frequency of exposure to ABT to a similar degree when compared with a control. Some studies had shown a significant reduction in the rate of ABT following the use of PAT systems [4,5,23–26]. Recently, Strümper et al. reported a significant reduction in the rate of ABT among patients treated with PAT [4,15]. Sinha et al. found that ABT was reduced by 80% in an autologous reinfusion group as compared with the standard suction group (RRs, 0.18; 95% CIs, 0.10 to 0.35; $P<0.00001$) [16]. Newman et al found that 3 of 35 patients in the PAT drain group required ABT, compared with 28 of 35 patients in the control group (RRs, 0.11; 95% CIs, 0.04 to 0.32; $P<0.0001$) [19]. A recent meta-analysis of RCTs found that PAT reduced the probability of receiving ABT for orthopedic surgery (RRs, 0.35, 95% CIs, 0.24 to 0.52) [27]. del Trujillo et al. found that PAT could decrease the exposure to ABT by 69% and could significantly reduce the units of allogeneic RBC required (MDs, −1.59; 95% CIs, −1.85 to −1.33; $P<0.00001$) in patients undergoing cemented or uncemented total arthroplasty [17]. The ABT rate has also been found to be significantly lower in patients receiving PAT after total knee arthroplasty [4,27,28]. Newman et al. also believed that PAT alone was safe and effective after unilateral total knee arthroplasty, as it is the least troublesome and the least expensive of the available methods of autologous transfusion [19]. Several studies previously showed that unwashed and filtered blood was of satisfactory quality and was safe to reinfuse [19,29].

Contrary to the above-mentioned results in which the use of a PAT system was shown to be advantageous, some authors have suggested insufficient efficiency for PAT [21,30]. Buzakuk et al. found that PAT transfusion failed to reduce the need for postoperative ABT following primary total knee arthroplasty (RRs, 1.08; 95% CIs, 0.55 to 2.15; $P=0.82$) [12]. Rollo reported no reduction in allogeneic RBC transfusions in total hip arthroplasty patients [31]. Ritter et al. and others failed to show a PAT system could reduce the need for ABT in patients scheduled for total hip and knee replacements [32]. Moreover, recent studies found that PAT after hip arthroplasty had a limited blood-conservation effect [3,4,33].

The pooled results of our study demonstrated significant decreases in the rate of homologous blood transfusion compared the PAT group with the control group (RRs, 0.65; 95% CIs, 0.42 to 1.00; $P=0.05$) (Figure 2). This meta-analysis identified statistically significant reduction in the number of patients receiving homologous transfusions and the overall red cell units of ABT among treatment groups. Thus, PAT in total hip or knee arthroplasty was found to be an effective way to significantly reduce the need for ABT.

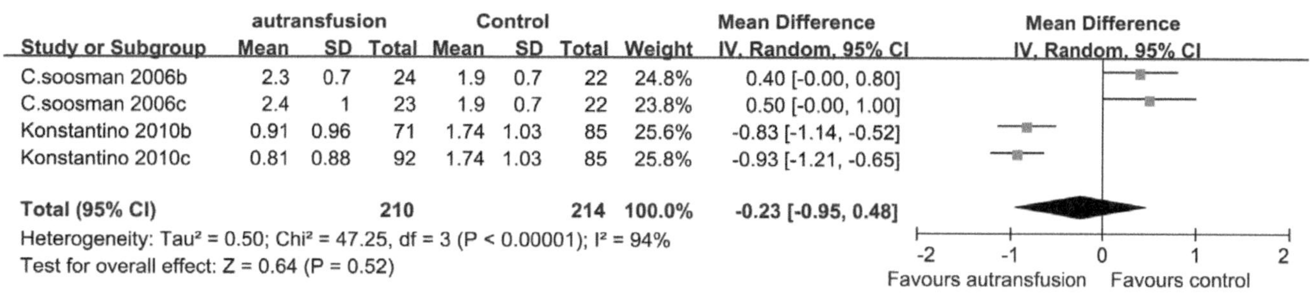

Figure 3. The MDs and 95% CIs for units of RBC per transfused patient among patients treated with vs. without PAT. The pooled result demonstrated that there was no significant difference of the ABT index between the PAT group and the control group.

Study or Subgroup	autotransfusion Mean	SD	Total	Control Mean	SD	Total	Weight	Mean Difference IV, Fixed, 95% CI
Newman 1997	896	545	35	891	401	35	31.6%	5.00 [-219.16, 229.16]
T.abuzakuk 2007	673	355	52	867	434	52	68.4%	-194.00 [-346.40, -41.60]
Total (95% CI)			**87**			**87**	**100.0%**	**-131.10 [-257.13, -5.07]**

Heterogeneity: Chi² = 2.07, df = 1 (P = 0.15); I² = 52%
Test for overall effect: Z = 2.04 (P = 0.04)

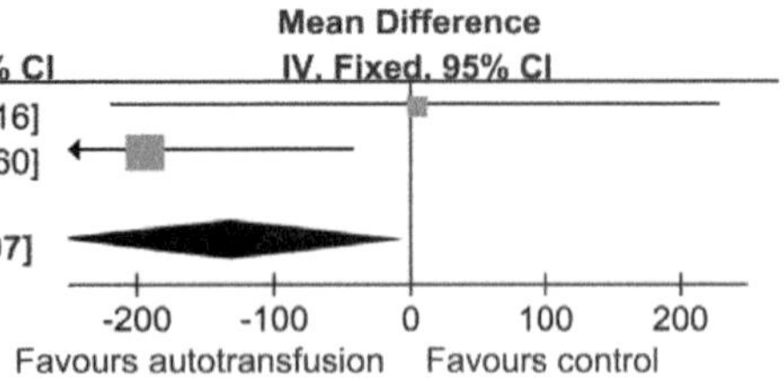

Figure 4. The MDs and 95% CIs for the volume of blood loss among patients treated with vs. without PAT. The result indicated significantly less volume of blood loss in the PAT group than in the control group.

Many potential factors such as tourniquet use, hypertension, cement, and surgical skill can lead to a difference in blood loss after joint surgery. The use of a tourniquet was found to decrease intra-operative blood loss but could not influence the postoperative blood loss in drains or affect transfusion rates [34]. Hypertension may lead to increased blood loss and increased transfusion requirements. However, no differences were found in the total calculated blood loss between patients with or without hyperten-

Study or Subgroup	autotransfusion Mean	SD	Total	Control Mean	SD	Total	Weight	Mean Difference IV, Fixed, 95% CI
8.1.1 post 1 day								
A.Amin 2008	10.5	1.49	92	10.4	1.59	86	7.8%	0.10 [-0.35, 0.55]
Adrianus 2007	10.5	1.1	80	10.1	0.96	80	15.7%	0.40 [0.08, 0.72]
C.soosman 2006b	10	1.45	23	10.5	1.45	22	2.2%	-0.50 [-1.35, 0.35]
C.soosman 2006c	10.3	1.61	24	10.5	1.45	22	2.1%	-0.20 [-1.08, 0.68]
Subtotal (95% CI)			**219**			**210**	**27.9%**	**0.20 [-0.04, 0.44]**
Heterogeneity: Chi² = 5.09, df = 3 (P = 0.17); I² = 41%								
Test for overall effect: Z = 1.62 (P = 0.10)								
8.1.2 post 2 day								
A.Amin 2008	10.5	1.48	92	10.2	1.49	86	8.4%	0.30 [-0.14, 0.74]
T.abuzakuk 2007	10.8	1.6	52	10.1	1.3	52	5.1%	0.70 [0.14, 1.26]
Subtotal (95% CI)			**144**			**138**	**13.6%**	**0.45 [0.11, 0.80]**
Heterogeneity: Chi² = 1.22, df = 1 (P = 0.27); I² = 18%								
Test for overall effect: Z = 2.57 (P = 0.01)								
8.1.3 post 3 day								
A.Amin 2008	11.1	1.4	92	10.8	1.58	86	8.3%	0.30 [-0.14, 0.74]
Adrianus 2007	9.9	1.2	80	9.6	1.2	80	11.6%	0.30 [-0.07, 0.67]
Konstantino 2010	9.7	1.5	92	9.8	1.2	85	10.1%	-0.10 [-0.50, 0.30]
Subtotal (95% CI)			**264**			**251**	**30.1%**	**0.17 [-0.07, 0.40]**
Heterogeneity: Chi² = 2.56, df = 2 (P = 0.28); I² = 22%								
Test for overall effect: Z = 1.40 (P = 0.16)								
8.1.4 post 5 day								
Adrianus 2007	10.1	1.2	80	9.9	1.1	80	12.6%	0.20 [-0.16, 0.56]
T.abuzakuk 2007	10.6	1.5	52	10.1	1.3	52	5.5%	0.50 [-0.04, 1.04]
Subtotal (95% CI)			**132**			**132**	**18.2%**	**0.29 [-0.01, 0.59]**
Heterogeneity: Chi² = 0.83, df = 1 (P = 0.36); I² = 0%								
Test for overall effect: Z = 1.92 (P = 0.06)								
8.1.5 post 7day								
C.soosman 2006b	10.6	1.13	23	10.6	1.13	22	3.7%	0.00 [-0.66, 0.66]
Konstantino 2010c	10.9	1.45	24	10.6	1.13	22	2.9%	0.30 [-0.45, 1.05]
Newman 1997	11.4	1.4	35	10.9	1.4	35	3.7%	0.50 [-0.16, 1.16]
Subtotal (95% CI)			**82**			**79**	**10.3%**	**0.27 [-0.13, 0.66]**
Heterogeneity: Chi² = 1.12, df = 2 (P = 0.57); I² = 0%								
Test for overall effect: Z = 1.32 (P = 0.19)								
Total (95% CI)			**841**			**810**	**100.0%**	**0.25 [0.12, 0.37]**

Heterogeneity: Chi² = 12.90, df = 13 (P = 0.46); I² = 0%
Test for overall effect: Z = 3.81 (P = 0.0001)
Test for subgroup differences: Chi² = 2.07, df = 4 (P = 0.72), I² = 0%

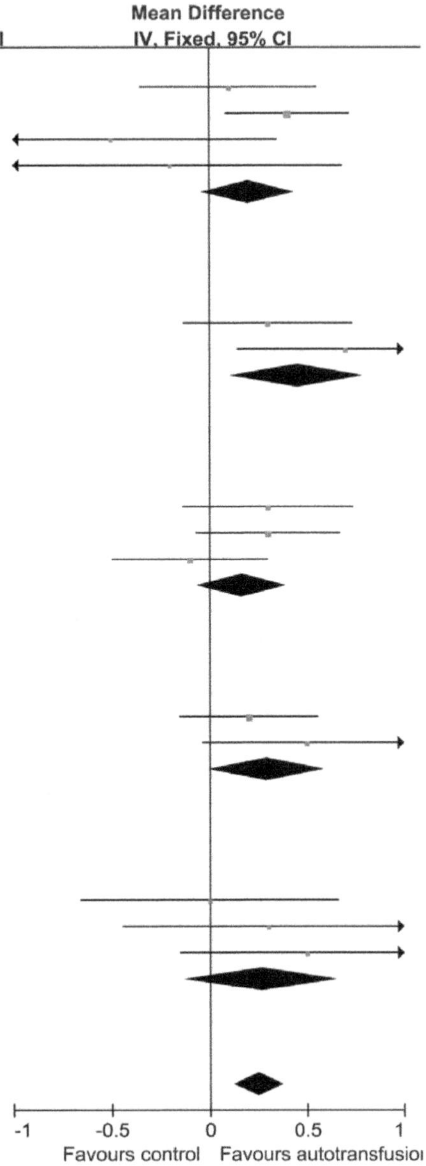

Figure 5. The MDs and 95% CIs for the post-operative Hb level among patients treated with vs. without PAT. It demonstrated that post-operative Hb was significantly higher in the PAT group than in the control group.

Study or Subgroup	Experimental Events	Experimental Total	Control Events	Control Total	Weight	Risk Ratio M-H, Fixed, 95% CI
11.1.1 PAT technique 1						
Adrianus 2007	14	80	16	80	24.2%	0.88 [0.46, 1.67]
C.soosman 2006c	1	23	1	22	1.5%	0.96 [0.06, 14.37]
Konstantino 2010	15	92	17	85	26.7%	0.82 [0.43, 1.53]
Newman 1997	4	35	16	35	24.2%	0.25 [0.09, 0.67]
Subtotal (95% CI)		**230**		**222**	**76.6%**	**0.66 [0.44, 0.98]**
Total events	34		50			
Heterogeneity: Chi² = 4.93, df = 3 (P = 0.18); I² = 39%						
Test for overall effect: Z = 2.07 (P = 0.04)						
11.1.2 PAT technique 2						
Konstantino 2010	9	71	17	85	23.4%	0.63 [0.30, 1.33]
Subtotal (95% CI)		**71**		**85**	**23.4%**	**0.63 [0.30, 1.33]**
Total events	9		17			
Heterogeneity: Not applicable						
Test for overall effect: Z = 1.20 (P = 0.23)						
Total (95% CI)		**301**		**307**	**100.0%**	**0.65 [0.46, 0.93]**
Total events	43		67			
Heterogeneity: Chi² = 4.96, df = 4 (P = 0.29); I² = 19%						
Test for overall effect: Z = 2.39 (P = 0.02)						
Test for subgroup differences: Chi² = 0.01, df = 1 (P = 0.93), I² = 0%						

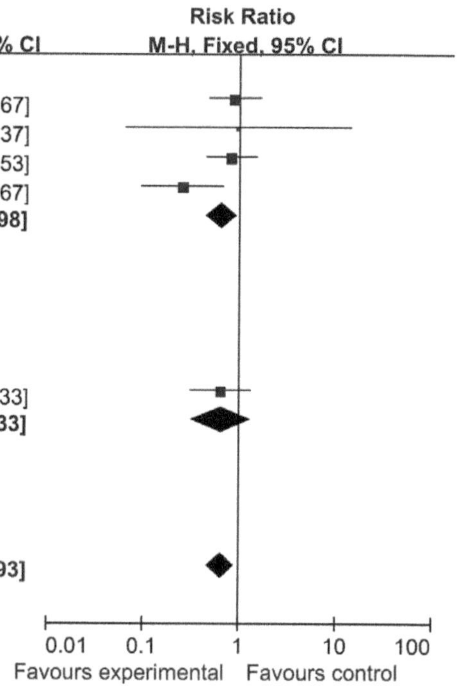

Figure 6. The RRs and 95% CIs for the incidence of febrile reaction among patients treated with vs. without PAT. It indicated that the febrile reaction rate in the PAT group decreased significantly compared with the control group.

sion [17]. In total hip replacement surgery, a significant portion of blood loss occurred during the intra-operative period, and there was a general consensus with regard to the nature of intra-operative blood loss [23,30]. Our meta-analysis found less blood loss in the PAT group than in the control group (MDs, −131.10; 95% CIs, −257.13 to −5.07; P = 0.04) (Figure 4). The exact mechanism underlying the reduced blood loss in PAT patients has yet to be determined, but it seems that blood loss can be reduced by preventing the use of banked blood [29,35–37]. It is therefore clearly preferable not to transfuse ABT if possible, especially in the context of orthopedic surgery.

The point at which to administer a blood transfusion is controversial. In the six studies included, the administration of banked blood was determined by the Hb value and/or clinical signs (e.g., blood pressure, pulse). The observed values were typical of those reported elsewhere. Recently, physicians have agreed that Hb value is a strong trigger for transfusion and that the clinical symptoms of anemia should always be considered when contemplating transfusion [35]. However, our understanding of human physiology, oxygen delivery and the safety and risks of ABT has changed considerably. Therefore, it was also suggested that decisions about transfusions should be based on an assessment of the patient's clinical needs and symptoms rather than laboratory values alone [38].

One of the trials included observed that 7 of the 13 patients in the study group that required ABT received it after day 5, when the Hb eventually fell below 9 g/dl [12]. In the control group, only one patient required ABT on day 5, whereas all of the others required ABT on day 2 after surgery. This effect was caused by a higher Hb level in the patients of the PAT group on day 2 (MDs, 0.45; 95% CIs, 0.11 to 0.80; P = 0.01) than in patients of the control group, which suggests that PAT prevents a rapid decrease in the Hb level during the early post-operative period. However, by day 5, this benefit disappeared (MDs, 0.29; 95% CIs, −0.01 to

Study or Subgroup	autotransfusion Events	autotransfusion Total	Control Events	Control Total	Weight	Risk Ratio M-H, Fixed, 95% CI
A.Amin 2008	3	92	2	86	14.8%	1.40 [0.24, 8.19]
Adrianus 2007	8	80	5	80	35.7%	1.60 [0.55, 4.68]
Konstantino 2010	5	163	3	85	28.1%	0.87 [0.21, 3.55]
Newman 1997	1	35	3	35	21.4%	0.33 [0.04, 3.05]
Total (95% CI)		**370**		**286**	**100.0%**	**1.09 [0.54, 2.21]**
Total events	17		13			
Heterogeneity: Chi² = 1.77, df = 3 (P = 0.62); I² = 0%						
Test for overall effect: Z = 0.25 (P = 0.80)						

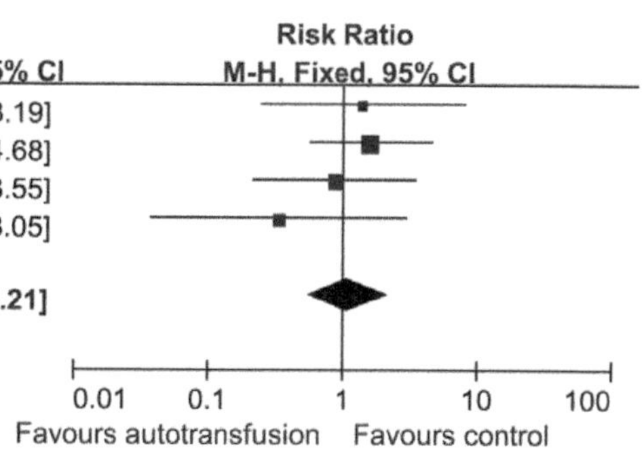

Figure 7. The RRs and 95% CIs for the incidence of infection among patients treated with vs. without PAT. The result revealed no significant difference between the treatment groups.

	autotransfusion			Control				Mean Difference
Study or Subgroup	Mean	SD	Total	Mean	SD	Total	Weight	IV, Fixed, 95% CI
C.soosman 2006b	7.8	4	23	9	2.8	22	13.7%	-1.20 [-3.21, 0.81]
C.soosman 2006c	7.9	3.1	24	9	2.8	22	19.1%	-1.10 [-2.81, 0.61]
Newman 1997	12.6	3.8	35	15.2	5.3	35	11.9%	-2.60 [-4.76, -0.44]
T.abuzakuk 2007	8.1	2.4	52	8.3	2.8	52	55.3%	-0.20 [-1.20, 0.80]
Total (95% CI)			**134**			**131**	**100.0%**	**-0.79 [-1.54, -0.05]**

Heterogeneity: Chi² = 4.31, df = 3 (P = 0.23); I² = 30%
Test for overall effect: Z = 2.09 (P = 0.04)

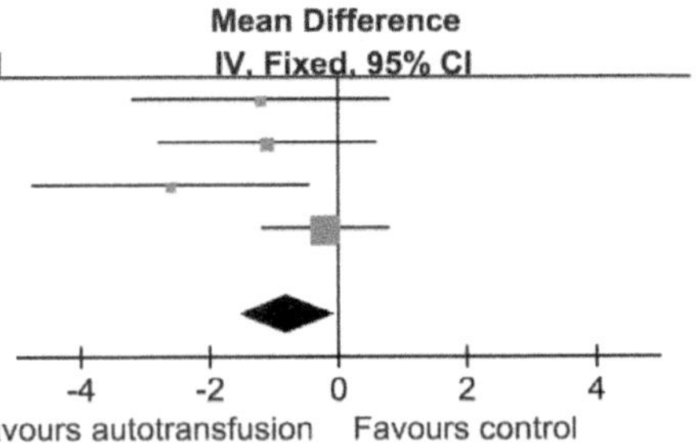

Figure 8. The MDs and 95% CIs for the length of hospital stay among patients treated with vs. without PAT. It demonstrated LOHS in the PAT patients was shorter than patients in the control group after surgery.

0.59; P = 0.06). This meta-analysis showed that PAT was effective in reducing ABT but not useful in achieving high postoperative Hb levels. These findings suggested that PAT was not useful in achieving high postoperative Hb levels to enhance recovery, which agreed with the findings of Adrianus [15].

The pooled results indicated significant differences between treatment groups with regard to the rate of febrile reactions (RRs, 0.65; 95% CIs, 0.46 to 0.93; P = 0.02) (Figure 6). The rate (30%) of mild febrile transfusion reactions was higher in Soosman's study [3] than in previous reports [39], which may have been the result of the inclusion of all mild febrile reactions (>1°C increase in temperature). A lower rate of re-infusion may prevent febrile reactions. It has been suggested that this rise in temperature was a response to the surgical procedure itself [25]. Therefore, postoperative febrile reactions are generally seen in the context of major orthopedic surgery. Some studies have indicated a lack of a difference in developing febrile reactions when using the PAT system or a regular postoperative low-vacuum drainage system. Nearly the same extent of patients with febrile reactions was found in both groups (RRs, 0.88; 95% CIs, 0.46 to 1.67; P = 0.69) [40,41]. Pooling these results with regard to the incidence of febrile reactions showed that adverse effects (chills and febricula) developed during PAT in some patients but less often than during ABT, which agreed with previous reports [18,23,25]. The exact mechanism underlying the higher rates of febrile episodes after ABT has yet to be determined, but it seems that this problem could be reduced by not using ABT [19].

Some reports [2,42,43] showed that the postoperative infection rate was significantly lower in PAT than in ABT patients. del Trujillo et al [17] observed no adverse effect of PAT return during the study but observed a tendency for a reduced rate of postoperative infections in patients receiving PAT. In contrast, an increased post-operative rate of infection was found in ABT patients [2]. The exact mechanism for this effect is not known; however, various theories exist, including one based on the immuno-depressant effects of ABT [44]. The observed effects also may be related to the immunostimulatory and anti-inflammatory effects of PAT [17,19]. Our meta-analysis finding indicated similar rates of infection in patients that received PAT compared with those that received ABT. However, because of the low incidence of infection, this systematic analysis was not sufficiently powered to compare the treatment groups with respect to postoperative infection rate. It is clearly preferable not to transfuse blood if possible, especially in the context of orthopedic surgery, in which deep infection is a devastating complication.

In a previous multivariate analysis, the re-infusion group remained an independent variable in LOHS. A reduction in LOHS was observed by Newman and Shulman [19,45], who found a reduction of 2 days, but this reduction was associated with a reduction in allogeneic RBCs. Newman also postulated that the use of a reinfusion technique after total knee arthroplasty could shorten the hospital stay by rendering the patients less febrile and infective [46]. Similar observations were made in other studies, in which each ABT-transfused patient stayed in the hospital for one additional day [35,47]. Similarly, the use of PAT blood after total knee arthroplasty appeared to decrease the LOHS and effectively reduce the postoperative requirements for ABT, as has been confirmed by recent studies [4,48]. It has recently been reported that hospitalization costs more for patients who undergo joint replacement when ABT is used. Therefore, the use of a PAT technique after total joint replacement can reduce costs by decreasing the ABT and decreasing the LOHS. This reduction in the hospital stay, which is probably related to decreased anxiety about the possibility of infection, is welcome by the hospital staff and patients. As a result, PAT following total joint arthroplasty not only reduces the need for ABT but also reduces the cost to the patient, as it is an inexpensive method. However, any reduction in the LOHS in patients receiving PAT versus ABT is difficult to evaluate, because without rigid criteria for discharge, standards may change slightly during the study period. Therefore, this connection between LOHS and cost should be interpreted cautiously because our study was not powered for this conclusion.

Conclusion

The use of PAT effectively reduces the demand for homologous banked blood transfusions in patients who have undergone total knee or hip arthroplasty. The LOHS and post-operative febrile reaction rate in the PAT groups were slightly reduced compared with the levels in the control group. Therefore, we would like to emphasize that the main benefit of this system was the ability to reduce banked blood utilization without compromising patient safety. We believe that in operations such as total knee arthroplasty, where a tourniquet is used intra-operatively and collection drains are used postoperatively and almost universally, PAT is the most appropriate method of autologous blood transfusion. The meta-analysis results suggest that there are clinical and economical advantages in avoiding the use of ABT blood. We therefore strongly recommend that PAT become more widely used, especially in operations such as total knee or hip arthroplasty where substantial blood loss is anticipated. Therefore, we conclude that PAT in total knee or hip arthroplasty is a safe and effective way to decrease ABT.

To our knowledge, this is the first meta-analysis to systematically compare the clinical results of PAT (postoperative auto-transfusion) with a control treatment in a population of patients undergoing total knee or hip arthroplasty who did not donate autologous blood pre-operatively. We found that the use of a PAT system significantly decreased the risk of ABT and LOHS. The use of PAT could also reduce the occurrence of wound complications and febrile reactions. This study, together with other previously published data, suggests that PAT drains are beneficial. A much larger study is required to confirm these results.

In summary, this meta-analysis has proven that the use of a PAT reinfusion system reduced significantly the demand for ABT, the number of patients who require ABT and the cost of hospitalization after total knee and hip arthroplasty. Larger, sufficiently powered studies are necessary to evaluate the presumed reduction in the incidence of infection as well as DVT after joint arthroplasty with the use of PAT.

Author Contributions

Designed and conceived the meta-analysis: MB FQ. Searched for the published results of relevant trials and analyzed the data: ZH. Wrote the manuscript and revised it: ZH JY GM. Conceived and designed the experiments: ZH JY FQ. Performed the experiments: ZH JY GM. Analyzed the data: ZH GM. Contributed reagents/materials/analysis tools: GM. Wrote the paper: ZH FQ.

References

1. Feagan BG, Wong CJ, Lau CY, Wheeler SL, Sue-A-Quan G, et al. (2001) Transfusion practice in elective orthopaedic surgery. Transfus Med 11: 87–95.
2. Cuenca J, García-Erce JA, Martínez F, Pérez-Serrano L, Herrera A, et al. (2006) Perioperative intravenous iron, with or without erythropoietin, plus restrictive transfusion protocol reduce the need for allogeneic blood after knee replacement surgery. Transfusion 46: 1112–1119.
3. So-Osman C, Nelissen RG, Eikenboom HC, Brand A (2006) Efficacy, safety and user-friendliness of two devices for postoperative autologous shed red blood cell re-infusion in elective orthopaedic surgery patients: a randomized pilot study. Transfus Med 16: 321–328.
4. Strümper D, Weber E, Gielen WS, Van Drumpt R, Bulstra S, et al. (2004) Clinical efficacy of postoperative autologous transfusion of filtered shed blood in hip and knee arthroplasty. Transfusion 44: 1567–1571.
5. Bursi F, Barbieri A, Politi L, Di Girolamo A, Malagoli A, et al. (2009) Perioperative red blood cell transfusion and outcome in stable patients after elective major vascular surgery. Eur J Vasc Endovasc Surg 37: 311–318.
6. Tobias JD (2004) Strategies for minimizing blood loss in orthopedic surgery. Semin Hematol 41: 145S–156S.
7. Grover M, Talwalkar S, Casbard A, Boralessa H, Contreras M, et al. (2006) Silent myocardial ischaemia and haemoglobin concentration: a randomized controlled trial of transfusion strategy in lower limb arthroplasty. Vox Sang 90: 105–112.
8. Rosencher N, Kerkkamp HE, Macheras G, Munuera LM, Menichella G, et al. (2003) Orthopedic surgery transfusion haemoglobin European overview (OSTHEO) study: blood management in elective knee and hip arthroplasty in Europe. Transfusion 43: 459–469.
9. Tsumara N, Yoshiya S, Chin T, Shiba R, Kohso K, et al. (2006) A prospective comparison of clamping the drain or post-operative salvage of blood in reducing blood loss after total knee arthroplasty. J Bone Joint Surg Br 88: 49–53.
10. Friederichs MG, Mariani EM, Bourne MH (2002) Perioperative blood salvage as an alternative to predonating blood for primary total knee and hip arthroplasty. J Arthroplasty 17: 298–303.
11. Steinberg EL, Ben-Galim P, Yaniv Y, Dekel S, Menahem A (2004) Comparative analysis of the benefits of autotransfusion of blood by a shed blood collector after total knee replacement. Arch Orthop Trauma Surg 124: 114–118.
12. Abuzakuk T, Senthil Kumar V, Shenava Y, Bulstrode C, Skinner JA, et al. (2007) Autotransfusion drains in total knee replacement. Are they alternatives to homologous transfusion? Int Orthop 31: 235–239.
13. Amin A, Watson A, Mangwani J, Nawabi D, Ahluwalia R, et al. (2008) A prospective randomised controlled trial of autologous retransfusion in total knee replacement. J Bone Joint Surg Br 90: 451–454.
14. Higgins JPT, Green S (editors). Cochrane handbook for systematic reviews of interventions version 5.1.0 [updated March 2011]. The Cochrane Collaboration, 2011. Available: http: www.cochrane-handbook.org. Accessed 2012 Dec 30.
15. Moonen AF, Knoors NT, van Os JJ, Verburg AD, Pilot P (2007) Retransfusion of filtered shed blood in primary total hip and knee arthroplasty: a prospective randomized clinical trial. Transfusion 47: 379–384.
16. Sinha A, Sinha M, Burgert S (2001) Reinfusion of drained blood as an alternative to homologous blood transfusion after total knee replacement. Int Orthop 25: 257–259.
17. del Trujillo MM, Carrero A, Munoz M (2008) The utility of the perioperative autologous transfusion system OrthoPAT in total hip replacement surgery: a prospective study. Arch Orthop Trauma Surg 128: 1031–1038.
18. Blatsoukas KS, Drosos GI, Kazakos K, Papaioakim M, Gioka T, et al. (2010) Prospective comparative study of two different autotransfusion methods versus control group in total knee replacement. Arch Orthop Trauma Surg 130: 733–737.
19. Newman JH, Bowers M, Murphy J (1997) The clinical advantages of autologous transfusion - A randomised, controlled study after knee replacement. J Bone Joint Surg Br 79: 630–632.
20. Spahn DR (2010) Anemia and Patient Blood Management in Hip and Knee Surgery: A Systematic Review of the Literature. Anesthesiology 113: 482–495.
21. Esler CNA, Blakeway C, Fiddian NJ (2003) The use of a closed-suction drain in total knee arthroplasty - A prospective, randomised study. J Bone Joint Surg Br 85: 215–217.
22. Holt BT, Parks NL, Engh GA, Lawrence JM (1997) Comparison of closed-suction drainage and no drainage after primary total knee arthroplasty. Orthopedics 20: 1121–1125.
23. Engelfriet CP, Reesink HW, Felfernig M, Sporn P, Kretschmer V, et al. (2006) Perioperative blood salvage. Vox Sang 91: 185–192.
24. Muñoz M, Ariza D, Garcerán MJ, Gómez A, Campos A (2005) Benefits of postoperative shed blood reinfusion in patients undergoing unilateral total knee replacement. Arch Orthop Trauma Surg 125: 385–389.
25. Muñoz M, Kühlmorgen B, Ariza D, Haro E, Marroquí A, et al. (2007) Which patients are more likely to benefit from postoperative shed blood salvage after unilateral total knee replacement? An analysis of 581 consecutive procedures. Vox Sang 92: 136–141.
26. Weatherall M, Maling TJ (2004) Oral iron therapy for anaemia after orthopaedic surgery: Randomized clinical trial. ANZ J Surg 74: 1049–1051.
27. Carless P, Moxey A, O'Connell D, Henry D (2004) Autologous transfusion techniques: a systematic review of their efficacy. Transfus Med 14: 123–144.
28. Thomas D, Wareham K, Cohen D, Hutchings H (2001) Autologous blood transfusion in total knee replacement surgery. Br J Anaesth 86: 669–673.
29. Faris PM, Ritter MA, Keating EM, Valeri CR (1991) Unwashed filtered shed blood collected after knee and hip arthroplasties - a source of autologous red-blood-cells. J Bone Joint Surg Am 73: 1169–1178.
30. Hansen E, Hansen MP (2004) Reasons against the retransfusion of unwashed wound blood. Transfusion 44: 45S–53S.
31. Rollo VJ, Hozack WJ, Rothman RH, Chao W, Eng KO (1995) Prospective randomized evaluation of blood salvage techniques for primary total hip-arthroplasty. J Arthroplasty 10: 532–539.
32. Ritter MA, Keating EM, Faris PM (1994) Closed wound drainage in total hip or total knee replacement - a prospective randomized study. J Bone Joint Surg Am 76: 35–38.
33. Muñoz M, García-Erce JA, Villar I, Thomas D (2009) Blood conservation strategies in major orthopaedic surgery: efficacy, safety and European regulations. Vox Sang 96: 1–13.
34. Smith TO, Hing CB (2009) A meta-analysis of tourniquet assisted arthroscopic knee surgery. Knee 16: 317–321.
35. Zacharopoulos A, Apostolopoulos A, Kyriakidis A (2007) The effectiveness of reinfusion after total knee replacement. A prospective randomised controlled study. Int Orthop 31: 303–308.
36. Fernandez MC, Gottlieb M, Menitove JE (1992) Blood-transfusion and postoperative infection in orthopedic patients. Transfusion 32: 318–322.
37. Triulzi DJ, Vanek K, Ryan DH, Blumberg N (1992) A clinical and immunological study of blood-transfusion and postoperative bacterial-infection in spinal surgery. Transfusion 32; 517–524.
38. NIH (1989) Summary of NIH consensus development conference on perioperative red-cell transfusion. Am J Hematol 31: 144.
39. Dalén T, Bengtsson A, Brorsson B, Engström KG (2003) Inflammatory mediators in autotransfusion drain blood after knee arthroplasty, with and without leucocyte reduction. Vox Sang 85: 31–39.
40. Andersson I, Tylman M, Bengtson JP, Bengtsson A (2001) Complement split products and pro-inflammatory cytokines in salvaged blood after hip and knee arthroplasty. Can J Anaesth 48: 251–255.
41. Handel M, Winkler J, Hörnlein RF, Northoff H, Heeg P (2001) Increased interleukin-6 in collected drainage blood after total knee arthroplasty-An association with febrile reactions during retransfusion. Acta Orthop Scand 72: 270–272.
42. Innerhofer P, Klingler A, Klimmer C, Fries D, Nussbaumer W (2005) Risk for postoperative infection after transfusion of white blood cell-filtered allogeneic or autologous blood components in orthopedic patients undergoing primary arthroplasty. Transfusion 45: 103–110.
43. Llewelyn CA, Taylor RS, Todd AA, Stevens W, Murphy MF, et al. (2004) The effect of universal leukoreduction on postoperative infections and length of hospital stay in elective orthopedic and cardiac surgery. Transfusion 44: 489–500.

44. Biedler AE, Schneider SO, Seyfert U, Rensing H, Grenner S, et al. (2002) Impact of alloantigens and storage-associated factors on stimulated cytokine response in an in vitro model of blood transfusion. Anesthesiology 97: 1102–1109.
45. Shulman G, Grecula MJ, Hadjipavlou AG (2002) Intraoperative autotransfusion in hip arthroplasty. Clin Orthop Relat Res 396: 119–130.
46. Gharehbaghian A, Haque KM, Truman C, Evans R, Morse R, et al. (2004) Effect of autologous salvaged blood on postoperative natural killer cell precursor frequency. Lancet 363: 1025–1030.
47. Murphy P, Heal JM, Blumberg N (1991) Infection or suspected infection after hip-replacement surgery with autologous or homologous blood-transfusions. Transfusion 31: 212–217.
48. Muñoz M, Ariza D, Garcerán MJ, Gómez A, Campos A (2005) Benefits of postoperative shed blood reinfusion in patients undergoing unilateral total knee relacement. Arch Orthop Trauma Surg 125: 385–389.

Timing Matters in Hip Fracture Surgery: Patients Operated within 48 Hours Have Better Outcomes. A Meta-Analysis and Meta-Regression of over 190,000 Patients

Lorenzo Moja[1,3]*, Alessandra Piatti[4], Valentina Pecoraro[2], Cristian Ricci[3], Gianni Virgili[5], Georgia Salanti[6], Luca Germagnoli[3], Alessandro Liberati[7†], Giuseppe Banfi[2,3]

1 Department of Biomedical Sciences for Health, University of Milan, Milan, Italy, **2** University of Milan, Milan, Italy, **3** Clinical Epidemiology Unit, IRCCS Galeazzi Orthopedic Institute, Milan, Italy, **4** Epidemiological Observatory, ASL Milano, Milan, Italy, **5** Department of Oto Specialised Surgical Sciences, University of Florence, Florence, Italy, **6** Clinical and Molecular Epidemiology Unit and Clinical Trials and Evidence-Based Medicine Unit, Department of Hygiene and Epidemiology, School of Medicine, University of Ioannina, Ioannina, Greece, **7** Department of Oncology, Hematology and Respiratory Diseases, University of Modena and Reggio Emilia, Modena, Italy

Abstract

Background: To assess the relationship between surgical delay and mortality in elderly patients with hip fracture. Systematic review and meta-analysis of retrospective and prospective studies published from 1948 to 2011. Medline (from 1948), Embase (from 1974) and CINAHL (from 1982), and the Cochrane Library. Odds ratios (OR) and 95% confidence intervals for each study were extracted and pooled with a random effects model. Heterogeneity, publication bias, Bayesian analysis, and meta-regression analyses were done. Criteria for inclusion were retro- and prospective elderly population studies, patients with operated hip fractures, indication of timing of surgery and survival status.

Methodology/Principal Findings: There were 35 independent studies, with 191,873 participants and 34,448 deaths. The majority considered a cut-off between 24 and 48 hours. Early hip surgery was associated with a lower risk of death (pooled odds ratio (OR) 0.74, 95% confidence interval (CI) 0.67 to 0.81; $P<0.000$) and pressure sores (0.48, 95% CI 0.38 to 0.60; $P<0.000$). Meta-analysis of the adjusted prospective studies gave similar results. The Bayesian probability predicted that about 20% of future studies might find that early surgery is not beneficial for decreasing mortality. None of the confounders (e.g. age, sex, data source, baseline risk, cut-off points, study location, quality and year) explained the differences between studies.

Conclusions/Significance: Surgical delay is associated with a significant increase in the risk of death and pressure sores. Conservative timing strategies should be avoided. Orthopaedic surgery services should ensure the majority of patients are operated within one or two days.

Editor: Roberta W. Scherer, Johns Hopkins Bloomberg School of Public Health, United States of America

Funding: This review was funded by the Istituto di Ricovero e Cura a Carattere Scientifico Galeazzi. Another source of institutional support was the Department of Public Health of the University of Milan. The funders had no role in study design, data collection and analysis, decision to publish, or preparation of the manuscript.

Competing Interests: The authors have declared that no competing interests exist.

* E-mail: moja@marionegri.it

† Deceased.

Introduction

Hip fractures are common and serious: they always cause short-term pain, disability and can lead to longer-term pain, disability and even deformity. Mortality rate is estimated to be 5–10% at one month and 12–27% at one year from surgery [1]. Recent data from the UK, USA and Canada show that patients are mostly older than 75 years and female [2,3,4]. Mortality in the elderly may reach 10% at one month, 20% at four months and 30% at one year [5]. These patients are the frailest among those who are admitted to hospital, and their outcomes are likely to depend closely on how their care is managed.

In the last decade efforts have been made to boost our knowledge of the prognostic factors influencing the course and management of hip fracture. As the majority are treated surgically, time to surgery may be decisive. Some studies report that pre-operative delay might lead to an increase in mortality and adversely influence other clinical outcomes such as infection and pressure sores [6,7,8,9]. Clinical guidelines recommend immediate reparative surgery, within 24–48 hours from hospital admission [10,11]. However, several observational studies found no association between time and mortality and concluded that further research is needed on whether functional outcomes are worsened by delaying surgery [12,13,14]. This approach is supported by

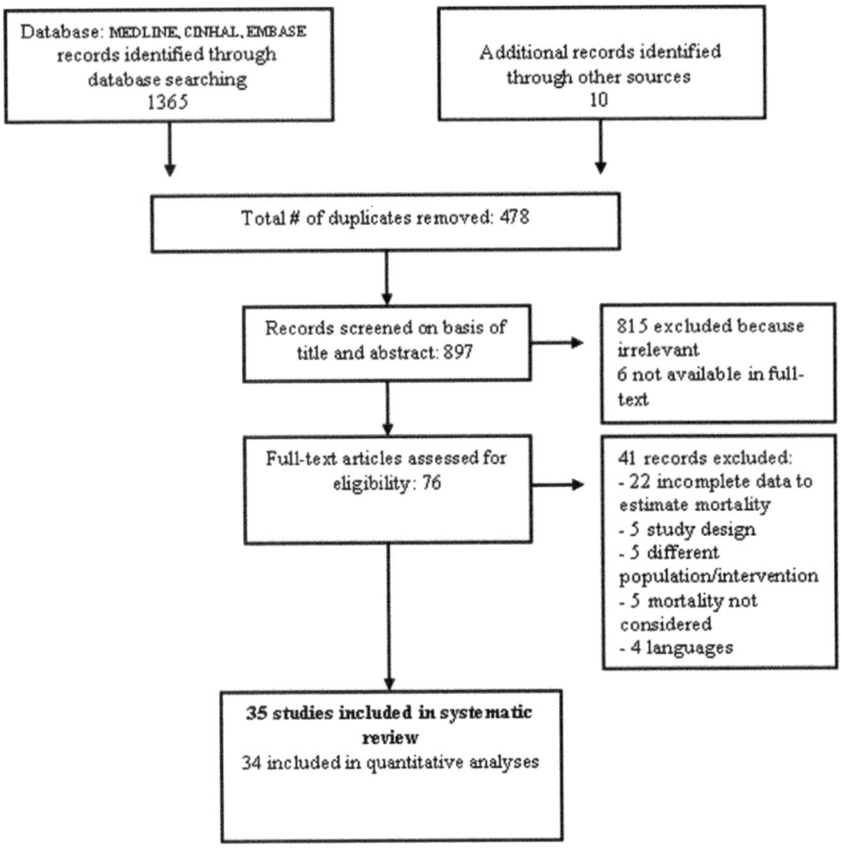

Figure 1. Selection for studies exploring the association between mortality and optimal time to surgery in patients with hip fractures.

geriatricians who offer an explicit rationale for postponing surgery: delay may be necessary and beneficial for stabilizing patients with co-morbidities [12].

A large number of observational studies have explored prognostic factors influencing hip fracture surgery, but with discordant results. Reasons might depend on the variability in adjusting for different confounders among studies, the lack of a consistent choice of the reference group and use of a common surgical delay cut-off.

A meta-analysis published in 2010 investigating the effect of surgical delay on mortality at different follow -up times, found significantly higher all-cause mortality for patients treated surgically more than 24, 48 and 72 hours from admission [15]. We moved from this high-quality meta-analysis to conduct a comprehensive meta-analysis which considered all prospective and retrospective evidence. The aims of this systematic review were: (i) to identify and describe all the studies which assessed whether surgical delay increases the mortality of elderly patients treated for hip fracture; (ii) to see whether delay is associated with increased mortality; (iii) to examine the influence of a wide range of *a priori* selected variables (age, sex, co-morbidities, etc.) using meta-regression; and (iv) to test the robustness of results using a Bayesian approach.

Methods

Eligibility

Studies were included if they met the following criteria: i) randomized, quasi-randomized (e.g. allocation based on date of admission), prospective and retrospective cohort and case-controlled studies; ii) patients with operated hip fractures; iii) patients aged 65 years or older (median or mean age per study); iv) reporting of timing of hip surgery; v) survival status adequately reported for meta-analysis; vi) published in English, French, Italian or Spanish after 1980. Evidence from controlled observational studies was included: it is unlikely that patients were randomized to receive immediate or postponed surgery to obtain evidence of the mortality-delay association because of ethical concerns. We did not define the optimal surgical delay from hospital admission to reparative surgery *a priori* but accepted what the authors claimed at face value. When authors did not give a cut-off, we arbitrarily selected 24 hours as optimal. Different time cut-offs were used as strata in our analyses.

Search strategy

Studies were identified by searching electronic databases and scanning reference lists of articles. This search was applied to Medline (1948 – /September 2011), and adapted for Embase (1974 – September 2011) and CINAHL (1982 – December 2011). The strategy was developed using the following key items: hip fracture, arthroplasty, and timing surgery (see Search strategy – *Table S1*) [16,17]. Manual searches of the reference lists of included studies, reviews, meta-analyses and guidelines on hip fracture surgery and prognostic factors were also done.

Study selection

The literature search was conducted independently and two reviewers (AP and LG) independently searched the literature who

Table 1. Characteristics of included studies.

Source	Design	Source of data	Data source for pre-operative time and confounding factor	Country	No of participants	Average age	% Female	Optimal Time (hours)	Methodology score
Al Ani 2008	Prospective	Two centres	Clinical records	Sweden	744	81	73	24	7
Bergeron 2006	Retrospective	One centre	Unclear	Canada	977	81	74	24	7
Bredahl 1992	Retrospective	One centre	Clinical records	Denmark	778	79	73	12	5
Carretta 2011	Retrospective	One centre	Administrative data	Italy	1320	83	77	48	7
Davis 1988	Prospective	Two centres	Clinical records	USA	230	81	82	48	6
Dorotka 2003	Prospective	One centre	Clinical records	Austria	182	78	76	24	7
Doruk 2003	Prospective	One centre	Clinical records	Turkey	65	76	64	120	7
Elliott 2003	Prospective	Two centres	Clinical Records	Ireland	1780	NR	77	24	9
Franzo 2005	Retrospective	18 centres	Administrative data	Italy	6629	82	81	48	8
Gdalevich 2004	Retrospective	One centre	Clinical records	Israel	651	NR	75	48	8
Grimes 2002	Retrospective	20 centres	Clinical records**	USA	8383	80	79	24	8
Hamlet 1997	Retrospective	One centre	Clinical records	USA	171	77	80	24	6
Holt 2008	Prospective	22 centres	Clinical records	UK	18692	NR	79	24	9
Kenzora 1986	Retrospective	One centre	Clinical records	USA	406	76	76	24	6
Maggi 2009	Prospective	Nine centres	Clinical records	Italy	2473	82	79	24	8
Majumdar 2006	Retrospective	Multicentre*	Administrative data	Canada	3864	82	71	24	8
Mc Guire 2004	Retrospective	Multicentre*	Administrative data	USA	18208	82	79	48	8
Moran 2005	Prospective	One centre	Clinical records	UK	2148	80	76	96	9
Mullen 1989	Prospective	One centre	Clinical records	USA	400	79	NR	24	6
Novack 2007	Retrospective	Seven centres	Administrative data	USA	3815	82	73	48	9
Orosz 2004	Prospective	Four centres	Clinical records	USA	1576	82	81	24	9
Parker 1992	Prospective	One centre	Clinical records	UK	468	81	83	48	7
Peleg 2011	Retrospective	Seven centres	Administrative data	Israel	6442	NR	NR	48	6
Radcliff 2008	Retrospective	181 centres	Administrative data	USA	5682	77	0	96	6
Rademakers 2007	Retrospective	One centre	Clinical records	Netherlands	722	82	76	12	5
Rae 2007	Prospective	One centre	Clinical records	Australia	222	79	72	48	8
Roos 1996	Retrospective	Multicentre*	Administrative data	USA	26213	81	79	48	5
Sexson 1988	Retrospective	One centre	Clinical records	USA	300	NR	77	24	8
Smektala 2008	Prospective	268 centres	Clinical records	German	2916	NR	80	48	8
Siegmeth 2005	Prospective	One centre	Clinical records	UK	3628	81	NR	48	8
Stoddart 2002	Retrospective	One centre	Clinical records	New Zealand	138	83	75	24	7
Sund 2005	Retrospective	Multicentre	Administrative data	Finland	16881	82	75	48	9
Swanson 1998	RCT	One centre	Clinical records	USA	71	79	78	48	NA
Verbeek 2007	Retrospective	One centre	Clinical records	Netherlands	192	80	77	24	9

Table 1. Cont.

Source	Design	Source of data	Data source for pre-operative time and confounding factor	Country	No of participants	Average age	% Female	Optimal Time (hours)	Methodology score
Weller 2005	Retrospective	One centre	Administrative data	Canada	57315	78	75	24	8

*Number of participating centres not reported. **Data already collected for other purpose. NR Not Reported. NA Not applicable.

then selected potentially eligible studies for inclusion. Disagreements between them were resolved by consensus; if no agreement could be reached, a third author (LM) was called in to decide. The fulltext of all eligible citations was examined in more detail.

Data Extraction

We developed a data extraction sheet, pilot-tested it on five randomly-selected studies, and refined it accordingly. One review author (AP) extracted the following data from studies included and entered in the data extraction form: study design, study year, participants (age, sex, case-mix and co-morbidities), country of origin and setting. A second author (CR) checked the extracted data to ensure quality. Disagreements were solved by discussion between the two review authors; if no agreement was reached, a third author (LM) could decide.

The primary outcome was unambiguous overall mortality. If applicable short- (<30 days) and long-term mortality (>30 days) were combined. Secondary outcomes were post-operative complications, i.e. infections, pressure sores, post-operative chronic pain, hospital length of stay, and readmission. If necessary, percentages of mortality or other outcomes were converted into frequencies.

For all studies that addressed mortality, we recorded the unadjusted matched odds ratios (OR) for: i) the comparison of early and delayed surgery; ii) whether any adjustment was made for covariates (e.g. age); iii) the adjusted estimate of the ORs and 95% confidence intervals (CIs). When univariate and multivariate adjusted models were available, both were abstracted. Since some studies reported only adjusted hazard ratios, we converted them to ORs using a formula to compute risk ratio from OR [18]. We used as control mortality risk the median control risk based on our primary meta-analysis.

If a study considered both young patients (<65 years or high-velocity injuries) and old patients, the data were extracted separately if possible, and only the elderly group was considered. If sorting was not possible and at least 90% of the patients in a study were classifiable as elderly, the study was included; if not it was excluded.

Methodological quality

Methodological quality was independently assessed by two review authors (AP and LG). For observational studies the Newcastle-Ottawa (NOS) scale for cohort and case-control studies was used [19,20]. This scale has three groups of items: selection, exposure/outcome and comparability. A study can be awarded a maximum of one star for each numbered item in 'patient selection' (four items) and 'exposure' (three items) and a maximum of two stars in the 'comparability of study groups' (two items), for a total of nine stars. Since we were interested in mortality of operated patients, we expected three items would be scored positively across all studies, specifically *Ascertainment of exposure (secure surgical record), Demonstration that outcome of interest was not present at start of study, Assessment of outcome (record linkage)*. In fact in our meta-analysis the NOS scale could have ranged between three and nine. For randomized controlled trials (RCTs) we summarized the risk of bias for mortality across the following specific domains within study: sequence generation, allocation concealment, and incomplete outcome data [21]. We decided *a priori* that only prospective observational studies that met eight or nine of the Newcastle-Ottawa Scale criteria were to be considered of high quality, whereas RCTs were considered of high quality if they satisfied two or more.

Table 2. Methodological Quality Assessment of Observational Studies Based on the Newcastle-Ottawa (NOS) scale.

Study ID	Selection		Comparability		Outcome		Total score*
	Representativeness of early cohort	Selection of delay cohort	Controlled for age	Controlled for co-morbidities	Follow- up length	Adequacy follow-up	
Al Ani 2008	*	*			*	*	7
Bergeon 2006	*	*	*	*			7
Bredahl 1992					*	*	5
Carretta 2011		*	*		*	*	7
Davis 1988	*	*			*		6
Dorotka 2003	*	*			*	*	7
Doruk 2003	*	*			*	*	7
Elliott 2003	*	*	*	*	*	*	9
Franzo 2005	*	*	*	*	*		8
Gdalevich 2004	*	*	*	*	*		8
Grimes 2002	*	*	*	*	*		8
Kenzora 1986	*	*			*		6
Hamlet 1997	*	*			*		6
Holt 2008	*	*	*	*	*	*	9
Maggi 2009	*	*	*	*	*		8
Majumdar 2006	*	*	*	*	*		8
Mc Guire 2004	*	*	*	*		*	8
Moran 2005	*	*	*	*	*	*	9
Mullen 1989	*	*			*	*	6
Novack 2007	*	*	*	*	*	*	9
Orosz 2004	*	*	*	*	*	*	9
Parker 1992	*	*			*	*	7
Peleg 2011			*		*	*	6
Radcliff 2008			*	*		*	6
Rademakers 2007	*	*					5
Rae 2007	*	*	*	*		*	8
Roos 1996			*			*	5
Sexson 1988	*	*		*	*	*	8
Siegmeth 2005	*	*		*	*	*	8
Smektala 2011	*	*	*		*	*	8
Stoddart 2002	*	*			*	*	7
Sund 2005	*	*	*	*	*	*	9
Verbeek 2007	*	*	*	*	*	*	9
Weller 2005	*	*	*	*	*		8

*Total score: sum of row totals plus 3 points scored positively across all studies (see methods section for details).

Data analysis

We did an overall quantitative synthesis using all ORs on mortality across all studies, with unadjusted data from each study. The results were pooled using the inverse variance method and ordered by study year. The random effects model described by DerSimonian and Laird [22] was used to synthesize data rather than the fixed effect model because it incorporates intra- and inter-study variability. This model was selected a priori as the meta-analysis was expected to include primarily observational studies with inherently more variability than RCTs. A Mantel-Haenszel OR was also computed using fixed effect and compared to the DerSimonian and Laird estimate to investigate any influence of small study effects on the pooled OR, since the DerSimonian and Laird methods tend to attribute greater weight to small studies with increasing heterogeneity [23]. The degree of heterogeneity between trials was assessed by the I-squared (I^2) statistic, with its 95% CI for each outcome. We accounted for heterogeneity in the results of our primary meta-analysis, using the prediction interval (estimated in a Bayesian setting) for the true effect in a new study, which describes the full distribution of effects in a random-effects meta-analysis [21].

Since meta-analyses of observational studies often give spuriously precise results, we tested the robustness of results with two approaches. First, we calculated the probability of the OR being

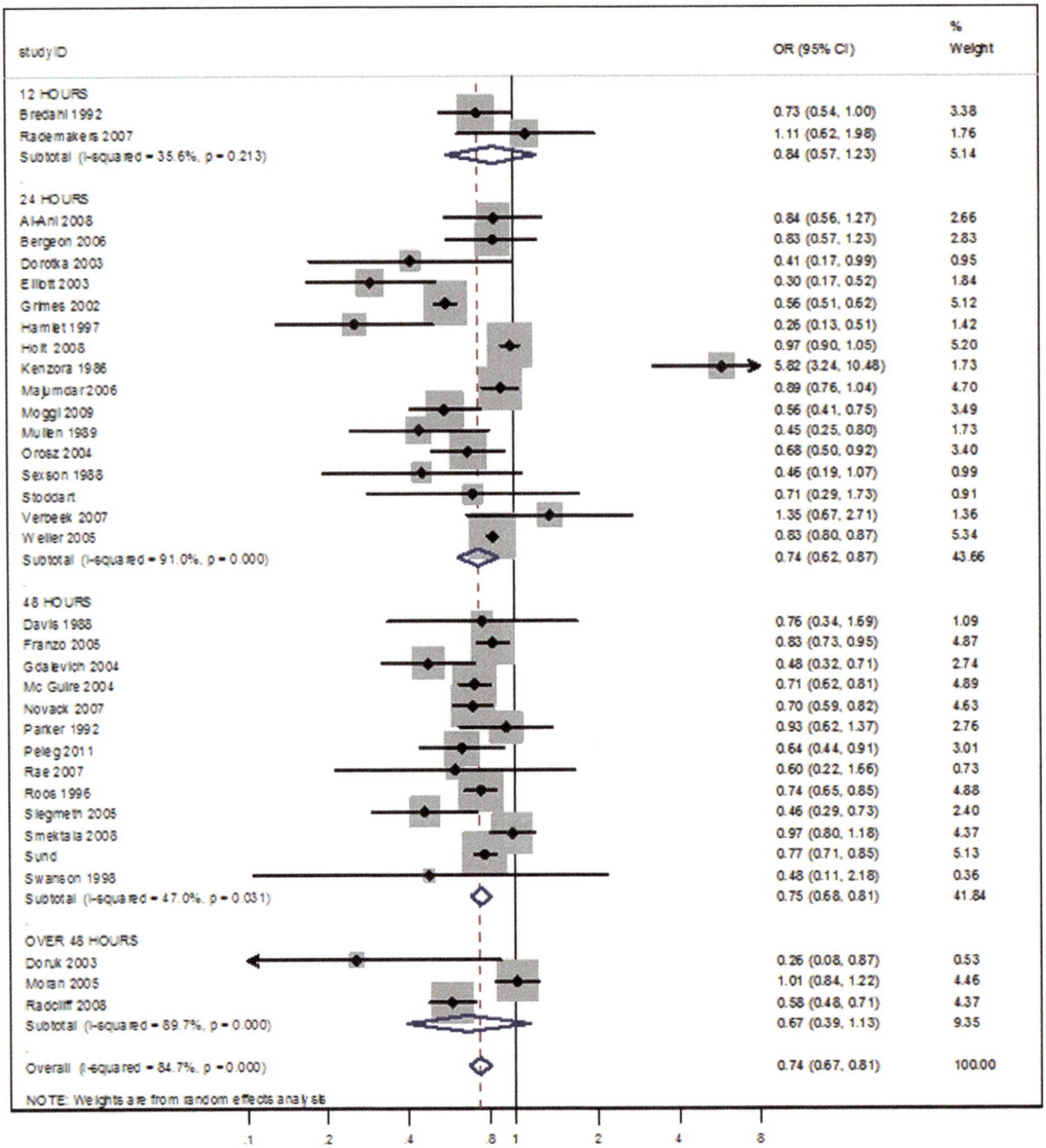

Figure 2. Meta-analysis of Early versus Delayed surgery time according to cut-off points (12, 24, 48, and over 48 hours). Outcome: overall mortality.

less than 1 from the predictive Bayesian interval. Second, we used credibility ceilings, a technique which assumes that methodological limitations implicit in included observational studies cannot give us more than a maximum certainty that an effect is in a particular direction and not null or in the other direction [24].

Sensitivity to prior assumptions was checked in the Bayesian estimation of the pooled OR as well as the predictive interval. We assumed different priors for the shape of the random effects distribution: Gamma (0.001, 0.001) on precision; uniform (0, 50) on inter-study variance tau2; uniform(0, 50) on inter-study standard deviation tau; and three functions of mean intra-study variance: uniform shrinkage on tau2, DuMouchel on tau, and half-normal on tau2.

Further sensitivity analysis was done to account for methodological differences between the studies. Data were synthesized for studies of high and low quality, using adjusted study-specific estimates, preferring the ones with the most extensive adjustment [25].

The extent to which study-level variables explained heterogeneity in predicting mortality was explored by fitting random effects

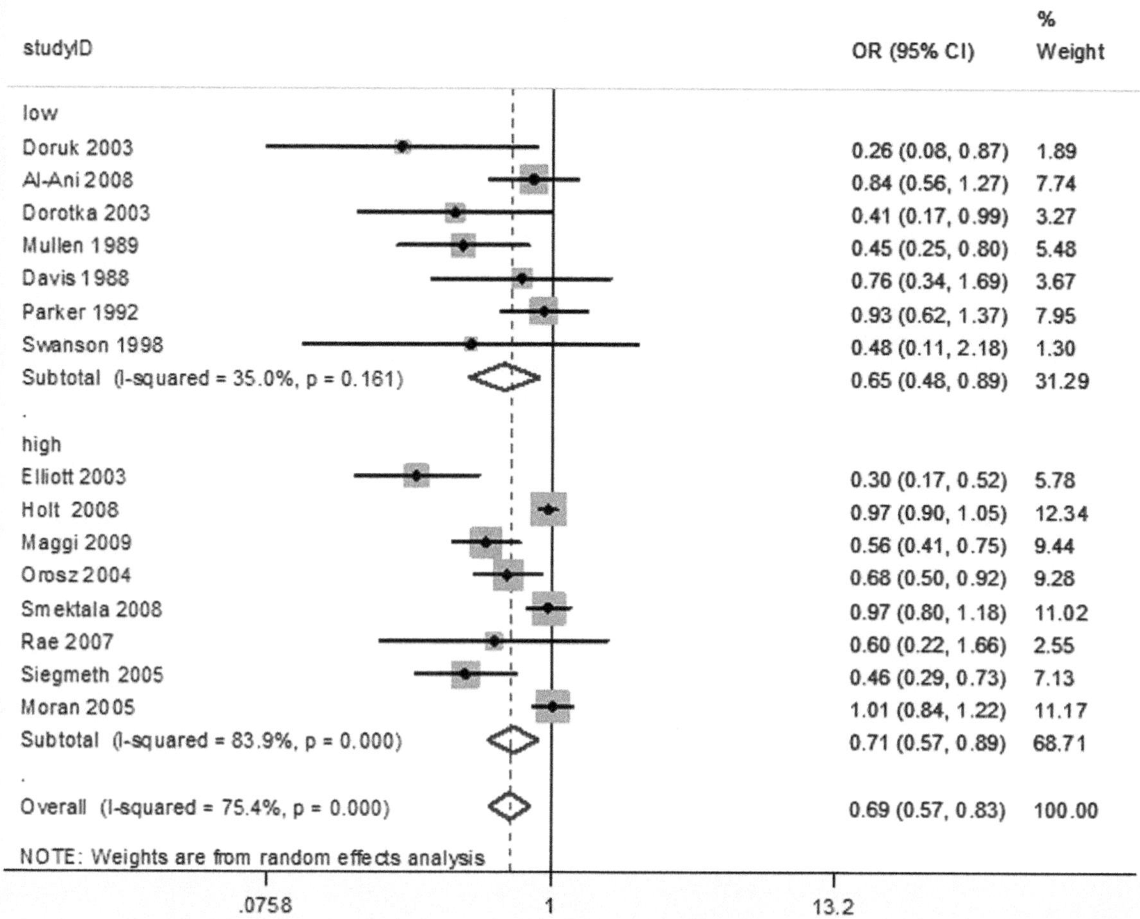

Figure 3. Meta-analysis of high and low-quality adjusted prospective studies comparing early versus delayed surgery time. Outcome: overall mortality.

meta-regression models to account for the design (prospective or retrospective), nature of data (administrative or clinical), methodological quality (8–9 stars or 1–7), health status or co-morbidities (to identify patients at high risk of mortality), location of study (United States or other), different optimal time cut-points, age, prevalence of females, study year, and optimal time treated as a continuous variable. The effect of mortality baseline risk was investigated in a Bayesian linear regression model.

We checked for potential publication and small study effects by the contour enhanced funnel plot [26,27] integrating visual inspection of the plot with the test proposed by Harbord [28].

Statistical analyses were done using Stata v.11 [29] and WinBUGS v.1.3 software [30] *P*-values less than 0.05 were considered statistically significant.

Results

Database searches yielded 1375 references. Hand-searching produced 10 more. Exclusion of duplicates and irrelevant references left 76 descriptive studies. We excluded 41 studies because of: incomplete data (n = 22), study design (n = 5), different population/intervention (n = 5), mortality not considered as an outcome (n = 5), language (n = 4). We included 35 studies fulfilling our inclusion criteria, all except one [31] providing data for our analyses (*Figure 1*) [6,7,13,31,32,33,34,35,36,37,38,39,40,41,42,-43,44,45,46,47,48,49,50,51,52,53,54,55,56,57,58]. This corresponds to 34 cohort studies, 14 using a prospective design and 20 a retrospective one, and one RCT. summarizes the main features of the 35 articles included, which included 191,873 participants. The number of participants in each trial ranged from 65 to 57,315 (*Table 1*). The mean age was 80 years (range 76–83 years). The mean proportion of women was 74% (0–83%) in the 32 studies reporting sex. Three studies were published in the 80's, six in the 90's and 26 (71.8%) after 2000. Twelve were from the USA, four from UK, three each from Canada and Italy, two each from Israel and Netherlands; Australia, Austria, Denmark, Finland, German, Ireland, New Zealand, Turkey and Sweden provided one study each.

Patient data were collected from clinical records in 24 studies, in ten from national or regional administrative databases, and in one the source was unclear. The optimal surgical delay was 12 hours in two studies, 24 hours in 16, 36 hours in one study, 48 in thirteen, and >72 in three. The quality measured through the

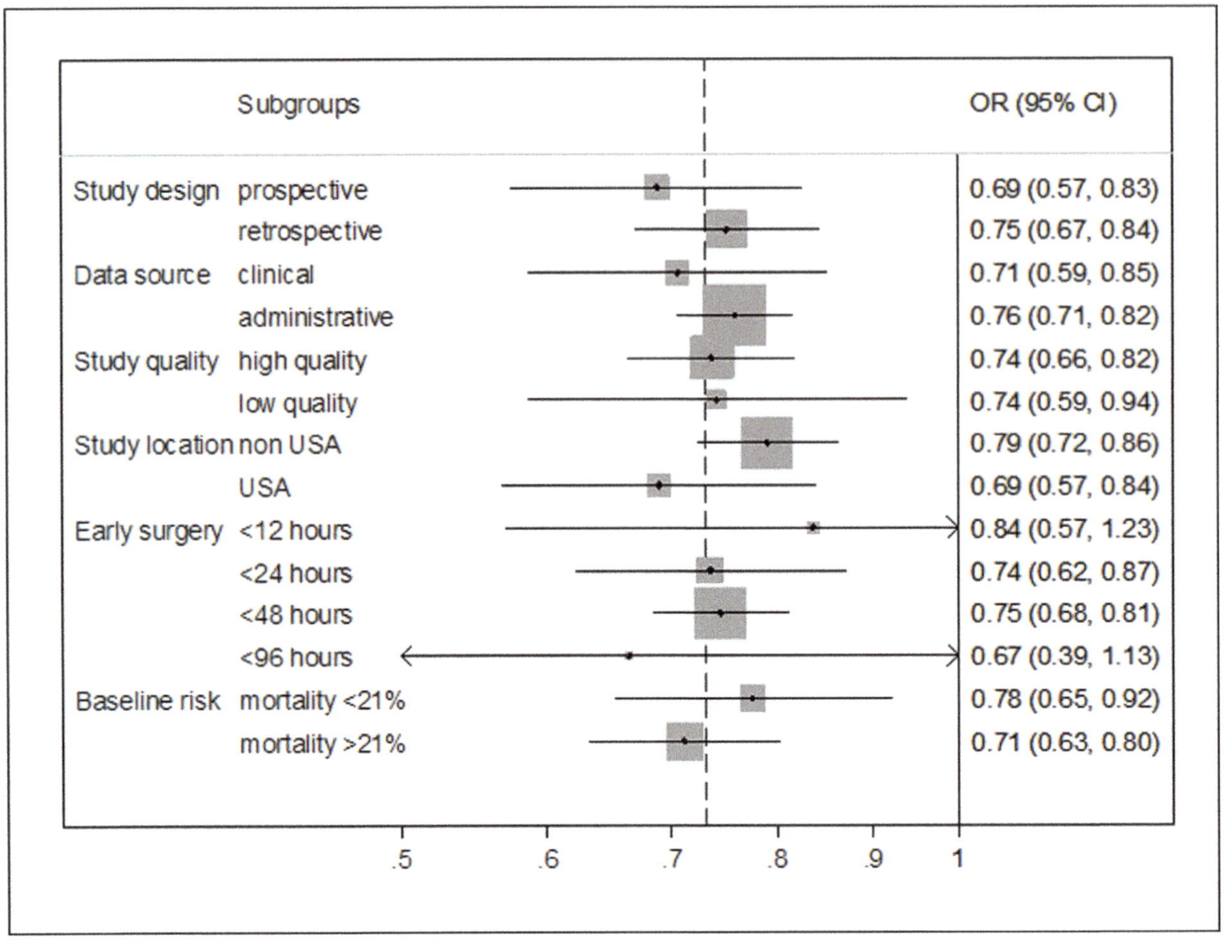

Figure 4. Subgroups analyses of Early and Delayed surgery time for overall mortality.

NOS scale ranged from five to nine points, with a median of seven (*Table 2*).

The only RCT was at high risk of bias [57]. Swanson randomized a limited number of patients (71) to a multifaceted intervention named 'early intervention'. Early surgery, early mobilization, and intensive support by health professionals were the main components, although it is difficult to evaluate their relative roles. The groups did not truly differ in terms of time to surgery: 90% of patients in the intervention group and 80% in the control group were operated within 48 hours. The generation of the randomization sequence and allocation concealment were likely to be inappropriate, possibly being affected by the time of hospital admission.

Time to surgery and mortality

Patients who underwent early surgery had significantly lower odds of death than those whose surgery was delayed (OR 0.74; 95% CI 0.67 to 0.81; p<0,0001.). Substantial heterogeneity ($I^2 = 84.7\%$) was detected as shown in the forest plots (*Figure 2*). The OR predictive interval was 0.48 to 1.13, meaning that no effect or an adverse effect of early surgery might be a plausible finding in a new study. The Mantel-Haenszel OR was 0.79 (95% CI 0.77 to 0.81; p<0.0001), suggesting a modest impact of small studies on the random effects estimate towards more beneficial values.

Bayesian meta-analysis yielded an OR of 0.72 and a 95% credible interval (0.61 to 0.84) the upper bound of which was relatively insensitive to assumptions about prior distribution for random effects. The likelihood of early surgery being found to be beneficial varied between 78% and 82% according to assumptions on priors, suggesting that no or an adverse effect of early surgery could be predicted in about 20% of future studies.

The benefit was resistant to conservative interpretation with sceptical credibility ceilings: only when we considered that there was no chance of any single study convincing us more than about 22% that the effect of early surgery was beneficial did the pooled estimate predict that early and delayed surgery were equivalent.

Meta-regression analyses

Risk of bias. Fourteen studies, seven of low quality [32,34,35,36,44,46,57] and eight of high quality [37,40,43,45,50,53,54], reported prospective adjusted measures of effect. The overall random effects meta-analysis of ORs yielded a pooled estimate favouring early surgery (OR: 0.69; 95% CI: 0.57–0.83; $I^2 = 75.4\%$). The test for differences between study quality subgroups was not statistically significant (random effects meta-regression $P = 0.42$). The results are reported in *Figure 3*.

Other confounders. *Table 3* summarizes meta-regression and *Figure 4* subgroup results on unadjusted data. In all studies the reporting of mortality stratified for comorbidity was incomplete and we were therefore unable to do a reliable meta-regression

Table 3. Random effects meta-regression analyses of Early and Delayed surgery time for overall mortality.

Characteristic	N. studies	N. participants	OR (95% CI)	p-value
Continuous variables				
Age (per 10 years)	28	159772	0.97 (0.36 to 2.63)	0.96
Female prevalence (per 10% more)	32	187885	1.03 (0.92 to 1.16)	0.55
Study year (per 10 years)	34	191873	0.90 (0.7 to 1.18)	0.46
Continuous time (per 24 hours)	34	191873	0.22 (0.00077 to 63.62)	0.59
Categorical variables				
Study design				
Prospective (reference)	15	35112	1	
Retrospective	20	156761	1.17 (0.82 to 1.66)	0.36
Data source category				
Clinical data (reference)	24	46843	1	
Administrative data	10	144053	1.05 (0.72 to 1.53)	0.78
Study quality				
8–9 stars (reference)	18	149228	1	
1–7 stars	17	42645	1.05 (0.73 to 1.5)	0.79
Study location				
Non-US study (reference)	23	129179	1	
US study	12	62694	0.94 (0.65 to 1.35)	0.74
Early surgery time cut-off definition				
<12 hours	2	1500	1.2 (0.55 to 2.65)	0.62
<24 hours (reference)	16	97100	1	
<48 hours	14	85378	0.97 (0.65 to 1.43)	0.87
<96–120 hours	3	7895	0.90 (0.46 to 1.78)	0.77
Baseline risk				
Risk<21%	17	85826	1	
Risk>21%	18	106047	0.86 (0.61 to 1.22)	0.40

analysis of this predictor. None of the covariates studied with meta-regression or subgroup analyses yielded any significant effects on mortality ($p \geq 0.05$). However, the power of these analyses is typically low and exploration of confounders may be possibly subject to aggregation bias.

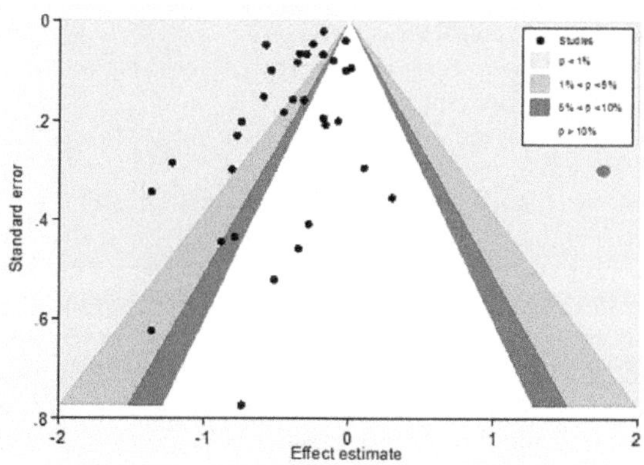

Figure 5. Contour enhanced funnel plot of studies comparing Early and Delayed surgery time for overall mortality. Caption: Kenzora 1986 (in red), while laying in the area of statistical significance favouring late surgery, may have interfered with the effect of small studies in the funnel plot.

The association between the OR for being operated earlier or later and study baseline risk approached statistical significance, but did not cross it (regression coefficient: −0.14; 95% Bayesian credible interval from −0.40 to 0.09) i.e., the decrease in mortality baseline risk corresponds to a decrease in the difference between early or late surgery (OR close to 1). The probability of the regression coefficient being different from nil was 0.88%.

Time to surgery and secondary outcomes

We were able to do additional meta-analyses for pressure sores (six studies, 4590 patients, random effects pooled OR 0.48, 95% CI, 0.38–0.60; $I^2 = 0\%$). The studies were extremely heterogeneous in terms of post-operative complications (i.e. different complications were grouped) and hospital length of stay. Considering the subsample of studies published since 2000, based on an arbitrary period focused on the last decade, mean length of stay varied between seven and 46 days, raising concern that studies differed in their postoperative pathways and hospital discharge policies. These health service differences prevented any meta-analysis of these outcomes. We found data from one study each for post-operative chronic pain and readmission.

Table 4. Similarities and differences between this systematic review and an independent one by Simunovic et al. 2010 [15].

Systematic review	Simunovic 2010	Moja 2012
Objectives	We conducted a systematic review and meta-analysis to determine the effect of early surgery on the risk of death and common postoperative complications among elderly patients with hip fracture.	The aims of this systematic review are: (i) to identify and describe all the studies which assessed whether operative delay increases the mortality of elderly patients treated surgically for hip fracture; (ii) to see whether delay is associated with increased mortality; and (iii) to examine the influence of *a priori* selected variables (age, sex, co-morbidities, etc.).
Results on mortality		
Overall	16 studies, 13 478 patients, RR 0.55, 95% CI 0.40–0.75, $p<0.001$, $I^2=71\%$.	34 studies, 191 873 patients, OR 0.74, 95% CI 0.67 to 0.81, $P<0.0001$, $I^2=85\%$.
High-quality studies	5 studies, 4 208 patients, RR 0.81, 95% CI 0.68–0.96, $p=0.01$, $I^2=0\%$.	8 studies, 33435 patients OR: 0.81; 95%CI: 0.71 to 0.59, $p=0.0001$, $I^2=86\%$.
Authors' conclusions on mortality	Earlier surgery was associated with a lower risk of death and lower rates of postoperative pneumonia and pressure sores among elderly patients with hip fracture. These results suggest that reducing delays may reduce mortality and complications.	Surgical delay is associated with a significant increase in the risk of death and pressure sores. Conservative timing strategies should be limited to patients who may benefit most. Orthopaedic surgery services should ensure the majority of patients are operated between one and two days.
Methods		
Outcomes	Mortality, pressure sores, pneumonia, deep vein thrombosis, pulmonary embolism	Mortality, pressure sores
Eligibility criteria	i) Patients 60 years of age or older; ii) who underwent surgery for a low-energy hip fracture; iii) evaluation of preoperative surgical delay; iv) consideration of all-cause mortality as an outcome; and v) prospective design.	i) Randomized, quasi-randomized (i.e. allocation based on date of admission), prospective and retrospective cohort and case-controlled studies; ii) inclusion of patients with operated hip fractures; iii) inclusion of timing of hip surgery; iv) inclusion of patients older than 65 years (median or mean age per study); v) survival status adequately reported for meta-analysis.
Study identification	No language and year restrictions.	Studies published in English, French, Italian or Spanish after 1980.
Risk of bias	Newcastle-Ottawa Scale criteria	Newcastle-Ottawa Scale criteria
Summary statistics	Relative Risk	Odds Ratio
Statistical approaches	Random-effects model of DerSimonian and Laird.	Primary: Random-effects model of DerSimonian and Laird, prediction interval. Secondary: fixed-effect model of Mantel-Haenszel and Bayesian.
Stratification for	Time according to follow-up mortality (short, medium and long-term).	Time according to cut-off points for surgery (12, 24, 48, and over 48 hours).
Strengths	Extensive study search Postoperative complications.	Meta-regression and Bayesian meta-analysis.

Small study effects

Visual inspection of the contour-enhanced funnel plot (*Figure 5*) indicated that pooled data did not appear to be heavily influenced by publication bias. This means that slight asymmetry of the plot is possible, with relatively few studies existing midway in the area of non-significance. It is also possible that others are 'missing' from this area. Nevertheless Harbord's test was not statistically significant ($P=0.173$).

Discussion

This meta-analysis of 35 studies showed that elderly patients operated for hip fracture sooner – i.e. within one or two days from hospital admission – have significantly less mortality than patients scheduled for surgery after the second day. After adjustment for age, female prevalence, location, and year, or after omitting low-quality and retrospective studies, this association remained consistently significant. This result was resistant to conservative approaches that increase the confidence attributed to significant effects based on nominal statistical significance. Observational study designs have limitations, but our results do indicate that there probably are differences in mortality outcomes between early and delayed hip fracture surgery, and may even be large in terms of patient benefits. Given the wide diversity of these studies and the frequent lack of control for clinically relevant confounders such as comorbidities, the quantitative results must be seen as merely strongly suggestive, not conclusive.

We observed substantial intra-study heterogeneity that was not explained by any of the study-level variables. Given the absolute majority of non-randomized studies and the variability in settings, health status and comorbidities, adjusting factors, and databases used, some heterogeneity is to be expected. Relying on quantitative inferences generated by observational studies, however, can lead to misleading claims when the overall data suffers from substantial heterogeneity that remains unexplained. On the other hand we explored and found no major differences between studies with adjustments for covariates or unadjusted studies and between studies using clinical or administrative data sources: This might limit the effects of confounders.

In patients immobilized for hip fractures, mortality is influenced by multiple risk factors. Less than half the studies considered comorbidity. Other covariates, such as the centre in multi-centre studies or cognitive impairment, were often ignored. Inadequacies in adjusting for important confounders is an important threat to this systematic review and it is very hard to make inferences or probe their exact depth *ex post*. This might reflect the excessive use of administrative databases rather than medical records to obtain a critical mass of data. Administrative databases are clearly a poor source of information on even major confounders and the rudimentary quality of this type of data has been questioned [25]. Another caveat is that large-scale studies based on administrative databases may have far more weight in a meta-analysis than smaller studies based on meticulous examination of full health records, even using methods to down-weight the spurious precision (i.e. random effects model).

Other threats to internal validity are plausible and relevant to this systematic review. Selection bias is the confounding of treatment effects with population differences: clinicians may without hesitation refer healthier patients for surgery, so differences in mortality tend to be confounded by the indication to surgery. This bias could be combined with another threat: in some studies patients were considered ineligible on the basis of acute medical conditions and surgical delays due to admission and pre-operative management. This builds in the plausible likelihood of group differences that can masquerade as treatment effect. If treatment improves the outcome and patients operated earlier are on average healthier, they could gain more from the treatment, returning to health faster than the controls, thus boosting the differences between groups.

There are other systematic reviews published in a short time on the relation between mortality and hip surgery [59,60]. Our results confirm the previous findings by Simunovic et al [15]. Although the large number of patients and studies increases the power of our meta-analysis, the precision of effect sizes should not be over-interpreted. Our meta-analysis reports the prediction interval that addresses the actual dispersion of effect sizes across studies and shows little change with more studies. The Bayesian meta-analysis predicts values of OR larger than 1 in about 20% of future studies. Thus, the mean benefit is unlikely to be found across all patients and clinical settings. Early surgery may not save lives, or can even cause more deaths. The interplay of clinical and organizational determinants of quality of care and the potential selection of patients at higher or lower risk of mortality at each hospital makes surgery and admission for hip fracture a complex procedure. In *Table 4* methods and results of the review by Simunovic are compared to this review to highlight the similar conclusions made by two independent groups.

Many different cut-off times have been used to distinguish early and late surgery: most studies used 24 and 48 hours while a few others used shorter (up to 6 hours) or longer (up to 72 hours) times. Although we grouped studies based on the cut-off time selected, it is difficult to draw a precise line between early and delayed surgery, and it is clear that all these observational comparison groups could still be unbalanced and give rise to significant biases. The optimal timing might be between 12 and 48 hours, identifying two time windows: an immediate timing strategy so that surgery is scheduled on the same or next calendar day after hospital admission and a rapid early timing strategy so that surgery is scheduled within two days of admission.

Although a randomized trial in this context has been opposed because it could be unethical [7], a stronger design such as a randomized trial evaluating the timing of surgery (immediate or rapid) is an attractive idea to reduce the threats supporting causal inferences. This approach is generally accepted in cardiology where there are several examples of randomized trials evaluating the optimal timing of invasive interventions [61,62]. In our systematic review we found only one RCT examining the effect of delayed hip surgery in the context of a multifaceted intervention [57]. Although this trial suffered by several shortcomings including poor intervention integrity, it can still be considered a key-milestone study because it offered patients a potential genuine equipoise. If observational designs are preferred, we invite investigators to use more quasi-experimental design elements: propensity scores based on medical records have been successfully used in some studies [41,45] and merit more attention.

In Italy, only one third of patients are operated within three days after admission (region ranges from 11% to 60%) [63]. The feasibility of operating sooner after the injury depends on the efficient use of hospital resources: key contextual elements are the number of surgeons, anaesthetists and operating rooms available and the absence of prolonged clinical assessments due to administrative delays or low-clinical-value investigations. The results of this study encourage hospitals to shorten the time from admission to hip fracture surgery: operating rooms available by night and day 33, 48, application of risk scores at admission [37], multi-disciplinary management 51, and timing as a quality indicator [56], have all been proposed to improve quality. Clearly, further economic analyses are needed to assess the cost-effectiveness of these strategies in various health care systems.

Early hip fracture surgery does appear to provide a survival benefit in comparison with later intervention; it was also associated with a significant reduction in pressure sores. Conservative timing strategies should be limited to patients who will benefit most (i.e. those requiring stabilization) because, besides consuming considerable resources, and physician and nursing time, they may severely affect a patient's health. Cardiac or renal failure is a compelling reason for delay: cardiologists or nephrologists are consulted to set the timing for surgery, and patients often require additional treatments and tests that take time. This unavoidable delay keeps the patient in bed, increasing the risk of pulmonary, skin and urinary infections and may erode the benefit brought by the specialist approach. Whenever possible the consultation should be completed in 24–48 hours. Administrative delays are unjustifiable. This strategy should be pursued in high- and low-volume hip fracture centres. The early surgery strategy is not intended as a race against time to operate patients in a few hours but everything possible should be done to ensure the majority of patients are operated within one to two days.

Acknowledgments

The authors wish to thank Judith Baggott, Haris Vasiliadis and Gustavo Zanoli who helped with translation or provided comments and editorial input to this review; Vanna Pistotti who revised the search strategy; Michela Cinquini and Rita Banzi who helped with data extraction from studies.

Author Contributions

Conceived and designed the experiments: LM AP GB. Performed the experiments: AP VP LG LM. Analyzed the data: AP CR GV GS. Wrote the paper: LM AP VP. Critical revision of the intellectual content of the manuscript: LM AP VP CR GV GS LG AL GB.

References

1. Parker M, Johansen A (2006) Hip fracture. Bmj 333: 27–30.
2. Improvement IfIa (2006) Delivering quality and value: focus on fractured neck of femur. NHS.
3. Brauer CA, Coca-Perraillon M, Cutler DM, Rosen AB (2009) Incidence and mortality of hip fractures in the United States. JAMA 302: 1573–1579.
4. Leslie WD, O'Donnell S, Jean S, Lagace C, Walsh P, et al. (2009) Trends in hip fracture rates in Canada. JAMA 302: 883–889.
5. Roberts SE, Goldacre MJ (2003) Time trends and demography of mortality after fractured neck of femur in an English population, 1968–98: database study. Bmj 327: 771–775.
6. Weller I, Wai EK, Jaglal S, Kreder HJ (2005) The effect of hospital type and surgical delay on mortality after surgery for hip fracture. Journal of Bone & Joint Surgery – British Volume 87: 361–366.
7. Novack V, Jotkowitz A, Etzion O, Porath A (2007) Does delay in surgery after hip fracture lead to worse outcomes? A multicenter survey. International Journal for Quality in Health Care 19: 170–176.
8. Bottle A, Aylin P (2006) Mortality associated with delay in operation after hip fracture: observational study. Bmj 332: 947–951.
9. Gdalevich M, Cohen D, Yosef D, Tauber C (2004) Morbidity and mortality after hip fracture: the impact of operative delay. Archives of Orthopaedic & Trauma Surgery 124: 334–340.
10. Mak JC, Cameron ID, March LM (2010) Evidence-based guidelines for the management of hip fractures in older persons: an update. Med J Aust 192: 37–41.
11. Scottish Intercollegiate Guideline Network (SIGN) (2009) SIGN 111: Management of hip fracture in older people. Edinburgh: Scottish Intercollegiate Guideline Network.
12. Orosz GM, Hannan EL, Magaziner J, Koval K, Gilbert M, et al. (2002) Hip fracture in the older patient: reasons for delay in hospitalization and timing of surgical repair. Journal of the American Geriatrics Society 50: 1336–1340.
13. Bergeron E, Lavoie A, Moore L, Bamvita J-M, Ratte S, et al. (2006) Is the delay to surgery for isolated hip fracture predictive of outcome in efficient systems? [see comment]. Journal of Trauma-Injury Infection & Critical Care 60: 753–757.
14. Grimes JP, Gregory PM, Noveck H, Butler MS, Carson JL (2002) The effects of time-to-surgery on mortality and morbidity in patients following hip fracture. American Journal of Medicine 112: 702–709.
15. Simunovic N, Devereaux PJ, Sprague S, Guyatt GH, Schemitsch E, et al. (2010) Effect of early surgery after hip fracture on mortality and complications: systematic review and meta-analysis. CMAJ 182: 1609–1616.
16. Handoll HH, Sherrington C (2007) Mobilisation strategies after hip fracture surgery in adults. Cochrane Database Syst Rev: CD001704.
17. Parker MJ, Handoll HH, Griffiths R (2004) Anaesthesia for hip fracture surgery in adults. Cochrane Database Syst Rev: CD000521.
18. Schunemann HJ, Oxman AD, Vist GE, Higgins JPT, Deeks JJ, et al. (2008) Chapter 12: Interpreting results and drawing conclusions. In: Higgins JPT, Green S, editors. Cochrane Handbook for Systematic Reviews of Interventions Version 5.0.1 [updated September 2008] The Cochrane Collaboration, 2008. Available from www.cochrane-handbook.org. Accessed 2010 Dec 15.
19. Higgins JPT, Altman DG (2008) Chapter 8: Assessing risk of bias in included studies. In: Higgins JPT, Green S, editors. Cochrane Handbook for Systematic Reviews of Interventions Version 5.0.1 [updated September 2008] The Cochrane Collaboration, 2008. Available from www.cochrane-handbook.org. Accessed 2010 Dec 15.
20. Wells GA, Shea B, O'Connell D, Peterson J, Welch V, et al. (2007) The Newcastle-Ottawa Scale (NOS) for assessing the quality of nonrandomised studies in meta-analyses. Ottawa: Ottawa Hospital Research Institute. Available at: http://www.ohri.ca/programs/clinical_epidemiology/oxford.asp Accessed: August 2012.
21. Higgins JP, Thompson SG, Spiegelhalter DJ (2009) A re-evaluation of random-effects meta-analysis. J R Stat Soc Ser A Stat Soc 172: 137–159.
22. DerSimonian R, Laird N (1986) Meta-analysis in clinical trials. Control Clin Trials 7: 177–188.
23. Sterne JAC, Egger M, Moher D (2008) Chapter 10: Addressing reporting biases. In: Higgins JPT, Green S, editors. Cochrane Handbook for Systematic Reviews of Interventions: Version 5.0.1 [updated September 2008] The Cochrane Collaboration, 2008. Available from www.cochrane-handbook.org. Accessed: 2010 Dec 15.
24. Salanti G, Ioannidis JP (2009) Synthesis of observational studies should consider credibility ceilings. J Clin Epidemiol 62: 115–122.
25. Papanikolaou PN, Christidi GD, Ioannidis JP (2006) Patient outcomes with teaching versus nonteaching healthcare: a systematic review. PLoS Med 3: e341.
26. Palmer TM, Peters JL, Sutton AJ, Moreno SG (2008) Contour-enhanced funnel plots for meta-analysis. Stata J 8: 242–254.
27. Peters JL, Sutton AJ, Jones DR, Abrams KR, Rushton L (2008) Contour-enhanced meta-analysis funnel plots help distinguish publication bias from other causes of asymmetry. J Clin Epidemiol 61: 991–996.
28. Harbord RM, Egger M, Sterne JA (2006) A modified test for small-study effects in meta-analyses of controlled trials with binary endpoints. Stat Med 25: 3443–3457.
29. StataCorp (2009) Stata Statistical Software: Release 11. College Station, TX: StataCorp LP.
30. Spiegelhalter DJ, Thomas A, Best NG (2000) WinBUGS Version 1.3 User Manual. Cambridge: MRC Biostatistics Unit. Available at: www.mrc-bsu.cam.ac.uk/bugs. Accessed: 2010 Dec 15.
31. Carretta E, Bochicchio V, Rucci P, Fabbri G, Laus M, et al. (2011) Hip fracture: effectiveness of early surgery to prevent 30-day mortality. Int Orthop 35: 419–424.
32. Al-Ani AN, Samuelsson B, Tidermark J, Norling A, Ekstrom W, et al. (2008) Early operation on patients with a hip fracture improved the ability to return to independent living. A prospective study of 850 patients. Journal of Bone & Joint Surgery – American Volume 90: 1436–1442.
33. Bredahl C, Nyholm B, Hindsholm KB, Mortensen JS, Olesen AS (1992) Mortality after hip fracture: results of operation within 12 h of admission. Injury 23: 83–86.
34. Davis TR, Sher JL, Porter BB, Checketts RG (1988) The timing of surgery for intertrochanteric femoral fractures. Injury 19: 244–246.
35. Dorotka R, Schoechtner H, Buchinger W (2003) The influence of immediate surgical treatment of proximal femoral fractures on mortality and quality of life. Operation within six hours of the fracture versus later than six hours [see comment]. Journal of Bone & Joint Surgery – British Volume 85: 1107–1113.
36. Doruk H, Mas MR, Yildiz C, Sonmez A, Kyrdemir V (2004) The effect of the timing of hip fracture surgery on the activity of daily living and mortality in elderly. Arch Gerontol Geriatr 39: 179–185.
37. Elliott J, Beringer T, Kee F, Marsh D, Willis C, et al. (2003) Predicting survival after treatment for fracture of the proximal femur and the effect of delays to surgery. J Clin Epidemiol 56: 788–795.
38. Holt G, Smith R, Duncan K, Finlayson DF, Gregori A (2008) Early mortality after surgical fixation of hip fractures in the elderly: an analysis of data from the scottish hip fracture audit. J Bone Joint Surg Br 90: 1357–1363.
39. Kenzora JE, McCarthy RE, Lowell JD, Sledge CB (1984) Hip fracture mortality. Relation to age, treatment, preoperative illness, time of surgery, and complications. Clin Orthop Relat Res: 45–56.
40. Maggi S, Siviero P, Wetle T, Besdine RW, Saugo M, et al. (2009) A multicenter survey on profile of care for hip fracture: predictors of mortality and disability. Osteoporos Int 21: 223–231.
41. Majumdar SR, Beaupre LA, Johnston DWC, Dick DA, Cinats JG, et al. (2006) Lack of association between mortality and timing of surgical fixation in elderly patients with hip fracture: results of a retrospective population-based cohort study [see comment]. Medical Care 44: 552–559.
42. McGuire KJ, Bernstein J, Polsky D, Silber JH (2004) The 2004 Marshall Urist award: delays until surgery after hip fracture increases mortality. Clinical Orthopaedics & Related Research: 294–301.
43. Moran CG, Wenn RT, Sikand M, Taylor AM (2005) Early mortality after hip fracture: is delay before surgery important? Journal of Bone & Joint Surgery – American Volume 87: 483–489.
44. Mullen JO, Mullen NL (1992) Hip fracture mortality. A prospective, multifactorial study to predict and minimize death risk. Clin Orthop Relat Res: 214–222.
45. Orosz GM, Magaziner J, Hannan EL, Morrison RS, Koval K, et al. (2004) Association of timing of surgery for hip fracture and patient outcomes. JAMA 291: 1738–1743.
46. Parker MJ, Pryor GA (1992) The timing of surgery for proximal femoral fractures. Journal of Bone & Joint Surgery – British Volume 74: 203–205.
47. Peleg K, Savitsky B, Yitzhak B, Avi I (2011) Different reimbursement influences surviving of hip fracture in elderly patients. Injury 42: 128–132.
48. Radcliff TA, Henderson WG, Stoner TJ, Khuri SF, Dohm M, et al. (2008) Patient risk factors, operative care, and outcomes among older community-dwelling male veterans with hip fracture. J Bone Joint Surg Am 90: 34–42.
49. Rademakers LMF, Vainas T, van Zutphen 2 SWAM, Brink PRG, van Helden SH (2007) Pressure Ulcers and Prolonged Hospital Stay in Hip Fracture Patients Affected by Time-to-Surgery. European Journal of Trauma and Emergency Surgery 33: 238–244.
50. Rae HC, Harris IA, McEvoy L, Todorova T (2007) Delay to surgery and mortality after hip fracture. ANZ Journal of Surgery 77: 889–891.
51. Roos LL, Walld RK, Romano PS, Roberecki S (1996) Short-term mortality after repair of hip fracture. Do Manitoba elderly do worse? Medical Care 34: 310–326.
52. Sexson SB, Lehner JT (1987) Factors affecting hip fracture mortality. Journal of Orthopaedic Trauma 1: 298–305.
53. Siegmeth AW, Gurusamy K, Parker MJ (2005) Delay to surgery prolongs hospital stay in patients with fractures of the proximal femur. Journal of Bone & Joint Surgery – British Volume 87: 1123–1126.
54. Smektala R, Endres HG, Dasch B, Maier C, Trampisch HJ, et al. (2008) The effect of time-to-surgery on outcome in elderly patients with proximal femoral fractures. BMC Musculoskelet Disord 9: 171.
55. Stoddart J, Horne G, Devane P (2002) Influence of preoperative medical status and delay to surgery on death following a hip fracture. ANZ J Surg 72: 405–407.
56. Sund R, Liski A (2005) Quality effects of operative delay on mortality in hip fracture treatment. Quality & Safety in Health Care 14: 371–377.
57. Swanson CE, Day GA, Yelland CE, Broome JR, Massey L, et al. (1998) The management of elderly patients with femoral fractures. A randomised controlled

trial of early intervention versus standard care. Medical Journal of Australia 169: 515–518.
58. Verbeek DOF, Ponsen KJ, Goslings JC, Heetveld MJ (2008) Effect of surgical delay on outcome in hip fracture patients: a retrospective multivariate analysis of 192 patients. International Orthopaedics 32: 13–18.
59. Shiga T, Wajima Z, Ohe Y (2008) Is operative delay associated with increased mortality of hip fracture patients? Systematic review, meta-analysis, and meta-regression. Can J Anaesth 55: 146–154.
60. Khan SK, Kalra S, Khanna A, Thiruvengada MM, Parker MJ (2009) Timing of surgery for hip fractures: a systematic review of 52 published studies involving 291,413 patients. Injury 40: 692–697.
61. Mehta SR, Granger CB, Boden WE, Steg PG, Bassand JP, et al. (2009) Early versus delayed invasive intervention in acute coronary syndromes. N Engl J Med 360: 2165–2175.
62. Montalescot G, Cayla G, Collet JP, Elhadad S, Beygui F, et al. (2009) Immediate vs delayed intervention for acute coronary syndromes: a randomized clinical trial. JAMA 302: 947–954.
63. Seccareccia F, D'Errigo P, Rosato S, Maraschini A, Badoni G, et al. (2010) Programma "Valutazione degli esiti per promuovere il miglioramento dell'efficacia nell'erogazione delle prestazioni ricomprese nei livelli essenziali di assistenza (LEA)". Istituto Superiore di Sanità; Rapporti ISTISAN 10/43.

Surgery-Induced Changes and Early Recovery of Hip-Muscle Strength, Leg-Press Power, and Functional Performance after Fast-Track Total Hip Arthroplasty: A Prospective Cohort Study

Bente Holm[1,2], Kristian Thorborg[2,3,4], Henrik Husted[1,4], Henrik Kehlet[1,5], Thomas Bandholm[2,4,6]*

1 The Lundbeck Centre for Fast-track Hip and Knee Arthroplasty, Copenhagen University Hospital, Hvidovre, Denmark, **2** Department of Physical Therapy, Physical Medicine and Rehabilitation Research – Copenhagen (PMR-C), Copenhagen University Hospital, Hvidovre, Denmark, **3** Arthroscopic Centre Amager, Copenhagen University Hospital, Amager, Copenhagen, Denmark, **4** Department of Orthopedic Surgery, Copenhagen University Hospital, Hvidovre, Denmark, **5** Section for Surgical Pathophysiology, Copenhagen University Hospital, Rigshospitalet, Copenhagen, Denmark, **6** Clinical Research Centre, Copenhagen University Hospital, Hvidovre, Copenhagen, Denmark

Abstract

Background: By measuring very early changes in muscle strength and functional performance after fast-track total hip arthroplasty (THA), post-operative rehabilitation, introduced soon after surgery, can be designed to specifically target identified deficits.

Objective(s): Firstly, to quantify changes (compared to pre-operative values) in hip muscle strength, leg-press power, and functional performance in the first week after THA, and secondly, to explore relationships between the muscle strength changes, and changes in hip pain, systemic inflammation, and thigh swelling.

Design: Prospective, cohort study.

Setting: Convenience sample of patients receiving a THA at Copenhagen University Hospital, Hvidovre, Denmark, between March and December 2011.

Participants: Thirty-five patients (65.9±7.2 years) undergoing THA.

Main outcome measures: Hip muscle strength, leg-press power, performance-based function, and self-reported disability were determined prior to, and 2 and 8 days after, THA (Day 2 and 8, respectively). Hip pain, thigh swelling, and C-Reactive Protein were also determined.

Results: Five patients were lost to follow-up. Hip muscle strength and leg press power were substantially reduced at Day 2 (range of reductions: 41–58%, $P<0.001$), but less pronounced at Day 8 (range of reductions: 23–31%, $P<0.017$). Self-reported symptoms and function (HOOS: Pain, Symptoms, and ADL) improved at Day 8 ($P<0.014$). Changes in hip pain, C-Reactive Protein, and thigh swelling were not related to the muscle strength and power losses.

Conclusion(s): Hip muscle strength and leg-press power decreased substantially in the first week after THA – especially at Day 2 – with some recovery at Day 8. The muscle strength loss and power loss were not related to changes in hip pain, systemic inflammation, or thigh swelling. In contrast, self-reported symptoms and function improved. These data on surgery-induced changes in muscle strength may help design impairment-directed, post-operative rehabilitation to be introduced soon after surgery.

Trial Registration: ClinicalTrials.gov NCT01246674.

Editor: François Hug, The University of Queensland, Australia

Funding: The study was supported by a grant from The Lundbeck Foundation, Hellerup, Denmark (www.lundbeckfonden.com). The funders had no role in study design, data collection and analysis, decision to publish, or preparation of the manuscript.

Competing Interests: The authors have declared that no competing interests exist.

* E-mail: thomas.bandholm@hvh.regionh.dk

Introduction

Total hip arthroplasty (THA) is commonly performed to relieve pain and improve functional performance in patients with end-stage hip osteoarthritis [1]. In many places, it is followed by out-patient physical rehabilitation, with the rehabilitation components sometimes differing between programs [2,3]. However, despite undergoing physical rehabilitation after THA, reduced muscle strength and functional performance have been reported at various time points when compared to the preoperative level [4–12], which may already have been reduced due to end-stage osteoarthritis [4,5,8,10–15].

Muscle strength losses have been reported for several muscle groups in the operated leg after THA, including those associated with hip abduction [4,14–19], adduction [4,5], flexion [4,5,8,14–19], and extension [4,5,8,14–19], as well as knee extension [4,5,12,14,19] and flexion [4]. With a few exceptions [20–22], these persisting multi-level strength deficits have primarily been reported in the later post-operative phase, that is, after the completion of out-patient physical rehabilitation, which is typically not well documented with respect to, for example, the applied strength training exercises (choice of exercises, intensity, volume, etc.) [23]. Hence, it is difficult to judge if persisting muscle strength deficits after THA appear to have been sufficiently targeted during the physical rehabilitation programs. In order to do so, early strength deficits induced by surgery need to be quantified, in order to design a specific, impairment-directed, postoperative rehabilitation program for implementation soon after surgery. This approach is an important initial step in the fast-track/enhanced recovery program methodology [24,25], which combines evidence from different peri-operative uni-modal interventions, including post-operative physical rehabilitation [23].

With respect to the mechanisms underlying the early loss of muscle strength after THA, failure of the central nervous system to activate muscles close to the operated hip joint due to intra-articular swelling may be involved [26]. This is also seen after total knee arthroplasty, and is commonly referred to as arthrogenic muscle inhibition [27,28]. Besides swelling, arthrogenic muscle inhibition has also been linked to inflammation, pain, joint laxity, and structural joint damage [28] – conditions that are known to occur soon after THA. Over time, atrophy of several muscles around the hip and knee joints in the operated leg seems to develop [29,30], which further contributes to the loss of muscle strength.

The primary objective of this study was to quantify changes (compared to preoperative values) in hip muscle strength, leg-press power, and functional performance within the first week after THA – before the start of out-patient physical rehabilitation. The secondary objective was to explore relationships between the muscle strength changes, and changes in hip pain, systemic inflammation, and thigh swelling. We hypothesized that muscle strength, power, and performance-based function would be substantially reduced in the first week after THA, compared to preoperative values.

Methods

Ethics statement

All patients were provided written information about the procedures of the study, and informed consent was obtained in strict accordance with the Declaration of Helsinki. The Ethics Committee in Copenhagen approved the study. (H-4-2010-FSP). ClinicalTrials.Gov-identifier: NCTO1246674, http://clinicaltrials.gov/ct2/show/NCT01246674.

Design

Patients, scheduled for a primary unilateral THA, were evaluated one week before surgery (Pre-surgery), one day post-surgery (Day 2), and 7 days post-surgery (Day 8). All three evaluations included assessments of muscle strength and power, as well as performance-based function, hip pain, and thigh swelling. In addition, blood sampling to assess systemic inflammation was conducted Pre-surgery and on Day 2, and self-reported disability was assessed Pre-surgery and on Day 8. All measurements were performed and recorded by the same experienced investigator, who was blinded to the results of all previous visits. The reporting of the study follows the recommendations of The Strengthening the Reporting of Observational Studies in Epidemiology (STROBE, [please see Supporting Information]) [31].

Participants

Between March and December 2011, patients awaiting a THA were included by convenience sampling from the pre-surgery program at the Department of Orthopedic Surgery at Copenhagen University Hospital, Hvidovre, Denmark, if they were one of the first three patients each day to receive a THA. To ensure sufficient reliability of the applied measurements, the same experienced investigator was used, which is why it was only possible to include a maximum of three patients per day. To reduce the risk of selection bias, the person responsible for assigning the patients' surgical times was kept unaware of the current study.

The inclusion criteria were: planned primary, unilateral THA due to end-stage osteoarthritis and age >18 years. The exclusion criteria were: inability to speak or understand Danish, inability to perform the outcome measures due to other diseases, such as rheumatoid arthritis, polyneuropathy, or extremity peripheral paresis.

Procedures

Peri-operative care. All patients were operated on using the posterior approach (standard, no minimally invasive surgery) with an uncemented THA. They followed a fast-track program for THA, which has been described in detail elsewhere [32]. Briefly, the program included standardized preoperative multidisciplinary education, multi-modal pain treatment for 6 days (a daily dose of gabapentin (900 mg/day), paracetamol (4 g/day), and celecoxib (400 mg/day) initiated on the morning of surgery, and continued for 6 days with morphine (10 mg) as a rescue analgesic for moderate or severe pain), and postoperative rehabilitation, including early ambulation but no progressive strength training. All patients were discharged to their homes, according to well-defined functional discharge criteria [33]. The length of hospital stay was counted as the number of nights hospitalized after the operation. Patients were told to continue with further daily analgesics and follow the 6-day prescribed pain treatment ordered by their general practitioner.

Outcome measures. Muscle strength of the hip actions: adduction, abduction and flexion in the operated leg was measured during isometric contractions, using a hand-held dynamometer (Chiroform ApS, Viborg, Denmark), according to Thorborg and co-workers [34]. After warm up and familiarization with the procedure, the muscle strength of hip flexion in sitting position, and hip abduction and adduction in the supine position, was determined. The hip action-order was randomized, and the order was the same for each patient for all evaluations. The patients performed four maximal contractions – separated by 60-sec pauses – and the contraction that elicited the largest force was used as the data point. Standardized verbal encouragement was provided during each trial (contraction). Muscle strength was subsequently expressed as maximal voluntary torque per kilogram of body mass (Nm/kg). The external lever-arm for hip flexion was the distance from the anterior superior iliac spine to 5 cm proximal to the patella border, for hip abduction it was the distance from the anterior superior iliac spine to 5 cm proximal to the proximal edge of the lateral malleolus, and for hip adduction it was the distance from the anterior superior iliac spine to 5 cm proximal to the proximal edge of the medial malleolus.

Leg-press power of the operated leg was estimated from a rapid extension of the operated leg from a flexed position, using a Nottingham Power Rig (Medical Physics and Clinical Engineering Department, Nottingham, United Kingdom), according to Short & Bassey [35]. Positioning of the patient was as follows: each patient sat in the rig with the knee and hip flexed in a self-selected comfortable position with the foot of the leg to be tested on the pedal, and secured on the seat with a seatbelt across the hips. The patient was then instructed to extend the leg to press the pedal as quickly as possible with maximum effort, with 60-sec pauses between trials. Standardized verbal encouragement was provided during each trial. The test was ended when leg press power decreased in two consecutive trials or ten trials had been performed. The press that had the highest power was identified, and power per kilogram of body mass was then used as the data point. For all evaluations, the patients used their available range of knee motion during the presses.

Performance-based function was assessed using The Timed Up & Go (TUG) [36] and 10-meter fast speed walking [37] tests, by measuring the time (in seconds using a stopwatch) required to rise from a chair, walk 3 meters, and return to the chair (TUG), and walk 10 meters as quickly and safely as possible (10-meter fast speed walking), using the habitual walking aid, if any was used. The trial that required the least number of seconds was used as the data point for each of the two performance-based functions. For details, see [22].

Hip pain was quantified at rest (supine), before the experimental protocol, and activity, using a 100-mm Visual Analog Scale (VAS), with endpoints – visible to the patients – of "no pain" (0) and "worst pain imaginable" (100). Activity-based recordings of hip pain were made during the tests of muscle strength/power and performance-based function, before which the patients were told to register hip pain during test performance and then rate it immediately after test termination. The pain recordings made during the trials that were subsequently selected as muscle strength, power, or performance-based function data points, were selected as the pain data points.

Self-reported disability was assessed using The Hip Disability and Osteoarthritis Outcome Score (HOOS) [38]. It is a 40-item questionnaire; constructed to assess patient-relevant outcomes in five separate subscales (Pain, Symptoms, Activities of daily living (ADL), Sport and recreational activities (Sport/rec), and Hip-related quality of life (QOL). For each subscale, a normalized score was then calculated with 100 indicating no symptoms and 0 indicating extreme symptoms.

Thigh volume was used as a surrogate measure of fluid accumulation around the operated hip joint, as intra-articular swelling could not be assessed, and because thigh swelling has been found to relate to knee-extension strength soon after hip fracture surgery [39]. Thigh volume was estimated using tape-measured circumferences of the upper and lower thigh with the patient lying in the supine position, using the Fustrum method [40]. It is based on the assumption that the thigh is approximately in the shape of a truncated cone, or frustum. The upper circumference was measured 25 cm proximal to the border of the patella, and the lower circumference, 5 cm proximal to the border of the patella. For details, see [40].

Systemic inflammation was measured by C-Reactive Protein (CRP) in venous blood preoperatively, and 24 hours after surgical incision. Concentrations of CRP were measured in blood samples drawn in 4 ml tubes with gel and lithium-heparin using a COBAS 6000 analyzer (Roche Diagnostics, Mannheim, Germany).

Statistical analyses

All variables, except hip pain, were normally distributed (Kolmogorov-Smirnoff). Normally distributed data are reported as means±1 standard deviation (SD), and non-normally distributed data as medians with inter-quartile ranges. Data from a pilot study indicated substantial strength, power, and functional performance losses at Days 2 and 8. Hence, the current study was powered (80% power) to detect changes of 30% or more for all strength, power and functional performance measurements, based on the measurement that required the greatest sample, which was 30 patients. These analyses were considered primary and powered to the primary objective of the study, while all secondary (correlation) analyses pertaining to the secondary objective of the study, were considered exploratory. A significance level of 5% ($P<0.05$) was used.

Changes in muscle strength and thigh volume over time (Pre-surgery, Day 2 and Day 8) were investigated using one-way repeated measures analyses of variance (ANOVAs). If a significant main effect of time was determined, pair-wise Bonferroni-corrected comparisons were used to identify differences between time points. Performance-based function are reported using descriptive statistics only, as a change in walking aid occurred between time points. Changes in hip pain over time (Pre-surgery, Day 2 and Day 8) were investigated using Friedman's Two-Way Analyses of Variance by Ranks. If a significant main effect of time was determined, Wilcoxons Signed Rank tests with Bonferroni corrections were used to identify differences between time points. Changes in self-reported disability (HOOS) and systemic inflammation from Pre-surgery were investigated using paired-samples t tests. Between-variable correlations were quantified using Pearson or Spearman correlation coefficients, depending on normal distribution or not. All analyses were performed for the 30 patients, who completed all follow-up visits (per-protocol-analyses).

Results

Participants

As the study used convenience sampling, eligibility was only examined on the days available for experimental work. Hence, the number of potentially eligible patients is unknown. The number of patients examined for eligibility was 40. Of these, 5 were excluded: 3 declined to participate, 1 had the surgery postponed due to suspicion of spinal disc herniation, and 1 had a planned bilateral, simultaneous THA instead of a unilateral THA. The number of patients confirmed eligible was 35, and these were included. Five dropped out after inclusion: three on post-operative Day 1 (1 due to hip dislocation twelve hours post-surgery, 1 due to proximal femoral fracture and hip dislocation two hours post surgery, 1 due to personal reasons), two between Day 2 and Day 8 (1 due to observation for acute myocardial infarction, 1 due to a hip fracture). The baseline characteristics of the remaining 30 patients, who attended all follow-up visits and had complete data sets, are shown in Table 1.

Table 1. Patient characteristics (n = 30).

Category	Result
Age, yrs	65.9±7.2
Women, number (%)	21 (70)
Height, cm	169.8±8.4
Body Mass, kg	81.0±17.1
Body Mass Index, kg/m^2	28.0±4.7
Length of stay*	1.9±1.0

Values are means±1SD, unless otherwise indicated. *postoperative nights.

Muscle strength and power

Changes in muscle strength and power are shown in Figure 1. Hip flexion, abduction, adduction, and leg-press power changed significantly over time, as ANOVA main effects were observed ($P<0.017$). The subsequent multiple comparisons revealed that muscle strength at Day 2 was reduced compared to Pre-surgery (hip flexion, abduction, adduction, and leg-press power $P<0.001$), that muscle strength at Day 8 was reduced compared to Pre-surgery (hip flexion, abduction, adduction, and leg-press power $P<0.017$), and that muscle strength increased from Day 2 to Day 8 (hip flexion, abduction, adduction, and leg-press power $P<0.006$). The muscle strength and power losses at Day 2 varied between 41% and 58%, with the greatest loss observed for leg-press power. The strength and power losses at Day 8 varied between 23% and 31%, with the greatest loss observed for hip-flexion strength. No correlations between hip muscle strength or leg press power and hip pain, reported during the tests of muscle strength and power, were observed.

Performance-based function

Performance-based function, assessed by the TUG and 10-meter fast speed walking tests, was indicated to have changed significantly over time, based on the descriptive statistics. Pre-surgery, where no patients used walking aids, the mean TUG-performance was 9.5±2.7 s, at Day 2, where all patients walked on two crutches, the mean TUG-performance was 18.3±6.5 s, and at Day 8, where 7 patients walked without walking aids, 10 walked with one crutch, and 13 with two crutches, the mean TUG-performance was 11.7±3.4 s. For the 10-meter fast speed walking test, the patients used the same walking aids as described above. The mean 10-meter fast speed walking test-performance was 1.40±0.31 m/s, 0.84±0.24 m/s, 1.14±0.32 m/s, at Pre-surgery, Day 2, and Day 8, respectively.

Self-reported disability

Self-reported disability, assessed by the HOOS, is shown in Figure 2. It improved from Pre-surgery to Day 8 for the subscales: Pain (pre: 53.9±16.6, post: 71.5±15.9, $P<0.001$), Symptoms (pre: 54.3±15.7, post: 70.8±15.8, $P<0.001$), ADL (pre: 53.1±16.2, post: 63.5±16.5, $P<0.014$), whereas it decreased for the subscale Sport/rec (pre: 59.6±25.5, post: 40.4±25.8, $P<0.002$) and did not change for QOL (pre: 61.5±19.0, post: 59.0±17.9, $P=0.679$).

Thigh volume, hip pain and systemic inflammation

Generally, thigh volume increased over time (Pre-surgery: 4167.1±808.2 cm^3, Day 2: 4376.1±834.1 cm^3, Day 8: 4489.1±861.8 cm^3), whereas hip pain at rest, maximal contractions, and performance-based function decreased over time, from mild to moderate Pre-surgery to mild at Days 2 and 8 (Table 2). Systemic inflammation (CRP) increased from 2.9±4.2 mg/l Pre-surgery to 84.3±35.0 mg/l at Day 2 ($P<0.001$). The increases in thigh volume and systemic inflammation did not correlate with any of the observed lower extremity strength or power losses.

Discussion

The main findings of the current study were (i) considerable loss of hip muscle strength and leg-press power postoperatively at Day 2, (ii) this loss was reduced but still lower at Day 8 compared with Pre-surgery, and (iii) changes in hip pain, thigh swelling or systemic inflammation were not associated with loss of hip muscle strength or leg-press power.

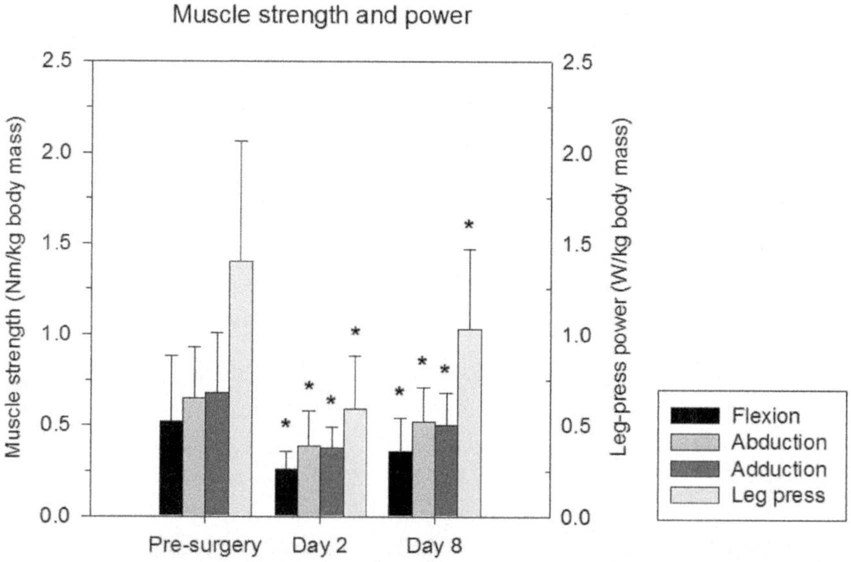

Figure 1. Changes in muscle strength/power over time in the operated leg. The secondary y-axis applies to the leg-press power measurement. *Day 2 statistically different from Pre-surgery, and Day 8 statistically different from Day 2 and Pre-surgery.

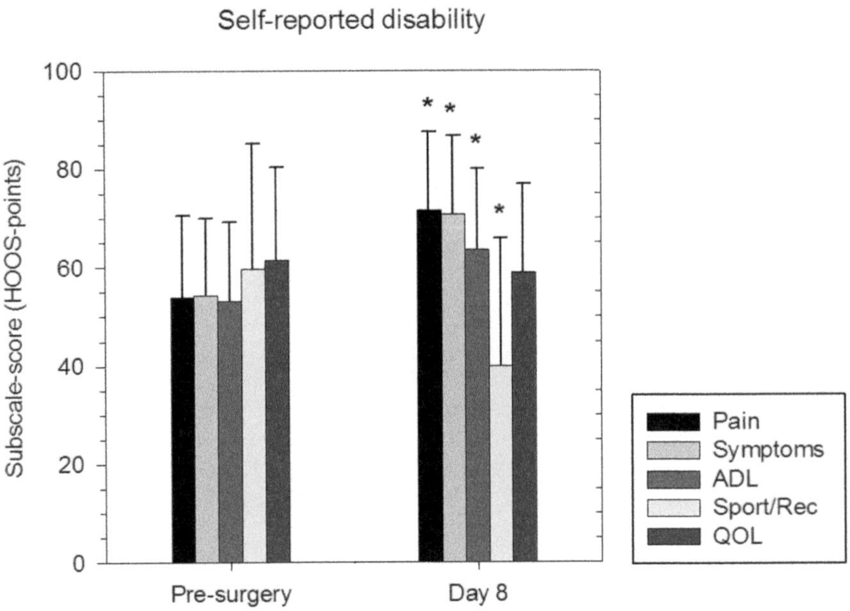

Figure 2. Changes in self-reported disability over time in the operated leg. *statistically different from Pre-surgery.

Loss of muscle strength and power after THA

The reasons for aiming to reach preoperative muscle strength values and, preferably, that of age-matched, healthy peers after THA are several. Firstly, muscle strength of the operated leg relates to functional performance soon after THA as well as much later [20]. Secondly, lower-extremity muscle weakness of the operated leg and asymmetric leg loading during sit-to-stands (healthy leg compensation) have been reported years after THA [41,42]. Finally, muscle strength decreases with increasing age [43]. Hence, surgery-induced reductions in muscle strength that are not addressed, may, theoretically, precipitate a loss of functional independence just a few years later. This is especially the case where strength values after surgery are close to cut points [44] for losing functional independence because of insufficient lower-extremity muscle strength.

Loss of hip muscle strength and leg-press power have been reported previously, at later time points – weeks to months – after surgery [4,5,8,14–19,22]. The current data more or less reflect surgery-induced muscle strength/power loss with spontaneous recovery soon after surgery, as previously no progressive strength training of these muscle groups had been instituted as early as this at our institution. The losses were pronounced at Day 2, but were generally returning towards values observed Pre-surgery. Acknowledging that values Pre-surgery may be reduced compared to those of age-matched, healthy peers due to end-stage osteoarthritis [4,5], it still indicates substantial spontaneous recovery of muscle strength in the first week after THA, which is in contrast to that observed after total knee arthroplasty [45,46]. One reason for this may be that the patients included in the current study entered a well-established fast-track post-surgery program [33], focusing on enhancing recovery by, for example, mobilization with full weight-bearing allowed within only a few hours of surgery. The use of opioid-sparing multimodal pain treatment – resulting in relatively little postoperative pain, nausea, and vomiting – also allows for earlier and maybe more extensive mobilization and time out of bed. These factors could explain the reduced losses.

The apparent rapid rate of recovery of muscle strength within the first week is supported by previous work, in which hip and

Table 2. Changes in hip pain at rest, and during maximal contractions and performance-based function.

Category	Pre-surgery (n = 30)	Day 2 (n = 30)	Day 8 (n = 30)
Resting pain, VAS-mm	10.0 (2.3–18.3)	11 (0–22.0)	1.5 (0–9.0)*‡$
Hip-flexion MVC pain, VAS-mm	21 (4.8–39.0)	21 (10.0–38.5)	14.5 (4.0–22.3)
Hip-abduction MVC pain, VAS-mm	20 (4.8–40.0)	20.5 (8.8–40.0)	10.5 (3.0–27.3)*‡$
Hip-adduction MVC pain, VAS-mm	18.5 (3.0–31.3)	21.5 (11.5–41.3)	8.5 (3.8–17.3)*$
Leg-press power pain, VAS-mm	23.5 (5.0–34.3)	20.0 (6.8–42.0)	10 (2.3–18.0)*‡$
"Timed Up & Go" pain, VAS-mm	21 (5.5–30.0)	15.5 (5.0–30.3)	5.0 (0–23.5)*‡$
"10 m walk" pain, VAS-mm	20.5 (6.0–40.0)	20.0 (3.8–33.0)	5.5 (1.5–18.3)*‡$

*Main effect of time, ‡Day 8 significantly different from Pre-surgery, and $Day 8 significantly different from Day 2. Data are medians (inter-quartile range). MVC, Maximal voluntary contraction; VAS, Visual Analog Scale

knee muscle strength 8 weeks after standard THA did not differ from pre-operative values [5]. However, authors have reported persisting hip-muscle atrophy [30] and strength deficits years after surgery, when compared to that of either the contra-lateral side [5,14], or age-matched peers [16,17], indicating a need for more intense types of physical rehabilitation. In many cases, the intensity of the rehabilitation provided after surgery seems sub-optimal, i.e. with too little intensity [23]. Pertaining to this notion, there are indications that both muscle strength and performance-based function recover more quickly after supervised rehabilitation introduced soon after surgery, including progressive strength training, compared to a lesser intensive, supervised rehabilitation control [21,29]. It therefore seems very relevant to investigate – on a larger scale – if the apparent rate of early recovery of muscle strength and functional performance following the operation can be accelerated further by a brief period of intensive and well-described rehabilitation introduced soon after surgery, including progressive strength training [47] of the hip muscles and leg extensors. Prior to this, it may be especially important to identify patients, who do not display the same rate of recovery, and hence, require more prolonged rehabilitation. It could be the case for patients with low(er) preoperative strength and functional performance [6]. Likewise, there may also be a proportion of patients with high(er) preoperative strength and functional performance, who require less or no supervised rehabilitation.

Acknowledging that the secondary analyses may have been underpowered (see methodological limitations), the current data do not lend much support for thigh swelling, systemic inflammation, or hip pain as candidates, underlying the initial losses of muscle strength after THA. However, failure of the central nervous system to activate muscles close to the operated hip joint due to intra-articular swelling warrants future investigation, as reduced neuromuscular activity of the hip muscles has been reported in healthy subjects after intra-articular injections [26]. The role of the inflammatory response for multi-level strength-losses after THA also warrants future investigation, as it has been indicated to affect early functional recovery (walking) after THA [48]. Post-operative hip pain, however, seems clinically insignificant. The reported pain intensities at Days 2 and 8 during rest, maximal contractions, and performance-based function were low and decreased over time, compared to Pre-surgery.

Loss of functional performance after THA

Loss of performance-based function soon after THA has been reported previously [22]. The current data seem to concur with this. We were only able to perform descriptive analyses of performance based function, as walking aids were self-selected and, thus, not controlled for. The reason for this was that we did not find it feasible to control for, this early after surgery. With this limitation in mind, performance-based function seems to reach preoperative values around 6–9 weeks after surgery [6], whereas self-reported function (WOMAC physical function) seems to reach preoperative values 1–2 weeks after surgery [6], depending on the applied outcome measure and type of post-operative rehabilitation. In the current study, self-reported function (HOOS ADL) improved from Pre-surgery to Day 8, while performance-based function was still markedly reduced. This discrepancy in the time courses of performance-based and self-reported function after THA is also observed in total knee arthroplasty [49,50]. The results underscore the importance of having both a performance-based and self-reported measure of function with acceptable psychometric properties, when quantifying changes in functional performance over time after THA, as these measures seem to capture different aspects of recovery after THA.

Generally, given the early loss of muscle strength and power, it is suggested that rehabilitation soon after THA should include progressive strength training [47] of both hip flexors, hip adductors, hip abductors, and leg extensors, as progressive strength training increases muscle strength of the operated leg when initiated early after THA [11,12,21], and appears safe [11,12,21]. Leg presses seem especially important, and they will also, to some degree, involve the hip adductors and abductors, in addition to all the leg extensors.

Study limitations

A few precautions should be made when interpreting the current data. Firstly, the study used a design with convenience sampling, which may, unintentionally, cause some selection bias. It was only possible to include a maximum of three patients per day, on days available for experimental work. However, the person responsible for assigning the patients' surgical times was kept unaware of the current study and, hence, did not know the distribution of experimental days, and that the maximum inclusion per experimental day was three patients. Secondly, the study was powered with respect to changes in muscle strength, power, and functional performance. All correlation analyses relating to the secondary objective were exploratory, which is why potential causes of the initial muscle strength loss and power loss may not have been indicated. Thirdly, as previously mentioned, some patients changed habitual walking aids during the course of the study, which may – in itself – have had an impact on their performance-based function. This is difficult to control for, so we performed these analyses using descriptive statistics only. Nevertheless, despite these limitations, the main finding of substantial strength loss and indications of performance-based function loss soon after THA in the current study is supported by previous related findings at later time points, which strengthens the external validity of these findings.

Conclusion

Hip muscle strength and leg-press power, decreased substantially in the first week after THA – especially at Day 2 – with some recovery evident at Day 8. In contrast, self-reported symptoms and function improved. Hip pain, thigh swelling, and systemic inflammation were not related to the observed muscle strength loss and power loss. These data on surgery-induced changes in lower extremity muscle strength may help in the design of impairment-directed, postoperative rehabilitation soon after THA, by serving as an indicator of muscle strength status prior to outpatient physical rehabilitation.

Supporting Information

Checklist S1 STROBE checklist of items that should be included in reports of cohort studies.

Author Contributions

Conceived and designed the experiments: BH KT HH HK TB. Performed the experiments: BH. Analyzed the data: BH TB KT. Contributed reagents/materials/analysis tools: TB KT HH HK. Wrote the paper: BH KT HH HK TB.

References

1. Gossec L, Paternotte S, Bingham CO 3rd, Clegg DO, Coste P, et al (2011) OARSI/OMERACT initiative to define states of severity and indication for joint replacement in hip and knee osteoarthritis. An OMERACT 10 Special Interest Group. J Rheumatol 38: 1765–1769. doi:10.3899/jrheum.110403.
2. Dauty M, Genty M, Ribinik P (2007) Physical training in rehabilitation programs before and after total hip and knee arthroplasty. Ann Readapt Med Phys 50: 462–468.
3. Minns Lowe CJ, Barker KL, Dewey ME, Sackley CM (2009) Effectiveness of physiotherapy exercise following hip arthroplasty for osteoarthritis: a systematic review of clinical trials. BMC Musculoskelet Disord 10: 98. doi:10.1186/1471-2474-10-98.
4. Holstege MS, Lindeboom R, Lucas C (2011) Preoperative quadriceps strength as a predictor for short-term functional outcome after total hip replacement. Arch Phys Med Rehabil 92: 236–241. doi:10.1016/j.apmr.2010.10.015.
5. Jensen C, Aagaard P, Overgaard S (2011) Recovery in mechanical muscle strength following resurfacing vs standard total hip arthroplasty-a randomised clinical trial. Osteoarthritis Cartilage 19: 1108–1116.
6. Kennedy D, Stratford P, Hanna S, Wessel J, Gollish J (2006) Modeling early recovery of physical function following hip and knee arthroplasty. BMC Musculoskelet Disord 7: 100.
7. Reardon K, Galea M, Dennett X, Choong P, Byrne E (2001) Quadriceps muscle wasting persists 5 months after total hip arthroplasty for osteoarthritis of the hip: a pilot study. Int Med J 31: 7–14.
8. Chou S-W, Ueng SWN, Lee MS (2008) Muscular recovery of hip flexors and extensors after two-incision total hip arthroplasty. Chang Gung Med J 31: 576–582.
9. Gilbey HJ, Ackland TR, Wang AW, Morton AR, Trouchet T, et al. (2003) Exercise improves early functional recovery after total hip arthroplasty. Clin Orthop Relat Res: 193–200.
10. Rossi MD, Brown LE, Whitehurst MA (2006) Assessment of hip extensor and flexor strength two months after unilateral total hip arthroplasty. J Strength Cond Res 20: 262–267. doi:10.1519/R-16234.1.
11. Suetta C, Andersen JL, Dalgas U, Berget J, Koskinen S, et al. (2008) Resistance training induces qualitative changes in muscle morphology, muscle architecture, and muscle function in elderly postoperative patients. J Appl Physiol 105: 180–186. doi:10.1152/japplphysiol.01354.2007.
12. Suetta C, Aagaard P, Rosted A, Jakobsen AK, Duus B, et al. (2004) Training-induced changes in muscle CSA, muscle strength, EMG, and rate of force development in elderly subjects after long-term unilateral disuse. J Appl Physiol 97: 1954–1961. doi:10.1152/japplphysiol.01307.2003.
13. Rasch A, Byström AH, Dalen N, Berg HE (2007) Reduced muscle radiological density, cross-sectional area, and strength of major hip and knee muscles in 22 patients with hip osteoarthritis. Acta Orthop 78: 505–510. doi:10.1080/17453670710014158.
14. Rasch A, Dalén N, Berg HE (2010) Muscle strength, gait, and balance in 20 patients with hip osteoarthritis followed for 2 years after THA. Acta Orthop 81: 183–188. doi:10.3109/17453671003793204.
15. Shih CH, Du YK, Lin YH, Wu CC (1994) Muscular recovery around the hip joint after total hip arthroplasty. Clin Orthop Relat Res: 115–120.
16. Frost KL, Bertocci GE, Wassinger CA, Munin MC, Burdett RG, et al. (2006) Isometric performance following total hip arthroplasty and rehabilitation. J Rehabil Res Dev 43: 435.
17. Bertocci GE, Munin MC, Frost KL, Burdett R, Wassinger CA, et al. (2004) Isokinetic performance after total hip replacement. Am J Phys Med Rehabil 83: 1–9. doi:10.1097/01.PHM.0000098047.26314.93.
18. Jan M-H, Hung J-Y, Lin JC-H, Wang S-F, Liu T-K, et al. (2004) Effects of a home program on strength, walking speed, and function after total hip replacement. Arch Phys Med Rehabil 85: 1943–1951.
19. Trudelle-Jackson E, Smith SS (2004) Effects of a late-phase exercise program after total hip arthroplasty: a randomized controlled trial. Arch Phys Med Rehabil 85: 1056–1062.
20. Vaz MD, Kramer JF, Rorabeck CH, Bourne RB (1993) Isometric hip abductor strength following total hip replacement and its relationship to functional assessments. J Orthop Sports Phys Ther 18: 526–531.
21. Husby VS, Helgerud J, Bjørgen S, Husby OS, Benum P, et al. (2009) Early maximal strength training is an efficient treatment for patients operated with total hip arthroplasty. Arch Phys Med Rehabil 90: 1658–1667. doi:10.1016/j.apmr.2009.04.018.
22. Holm B, Kristensen MT, Husted H, Kehlet H, Bandholm T (2011) Thigh and knee circumference, knee-extension strength, and functional performance after fast-track total hip arthroplasty. PM R 3: 117–124; quiz 124. doi:10.1016/j.pmrj.2010.10.019.
23. Bandholm T, Kehlet H (2012) Physiotherapy exercise after fast-track total hip and knee arthroplasty: time for reconsideration? Arch Phys Med Rehabil 93: 1292–1294. doi:10.1016/j.apmr.2012.02.014.
24. Kehlet H, Dahl JB (2003) Anaesthesia, surgery, and challenges in postoperative recovery. Lancet 362: 1921–1928. doi:10.1016/S0140-6736(03)14966-5.
25. Kehlet H, Wilmore DW (2008) Evidence-based surgical care and the evolution of fast-track surgery. Ann Surg 248: 189–198. doi:10.1097/SLA.0-b013e31817f2c1a.
26. Freeman S, Mascia A, McGill S (n.d.) Arthrogenic neuromusculature inhibition: A foundational investigation of existence in the hip joint. Clin Biomech (Bristol, Avon). Available: http://www.sciencedirect.com/science/article/pii/S0268003312002719. Accessed 22 January 2013.
27. Mizner RL, Petterson SC, Stevens JE, Vandenborne K, Snyder-Mackler L (2005) Early quadriceps strength loss after total knee arthroplasty. The contributions of muscle atrophy and failure of voluntary muscle activation. J Bone Joint Surg Am 87: 1047–1053. doi:10.2106/JBJS.D.01992.
28. Rice DA, McNair PJ (2010) Quadriceps Arthrogenic Muscle Inhibition: Neural Mechanisms and Treatment Perspectives. Semin Arthritis Rheum 40: 250–266. doi:10.1016/j.semarthrit.2009.10.001.
29. Suetta C, Magnusson SP, Rosted A, Aagaard P, Jakobsen AK, et al. (2004) Resistance Training in the Early Postoperative Phase Reduces Hospitalization and Leads to Muscle Hypertrophy in Elderly Hip Surgery Patients-A Controlled, Randomized Study. J Am Geriatr Soc 52: 2016–2022. doi:10.1111/j.1532-5415.2004.52557.x.
30. Rasch A, Bystrom AH, Dalen N, Martinez-Carranza N, Berg HE (2009) Persisting muscle atrophy two years after replacement of the hip. J Bone Joint Surg Br 91: 583–588.
31. Von Elm E, Altman DG, Egger M, Pocock SJ, Gøtzsche PC, et al. (2007) The Strengthening the Reporting of Observational Studies in Epidemiology (STROBE) statement: guidelines for reporting observational studies. PLoS Med 4: e296. doi:10.1371/journal.pmed.0040296.
32. Husted H, Lunn TH, Troelsen A, Gaarn-Larsen L, Kristensen BB, et al. (2011) Why still in hospital after fast-track hip and knee arthroplasty? Acta Orthop 82: 679–684. doi:10.3109/17453674.2011.636682.
33. Husted H, Holm G, Jacobsen S (2008) Predictors of length of stay and patient satisfaction after hip and knee replacement surgery: fast-track experience in 712 patients. Acta Orthop 79: 168–173. doi:10.1080/17453670710014941.
34. Thorborg K, Petersen J, Magnusson SP, Hölmich P (2010) Clinical assessment of hip strength using a hand-held dynamometer is reliable. Scand J Med Sci Sports 20: 493–501. doi:10.1111/j.1600-0838.2009.00958.x.
35. Bassey EJ, Short AH (1990) A new method for measuring power output in a single leg extension: feasibility, reliability and validity. Eur J Appl Physiol Occup Physiol 60: 385–390.
36. Podsiadlo D, Richardson S (1991) The timed "Up & Go": a test of basic functional mobility for frail elderly persons. J Am Geriatr Soc 39: 142–148.
37. Watson MJ (2002) Refining the ten-metre walking test for use with neurologically impaired people. Physiotherapy 88: 386–397.
38. Nilsdotter AK, Lohmander LS, Klässbo M, Roos EM (2003) Hip disability and osteoarthritis outcome score (HOOS)-validity and responsiveness in total hip replacement. BMC Musculoskelet Disord 4: 10. doi:10.1186/1471-2474-4-10.
39. Kristensen MT, Bandholm T, Bencke J, Ekdahl C, Kehlet H (2009) Knee-extension strength, postural control and function are related to fracture type and thigh edema in patients with hip fracture. Clin Biomech (Bristol, Avon) 24: 218–224. doi:10.1016/j.clinbiomech.2008.10.003.
40. Kazmi SSH, Stranden E, Kroese AJ, Slagsvold C-E, Diep LM, et al. (2007) Edema in the lower limb of patients operated on for proximal femoral fractures. J Trauma 62: 701–707. doi:10.1097/01.ta.0000196968.45151.7f.
41. Talis VL, Grishin AA, Solopova IA, Oskanyan TL, Belenky VE, et al. (2008) Asymmetric leg loading during sit-to-stand, walking and quiet standing in patients after unilateral total hip replacement surgery. Clin Biomech (Bristol, Avon) 23: 424–433. doi:10.1016/j.clinbiomech.2007.11.010.
42. Sicard-Rosenbaum L, Light KE, Behrman AL (2002) Gait, Lower Extremity Strength, and Self-Assessed Mobility After Hip Arthroplasty. J Gerontol A Biol Sci Med Sci 57: M47–M51. doi:10.1093/gerona/57.1.M47.
43. Lauretani F, Russo CR, Bandinelli S, Bartali B, Cavazzini C, et al. (2003) Age-associated changes in skeletal muscles and their effect on mobility: an operational diagnosis of sarcopenia. J Appl Physiol 95: 1851–1860. doi:10.1152/japplphysiol.00246.2003.
44. Manini TM, Visser M, Won-Park S, Patel KV, Strotmeyer ES, et al. (2007) Knee Extension Strength Cutpoints for Maintaining Mobility. J Am Geriatr Soc 55: 451–457. doi:10.1111/j.1532-5415.2007.01087.x.
45. Holm B, Kristensen MT, Bencke J, Husted H, Kehlet H, et al. (2010) Loss of knee-extension strength is related to knee swelling after total knee arthroplasty. Arch Phys Med Rehabil 91: 1770–1776. doi:10.1016/j.apmr.2010.07.229.
46. Mizner RL, Petterson SC, Snyder-Mackler L, others (2005) Quadriceps strength and the time course of functional recovery after total knee arthroplasty. J Orthop Sports Phys Ther 35: 424.
47. Delorme T (1945) Restoration of muscle power by heavy-resistance exercises. J Bone Joint Surg Am 27: 645–667.
48. Hall GM, Peerbhoy D, Shenkin A, Parker CJ, Salmon P (2001) Relationship of the functional recovery after hip arthroplasty to the neuroendocrine and inflammatory responses. Br J Anaesth 87: 537–542.
49. Stevens-Lapsley JE, Schenkman ML, Dayton MR (2011) Comparison of self-reported knee injury and osteoarthritis outcome score to performance measures in patients after total knee arthroplasty. PM R 3: 541–549; quiz 549. doi:10.1016/j.pmrj.2011.03.002.
50. Mizner RL, Petterson SC, Clements KE, Zeni JA Jr, Irrgang JJ, et al. (2011) Measuring functional improvement after total knee arthroplasty requires both performance-based and patient-report assessments: a longitudinal analysis of outcomes. J Arthroplasty 26: 728–737. doi:10.1016/j.arth.2010.06.004.

Identification of Quantitative Trait Loci (QTL) for Canine Hip Dysplasia and Canine Elbow Dysplasia in Bernese Mountain Dogs

Sophia Pfahler, Ottmar Distl*

Institute for Animal Breeding and Genetics, University of Veterinary Medicine Hannover, Hannover, Germany

Abstract

A genome-wide association study for canine hip dysplasia (CHD) and canine elbow dysplasia (CED) using the Illumina canine high density bead chip had been performed for 174 Bernese mountain dogs. General and mixed linear model analysis identified two different regions with single nucleotide polymorphisms (SNPs) on dog chromosome (CFA) 14 significantly associated with CHD and a further significantly CHD-associated region on CFA37. For CED, four SNPs on CFA11 and 27 were significantly associated. The identified SNPs of four associated regions included nearby candidate genes. These possible positional candidates were the genes *PON2* on CFA14 and *FN1* on CFA37 for CHD and the genes *LMNB1* on CFA11 and *WNT10B* on CFA27 for CED.

Editor: Stephen Moore, University of Queensland, Australia

Funding: The study was supported by a grant of the German Breeding Association for Swiss Mountain Dogs (SSV-DI/1-2). The funders had no role in study design, data collection and analysis, decision to publish, or preparation of the manuscript.

Competing Interests: The authors have declared that no competing interests exist.

* E-mail: ottmar.distl@tiho-hannover.de

Introduction

Hip dysplasia (CHD) and elbow dysplasia (CED) are common orthopedic conditions of the dog. These diseases affect dogs of all breeds with different prevalences. CHD is characterized by instability and subluxation or luxation of hips causing erosion of the articular cartilage and synovitis. CED results in osteoarthrotic changes, incongruity of the joint and lameness. Radiographic diagnosis of CED includes osteoarthrotic changes and the primary lesions incongruity of the elbow joint, fragmented medial coronoid process, osteochondrosis dissecans of the trochlea humeri and an ununited anconeal process. Genetic and environmental factors influence the expression of CHD and CED [1–4]. The Bernese mountain dogs (BMD) are affected by both diseases. Prevalences between 23 and 32% were reported for CHD in this breed, with the highest prevalence of CHD-affected dogs in Germany [5–8]. Among 20 and 37% dogs, CED was found in the various European BMD populations [5–7,9–10]. Heritabilities were estimated at 0.26–0.42 for CHD and at 0.17–0.38 for CED in BMD populations from Finland, Sweden and Germany [5,7,10].

BMD belong to the large dog breeds officially recognized by the FCI (Fédération Cynologique Internationale) under the FCI-standard number 45. This breed has an ancestral origin in the area of the Canton Berne in the Switzerland and after breed foundation as early as 1907, this breed became worldwide popular as a companion, family and multi-purpose dog. Originally, BMD were used for cattle driving and as guard and draught dogs on farms in Switzerland and South Germany. Like the other three Sennenhund breeds, the BMD has a distinctive tricolored hair coat, but is the only Sennenhund breed with a long haircoat (http://www.nmbe.ch/research/vertebrates/research/kynologie/swiss-dog-breeds/bernese-mountain-dog).

Quantitative trait loci (QTL) controlling CHD were identified on 19 chromosomes using genome-wide microsatellite sets for linkage analysis in German shepherd dogs [11], on twelve chromosomes for a Labrador Greyhound crossbreeding pedigree [12–14] and on two chromosomes for Portuguese water dogs [15–16]. A genome-wide association study, using the Labrador Greyhound crossbreeding pedigree and six dog breeds, revealed four CHD-associated SNPs on three chromosomes and two osteoarthritis-associated SNPs on two chromosomes [14]. An association of a *fibrillin 2*-haplotype with hip osteoarthritis and an increased expression of *MIG-6* and *fibronectin* in osteoarthritic cartilage were shown in dogs [17–19].

The collagen genes *COL1A1, COL1A2, COL2A1, COL3A1, COL5A1, COL5A2, COL6A3, COL9A1, COL9A2, COL9A3, COL10A1, COL11A1, COL11A2*, and *COL24A1* were eliminated as candidates for fragmented coronoid process in Labrador retrievers [20].

The objectives of the present study were to identify SNPs associated with CHD and CED using the Illumina high density canine bead chip (Illumina, San Diego, CA, USA) for BMD. In the genomic regions identified through the genome-wide association study (GWAS), we determined positional candidate genes by their involvement in the human or murine development of cartilage and the pathophysiology of human osteoarthritis (OA).

Results

The GWAS using a general linear model (GLM) identified three QTL for CHD (Figure 1) and two QTL for CED (Figure 2) on four different chromosomes harbouring significantly associated SNPs. The quantile-quantile (Q–Q) plots illustrated that inflation due to stratification effects had been removed by the general linear models employed for CHD and CED (Figures 3, 4). We determined the threshold for significance at a $-\log_{10}$P-value of 4.97 which corresponds to a P-value of 0.05 after applying the Benjamini-Hochberg-FDR correction for multiple testing. The $-\log_{10}$P-values corrected for multiple testing were at 2.0 (BICF2P1089246 on CFA14), 1.51 (BICF2P1282232 on CFA14) and 3.27 (BICF2S23052396 on CFA37) for CHD and 1.55 (BICF2G630294653 on CFA11), 1.73 (BICF2G630294836 on CFA11), 1.41 (BICF2P1025413 on CFA27) and 2.11 (BICF2G630140058 on CFA27) for CED. Mixed linear model (MLM) analyses confirmed the associations of the same SNPs as found by the GLM analysis (Table S1).

In order to show the impact of the significantly associated SNPs on disease occurrence of CHD and CED, the variance explained by the significantly associated SNPs in the GLM and odds ratios (ORs) were estimated using sex as strata (Table 1). The ORs for the CHD-SNPs were at 2.08–3.45 and for the CED-SNPs at 2.94–3.21.

For all five QTL and their flanking genomic regions, the $-\log_{10}$P-values and all genes annotated on the dog genome assembly build 2.1 are shown in Figures 5, 6, 7, 8, 9. Then, we analysed the haplotype structure and haplotype association for these genomic regions surrounding the significantly associated SNPs and containing CHD- or CED-SNPs with $-\log_{10}$P-values>2.0–3.0 using GLM analyses. For the haplotype association analyses, CHD and CED were treated as binary traits considering CHD- or CED-affected dogs as cases and dogs free from CHD and CED as controls. Haplotype blocks with significantly CHD- or CED-associated SNPs were identified within two of the five associated genomic regions (Table S2). On CFA37, there was one significantly CHD-associated haplotype at 25.0–25.2 Mb and this haplotype block contained the CHD-associated SNP BICF2S23052396. The chromosomal region on CFA11 at 17–24 Mb contained 44 haplotype blocks. In this region haplotypes from seven blocks were significantly associated with CED after applying permutation tests. The significantly CED-associated SNPs BICF2G630294653 and BICF2G630294836 on CFA11 were located within associated haplotype blocks at 18.80–19.07 and 19.11–19.13 Mb, respectively.

Discussion

In the present study using the Illumina canine high density bead chip for 174 BMD, we identified three SNPs significantly associated with CHD on CFA14 and 37 and each two SNPs significantly associated with CED on CFA11 and 27. The results of the GWAS were consistent for the GLM and MLM even when the inbreeding coefficients and the first two to six principal components (PCA) were regarded as additional covariates. Two of the three significantly CHD-associated SNPs were located in intergenic regions. The CHD-associated SNP BICF2P1282232 was located within intron 9 of *CTTNBP2* (*cortactin-binding protein 2*). An obvious functional relationship of CTTNBP2 with CHD could not be found. An intron of the gene *MARCH3* on CFA11 harboured the CED-associated SNP BICF2G630294836. There was no obvious relation between this gene and the pathogenesis of CED. Similarly, the SNP BICF2G630294653 was located within intron 2 of *C5orf48* which encodes an uncharacterized protein. The further CED-associated SNPs on CFA27 were intergenic.

The human homologues of the genes *PON1*, *PON2* and *PON3* (*paraoxonase*) on CFA14 are part of the gamma-hexachlorocyclohexane degradation pathway that was associated with low bone mineral density of hips [21]. The *paraoxonase* 2 gene is nearest to the CHD-associated SNP BICF2P1089246 on CFA14, approximately 183 kb upstream of this SNP, and with this SNP located in the same haplotype block. The *protein phosphatase 1, regulatory subunit 9A* (*PPP1R9A*) gene that is imprinted in human and mouse was shown to be involved in the development of skeletal muscles [22]. A reduced muscle tonus can destabilize the hip joint and thereby possibly be a part of CHD pathogenesis. This gene is located approximately 609 kb upstream of the CHD-associated SNP on CFA14.

On CFA37, *FN1* (*fibronectin*), is located approximately 361 kb downstream of the CHD-associated SNP. FN1 is a component of the extracellular matrix in cartilage and an important function in

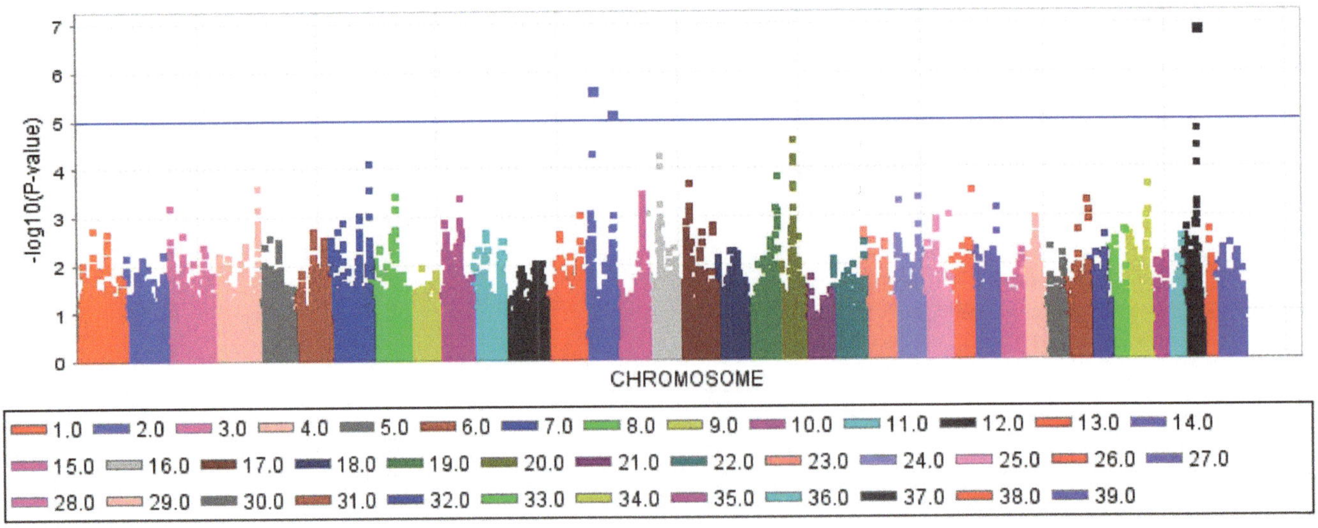

Figure 1. Manhattan plot of $-\log_{10}$P-values of the genome-wide association study for the canine hip dysplasia score in Bernese mountain dogs using a general model analysis. On the X-axis, the SNPs are given by dog chromosome number. The $-\log_{10}$P-values for each SNP genotype effect are plotted against the SNP position on each chromosome. Chromosomes are differentiated by colors. The color keys are given below the plot. The blue line indicates the threshold of the $-\log_{10}$P-values for genome-wide significance after correcting for multiple testing.

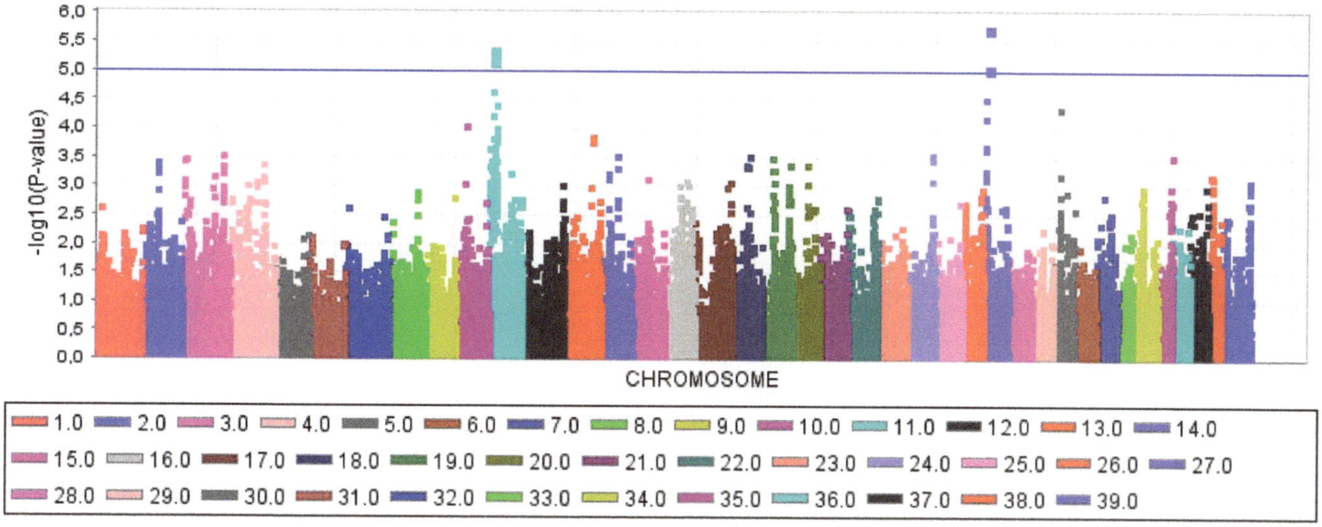

Figure 2. Manhattan plot of $-\log_{10}$P-values of the genome-wide association study for the canine elbow dysplasia score in Bernese mountain dogs using a general model analysis. On the X-axis, the SNPs are given by dog chromosome number. The $-\log_{10}$P-values for each SNP genotype effect are plotted against the SNP position on each chromosome. Chromosomes are differentiated by colors. The color keys are given below the plot. The blue line indicates the threshold of the $-\log_{10}$P-values for genome-wide significance after correcting for multiple testing.

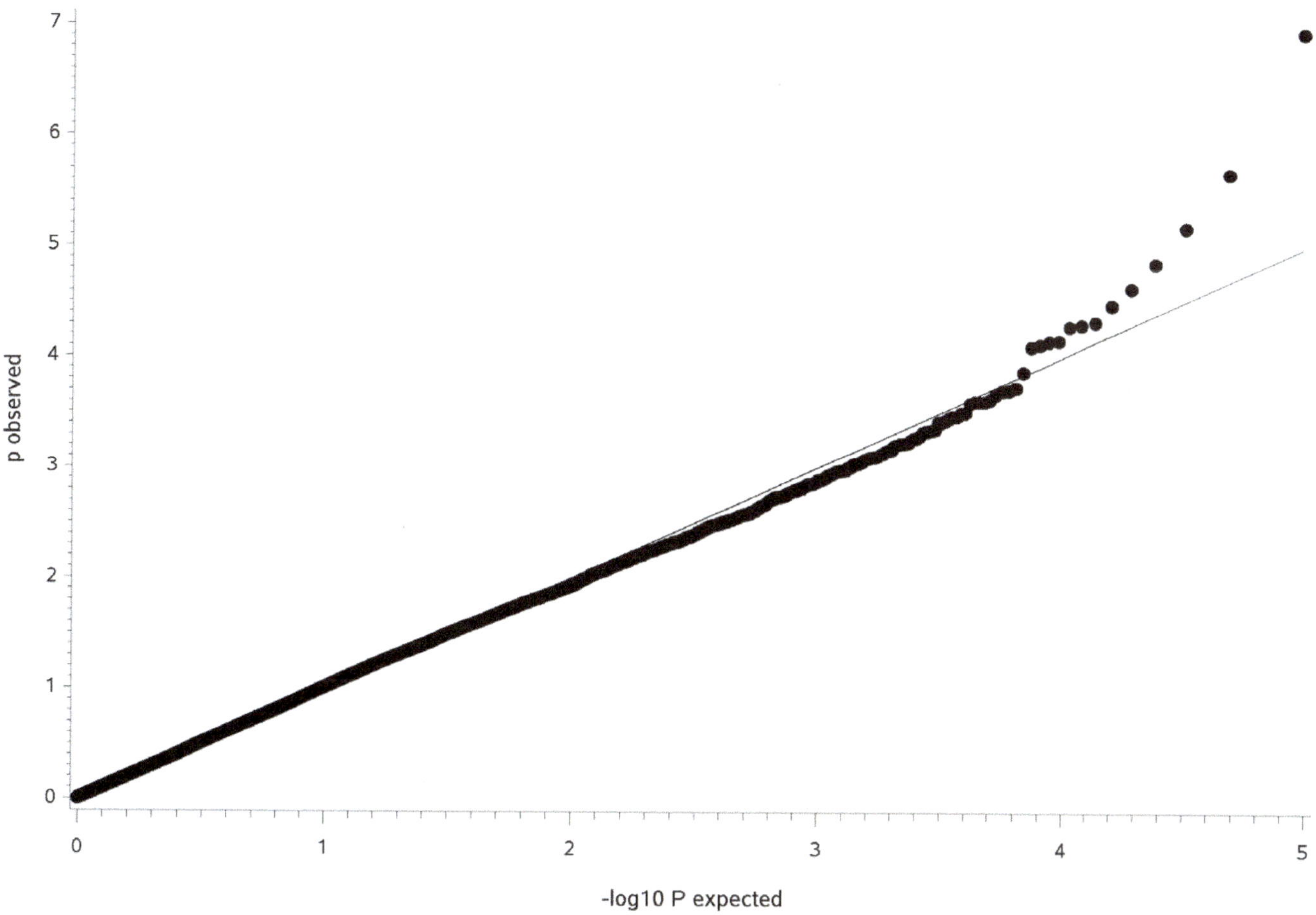

Figure 3. Q-Q-plot of expected $-\log_{10}$P-values versus observed$-\log_{10}$P-values from the general model analysis for canine hip dysplasia score in Bernese mountain dogs. Shown are all 96,412 SNPs included in the genome-wide association analysis with the grey line corresponding to the null hypothesis of no association.

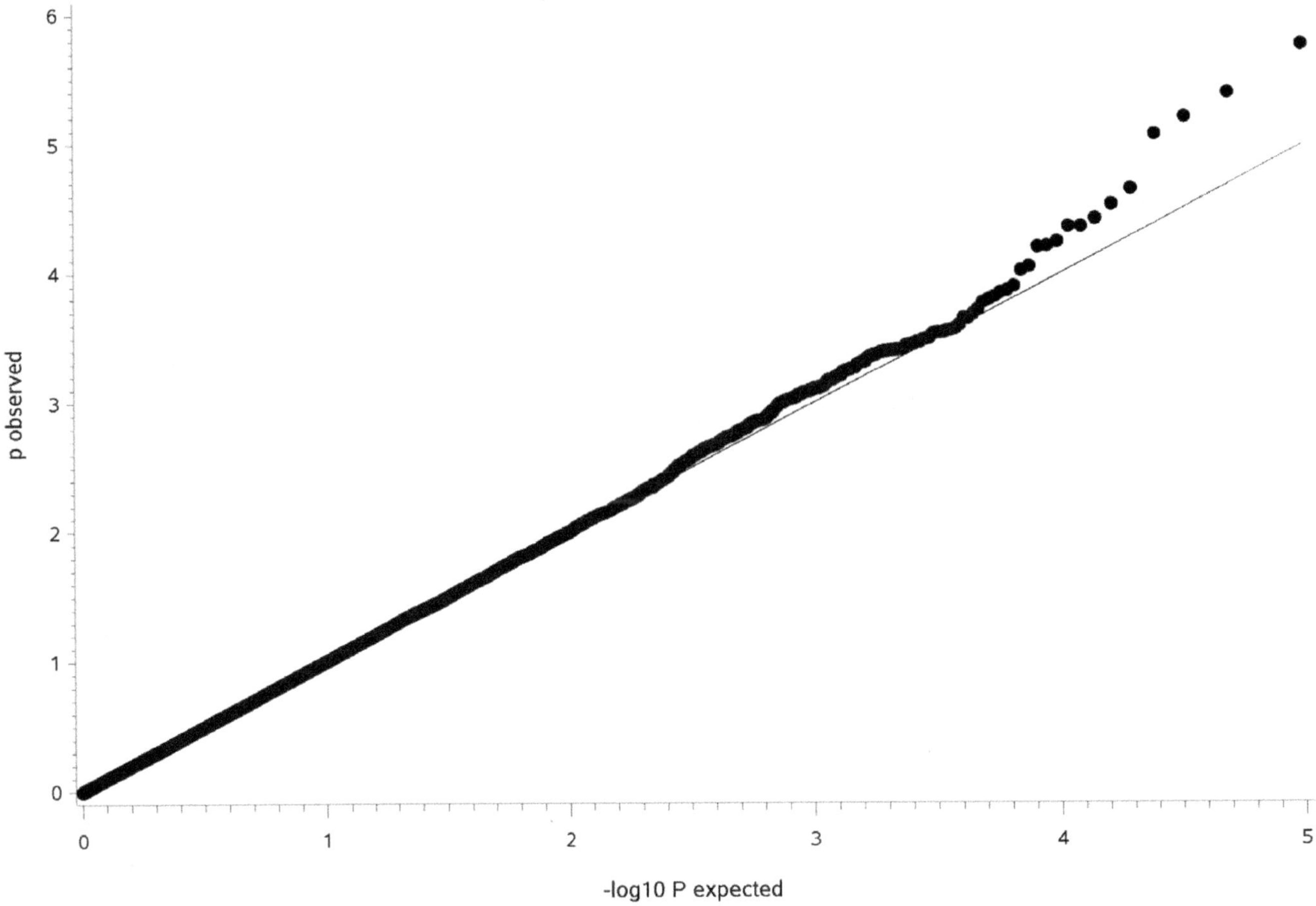

Figure 4. Q-Q-plot of expected $-\log_{10}$P-values versus observed$-\log_{10}$P-values from the general model analysis for canine elbow dysplasia score in Bernese mountain dogs. Shown are all 96,412 SNPs included in the genome-wide association analysis with the grey line corresponding to the null hypothesis of no association.

Table 1. Summary of results for the genome-wide association study using a general linear model analysis and sex-stratified case-control analysis for canine hip and elbow dysplasia in Bernese mountain dogs.

Trait CFA	Position	SNP-ID	Minor allele	MAF	MAF_a	MAF_u	V_{SNP}	OR	CI-L	CI-U	$-\log_{10}P$	Candidate gene	Distance to the nearest candidate gene in kb
Canine hip dysplasia													
14	23,811,133	BICF2P1089246	C	0.32	0.46	0.29	0.14	2.08	1.22	3.57	5.66	*PON2*	183
14	59,537,633	BICF2P1282232	T	0.15	0.29	0.11	0.12	3.08	1.63	5.85	5.17	–	–
37	25,095,511	BICF2S23052396	A	0.12	0.25	0.09	0.15	3.45	1.75	6.67	6.93	*FN1*	361
Canine elbow dysplasia													
11	18,913,755	BICF2G630294653	T	0.21	0.36	0.16	0.12	2.98	1.68	5.29	5.21	*LMNB1*	89
11	19,114,139	BICF2G630294836	A	0.22	0.38	0.17	0.13	2.94	1.67	5.26	5.39	*LMNB1*	55
27	7,848,483	BICF2P1025413	T	0.15	0.29	0.11	0.12	3.20	1.68	6.08	5.08	*WNT10B*	763
27	7,956,078	BICF2G630140058	G	0.16	0.31	0.12	0.13	3.21	1.74	5.93	5.76	*WNT10B*	655

The SNP-ID, the position on dog chromosome (CFA) in base pairs (bp), minor allele, minor allele frequency (MAF) for all, affected (MAF_a) and unaffected (MAF_u) dogs (controls), variance explained by the single SNPs (V_{SNP}) and $-\log_{10}$P-values ($-\log_{10}P$) of the general model analysis are given. Odds ratios (OR) with 95% confidence intervals (CI) are from a sex-stratified case-control analysis for CHD- and CED-affected dogs. Positional candidate genes with their distance to the associated SNP are shown according to the dog genome assembly build 2.1.

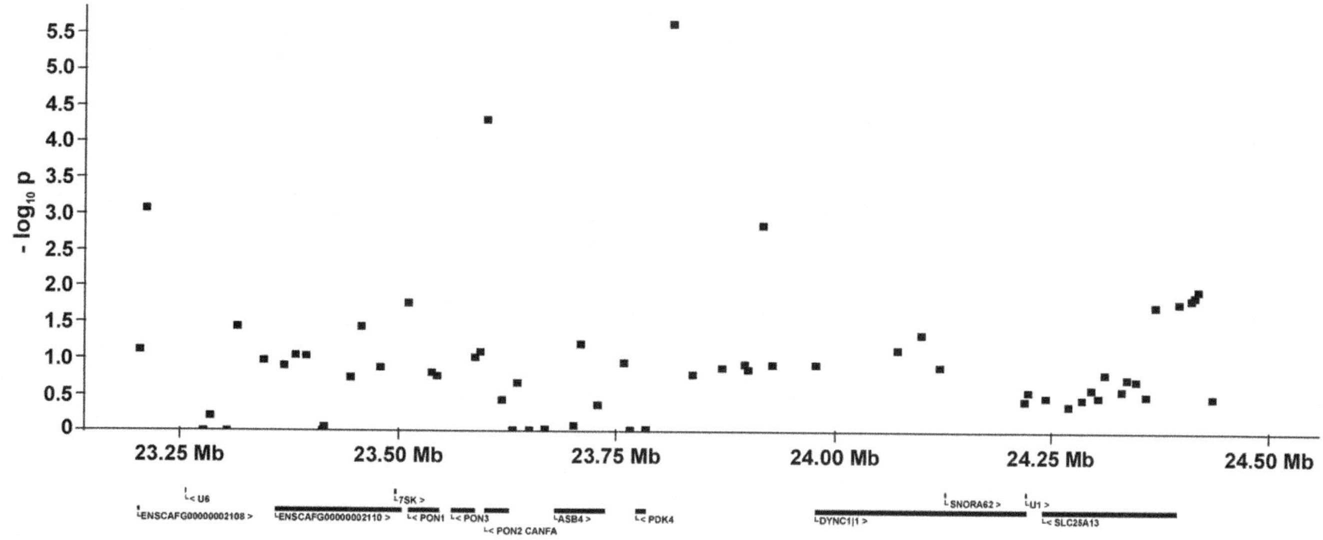

Figure 5. Genomic region with a significant association for canine hip dysplasia on dog chromosome (CFA) 14 at 23.25–24.5 Mb. The $-\log_{10}$P-values of all 62 SNPs in this region and the genes annotated according to the dog genome assembly build 2.1 are shown.

matrix organization of cartilage had been suggested [23]. The fibronectin concentrations from canine femoral head cartilage with lesions were higher than from cartilage surrounding these regions [19]. In addition, in dogs with high risk to OA, fibronectin concentrations from explanted cartilage were higher in comparison to dogs with low OA risk [19].

The canine *lamin B1* (*LMNB1*) gene resides in a significantly CED-associated haplotype block at 18.80–19.07 Mb. Mice with a homozygous mutation causing the functional loss of *lamin B1* were nonviable because of respiratory problems and bone malformations. Growth and ossification of long bones were disturbed [24].

For the CED-QTL on CFA27, a candidate gene involved in chondrocyte metabolism, OA and osteoblast differentiation was found. The *wingless-type MMTV integration site family, member 10B* (*WNT10B*) gene approximately 655 kb downstream of the SNP BICF2G630140058 is associated with the bone mass and the bone mineral density in the human hip [25].

The SNP BICF2P1089246 on CFA14 is located within a CHD-QTL identified in a genome-wide linkage analysis using 261 microsatellites for German shepherd dogs [11]. The CHD-associated SNP on CFA37 at 25.0 Mb of the present study is on the same chromosome, but in far distance to the CHD-QTL found in the Labrador-Greyhound crossbreeding pedigree at 42.1–44.6 Mb [12], however, in the neighbourhood of a SNP associated with hip OA at 17.2 Mb detected in an across-breed GWAS [13]. As the FCI grading uses osteoarthrotic changes as criteria for the CHD-status, joint QTL for the CHD-status and OA may exist.

Genetic correlations among CHD and CED were close to zero in Swedish [7], at 0.26 in Finnish [10] and at 0.31 in German

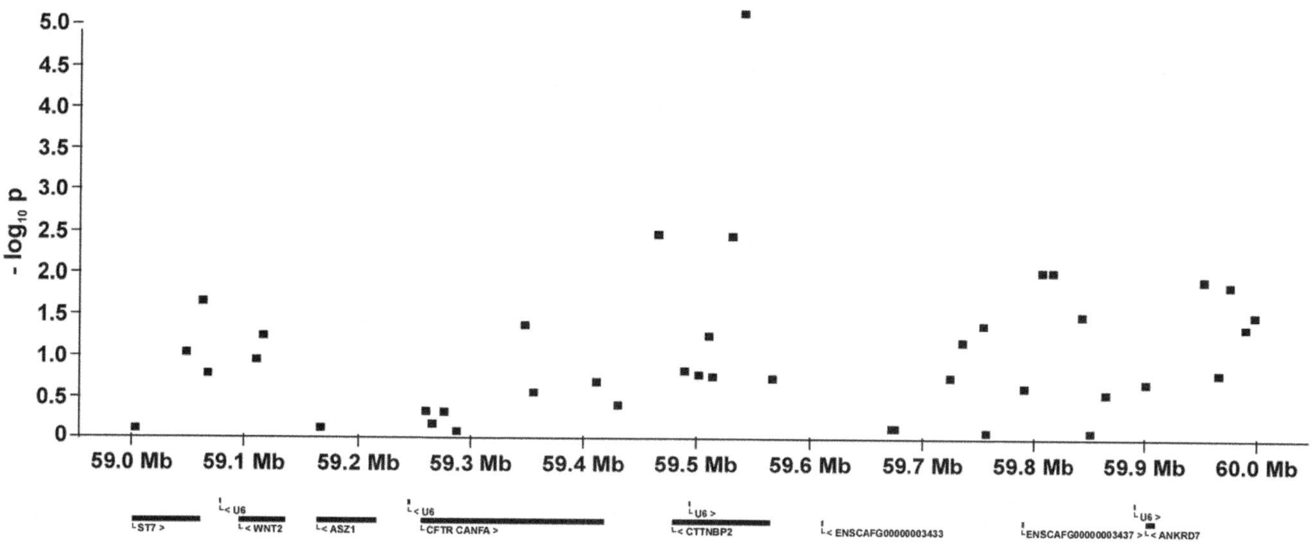

Figure 6. Genomic region with a significant association for canine hip dysplasia on dog chromosome (CFA) 14 at 59.5–60.0 Mb. The $-\log_{10}$P-values of all 41 SNPs in this region and the genes annotated according to the dog genome assembly build 2.1 are shown.

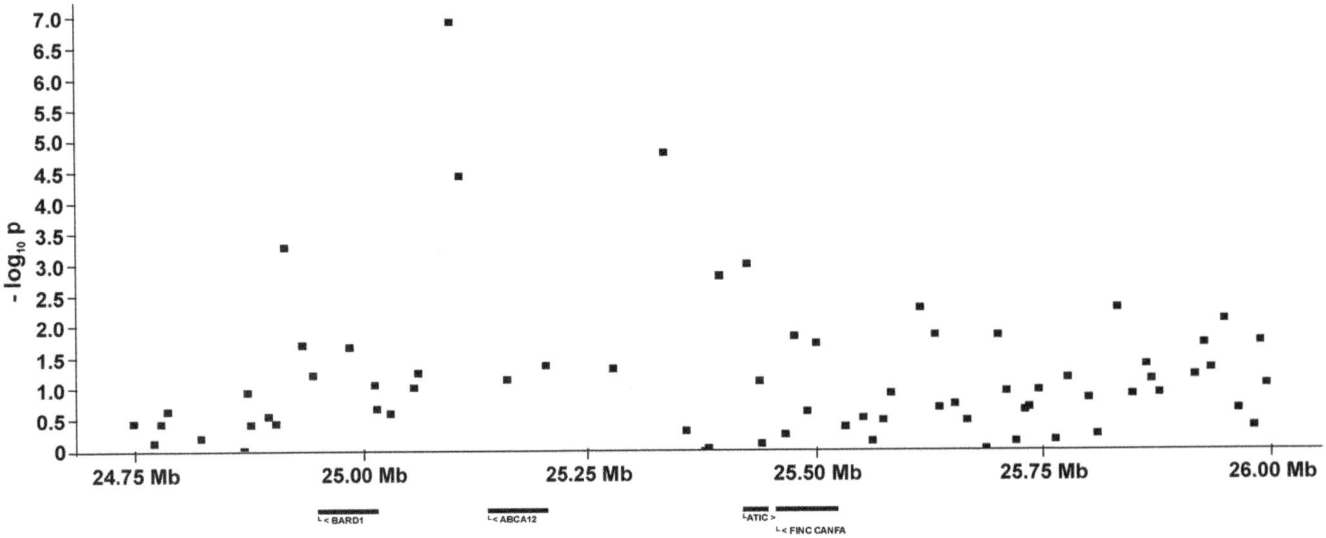

Figure 7. Genomic region with a significant association for canine hip dysplasia on dog chromosome (CFA) 37 at 24.75–26.0 Mb. The $-\log_{10}$P-values of all 58 SNPs in this region and the genes annotated according to the dog genome assembly build 2.1 are shown.

population genetic analyses for BMD [5]. No overlap was found between QTL for CHD and CED in the present GWAS and no common metabolic pathway was detected among genes located in CHD- and CED-associated chromosomal regions of the present GWAS. Thus, our study supports the assumption that CHD and CED are different genetic traits that may not share many common loci.

In summary, we mapped three loci on dog chromosomes (CFA) 14 and 37 significantly associated with CHD and two loci on CFA11 and 27 significantly associated with CED. The effects of the SNPs had ORs at 2.1–3.5 for disease occurrence. The SNPs with higher ORs had lower MAFs indicating that the alleles with higher risk to CHD and CED had a lower prevalence in BMD analysed here. Four of the five identified CHD- and CED-loci had nearby candidate genes.

Materials and Methods

Ethics Statement

All animal work has been conducted according to the national and international guidelines for animal welfare. The dogs in this

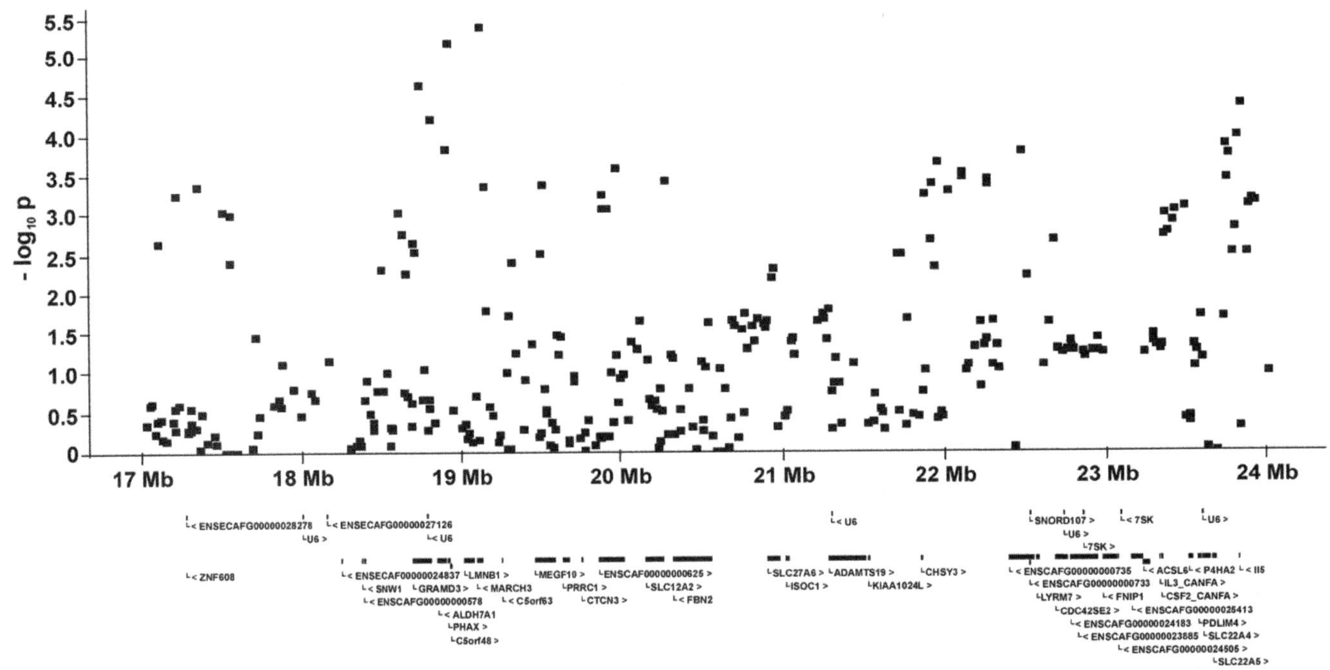

Figure 8. Genomic region with a significant association for canine elbow dysplasia on dog chromosome (CFA) 11 at 17.0–24.0 Mb. The $-\log_{10}$P-values of all 314 SNPs in this region and the genes annotated according to the dog genome assembly build 2.1 are shown.

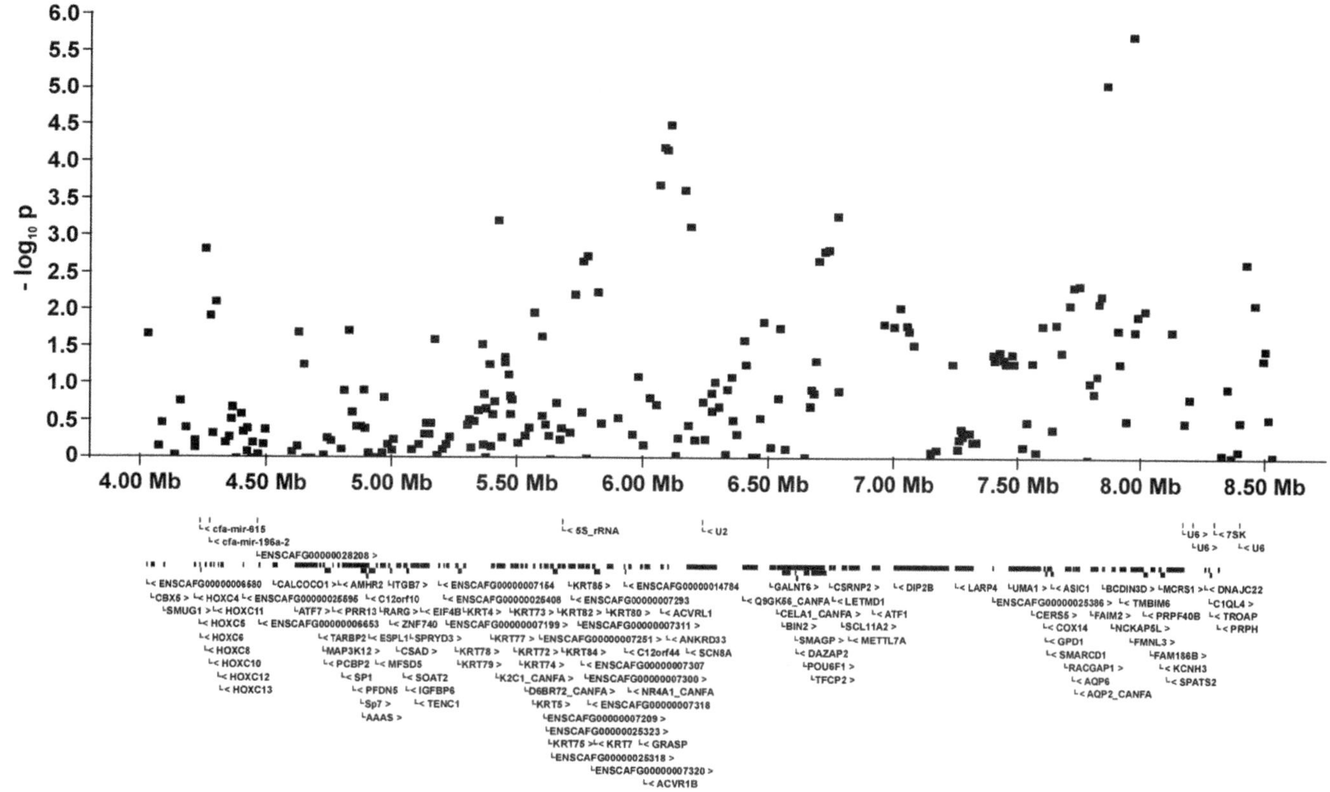

Figure 9. Genomic region with a significant association for canine elbow dysplasia on dog chromosome (CFA) 27 at 4.0–8.5 Mb. The $-\log_{10}$P-values of all 241 SNPs in this region and the genes annotated according to the dog genome assembly build 2.1 are shown.

study were included with the consent of their owners. The blood samples were collected by veterinarians during the routine examination for CHD and CED regarding principles of good veterinary practice. These diagnostic procedures had to be carried out anyway. All blood-sampling of dogs was done in veterinary practices for small animals by trained staff. CHD and CED examinations are compulsory for all dogs intended for breeding and these examinations were performed in veterinary clinics and practices according to the rules for hip screening of the FCI and the International Elbow Working Group (IEWG). Approval from the ethics committee was not obtained because blood sampling was done during a diagnostic veterinary procedure according to the German Animal Welfare Law (released on 05/18/2006, last changes on 12/09/2010).

Animals

The sample genotyped included 174 purebred Bernese mountain dogs born in the years 1996 to 2010 (Table 2). In order to reduce the influence of the population structure for the GWAS, we chose only one descendent of each paternal grandsire from all dogs presented for X-raying of the hips and elbows from the birth year cohorts of 1996–2010.

All animals genotyped were screened for CHD according to the rules of the FCI and for CED according to the rules of the IEWG (http://www.vet-iewg.org/joomla/index.php/archive/23-2001-international-elbow-protocol-vancouver). The minimum age at the time of examination was twelve months for all dogs. A ventrodorsal X-ray of the hips and a flexed mediolateral projection of the elbow had to be taken by an accredited veterinarian with the dog in general anaesthesia. A breed specific expert evaluation report was provided for the X-rays scoring hip joints as normal (A), borderline (B), mild (C), moderate (D) or severe CHD (E) [26–27]. Elbows were categorized as free (ED 0) or mild to severe CED (ED I–ED III) based on the presence of primary lesions and secondary arthrotic changes. In Germany, presence of a primary elbow lesion (fragmented medial coronoid process, ununited anconeal process, osteochondrosis of the medial humeral condyle, radio-ulnar length

Table 2. Number of Bernese mountain dogs genotyped on the Illumina high density beadchip.

CED-score	Female dogs	Male dogs	All dogs
Free	93	47	140
I	22	9	31
II	2	0	2
III	0	1	1
CHD-score			
A	87	49	136
B	4	1	5
C	26	7	33
Total	117	57	174

Number of dogs stratified by sex, canine hip dysplasia (CHD) and canine elbow dysplasia (CED) scores are given. Controls include dogs free from CHD and CED. Cases for CHD or CED are dogs classified with CHD-scores B or C or dogs classified with CED scores I, II or III. All dogs affected by CED, but three dogs were free from CHD.

discrepancy) leads to the classification of severe CED. Dogs classified as free form CHD and CED were used as controls and the other dogs as cases according to their scores for CHD or CED. The disease conditions for GWAS were treated as quantitative traits encoding CHD- and CED-unaffected dogs with one and the other conditions with 2–5 (CHD) or 2–4 (CED) for borderline (CHD) or mild (CED) to severe affection status.

DNA Extraction

Extraction of genomic DNA from Na-EDTA blood samples was performed through a standard ethanol fractionation with concentrated sodiumchloride (6 M NaCl) and sodium dodecyl sulphate (10% SDS). Concentration of DNA was adjusted to 50 ng/µl in the samples used for genotyping.

SNP Genotyping

Genotyping of the 174 BMD for the GWAS was done on the canine Illumina high density beadchip (Illumina) containing 173,662 SNPs. Quality criteria for further analyses were minor allele frequencies (MAF) >0.05, genotyping rate per SNP>0.90 and tests for Hardy-Weinberg equilibrium (p-value<0.000001). After filtering for quality criteria, 96,412 SNPs had been left for analysis. The mean genotyping rate per individual was 99 per cent.

Statistical Analysis

The ALLELE procedure of SAS/Genetics, version 9.3 (SAS Institute, Cary, NC, USA) was used to calculate polymorphism information content, heterozygosity, allelic diversity, allele and genotype frequencies and χ^2-tests for Hardy-Weinberg-Equilibrium for the SNPs genotyped. The GWAS was performed using both a general (GLM) and a mixed (MLM) linear model. CHD- and CED-scores were treated as quantitative traits (1 = CHD-A to 5 = CDH-E, 1 = ED free to 4 = ED III). The analyses were run using TASSEL, version 3.0.88 [28]. The GLM explained for sex effects and the respective SNP genotypes. The MLM included an additional random animal effect via the identity-by-state-kinship (IBS) matrix. The IBS matrix reflects the genomic relationship matrix among all individuals genotyped and captures the relatedness among animals as well as the cryptic family structure. Cryptic relatedness is due to distant relationships and therefore, may not be displayed through the pedigrees of the animals. Further GLM and MLM models with the inbreeding coefficients and the first two to six PCAs using as linear covariates had been run to test the robustness of the models. PCAs were parameterized to infer possible population stratification due to genetic ancestry. In order to avoid that blocks with long-range linkage disequilibria (LD) influence PCAs, we used a pruned set of SNPs in approximate linkage equilibria. Thus, PCAs and IBS-kinship coefficients were derived from a pruned set of 10,075 genome-wide and equidistantly distributed SNPs at pair-wise LD (r^2) <0.3. The results for the extended models were consistent with the GLM and MLM analyses omitting PCAs and the inbreeding coefficient. Therefore, the results reported refer to GLM and MLM analyses with sex and the respective SNP genotypes as fixed effects and in the MLM with an additional random animal effect parameterized via the genomic relationship matrix. The reason for this consistency across the different models employed stems from the fact that PCAs, inbreeding coefficients and relatedness were rather equally distributed among affected and controls. We applied the Benjamini-Hochberg-FDR correction using the MULTIPLE TEST procedure of SAS, version 9.3, to determine the threshold for genome-wide significance.

Genotypic and allelic associations and allelic trends as well as ORs with their 95% confidence intervals for CHD- and CED-SNPs were calculated using the CASECONTROL procedure of SAS/Genetics and sex as strata.

We analysed the haplotype structure of the identified genomic regions and tested the associations of haplotype blocks using Haploview 4.0 [29]. CHD- and CED-scores had to be treated as binomial traits (CHD-A vs. CHD-B-E and ED free vs. ED I-ED III) in these analyses and a permutation rate of 10,000 was chosen.

Supporting Information

Table S1 Results for the genome-wide association study using a mixed linear model (MLM) analysis for canine hip dysplasia (CHD) and canine elbow dysplasia (CED) in Bernese mountain dogs. The SNP-ID, the position on dog chromosome (CFA) in base pairs (bp) according to the dog genome assembly build 2.1, the variance explained by the single SNPs ($V_{SNP-MLM}$) and $-\log_{10}$P-values ($-\log_{10}$P-MLM) of the MLM analysis are given.

Table S2 Association tests for haplotype blocks using Haploview for canine hip dysplasia and canine elbow dysplasia. The test statistics including χ^2– and P-values (P) using 10,000 permutations for significantly associated haplotypes containing significantly associated SNPs from the general model analysis are shown. For these significantly associated SNPs, the SNP-ID and their chromosomal position are given.

Acknowledgments

The authors thank the German Breeding Association for Swiss Mountain Dogs (Schweizer Sennenhund Verein Deutschland e.V., SSV) for providing EDTA-blood samples, pedigree data and diagnoses for hip and elbow dysplasia.

Author Contributions

Conceived and designed the experiments: OD SP. Performed the experiments: SP OD. Analyzed the data: SP OD. Contributed reagents/materials/analysis tools: OD. Wrote the paper: SP OD.

References

1. Janutta V, Hamann H, Distl O (2006) Complex segregation analysis of canine hip dysplasia in German shepherd dogs. J Hered 97: 13–20.
2. Comhaire FH, Snaps F (2008) Comparison of two canine registry databases on the prevalence of hip dysplasia by breed and the relationship of dysplasia with body weight and height. Am J Vet Res 69: 330–333.
3. Stock KF, Klein S, Tellhelm B, Distl O (2011) Genetic analyses of elbow and hip dysplasia in the German shepherd dog. J Anim Breed Genet 128: 219–229.
4. Guthrie S, Pidduck HG (1990) Heritability of elbow osteochondrosis within a closed population of dogs. JSAP 31: 93–96.
5. Hartmann P, Stock KF, Distl O (2010) Multivariate genetische Analyse der Hüft- und Ellenbogengelenkdysplasie sowie der Osteochondrose des Schultergelenks beim Berner Sennenhund. Berl Münch Tierärztl Wochenschr 123: 488–495.
6. Coopman F, Verhoeven G, Saunders J, Duchateau L, van Bree H (2008) Prevalence of hip dysplasia, elbow dysplasia and humeral head osteochondrosis in dog breeds in Belgium. Vet Rec 163: 654–658.
7. Malm S, Fikse WF, Danell B, Strandberg E (2008) Genetic variation and genetic trends in hip and elbow dysplasia in Swedish Rottweiler and Bernese Mountain Dog. J Anim Breed Genet 125: 403–412.
8. Genevois JP, Remy D, Viguier E, Carozzo C, Collard F, et al. (2008) Prevalence of hip dysplasia according to official radiographic screening, among 31 breeds of dogs in France. Vet Comp Orthopaed 21: 21–24.

9. Sturaro E, Ojala M, Mäki K, Bittante G, Carnier P, et al. (2005) Results from an explorative screening program for elbow dysplasia in some breeds of dogs in Italy. Ital J Anim Sci 4: 233–240.
10. Mäki K, Groen AF, Liinamo A-E, Ojala M (2002) Genetic variances, trends and mode of inheritance for hip and elbow dysplasia in Finnish dog populations. Anim Sci 75: 197–207.
11. Marschall Y, Distl O (2007) Mapping quantitative trait loci for canine hip dysplasia in German Shepherd dogs. Mamm Genome 18: 861–870.
12. Todhunter RJ, Mateescu R, Lust G, Burton-Wurster NI, Dykes NL, et al. (2005) Quantitative trait loci for hip dysplasia in a cross-breed canine pedigree. Mamm Genome 16: 720–730.
13. Zhu L, Zhang Z, Feng F, Schweitzer P, Phavaphutanon J, et al. (2008) Single nucleotide polymorphisms refine QTL intervals for hip joint laxity in dogs. Anim Genet 39: 141–146.
14. Zhou Z, Sheng X, Zhang Z, Zhao K, Zhu L, et al. (2010) Differential genetic regulation of canine hip dysplasia and osteoarthritis. PLoS One 5: e13219.
15. Chase K, Lawler DF, Adler FR, Ostrander EA, Lark KG (2004) Bilaterally asymmetric effects of quantitative trait loci (QTLs): QTLs that affect laxity in the right versus left coxofemoral (hip) joints of the dog (Canis familiaris). Am J Med Genet A 124A: 239–247.
16. Chase K, Lawler DF, Carrier DR, Lark KG (2005) Genetic regulation of osteoarthritis: A QTL regulating cranial and caudal acetabular osteophyte formation in the hip joint of the dog (Canis familiaris). Am J Med Genet A 135: 334–335.
17. Friedenberg SG, Zhu L, Zhang Z, van den Berg Foels W, Schweitzer PA, et al. (2010) Evaluation of a fibrillin 2 gene haplotype associated with hip dysplasia and incipient osteoarthritis in dogs. Am J Vet Res 72: 530–540.
18. Mateescu RG, Todhunter RJ, Lust G, Burton-Wurster N (2005) Increased MIG-6 mRNA transcripts in osteoarthritic cartilage. Biochem Biophys Res Commun 332: 482–486.
19. Burton-Wurster N, Farese JP, Todhunter RJ, Lust G (1999) Site-specific variation in femoral head cartilage composition in dogs at high and low risk for development of osteoarthritis: insights into cartilage degeneration. Osteoarthritis Cartilage 7: 486–497.
20. Salg KG, Temwitchitr J, Imholz S, Hazewinkel HA, Leegwater PA (2006) Assessment of collagen genes involved in fragmented medial coronoid process development in Labrador Retrievers as determined by affected sibling-pair analysis. Am J Vet Res 67: 1713–1718.
21. Lee YH, Choi SJ, Ji JD, Song GG (2012) Pathway analysis of genome-wide association study for bone mineral density. Mol Biol Rep 39: 8099–8106.
22. Nakabayashi K, Makino S, Minagawa S, Smith AC, Bamforth JS, et al. (2004) Genomic imprinting of PPP1R9A encoding neurabin I in skeletal muscle and extra-embryonic tissues. J Med Genet 41: 601–608.
23. MacLeod JN, Burton-Wurster N, Gu DN, Lust G (1996) Fibronectin mRNA splice variant in articular cartilage lacks bases encoding the V, III-15, and I-10 protein segments. J Biol Chem 271: 18954–18960.
24. Vergnes L, Peterfy M, Bergo MO, Young SG, Reue K (2004) Lamin B1 is required for mouse development and nuclear integrity. Proc Natl Acad Sci USA 101: 10428–10433.
25. Zmuda JM, Yerges LM, Kammerer CM, Cauley JA, Wang X, et al. (2009) Association analysis of WNT10B with bone mass and structure among individuals of African ancestry. J Bone Miner Res 24: 437–447.
26. Brass W (1993) Hüftgelenkdysplasie und Ellbogenerkrankung im Visier der Fédération Cynologique Internationale. Kleintierpraxis 38: 191–266.
27. Flückiger M (2007) Scoring radiographs for canine hip dysplasia – the big three organizations in the world. EJCAP 17: 135–140.
28. Bradbury PJ, Zhang Z, Kroon DE, Casstevens TM, Ramdoss Y, et al. (2007) TASSEL: software for association mapping of complex traits in diverse samples. Bioinformatics 23: 2633–2635.
29. Barrett JC, Fry B, Maller J, Daly MJ (2005) Haploview: analysis and visualization of LD and haplotype maps. Bioinformatics 21: 263–265.

17

The Geometry of the Bone Structure Associated with Total Hip Arthroplasty

Zhang Yang, Wang Jian, Li Zhi-han, Xiao Jun, Zhao Liang, Yan Ge, Shi Zhan-jun*

Department of Orthopaedic Surgery, Nanfang Hospital, Southern Medical University, Guangzhou, Guangdong, China

Abstract

Close adaptation of the prosthesis to the bone is the key to achieving optimal stability and fixation for total hip arthroplasty (THA). However, there have been no adequate studies of bone morphology, especially in different races. The aim of this study was to analyze the geometry of the acetabulum and proximal femur of people from South China, based on three-dimensional reconstruction, and to detect differences between different population subsets. CT scans were performed on 80 healthy volunteers (160 hips) from South China, comprising 40 males (80 hips) and 40 females (80 hips). The images were imported into Mimics 10.01 to perform 3D reconstruction. THA-associated anatomical parameters were measured and compared with other published data. In comparison with published data, it seemed that people from South China have smaller acetabular abduction angle, larger acetabular supro-inferior diameter, larger neck-shaft angle, smaller offset, thinner femoral shaft and more proximal isthmus, which needed to be further confirmed. There were significant differences between the genders in most parameters. As significant differences in canal flare index (CFI) and distal canal flare index (DCFI) were found between genders, it was concluded the most significant differences lay in the isthmus of the femur. Among the femora, according to Noble's classification we identified more normal types and fewer stovepipe and champagne-flute types than expected from the literature, indicating that uncemented prostheses would be suitable for most people from South China. Our findings reveal that simply choosing the smallest of a series of prostheses would not necessarily provide a good fit, due to the different trends from the proximal to the distal part of the femur. Significant variation exists in THA-associated anatomy between genders and population subsets. It is therefore imperative that each patient receives individual consideration rather than assuming all patients have the same anatomy, especially for different races.

Editor: Carlos Eduardo Ambrosio, Faculty of Animal Sciences and Food Engineering, University of São Paulo, Pirassununga, SP, Brazil, Brazil

Funding: The authors have no support or funding to report.

Competing Interests: The authors have declared that no competing interests exist.

* E-mail: mariaresearcher@hotmail.com

Introduction

Total hip arthroplasty (THA) has been proven to be a good choice for many disorders of the hip [1]. During development of hip prostheses, a variety of implants have been designed for THA. As a result a consensus has been reached among surgeons that close adaptation of the prosthesis to the bone geometry is required to achieve optimal primary stability and secondary biologic fixation [2]. Therefore, the key to successful THA is sound knowledge of the geometry of the associated bone structures, the acetabulum and proximal femur. The geometry of the bone varies from individual to individual, thus implants are made in a range of sizes to match bone geometry. However, these prostheses would fit only common anatomies, rather than taking into account variations between different genders, ages and races [3]. Despite the importance of morphological study, no adequate research has been carried out to investigate the shape of the bone, especially the endosteal geometry. On the contrary, it has been reported that periosteal femoral geometry should be used to design the implant, because of its association with the medullary cavity [4].

As part of the development of surgical technique, a series of related studies have been carried out. Noble *et al.* [4] demonstrated the presence of both endosteal and periosteal variation, and the need for multiple stem designs to achieve close fit. Walker and Robertson [5] designed a femoral stem to fit an average femoral cavity based on a three-dimensional analysis, and observed considerable variation in the shape and angulation of the femoral cavity at the osteotomy level. Husmann *et al.* [6] described the endosteal morphology of the proximal femur focusing on the variation of the metaphyseal region, implying that a single cementless stem design, even if several sizes were available, would not fit all femoral cavities [7].

Yet, despite the published data, there are no adequate data on bone morphology, especially in different races. We found that, in our clinical practice using imported prostheses, the two adjacent sizes of prosthesis may be too large and too small, or in some cases the distal component may be suitable while the proximal component was too small. We hypothesized that the THA-associated geometry was different between genders, and that of people from South China, especially enlargement of the endosteal dimensions, differed significantly from the Caucasian model according to which the implants were designed. The aims of this study were to (1) investigate and describe the geometry of the acetabulum and proximal femur of people from South China, (2) investigate variations in the acetabulum and proximal femur among different individuals, and (3) determine whether the sizes of the acetabulum and proximal femur were related to demographic

Table 1. Results of measurement of the acetabula of healthy adults in South China.

	Total	Male	Female
AAVA (°)	20.09±2.56	19.82±2.50	20.35±2.62
AABA (°)	49.32±3.77	50.79±3.15	47.85±3.79*
ASD (mm)	58.74±4.20	61.47±3.50	56.03±2.89*

AAVA: acetabular anteversion angle, AABA: acetabular abduction angle, ASD: acetabular suprainferior diameter.
*There was significant difference between the male and the female (P<0.05).

data, such as gender and age, based on three-dimensional (3D) reconstruction which was a more credible method.

Materials and Methods

Selection of Study Population

This study was approved by the ethics committee of Nanfang Hospital and signed informed consent was obtained from each patient. In this study, the included population was a nonrandomized, healthy group of volunteers. The inclusion criteria were as follows: people from Guangdong and Guangxi province of China (whose last five generations also lived in the two provinces), having no hip disorders. Pregnant women and people with the following signs of the hip were excluded: pain, deformity, abnormal movement, claudication, rheumatic fever, rickets, rheumatoid arthritis, osteoarthritis, osteonecrosis of the femoral head, fracture or previous surgery.

Eighty individuals (40 males and 40 females) were recruited in this study. One hundred and sixty scanned hips were available for analysis. The average age was 31.38 (20–45) years, the average height was 167.25 (151–185) cm, and the average weight was 59.99 (40–80) kg. The procedures followed were in accordance with the Helsinki Declaration of 1975, as revised in 2000.

CT Evaluation

All patients were scanned following an identical protocol using a 64-slice multi slice spiral CT (GE Crop. Fairfield, CT). Patients were placed in the supine position. The lower limbs were fully extended, fixed in neutral rotation with toes pointed up, and strapped to prevent movements during acquisition. CT scans were taken with a contiguous thickness of 0.625 mm, from the anterior superior spine to the top of the patella, with settings of 120 kV and 80 mA. Images from each CT scan were saved as DICOM images and recorded on a separate CD-ROM.

3D Reconstruction and Measurement

The DICOM images were imported into Mimics 10.01 software (Materialise, Leuven, Belgium) to perform 3D reconstruction. The bone geometry was calculated automatically based on radiodensity and stored as a contour map. The contours from sequential images

Table 2. Results of measurement of dimensions at different levels of the proximal femur and femoral indices.

	Total	Male	Female
FAVA (°)	16.47±2.72	15.52±2.51	17.41±2.61*
NSA (°)	130.24±4.34	129.98±3.66	130.49±4.93
FHD (mm)	45.22±3.61	48.06±1.97	42.37±2.43*
Offset (mm)	37.16±3.85	39.33±3.18	35.00±3.20*
MLD+20 (mm)	41.69±4.43	43.12±4.72	40.26±3.61*
APD+20 (mm)	31.00±3.29	32.03±3.39	29.98±2.86*
MLD (mm)	25.62±4.02	25.61±4.10	25.63±3.96
APD (mm)	23.91±3.46	24.69±3.41	23.13±3.35*
MLD−20 (mm)	19.78±2.43	20.21±2.45	19.36±2.35*
APD−20 (mm)	17.50±3.05	18.19±2.60	16.80±3.31*
IID (mm)	11.34±1.68	12.10±1.37	10.58±1.62*
IED (mm)	25.50±2.32	26.48±2.10	24.52±2.11*
IP (mm)	106.60±5.61	106.93±6.24	106.26±4.90
CFI	3.74±0.57	3.60±0.49	3.88±0.60*
MCFI	2.12±0.24	2.15±0.26	2.10±0.22
DCFI	1.56±0.28	1.51±0.21	1.61±0.34*

FAVA: femoral anteversion angle, NSA: neck-shaft angle, FHD: diameter of the femoral head, Offset: femoral offset, MLD+20 and APD+20: medial-lateral diameter and antero-posterior diameter of bone medullary cavity at a plane of 20 mm above the lesser trochanter, MLD and APD: medial-lateral diameter and antero-posterior diameter of bone medullary cavity at the midpoint of the lesser trochanter, MLD−20 and APD−20: medial-lateral diameter and antero-posterior diameter of bone medullary cavity at a plane of 20 mm below the lesser trochanter, IID: internal diameter of the isthmus, IED: external diameter of the isthmus, IP: distance from the midpoint of the lesser trochanter to the isthmus. CFI: Canal flare index. MCFI: Metaphyseal canal flare index. DCFI: Distal canal flare index.
*There was significant difference between the male and the female (P<0.05).

Table 3. Comparison of acetabular measurements between this study and other published data.

Author	Tallroth [23]	Vandenbussche [27]	Murphy [28]
Country	Finland	NR	U.S.A
Measuring method	CT	CT reconstruction	CT reconstruction
Sample size	40	100	34
AAVA (°)	21.00±7.00	16.90±5.50*	20.40±7.10
P	0.30	0.00	0.73
AABA (°)		38.70±4.80*	53.00±6.30*
P		0.00	0.00
ASD (mm)		48.50±4.40*	
P		0.00	

AAVA: acetabular anteversion angle, AABA: acetabular abduction angle, ASD: acetabular suprainferior diameter.
*Significantly different compared with our study ($P<0.05$).
NR: not reported.

were connected using triangular surface tiles to create 3D models, which could then be displayed in any position or orientation. Using the software, the following steps were performed to create 3D bone reconstructions: contrast adjustment (0–350), thresholding (226–1821), region growing, editing masks, editing masks in 3D, calculating polylines, cavity filling, boolean operations, morphology operations and 3D calculations. Images in the horizontal, coronal and sagittal planes were defined. The center of the acetabulum and femoral head rotation was deduced in the software by fitting a sphere through the surface of the femoral head.

The following parameters were measured: anteversion angle (AAVA), abduction angle (AABA) and supro-inferior diameter (ASD) of the acetabula; the femoral anteversion angle (FAVA), neck-shaft angle (NSA), diameter of the femoral head (FHD), offset, medial-lateral diameter and antero-posterior diameter of the bone medullary cavity at a plane 20 mm above (MLD+20,APD+20), at the midpoint (MLD,APD), and 20 mm below the lesser trochanter (MLD−20, APD−20), the internal (IID) and external diameter (IED) of the isthmus, and the position of the isthmus (IP). Canal flare index (CFI) was calculated as the ratio between the medial-lateral canal width 20 mm above the midpoint of the lesser trochanter and the isthmus width [4]. Metaphyseal canal flare index (MCFI) was determined to specify the variability of the proximal femoral opening (the ratio between mediolateral canal width 20 mm above and 20 mm below the midpoint of the lesser trochanter). Distal canal flare index (DCFI) was defined as the ratio between mediolateral canal width 20 mm below the midpoint of the lesser trochanter and isthmus width, to specify the opening of the femoral diaphysis.

To perform the above measurement, several key points need to be located. Spherical fitting was performed to the femoral head, and the center of the sphere was regarded as the center of the femoral head. The axes of the femoral shaft and neck were calculated as the center of polylines of the endosteal cavity, and the intersection of the two axes was regarded as the break point between the shaft and neck. Other points were located according to their coordinates along certain axes, which meant the points with minimum or maximum coordinates were chosen. For example, when measuring the internal diameter of the isthmus, all coordinates of points on the medullary cavity were exported, and the two points with maximum and minimum coordinates along the X axis were chosen.

Statistical Analysis

The intraclass correlation coefficient (ICC) was applied to assess the reliability: 0.00 to 0.20, poor; 0.21 to 0.40, fair; 0.41 to 0.60, moderate; 0.61 to 0.80, substantial; and 0.81 to 1.00, perfect. In order to ensure the reliability of the results, 40 cases (20 males and 20 females) were selected randomly, and two authors performed the measurements on these cases twice each with an interval of one month.

Distribution of the values was assessed using descriptive statistical analysis. Normally-distributed data were compared using Student's *t* test, otherwise a non-parametric test was applied. Pearson correlations were used to determine the relationships between different anatomic parameters. In correlation analysis, the data of only one side was selected randomly. Results of different studies were compared by ANOVA. *P*-values <0.05 were considered significant.

Results

Measurement reliability was satisfactory with ICC varying from 0.72–0.93 for different indicators. The measurement results were characterized by a normal distribution after normality testing. The acetabulum was anteverted 20.09° (2.56°) and abducted 49.32° (3.77°), with an average supro-inferior diameter of 58.74 mm (4.20 mm). These findings are summarized in Table 1. The means and standard deviations (SDs) of the dimensions at different levels of the proximal femur are presented in Table 2. There were significant differences in most parameters between males and females.

Several studies have been performed to analyze the bone structure (Table 3 and Table 4). Through comparison with previously-reported findings we conclude that people from South China who were the subjects of this study have a larger neck-shaft angle, smaller offset, thinner shaft and more proximal isthmus. The abduction angle of the acetabulum was smaller and the supro-inferior diameter was larger, while there was no significant difference in the anteversion angle. Taking into the consideration of different methodologies, the comparison need to be further confirmed.

Considering the correlation between diameters at different levels of the proximal femur with age and height (Table 5), the correlation coefficients varied from −0.010 (internal diameter of isthmus *vs.* offset, $P=0.908$) to 0.833 (internal diameter of isthmus *vs.* medial-lateral diameter of bone medullary cavity 20 mm above

Table 4. Comparison of femoral measurements between this study and other published data.

Author	Massin [2]	Blaimont [3]	Rubin [25]	Noble [4]	Laine [7]
Country	France	NR	NR	U.S.A	NR
Measurement method	X-ray	X-ray	Cadaver	Cadaver	CT of cadaver
Sample size	400	166	32	200	50
NSA(°)	123.1±8.2*	124±8*	122.9±7.6*	124.7±7.4*	
P	0.00	0.00	0.00	0.00	
FHD (mm)	45.6±4.2		43.4±2.6*	46.1±4.8	
	0.45		0.01	0.14	
Offset (mm)	41.0±6.2*	46.6±7*	47.0±7.2*	43.0±6.8*	
		0.00	0.00	0.00	
MLD+20 (mm)	44.1±6.0*		43.1±5.0	45.4±5.3*	45.42±4.46*
			0.15	0.00	
APD+20 (mm)					31.39±3.45
P					0.52
MLD (mm)	26.5±3.6		27.9±3.6*	29.4±4.6*	28.73±3.21*
	0.05		0.01	0.00	
APD (mm)					25.58±2.86*
P					
			21.0±2.7*	20.9±3.5*	20.41±2.14
			0.02	0.01	0.14
APD−20 (mm)					20.71±2.47*
P					0.00
IID (mm)	12.4±2.3*	14.8±3*	13.1±2.1*		11.06±1.88*
P	0.00	0.00	0.00		
IED (mm)	27.6±3.0*		26.7±1.8*		
P	0.00		0.00		
IP (mm)			105.7±17.9	113.4±16.4*	
P			0.69	0.00	
CFI	3.6±0.8		3.36±0.75*		
P	0.06		0.01		

NSA: neck-shaft angle, FHD: diameter of the femoral head, MLD+20 and APD+20: medial-lateral diameter and antero-posterior diameter of bone medullary cavity at a plane of 20 mm above the lesser trochanter, MLD and APD: medial-lateral diameter and antero-posterior diameter of bone medullary cavity at the midpoint of the lesser trochanter, MLD−20 and APD−20: medial-lateral diameter and antero-posterior diameter of bone medullary cavity at a plane of 20 mm below the lesser trochanter, IID: internal diameter of the isthmus, IED: external diameter of the isthmus, IP: distance from the midpoint of the lesser trochanter to the isthmus. CFI: Canal flare index.
*Significantly different compared with our study ($P<0.05$).
NR: not reported.

lesser trochanter, $P=0.000$). Weaker correlations were generally observed between most of the parameters. Significant correlations were detected between variables describing the canal width in the vicinity of the lesser trochanter, consistent with the studies of Dai *et al.* [8] and Noble *et al.* [4]. The dimensions of the femoral neck did not correlate or correlated weakly with the size of the femur (Table 6). There was no strong correlation between the dimensions of the femoral neck and the acetabulum (Table 7).

Discussion

In addition to relieving pain, the objective of THA is to achieve good reconstruction of the hip [9] and thus diminish the risk of future degenerative changes and dislocation, accomplished by reorienting the acetabulum to achieve improved loading conditions at the joint surface [10]. A series of clinical and experimental studies of THA have demonstrated that it is essential to achieve a close geometric fit between the prosthetic component and the supporting bone for primary and durable fixation. Malposition of the acetabular cup results in increased risk of dislocation, limited range of motion, and impingement [11]. The stability of the femoral component depends on a balance of proximal and distal load transfer from the implant to the femur [12]. The relative contributions of the proximal and distal support depend mainly on the fit of the prosthesis to the bone. Experiments have suggested that relative motion between the implant and bone more than 14 micra before bone ingrowth will lead to inadequate implant fit and fibrous encapsulation of the implants. Thus to achieve a satisfactory outcome of THA, detailed knowledge of the associated anatomy is required [4].

Anatomy in Different Races

Given the wide individual variability in THA-associated anatomical bone structure, it should be noted that one procedure/implant could cure one patient's hip disorders but

Table 5. Correlation between diameters at different levels of the proximal femur with age and height.

e	MLD+20	APD+20	MLD	APD	MLD−20	APD−20	IID	IED	IP	CFI	MCFI	DCFI
Age	0.230*	0.063	−0174*	0.049	0.142	−0.064	−0.153*	0.193	0.065	−0.075	−0.122	−0.067
Height	0.157	0.091	−0.195*	−0.110	0.068	−0.040	−0.098	0.146	−0.200	−0.102	−0.026	−0.112
MLD+20		0.132	0.253*	−0.099	−0.104	0.046	0.833*	−0.187*	−0.134	0.937*	0.981*	−0.073
APD+20			0.258*	0.367*	0.080	−0.091	−0.141	0.253*	−0.122	−0.081	0.048	−0.084
MLD				0.105	0.391*	−0.113	−0.122	0.022	0.069	−0.148	−0.024	−0.009
APD					0.169*	0.223	0.175*	−0.237*	0.072	0.127	0.075	0.054
MLD−20						0.290*	0.224*	0.072	−0.159	0.147	−0.979*	0.070
APD−20							0.059	−0.045	−0.045	0.038	−0.012	0.978*
IID								0.211*	0.241	−0.973*	0.060	−0.970*
IED									0.084	0.186*	0.050	0.163
IP										0.248*	−0.046	0.181
CFI											−0.020	0.770*
MCFI												−0.242*

MLD+20 and APD+20: medial-lateral diameter and antero-posterior diameter of bone medullary cavity at a plane of 20 mm above the lesser trochanter, MLD and APD: medial-lateral diameter and antero-posterior diameter of bone medullary cavity at the midpoint of the lesser trochanter, MLD−20 and APD−20: medial-lateral diameter and antero-posterior diameter of bone medullary cavity at a plane of 20 mm below the lesser trochanter, IID: internal diameter of the isthmus, IED: external diameter of the isthmus, IP: distance from the midpoint of the lesser trochanter to the isthmus. CFI: Canal flare index. MCFI: Metaphyseal canal flare index.
**P*<0.05.

Table 6. Correlation between dimensions of the femoral neck and femoral sizes.

	FAVA	NSA	FHD	Offset
Age	0.179*	0.252*	0.144	0.150
Height	0.247*	0.183*	0.532*	0.247*
FAVA		−0.039	−0.167*	−0.100
NSA			−0.107	−0.094
FHD				−0.094
offset				
MLD+20	−0.201*	0.120	−0.072	0.105
APD+20	0.067	−0.269*	0.003	0.171*
MLD	0.244*	0.056	0.089	−0.175*
APD	−0.043	0.162	0.095	−0.125
MLD−20	−0.032	−0.026	0.058	0.031
APD−20	0.145	−0.113	0.164*	0.050
IID	0.157	−0.080	0.156	−0.010
IED	−0.058	0.038	0.006	0.066
IP	0.060	−0.120	0.007	0.037

FAVA: femoral anteversion angle, NSA: neck-shaft angle, FHD: diameter of the femoral head, MLD+20 and APD+20: medial-lateral diameter and antero-posterior diameter of bone medullary cavity at a plane of 20 mm above the lesser trochanter, MLD and APD: medial-lateral diameter and antero-posterior diameter of bone medullary cavity at the midpoint of the lesser trochanter, MLD−20 and APD−20: medial-lateral diameter and antero-posterior diameter of bone medullary cavity at a plane of 20 mm below the lesser trochanter, IID: internal diameter of the isthmus, IED: external diameter of the isthmus, IP: distance from the midpoint of the lesser trochanter to the isthmus.
*$P<0.05$.

worsen another's. Small changes during osteotomy or in implant design could either drastically improve or worsen the outcome of the procedure. The variability in bone morphology is consistent with the consensus that the geometry of the femur is determined by a series of genetic and environmental factors, such as race, sex, age, and life-style. These influences appear to lead to unique bone geometries, as characteristic of each individual as any other feature of human anatomy [4]. Based on the classification of CFI described by Noble *et al.* [4], the shape distribution of the femoral cavity is shown in Figure 1. Compared with the report by Noble *et al.*, there were more normal types (85% *vs.* 83%) but fewer stovepipe types (7.5% vs. 9%) or champagne-flute types (7.5% *vs.* 8%).

Good clinical results and midterm survival rates of cementless THA have been published [13], but failures of prosthetic design still occur, even in the short-term [14], caused by micromotion of the prosthesis. An implant which perfectly fills both the proximal and distal femoral canal would be difficult to insert without breaking the femur [15]. Finite-element studies [16] and photoelastic coating strain analysis [5] have demonstrated the importance of metaphyseal fit in achieving physiologic-like implant–bone load transfer and in minimizing stress shielding and disadvantageous bone remodeling. Femoral stem micromotion studies have also emphasized the importance of metaphyseal endosteal stem fit in the reduction of torsional motion [17]. Thus a good metaphyseal fit is considered to be one of the major goals in cementless femoral stem design. With this objective in mind, the femoral stem should be selected according to the metaphyseal shape, which is described by MCFI rather than CFI, which depicts the entire proximal bone. This is also demonstrated in this study, in which MCFI was found to correlate with the medullary cavity width 20 mm above and below the lesser trochanter, while CFI correlates with the medullary cavity width 20 mm above the lesser trochanter and the dimensions of the isthmus. Thus, it was found that simply choosing the smallest size of a series of prostheses would not provide a good fit, due to the different trends from the proximal to the distal part of the femur.

Surgeons are always trying to restore the original position of the center of the femoral head to ensure maintenance of leg length and reestablishment of the original balance joint forces. Thus femoral components must be available in a range of neck lengths (neck-shaft angle, offset) for each separate stem size. Improving the design of the epiphyseal section of the implant becomes a necessity. Observations in this study showed variation of the neck shaft angle of 27.53°, which is consistent with the results of Clark *et al.* [18]. Neck shaft angle did not correlate with the size of the femur, implying that it would be logical to propose several neck shaft angles for each stem [2]. Custom-made [19] and modular [20] femoral prostheses have been designed to overcome such problems. Early radiologic and clinical results using modular prostheses have been promising, but some problems, for example intraoperative femoral fractures [21], still remain to be overcome. However poor results have also been reported with nonporous custom-made components [22].

Gender Differences

It was noteworthy that, in this study as well as those discussed above, gender differences existed in most of the parameters, and were of the same magnitude, implying that surgeons should take the slight variations between male and female geometry into account when planning and performing THA. The results highlight the importance of determining normal values for the acetabular orientation of the different genders [23]. Furthermore, as the CFI and DCFI differ significantly between the two genders, we found that the most significant differences lay in the isthmus of the femur. Some knee implants have been designed to be gender-specific ostensibly to provide a better anatomic fit and improved

Table 7. Correlation between dimensions of the femoral neck and the acetabulum.

	AAVA	AABA	ASD	FAVA	NSA	FHD	Offset
AAVA		0.142	−0.100	−0.156	0.026	−0.104	0.030
AABA			−0.209*	0.071	0.021	0.019	−0.002
ASD				−0.031	0.097	0.206*	−0.114

AAVA: acetabular anteversion angle, AABA: acetabular abduction angle, ASD: acetabular suprainferior diameter.
FAVA: femoral anteversion angle, NSA: neck-shaft angle, FHD: diameter of the femoral head.
*$P<0.05$.

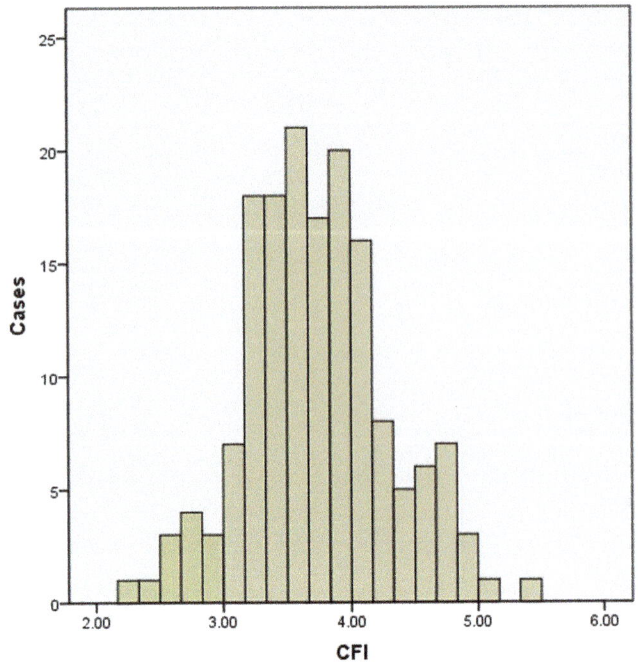

Figure 1. Distribution of the CFI of the proximal femur.

bone coverage. Such implants are expected to be developed for use in THA to reduce the incidence of post-operative dislocation.

Measurement Methods

Anatomic measurements based on CT images are reported to be convenient and rapid for routine diagnosis, as well as for preoperative analysis if necessary [24]. Additionally, CT evaluations provide surgeons with the information they need to choose suitable candidates for surgery. The ability to define the goals of surgery and to plan appropriate adjustments are of paramount importance. Also, it can be concluded from our study that CT reconstruction is a precise but expensive investigation which is not always easily available to the surgeon. Conventional radiographs provide an acceptable level of accuracy in the distal femur, but not the proximal. Their imprecision is increased in clinical practice by other factors, such as incorrect positioning of the patient because of pain or contracture, or small variations in leg rotation, which significantly alter neck-shaft angle and isthmus width [25]. Conventional 2D radiology thus remains the most convenient method available for routine THA. However, the absence of precise radiological data may result in insufficient accuracy to perform pre-operative design for custom-made prostheses.

The application of 3D reconstruction in studies has numerous advantages over cadaver specimens: greater number of cases, accessible demographic data, ideal magnification and spatial orientation of the bone structure. By means of digitization, points can be clearly marked and their placement may be corrected a posteriori, if needed.

The characteristics of this study can be summarized as aiming at different races and precision of measurements. The availability of THA-associated geometric data allows guidelines to be developed for the procedure and assessment of the match between the bone and the prosthesis. It is imperative that each patient should be considered individually even while assumed to have the same anatomy [26], especially for different races. Failure to understand individual characteristics may lead to incorrect surgical performance.

Author Contributions

Conceived and designed the experiments: SZ. Performed the experiments: ZY WJ. Analyzed the data: XJ ZL. Contributed reagents/materials/analysis tools: XJ ZL. Wrote the paper: ZY LZ. Revised the manuscript: ZY YG.

References

1. Higashi H, Barendregt JJ (2011) Cost-effectiveness of total hip and knee replacements for the Australian population with osteoarthritis: discrete-event simulation model. PLoS One 6: e25403.
2. Massin P, Geais L, Astoin E, Simondi M, Lavaste F (2000) The anatomic basis for the concept of lateralized femoral stems: a frontal plane radiographic study of the proximal femur. J Arthroplasty 15: 93–101.
3. Blaimont P, Delronge G, Smeyers B, Halleux P, Lasudry N, et al. (1993) Anatomical and extensometric study concerning the collar support and the prosthetic sleeve. Basis of the conception of an anatomic prosthesis. Acta Orthop Belg 59: 170–181.
4. Noble PC, Alexander JW, Lindahl LJ, Yew DT, Granberry WM, et al. (1988) The anatomic basis of femoral component design. Clin Orthop 235: 148–165.
5. Walker PS, Robertson DD (1988) Design and fabrication of cementless hip stems. Clin Orthop 235: 25–34.
6. Husmann O, Rubin PJ, Leyvraz PF, de Roguin B, Argenson JN (1997) Three-dimensional morphology of the proximal femur. J Arthroplasty 12: 444–450.
7. Laine HJ, Lehto MU, Moilanen T (2000) Diversity of proximal femoral medullary canal. J Arthroplasty 15: 86–92.
8. Dai KR, An KN, Hein Tl (1985) Geometric and biomechanical analysis of the human femur. Trans Orthop Res Soc 10: 99–102.
9. Xu CP, Li X, Song JQ, Cui Z, Yu B (2013) Mini-incision versus standard incision total hip arthroplasty regarding surgical outcomes: a systematic review and meta-analysis of randomized controlled trials. PLoS One 8: e80021.
10. Hipp JA, Sugano N, Millis MB, Murphy SB (1999) Planning acetabular redirection osteotomies based on joint contact pressures. Clin Orthop Relat Res 364: 134–143.
11. Aydogan M, Burç H, Saka G (2013) A new method for the measurement of anteversion of the acetabular cup after total hip arthroplasty. Eur J Orthop Surg Traumatol 20. [Epub ahead of print].
12. Lennon AB, Prendergast PJ (2001) Evaluation of cement stresses in finite element analyses of cemented orthopaedic implants. J Biomech Eng 123: 623–628.
13. Sotereanos NG, Engh CA, Glassman AH, Macalino GE, Engh CA Jr (1995) Cementless femoral components should be made from cobalt chrome. Clin Orthop Relat Res 313: 146–153.
14. Havelin LI, Espehaug B, Vollset SE, Engesaeter LB (1995) Early aseptic loosening of uncemented femoral components in primary total hip replacement. A review based on the Norwegian Arthroplasty Register. J Bone Joint Surg Br 77: 11–17.
15. Delaunay C, Kapandji AI (1998) 10-year survival of Zweymüller total prostheses in primary uncemented arthroplasty of the hip. Rev Chir Orthop Reparatrice 84: 421–432.
16. Huiskes R, van Rietbergen B (1995) Preclinical testing of total hip stems. The effects of coating placement. Clin Orthop Relat Res 319: 64–76.
17. Hua J, Walker PS (1994) Relative motion of hip stems under load. An in vitro study of symmetrical, asymmetrical, and custom asymmetrical designs. J Bone Joint Surg Am 76: 95–103.
18. Clark JM, Freeman MA, Witham D (1987) The relationship of neck orientation to the shape of the proximal femur. J Arthroplasty 2: 99–109.
19. Bargar WL, Taylor JK, Kay JF (1993) Custom femoral components: porous hydroxyapatite. J Bone Joint Surg Br 75: 255.
20. Whiteside LA, Arima J, White SE, Branam L, McCarthy DS (1994) Fixation of the modular total hip femoral component in cementless total hip arthroplasty. Clin Orthop Relat Res 298: 184–190.
21. Simonet JY, Argenson JN, Aubaniac JM (1993) The use of uncemented custom-made prostheses in high congenital dislocation of the hip. J Bone Joint Surg Br 75: 257.
22. Lombardi AV Jr, Mallory TH, Eberle RW, Mitchell MB, Lefkowitz MS, et al. (1995) Failure of intraoperatively customized non-porous femoral components inserted without cement in total hip arthroplasty. J Bone Joint Surg Am 77: 1836–1844.
23. Tallroth K, Lepistö J (2006) Computed tomography measurement of acetabular dimensions: normal values for correction of dysplasia. Acta Orthop 77: 598–602.
24. Haddad FS, Garbuz DS, Duncan CP, Janzen DL, Munk PL (2000) CT evaluation of periacetabular osteotomies. J Bone Joint Surg Br 82: 526–531.
25. Rubin PJ, Leyvraz PF, Aubaniac JM, Argenson JN, Estève P, et al. (1992) The morphology of the proximal femur. A three-dimensional radiographic analysis. J Bone Joint Surg Br 74: 28–32.
26. Klaue K, Wallin A, Ganz R (1988) CT evaluation of coverage and congruency of the hip prior to osteotomy. Clin Orthop Relat Res 232: 15–25.
27. Vandenbussche E, Saffarini M, Taillieu F, Mutschler C (2008) The asymmetric profile of the acetabulum. Clin Orthop Relat Res 466: 417–423.
28. Murphy SB, Kijewski PK, Millis MB, Harless A (1990) Acetabular dysplasia in the adolescent and young adult. Clin Orthop Relat Res 261: 214–223.

Effects of Home-Based Interval Walking Training on Thigh Muscle Strength and Aerobic Capacity in Female Total Hip Arthroplasty Patients: A Randomized, Controlled Pilot Study

Yutaka Morishima[1,2], Takashi Mizushima[2], Katsuya Yamauchi[2], Mayuko Morikawa[1,3], Shizue Masuki[1], Hiroshi Nose[1,3]*

1 Department of Sports Medical Sciences, Shinshu University Graduate School of Medicine, Matsumoto, Japan, **2** Department of Rehabilitation, Hamamatsu University School of Medicine, Hamamatsu, Japan, **3** Jukunen Taiikudaigaku Research Center, Matsumoto, Japan

Abstract

Due to the reduced physical activity of patients who have undergone total hip arthroplasty (THA), there are no home-based exercise training regimens for preventing muscle atrophy and aerobic capacity impairment in these patients. We examined whether interval walking training (IWT) could prevented these issues. Twenty-eight female patients (~60 years of age) who had undergone THA more than 2 months prior were randomly divided into IWT (n = 14) and control (CNT, n = 14) groups. The IWT subjects trained at a target of 60 min of fast walking at >70% peak aerobic capacity for walking (VO_{2peak}) per wk for 12 wk, while those in the CNT maintained their previous sedentary life during the same period. We measured the energy expenditure of the daily physical activity, except during sleeping and bathing, every minute and every day during the intervention. We also measured the isometric knee extension (F_{EXT}) and flexion (F_{FLX}) forces, VO_{2peak}, and anaerobic threshold during the graded cycling exercise (VO_{2AT}) before and after the intervention. All subjects, except for one in IWT, completed the protocol. F_{FLX} increased by 23% on the operated side ($P = 0.003$) and 14% on the non-operated side of IWT ($P = 0.006$), while it only increased on the operated side of CNT ($P = 0.03$). The VO_{2peak} and VO_{2AT} in IWT increased by 8% ($P = 0.08$) and 13% ($P = 0.002$), respectively, and these changes were significantly higher in the IWT than in CNT group (both, $P<0.05$). In conclusion, IWT might be an effective home-based training regimen for preventing the muscle atrophy from reduced daily physical activity in THA patients.

Trial Registration: UMIN-CTR UMIN000013172

Editor: Naoyuki Hayashi, Tokyo Institute of Technology, Japan

Funding: This study was supported in part by grants from the Ministry of Health, Labor, and Welfare (Comprehensive Research on Aging and Health) and the Japan Society for the Promotion of Science. The funders had no role in study design, data collection and analysis, decision to publish, or preparation of the manuscript.

Competing Interests: The authors have declared that no competing interests exist.

* Email: nosehir@shinshu-u.ac.jp

Introduction

Total hip arthroplasty (THA) is a broadly prescribed surgical treatment for patients with advanced arthritic disorders of the joint. [1] However, THA patients are thought to suffer from muscular atrophy and weakness on the operated limb side more than 2 years after surgery; [2,3] these changes might be accompanied by joint instability, prosthesis loosening, risk of falls, and other complications, [4–7] and they might advance to impaired mobility of the joint, [1,8–11] resulting in reduced daily physical activity and aerobic capacity in a vicious cycle.

To prevent these problems, exercise training for rehabilitation is performed immediately after surgery under the supervision of medical staff while the patient stays in the hospital with financial support from national insurance; however, a maximum period of 2 wk is recommended for hospital management reasons, and this period is too short for recovering muscle strength. Patients are allowed to visit a hospital for rehabilitation up to several months following discharge, and resistance training using machines has also been reported to be effective; [12] however, limited financial support from insurance, impaired mobility, and the inconvenience of the transportation options for travelling to the hospital might discourage patients from continuing exercise training [13–16].

Therefore, the development of a home-based exercise regimen is needed so that THA patients can perform habitual exercise to increase their muscle strength on the side of the treated limb. Recently, we developed an exercise training system for middle-aged and older people featuring 1) interval walking training (IWT), 2) the use of a portable calorimeter, and 3) the e-Health Promotion System. Using the system, we found that middle-aged and older people who performed IWT for 5 months had ~10% increased thigh muscle strength and peak aerobic capacity for walking ($\dot{V}O_{2peak}$) [17,18] with a much higher adherence rate to IWT (94%) than for a standard walking training regimen (~60%); however, there have been no studies on THA patients [19].

Therefore, the purpose of this pilot study was to examine whether the training system is helpful for increasing thigh muscle strength and aerobic capacity as well as improving daily physical activity in THA patients.

Methods

The protocol for this trial and supporting CONSORT checklist are available as supporting information; see Checklist S1 and Protocol S1.

Ethics Statement

This study was approved by the Ethics Committee of Hamamatsu University School of Medicine and was in accordance with the Declaration of Helsinki. All participants provided written informed consent for participation.

Trial registration

The clinical trial was registered after participant recruitment for this study. However, we recruited the first participant for this study after approval by the ethics committee of Hamamatsu University School of Medicine. Additionally, all ongoing and related trials for the exercise training of THA patients are registered.

Participants

The criteria for subjects with total hip arthroplasty were that they were able to walk independently without any assistive devices. The exclusion criteria were suffering from any acetabular and/or femoral prosthesis failure or other comorbidities or the presence of any cardiopulmonary, neurologic, or cognitive diseases.

Figure 1 shows the flow profile of subjects in the present study. Recruitment and screening began on August 1. To recruit subjects for this study, we mailed leaflets to female patients who had undergone THA at Hamamatsu University Hospital and who visited the hospital for rehabilitation before June 2009. As a result, 28 of 98 respondents met the criteria, and all provided written informed consent before participating in the study. They were randomly divided [20] into interval walking training (IWT, $n = 14$) and control (CNT, $n = 14$) groups such that there were no significant differences in the medical history, current physical characteristics (**Table 1**), and other measurements before training.

Randomization

Allocation was performed using permuted-block randomization (block of 4). YM generated the random allocation sequence. Each eligible and consenting subject was assigned to one of the groups. Only known one researcher (YM) knew of the exact allocation.

Intervention Protocols

The training experiments were conducted from September 6, 2009 to December 20, 2009. The subjects were instructed to visit the gym at 8:30 am on the assigned day in September after overnight fasting. After interviewing the subjects about their current hip joint pain, their subjective feeling of satisfaction with walking using the visual analogue scale (VAS) and their quality of life with the Medical Outcomes Study 36-item short-form health survey (SF-36), [21,22] we measured their height and body weight. After allowing them to eat a light breakfast and rest for an hour, we measured the thigh muscle strength and $\dot{V}O_{2peak}$. Within a week, the subjects were invited to our laboratory in the hospital an hour or more after breakfast or lunch and were asked to participate in a measurement of the anaerobic threshold by graded cycling exercise ($\dot{V}O_{AT}$). [23] When they left the laboratory after the measurement, we provided them with a portable calorimeter with a tri-axial accelerometer (JD-Mate; Kissei Comtec, Matsumoto, Japan) and instructed them to measure their energy expenditure due to physical activity every minute during the day, except during sleeping and bathing periods, for 7 consecutive days before the start of training.

Before IWT, the subjects visited a gym near the hospital and received instructions about the exercise program. They were told to repeat 5 or more sets of 2- to 3-minute low-intensity walking intervals at ~40% of the pre-training $\dot{V}O_{2peak}$, followed by a 3-minute interval of high-intensity walking at >70% but <85% $\dot{V}O_{2peak}$, ≥4 days/wk; the total fast walking time per week reached ≥60 min. The intensity and steps were monitored with JD-Mate, which was worn on the mid-clavicular line of the right or left waist. A beeping signal alerted subjects when a change of intensity was scheduled, and another sound told them when their walking intensity had reached the target level. Once subjects had learned the program, they were allowed to choose their training time. Additionally, in IWT, the energy expenditure (oxygen consumption rate) due to physical activity other than IWT and steps was measured with JD-Mate during the day, except for during bathing and sleeping periods, while the beeping signal and sounds of the device were switched off. The total energy expenditure due to physical activity is presented in **Table 2**, including that for IWT.

Every 2 weeks, the subjects visited the hospital, and data from the tracking devices were transferred over the internet to a central server in the administrative center for automatic analysis and reporting of the IWT effects from a database of more than 3,000 middle-aged and older people without THA; we call this system the e-Health Promotion System (Kissei Comtec). [24] Physical therapists used these reports to track the daily walking intensity and the other parameters given in **Table 2** to instruct subjects on how best to achieve the target levels. If the targets were not met, they encouraged subjects to increase their efforts to achieve them.

Subjects in CNT were instructed to maintain the same lifestyle as before training. Every 2 weeks during the training period for IWT, they visited the hospital, and the energy expenditure due to daily physical activity and steps during the day, except during sleeping and bathing periods, was transferred over the internet from the tracking devices to the central server in the administrative center, but, unlike in IWT, there was no automatic analysis and reporting.

After the 12-wk training period, we measured the same variables as before training for both groups. After the post-training measurements, we instructed the subjects in both groups to continue measuring their energy expenditure from daily physical activity and steps during the day, except during the sleeping and bathing periods, for 7 consecutive days after the end of training. The data were then transferred to the server after measurements.

Number of subjects for the analyses

In IWT, one subject was excluded from the following analyses because she was absent on one of the measurement days assigned after training. Therefore, we analyzed 13/14 and 14/14 subjects in IWT and CNT, respectively.

Measurements

Thigh muscle strength. Isometric bilateral knee extension (F_{EXT}) and flexion (F_{FLX}) forces were measured with an isometric dynamometer (GT-330; OG Giken, Tokyo, Japan). The higher value from 2 trials each for extension and flexion forces, which were displayed on the screen of the dynamometer, was adopted for

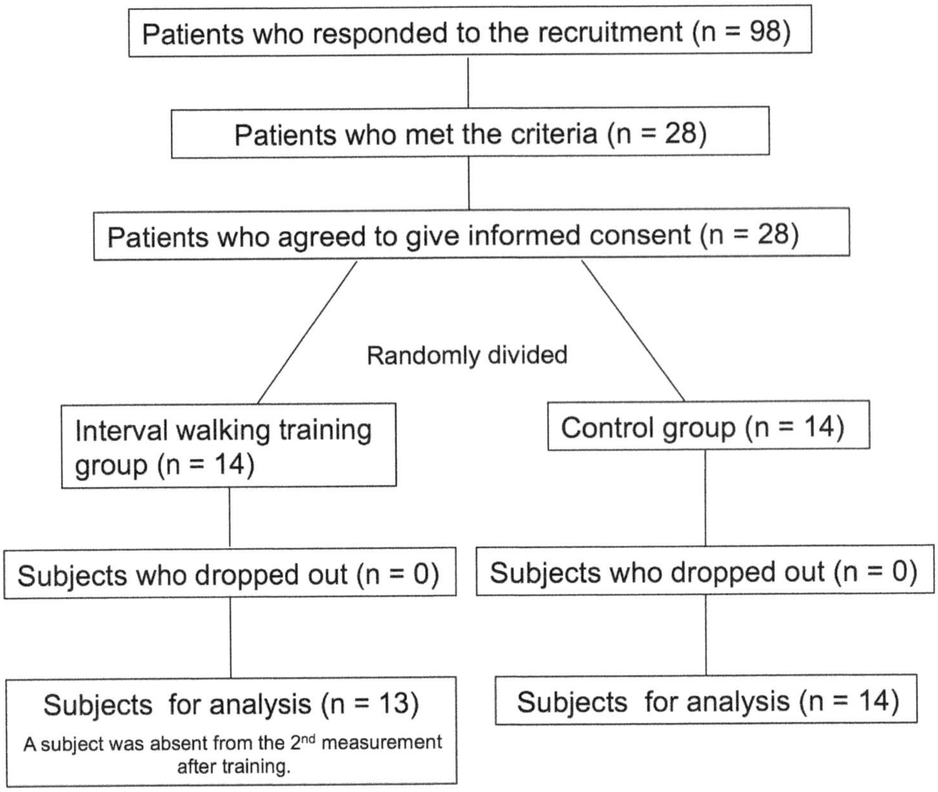

Figure 1. CONSORT flow diagram. Flow profile of the subjects.

analysis. Similarly, we measured the strength of the other knee joint.

Because 3/13 subjects in IWT underwent THA on both hip joints and the remaining 10 subjects underwent THA on one side, we analyzed the effect of IWT on the thigh muscle strength on 16 operated sides and 10 non-operated sides in this group. Similarly, in CNT, 3/14 subjects underwent THA on both hip joints, and the remaining 11 subjects underwent THA on one side. Therefore, we analyzed the thigh muscle strength before and after training for 17 operated sides and 11 non-operated sides in this group.

***$\dot{V}O_{2peak}$*.** Subjects with the accelerometer on their back walked for 3 minutes on a flat floor at 3 graded, subjective velocities (slow, moderate, and fast) with ~25°C room temperature and ~60% relative humidity. At the same time, the heart rate was recorded with an electrocardiogram, and 3-dimensional acceleration was measured at 10-millisecond intervals and recorded as averaged values of the 5-second memories. [25,26] The total impulse from the accelerometer was transferred to a computer and converted to the oxygen consumption rate ($\dot{V}O_2$) using a previously reported equation. [25,26] The $\dot{V}O_{2peak}$ and peak heart rate (HR_{peak}) for walking values are those for the last 30 seconds at the maximal walking speed.

$\dot{V}O_{2AT}$. We determined the $\dot{V}O_{2AT}$ at ~25°C room temperature and ~60% relative humidity with an expired gas analysis system (AE-310S; Minato, Tokyo, Japan). The $\dot{V}O_2$ and carbon dioxide production ($\dot{V}CO_2$) were measured for every breath. The exercise intensity was increased by 10 watts per minute and stopped when the anaerobic threshold was judged to have been

Table 1. Physical characteristics of the subjects.

	CNT (n = 14)	IWT (n = 13)	*P* (Group)
Age (years)	59.9±5.4 (52–68)	60.3±7.4 (52–74)	NS
Height (cm)	151.9±5.8 (144–166)	153.3±3.4 (146.8–159.4)	NS
Body mass (kg)	57.0±9.6 (48.0–69.8)	54.0±5.3 (43.3–80.6)	NS
BMI (kg/m^2)	24.7±4.1 (20.1–35.4)	23.0±2.6 (19.4–28.5)	NS
Reason for operation	OA: 13; ANFH: 1	OA: 13	NA
Operated side (left/right/bilateral)	7/4/3	5/5/3	NA
Postoperative period (months)	34±46 (2–170)	58±58 (9–181)	NS

Values are given as the means ± SD (range). CNT, control group; IWT, interval walking group; OA, osteoarthritis; ANFH, avascular necrosis of femoral neck head; BMI, body mass index; and NA, not applicable.

Table 2. Total energy expenditure for IWT and physical activity.

	CNT (n = 14)			IWT (n = 13)					
	Before	**During**	**After**	**Before**	**During**	**After**	*P*	*P*	*P*
	(1 wk)	**(12 wk)**	**(1 wk)**	**(1 wk)**	**(12 wk)**	**(1 wk)**	**(Group)**	**(Time)**	**(Group×Time)**
§Total energy expenditure (O_2 ml/kg/wk)	14614±1496	13616±1361	10258±1827	14032±1133	14744±1012	13824±1495	NS	NS	NS
Total steps (steps/wk)	50537±5411	51636±5411	40159±6749	50693±5845	53016±5845	44619±6105	NS	NS	NS
Fast walking									
§Intensity (O_2 ml/kg/min)	10.6±0.6	12.0±1.4	9.7±1.3	9.7±0.6	8.9±0.9	10.2±0.8	NS	NS	NS
Time (min/wk)	76±16	69±15	75±17	100±27	156±15*†	127±18†	<0.0001	<0.0001	<0.0001
§Energy expenditure (O_2 ml/kg/wk)	786±196	805±153	710±176	828±211	1363±157†	1221±169†	.013	NS	NS

Values are given as the means ± SE. Before, for 1 wk before training; During, for 12 wk during training; and After, for 1 wk after training.
§Resting oxygen consumption is not included.
*Significant difference from the value before training, $P<0.05$;
†Significant difference from the corresponding value in CNT, $P<0.05$. The other abbreviations are the same as in **Table 1**.

reached according to the standard method [23,27,28] by viewing the $\dot{V}O_2$ vs. VCO_2 relationship displayed on the screen of the system during exercise. We also determined the heart rate at $\dot{V}O_{2AT}$ (HR_{AT}).

Total energy expenditure due to IWT and physical activity in daily life. As shown in Table 2, the total energy expenditure due to physical activity was determined by adding the $\dot{V}O_2$ (O_2 ml/kg/min) before (1 wk), during (12 wk), and after (1 wk) the training periods after excluding the energy expenditure at rest, which was assumed to be constant during these periods, and this energy is presented as the O_2 ml/kg/wk. Similarly, the walking steps were determined by summing the steps for the respective periods and are presented as steps/wk. A $\dot{V}O_2$ above 70% $W\dot{V}O_{2peak}$ for individuals was regarded as the intensity for fast walking (O_2 ml/kg/min), and the total energy used for fast walking was determined by summing the $\dot{V}O_2$ for the respective periods, after excluding the rate during rest, and this energy is presented as O_2 ml/kg/wk.

Questionnaires. Hip joint pain was evaluated with the 100-mm VAS scale, where 0 represents "no pain" and 100 represents the "worst pain". Similarly, walking satisfaction was evaluated using 0 as "no satisfaction" and 100 as "full satisfaction". The SF-36 was used to evaluate the quality of daily life [21,22].

Statistical Analysis

The Mann-Whitney *U* test was used to test for differences in the physical characteristics between the IWT and CNT groups (**Table 1**). Two-way analysis of variance (ANOVA) [group (CNT vs IWT)×time (before vs. after training)] for repeated measures was also used to examine any significant differences in the variables before and after training between groups (**Tables 2–4** and the questionnaires). The model was also used to examine any significant changes in the variables after training with an interactive effect of (group×time) on the variables (**Tables 2–4** and the questionnaires). After confirmation of the significance by ANOVA, the Tukey-Kramer method was used as a post-hoc test to examine any significant differences in variables in specific comparisons between groups before and after training (**Tables 2–4** and the questionnaires). We determined significant differences in the changes of the variables after training between groups by ANCOVA after correcting for their pre-training values as covariates (**Figure 2 & 3**). We present the statistical power (1-β) in the text at $\alpha = 0.05$ in both groups when the variables increased significantly after training or when the increases were significantly greater in IWT than in CNT with the minimum sample sizes to detect the greater increases (**Figures 2 & 3**). All data are reported as the mean±standard error (SE), unless otherwise indicated. The null hypothesis was rejected at $P<0.05$.

Results

The adherence to the program was 100% in IWT (including one subject who was excluded from the analysis). Additionally, there were no adverse events, including musculoskeletal injuries and falling, during the training period.

Table 1 shows the physical characteristics of subjects in the IWT and CNT with no significant differences between groups.

Table 2 shows the total energy expenditure due to physical activity in both groups. We found that the fast walking time was two-fold higher in IWT than in CNT during and after training periods (both, $P=0.001$). Additionally, the energy expenditure for fast walking was higher in IWT than in CNT during the training periods ($P=0.018$ and $P=0.047$, respectively).

The body mass after training was 57.6±2.6 kg in CNT and 54.1±1.5 kg in IWT and it did not significantly differ from the mass before training in either of the two groups ($P=0.20$ and $P=0.90$, respectively).

Table 3 shows the thigh muscle strength before and after training in both groups. F_{EXT} and F_{FLX} before and after training in both groups tended to be lower on the operated side than on the non-operated side in each group, but there were no significant differences (all, $P>0.05$). We found that F_{FLX} (Nm/kg) increased on the operated and non-operated sides of IWT ($P=0.0031$, (1-β) = 0.95, and $P=0.0063$, (1-β) = 0.95, respectively), while it only increased on the operated side of CNT ($P=0.028$, (1-β) = 0.62) with an interactive effect of group (CNT and IWT)×time (before and after training) for F_{FLX} on the operated side ($P=0.023$). This result suggests that the increase in F_{FLX} on the operated side was significantly higher in IWT than in CNT.

Table 4 shows the aerobic capacity before and after training in both groups. $\dot{V}O_{2peak}$ tended to increase in IWT ($P=0.080$), while it remained unchanged in CNT ($P=0.13$), with an interactive effect of (group×time) on the change ($P=0.018$), suggesting that the increase in IWT was significantly higher than that in CNT. Similarly, $\dot{V}O_{2AT}$ increased in IWT ($P=0.0021$, (1-β) = 0.96), while it remained unchanged in CNT ($P=0.38$) and there was an interactive effect of (group×time) on the change ($P=0.0016$), suggesting that the increase was significantly higher in IWT than in CNT. The HR_{peak} remained unchanged after training in both groups, but HR_{AT} increased after the training in IWT ($P=0.045$, (1-β) = 0.53).

Figure 2 summarizes the changes in the F_{EXT} and F_{FLX} on the operated and non-operated sides after training in both groups and after correcting for the values before training by ANCOVA. Although F_{EXT} on both sides remained unchanged after the training in both groups, F_{FLX} increased by 23% ($P=0.0031$) and 14% ($P=0.0063$) on the operated and non-operated sides, respectively, after the training in IWT, while it increased only on the operated side of CNT ($P=0.028$). The increase on the operated side was significantly higher in IWT than in CNT (ANCOVA, $P=0.002$, (1-β) = 0.95). The minimum sample size for detecting the difference in the increases in F_{FXT} between group at $\alpha = 0.05$ and (1-β) = 0.9 was 12 for each group, which is smaller than the size in the present study.

Figure 3 shows the changes in $\dot{V}O_{2peak}$ and $\dot{V}O_{2AT}$ after training in both groups. Although both remained unchanged in CNT (both, $P>0.10$), the increases in the $\dot{V}O_{2peak}$ and $\dot{V}O_{2AT}$ in IWT were 8% ($P=0.08$) and 13% ($P=0.0021$), respectively, which were significantly higher in IWT than in CNT (ANCOVA, $P=0.018$, (1-β) = 0.68 and $P=0.0016$, (1-β) = 0.94, respectively). The minimum sample size for detecting the differences in the changes in the $\dot{V}O_{2peak}$ and $\dot{V}O_{2AT}$ between groups at $\alpha = 0.05$ and (1-β) = 0.9 were 23, which is more than in the present study, and 12, which is less than in the present study, for each group, respectively.

The hip pain score was not significantly different between the groups before training ($P>0.55$). After training, the score remained unchanged in both groups on the operated side ($P>0.06$) and on the non-operated side ($P>0.06$).

The walking satisfaction score significantly increased in IWT from 44±9 to 55±8 ($P=0.047$, (1-β) = 0.53) but not in CNT, whose values changed from 55±10 to 43±10 ($P=0.24$) with no significant interactive effect of (group×time) ($P=0.27$).

The "vitality" score in SF-36 significantly increased in IWT from 45±3 to 52±2 ($P=0.005$, (1-β) = 0.87) but not in CNT, whose values changed from 48±3 to 52±3 ($P=0.19$). However, there was no significant interactive effect of (group×time)

Table 3. Thigh muscle strength before and after training.

	CNT (n = 14)			IWT (n = 13)			P
	Before	After	P (Time)	Before	After	P (Time)	(Group × time)
Operated side							
n	17	17		16	16		
F_{EXT} (Nm)	74.6±7.7	74.5±7.5	NS	83.8±5.2	92.5±4.9	NS	NS
(Nm/kg)	1.36±0.15	1.35±0.14	NS	1.56±0.11	1.73±0.12	NS	NS
F_{FLX} (Nm)	36.3±2.3	39.3±2.3*	0.022	37.7±3.3	46.2±2.4**	0.0021	0.036
(Nm/kg)	0.65±0.04	0.70±0.03*	0.028	0.69±0.06	0.85±0.04**	0.0031	0.023
Non-operated side							
n	11	11		10	10		
F_{EXT} (Nm)	96.4±6.5	102.9±11.3	NS	93.3±9.1	88.5±10.1	NS	NS
(Nm/kg)	1.67±0.13	1.72±0.17	NS	1.78±0.19	1.64±0.19	NS	NS
F_{FLX} (Nm)	38.1±4.1	43.4±4.1	NS	40.8±2.1	46.6±2.5**	0.0032	NS
(Nm/kg)	0.64±0.06	0.74±0.07	NS	0.77±0.04	0.87±0.05**	0.0063	NS

Values are given as the means ± SE. F_{EXT}, knee extension force; F_{FLX}, knee flexion force. Significant differences compared to the value before training, *$P<0.05$ and **$P<0.01$.

Table 4. Aerobic capacities before and after training.

	CNT (n = 14)			IWT (n = 13)			P
	Before	After	P (Time)	Before	After	P (Time)	(Group × Time)
$\dot{V}O_{2peak}$ (ml/kg/min)	16.6±0.8	15.7±0.6	NS	15.8±0.8	17.0±1.1	NS	0.018
HR_{rest}^{1} (beats/min)	81±4	81±3	NS	81±2	79±2	NS	NS
HR_{peak} (beats/min)	141±4	143±4	NS	139±4	138±6	NS	NS
$\dot{V}O_{2AT}$ (ml/kg/min)	13.8±0.6	13.5±0.6	NS	13.7±0.4	15.5±0.5**	0.0021	0.0016
HR_{rest}^{2} (beats/min)	77±2	79±2	NS	77±2	78±2	NS	NS
HR_{AT} (beats/min)	108±2	109±2	NS	110±2	114±2*	0.045	NS

Values are given as the mean ± SE. $\dot{V}O_{2peak}$, peak aerobic capacity for walking; HR_{rest}^{1}, heart rate at rest before starting the exercise for the $\dot{V}O_{2peak}$ measurement; HR_{peak}, peak heart rate at $\dot{V}O_{2peak}$; $\dot{V}O_{2AT}$, anaerobic threshold for cycling; HR_{rest}^{2}, heart rate at rest before starting the exercise for the $\dot{V}O_{2AT}$ measurement; and HR_{AT}, heart rate at $\dot{V}O_{2AT}$. Significant differences compared to the value before training, *$P<0.05$ and **$P<0.01$.

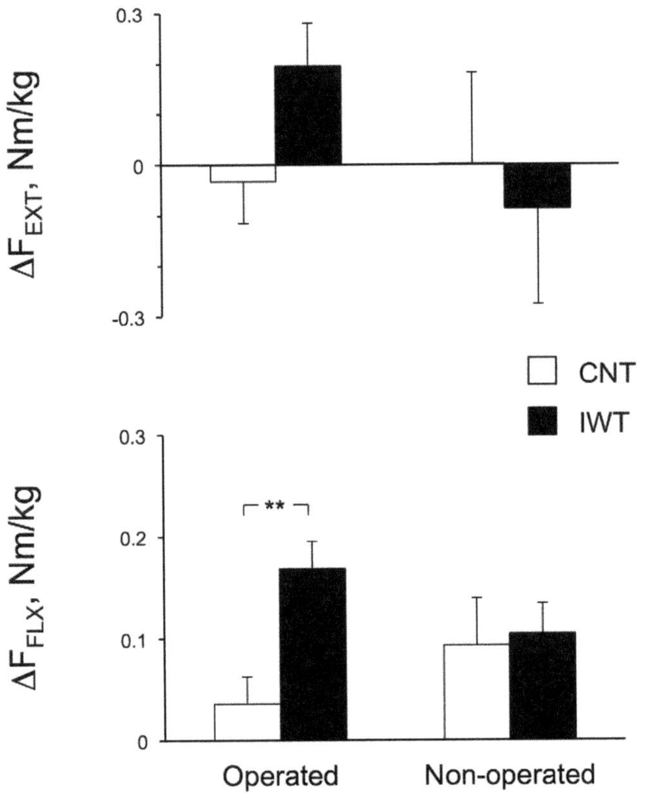

Figure 2. Changes in the thigh muscle strength after training on the operated and non-operated sides. The isometric knee extension (F_{EXT}) and flexion force (F_{FLX}) are shown as the means with SE bars for 17 and 16 measurements on the operated side and 11 and 10 measurements on the non-operated side in 14 and 13 subjects in the control (CNT) and interval walking training (IWT) groups, respectively. Significant difference between the CNT and IWT groups, $^{**}P<0.01$.

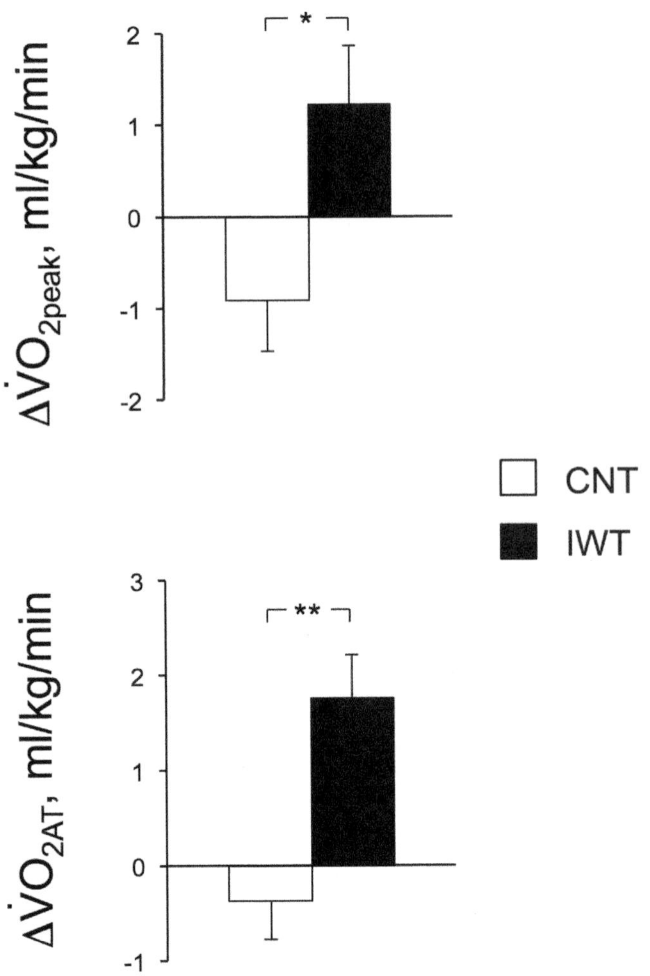

Figure 3. Changes in the aerobic capacities after training. The peak aerobic capacity for walking (VO_{2peak}) and anaerobic threshold by graded cycling exercise (VO_{2AT}) are shown as the means with SE bars for 14 and 13 subjects in the CNT and IWT groups, respectively. Significant differences between the CNT and IWT groups, $^{*}P<0.05$ and $^{**}P<0.01$.

($P = 0.24$). There were no significant changes in the other items of SF-36 before and after training in either group ($P = 0.07$–1.0).

Discussion

In the present study, all THA patients in IWT performed fast walking for more than an average of 60 min per week during the 12-wk training period, leading to increased F_{FLX} on the operated side and increased aerobic capacity, which were accompanied by a lack of hip pain.

We compared the $\dot{V}O_{2peak}$, F_{EXT}, and F_{FLX} before training in CNT and IWT in the present study with those in each of 3 groups that were divided equally according to $\dot{V}O_{2peak}$ (n = 156, each) in the previous study; [18] in that study, we examined the effects of 4-month IWT in 468 middle-aged and older women without THA and with an average age of ~65 years, which was ~5 years older than in the present study. We found that the $\dot{V}O_{2peak}$ and F_{EXT} in the present study were not significantly different from those in the lowest $\dot{V}O_{2peak}$ group ($P>0.05$), while they were significantly lower than those in the middle $\dot{V}O_{2peak}$ group ($P<0.01$). In contrast, the F_{FLX} was significantly lower than that in the lowest $\dot{V}O_{2peak}$ group ($P<0.01$). Therefore, the $\dot{V}O_{2peak}$ and F_{EXT} in the subjects in the present study belong to the bottom 30% group of the age-matched healthy population [20] with a significantly lower F_{FLX} than in that group.

As indicated in **Table 2**, the fast walking time was 87 min/wk higher in IWT than in CNT. Nemoto et al. [17] examined the effects of 5-month IWT on $\dot{V}O_{2peak}$, F_{EXT}, and F_{FLX} in 31 middle-aged women and older women with an average age of ~65 years and no THA, using a target similar to that of the present study, and the researchers reported that the total fast walking time was 32 min/day, the number of walking days was 4.5 days/wk, and the total fast walking time was 144 min/wk. Additionally, Morikawa et al. [18] examined the effects of 4-month IWT on lifestyle-related diseases in 468 middle-aged and older women with an approximate age of ~65 years lacking THA, and the authors reported that the total fast walking time was 22 min/day, the number of walking days was 3.9 day/wk, and the total fast walking time was 85.8 min/wk. Similarly, Okazaki et al. [29] examined the effects of macronutrient supplementation during 5-month IWT on the thigh muscle strength in 35 middle-aged and older women with an approximate age of ~61 years and reported that the total fast walking time was 21.5 min/day, the number of walking days was 4.1 days/wk, and the total fast walking time was

88.2 min/wk. Therefore, the IWT subjects likely accomplished the target of more than 60 min/wk of fast walking at an intensity of more than 70% $\dot{V}O_{2peak}$ as in the previous studies [17,18].

As shown in **Table 3** and **Figure 2**, F_{FLX} in IWT increased significantly by 23% on the operated side and by 14% on the non-operated side, while F_{EXT} remained unchanged after training.

Previous studies have suggested that the response of F_{FLX} to IWT is more sensitive than that of F_{EXT}. [17,18] Nemoto et al. [17] reported that after 5-month IWT, the increase in F_{FLX} was 16% higher than the 12% increase in F_{EXT}. Similar results were also reported in previous studies. [17,27] The precise reasons for the less sensitive response of F_{EXT} remain unclear; however, it might be because the F_{FLX} value is lower than the F_{EXT} value before training. According to the current American College of Sports Medicine guidelines, [30] repetitive contractions above a given percent of maximal force are recommended for increasing muscle strength. In other words, if muscles generate more than a given force in repetitive contractions during training, the strength will increase, but the strength will not otherwise increase. Indeed, Nemoto et al. [17] suggested that the thigh muscle strength remained unchanged after a 5-month moderate-intensity (50% $\dot{V}O_{2peak}$) continuous walking training regimen, while it increased after IWT, which is similar to the results for IWT in the present study. Therefore, the higher sensitivity of F_{FLX} to IWT compared that of F_{EXT} was because the relative exercise intensity was sufficiently high to increase the strength in F_{FLX} but not in F_{EXT}.

As shown in **Table 4** and **Figure 3**, the $\dot{V}O_{2peak}$ and $\dot{V}O_{2AT}$ in IWT increased by 8% and 13%, respectively, while both remained unchanged in CNT.

Nemoto et al. [17] suggested that the $\dot{V}O_{2peak}$ in individual subjects was significantly correlated with their thigh muscle strength and that the increase after 5-month IWT was accompanied by an increase in thigh muscle strength, suggesting that the changes in $\dot{V}O_{2peak}$ and $\dot{V}O_{2AT}$ were caused by the increased oxygen extraction rate in the muscle tissue due to increases in muscle mass, capillary density, and cellular oxidative capacity.

In the present study, the hip pain score remained unchanged in IWT. Generally, THA patients tend to be physically inactive, fearing acetabular cap wear of the implanted joints due to more frequent friction on the surface during walking; [31] however, recent studies have suggested that the wear is not related to the daily physical activity level [32] and, furthermore, the incidence of joint replacement was much higher in patients with less regular exercise, which is most likely due to the reduction in the surrounding muscle mass supporting the joint. [33] We found that the walking satisfaction score, "vitality" in SF-36 in IWT, was improved as the thigh muscle strength increased after training (**Table 3**), which is consistent with the results in the previous study [33].

Limitations

In the present study, we did not measure the hip muscle strength; however, Judd et al. [33] suggested that the hip flexor and abductor forces recovered to those in the age-matched healthy older women within 12 months after surgery in THA patients, while the hip extensor and knee flexor and extensor forces remained ~20% lower than in those in healthy women. In the present study, we confirmed that the F_{EXT} and F_{FLX} before training in both groups were ~20% lower than those in the age-matched total population of healthy women; [18] therefore, the hip and thigh muscle strength likely matched those that were previously reported for THA patients [33].

We only monitored the improvement in daily physical activity for one week after training. Therefore, it is unclear whether the patients would continue IWT afterwards; however, it has been suggested that the adherence rate of 4 months of IWT was 94% in age-matched healthy women, which was due to the instruction service that provided achievement-based feedback over the internet. [18] Therefore, we surmised that most THA patients would continue IWT if the service was provided afterwards.

In the present study, a mild exercise control group was not included; however, Nemoto et al. [17] reported in middle-aged and older people, the F_{EXT} and F_{FLX} significantly increased after high intensity interval walking training for 5 months, while it did not increase after moderate intensity continuous walking training, although the time and steps for training were less in high intensity interval walking training group than in the moderate intensity continuous walking training group. Accordingly, they suggested that high intensity interval walking training increased the thigh muscle strength as resistance training by using machines recommended by the ACSM. [30] We confirmed this in THA patients in the present study.

The subjects in the present study had relatively low BMIs and were middle-aged and older Japanese women. Because this is the first study to evaluate the effects of IWT on THA patients, further studies are needed to assess whether our findings are true for a fatter, Western population.

As mentioned previously, the physical fitness in the subjects in the present study belongs to the bottom 30% group of the age-matched healthy population. [18] Morikawa et al. [18] suggested that the symptoms of life-style related diseases, including hypertension, hyperglycemia, obese, and dyslipidemia, were the worst in the group, but the symptoms improved the most with most increased physical fitness after 5-month interval waling training. Future studies are needed to evaluate the effects of interval walking training on life-style related diseases in THA patients.

Conclusion

IWT might be an effective home-based training regimen for preventing muscle atrophy due to reduced daily physical activity in THA patients.

Supporting Information

Check list S1 CONSORT checklist.

Protocol S1 Trial Protocol.

Protocol S2 Trial Protocol in original language (in Japanese).

Medical Research Ethics Review Application Form S1 Medical Research Ethics Review Application Form.

Medical Research Ethics Review Application Form S2 Medical Research Ethics Review Application Form in original language (in Japanese).

Author Contributions

Conceived and designed the experiments: HN. Performed the experiments: YM TM KY. Analyzed the data: YM SM MM. Contributed reagents/materials/analysis tools: HN. Wrote the paper: YM SM HN.

References

1. Nilsdotter AK, Roos EM, Westerlund JP, Roos HP, Lohmander LS (2001) Comparative responsiveness of measures of pain and function after total hip replacement. Arthritis and rheumatism 45: 258–262.
2. Rasch A, Dalén N, Berg HE (2010) Muscle strength, gait, and balance in 20 patients with hip osteoarthritis followed for 2 years after THA. Acta Orthopaedica 81: 183–188.
3. Rasch A, Byström AH, Dalén N, Martinez-Carranza N, Berg HE (2009) Persisting muscle atrophy two years after replacement of the hip. The Journal of bone and joint surgery British volume 91: 583–588.
4. Long WT, Dorr LD, Healy B, Perry J (1993) Functional recovery of noncemented total hip arthroplasty. Clinical orthopaedics and related research: 73–77.
5. Perrin T, Dorr LD, Perry J, Gronley J, Hull DB (1985) Functional evaluation of total hip arthroplasty with five- to ten-year follow-up evaluation. Clinical orthopaedics and related research: 252–260.
6. Dorr LD, Wan Z (1998) Causes of and treatment protocol for instability of total hip replacement. Clinical orthopaedics and related research: 144–151.
7. Lachiewicz PF, Soileau ES (2002) Stability of total hip arthroplasty in patients 75 years or older. Clinical orthopaedics and related research: 65–69.
8. Murray MP, Gore DR, Brewer BJ, Gardner GM, Sepic SB (1979) A comparison of the funtional performance of patients with Charnley and Müller total hip replacement. A two-year follow-up of eighty-nine cases. Acta orthopaedica Scandinavica 50: 563–569.
9. Victor CR (1987) Rehabilitation after hip replacement: a one year follow up. International journal of rehabilitation research Internationale Zeitschrift für Rehabilitationsforschung Revue internationale de recherches de réadaptation 10: 162–167.
10. Sicard-Rosenbaum L, Light KE, Behrman AL (2002) Gait, lower extremity strength, and self-assessed mobility after hip arthroplasty. The journals of gerontology Series A, Biological sciences and medical sciences 57: M47–51.
11. Madsen MS, Ritter MA, Morris HH, Meding JB, Berend ME, et al. (2004) The effect of total hip arthroplasty surgical approach on gait. Journal of orthopaedic research: official publication of the Orthopaedic Research Society 22: 44–50.
12. Trudelle-Jackson E, Smith SS (2004) Effects of a late-phase exercise program after total hip arthroplasty: a randomized controlled trial. Archives of Physical Medicine and Rehabilitation 85: 1056–1062.
13. Mossey JM, Mutran E, Knott K, Craik R (1989) Determinants of recovery 12 months after hip fracture: the importance of psychosocial factors. American journal of public health 79: 279–286.
14. Magaziner J, Simonsick EM, Kashner TM, Hebel JR, Kenzora JE (1990) Predictors of functional recovery one year following hospital discharge for hip fracture: a prospective study. Journal of gerontology 45: M101–7.
15. Sashika H, Matsuba Y, Watanabe Y (1996) Home program of physical therapy: effect on disabilities of patients with total hip arthroplasty. Archives of physical medicine and rehabilitation 77: 273–277.
16. Jan M-H, Hung J-Y, Lin JC-H, Wang S-F, Liu T-K, et al. (2004) Effects of a home program on strength, walking speed, and function after total hip replacement. Archives of physical medicine and rehabilitation 85: 1943–1951.
17. Nemoto K, Gen-no H, Masuki S, Okazaki K, Nose H (2007) Effects of high-intensity interval walking training on physical fitness and blood pressure in middle-aged and older people. Mayo Clinic proceedings Mayo Clinic 82: 803–811.
18. Morikawa M, Okazaki K, Masuki S, Kamijo Y, Yamazaki T, et al. (2011) Physical fitness and indices of lifestyle-related diseases before and after interval walking training in middle-aged and older males and females. British journal of sports medicine 45: 216–224.
19. Sakai A, Terasawa K, Inaki M (2000) Physical effects of" The Matsumoto physical training program for senior citizens." Shinshu Medical Journal 48: 89–96.
20. Schulz KF, Altman DG, Moher D (2011) CONSORT 2010 statement: updated guidelines for reporting parallel group randomised trials. International journal of surgery (London, England) 9: 672–677.
21. Fukuhara S, Bito S, Green J, Hsiao A, Kurokawa K (1998) Translation, adaptation, and validation of the SF-36 Health Survey for use in Japan. Journal of clinical epidemiology 51: 1037–1044.
22. Fukuhara S, Ware J, Kosinski M (1998) Psychometric and clinical tests of validity of the Japanese SF-36 Health Survey. Journal of clinical epidemiology 51: 1045–1053.
23. Wasserman K, Whipp BJ, Koyl SN, Beaver WL (1973) Anaerobic threshold and respiratory gas exchange during exercise. Journal of applied physiology 35: 236–243.
24. Nose H, Morikawa M, Yamazaki T, Nemoto K-I, Okazaki K, et al. (2009) Beyond epidemiology: field studies and the physiology laboratory as the whole world. The Journal of physiology 587: 5569–5575.
25. Iwashita S, Takeno Y, Okazaki K, Itoh J, Kamijo Y, et al. (2003) Triaxial accelerometry to evaluate walking efficiency in older subjects. Medicine and science in sports and exercise 35: 1766–1772.
26. Yamazaki T, Gen-No H, Kamijo Y-I, Okazaki K, Masuki S, et al. (2009) A new device to estimate VO2 during incline walking by accelerometry and barometry. Medicine and science in sports and exercise 41: 2213–2219.
27. Davis JA, Frank MH, Whipp BJ, Wasserman K (1979) Anaerobic threshold alterations caused by endurance training in middle-aged men. Journal of applied physiology: respiratory, environmental and exercise physiology 46: 1039–1046.
28. Beaver WL, Wasserman K, Whipp BJ (1986) A new method for detecting anaerobic threshold by gas exchange. Journal of applied physiology (Bethesda, Md: 1985) 60: 2020–2027.
29. Okazaki K, Yazawa D, Goto M, Kamijo Y-I, Furihata M, et al. (2013) Effects of macronutrient intake on thigh muscle mass during home-based walking training in middle-aged and older women. Scandinavian journal of medicine & science in sports.
30. Armstrong LE, GJ B, MJ B, SE D, KP D, et al. (2006) General principles of exercise prescription. In: Whayley MH, Brubaker PH, Otto RM, eds. ACSM's guidelines for exercise testing and prescription. 7th ed. Philadelphia: Lippincott Williams & Wilkins.
31. Dowson D (2001) New joints for the Millennium: wear control in total replacement hip joints. Proceedings of the Institution of Mechanical Engineers Part H, Journal of engineering in medicine 215: 335–358.
32. Bennett D, Humphreys L, O'Brien S, Kelly C, Orr J, et al. (2008) Activity levels and polyethylene wear of patients 10 years post hip replacement. Clinical biomechanics (Bristol, Avon) 23: 571–576.
33. Judd DL, Dennis DA, Thomas AC, Wolfe P, Dayton MR, et al. (2013) Muscle Strength and Functional Recovery During the First Year After THA. Clinical orthopaedics and related research.

Comparative Study of W-Shaped Angular Plate and Reconstruction Plate in Treating Posterior Wall Fractures of the Acetabulum

Qi Zhang[1]⁹, Wei Chen[1]⁹, Xiaobo Wu[2]⁹, Yanling Su[1], Zhiyong Hou[1], Yingze Zhang[1]*

1 Department of Orthopaedic Surgery, The Third Hospital of Hebei Medical University, Shijiazhuang, Hebei, P.R. China, **2** Department of Orthopaedic Surgery, The Second Hospital of Tangshan, Tangshan, Hebei, P.R. China

Abstract

Objective: This study aims to assess the medium-term results of the reconstruction of posterior wall fractures using a W-shaped acetabular angular plate (WAAP) compared to those fixed using a reconstruction plate.

Methods: Between July 2006 and March 2009, we performed a retrospective study, which collected data for any patient treated for a posterior acetabular wall fracture. At the time of treatment, patients were either treated using a WAAP or a pelvic reconstruction plate. The intraoperative fluoroscopic images for both groups were compared. The quality of reduction and radiological grading were assessed according to the criteria developed by Matta. The clinical assessment was based on a modified Merle d'Aubigne and Postel scoring.

Results: 53 patients met the inclusion criteria and were followed up for an average of 38 months. 25 patients were treated with a WAAP (study group), and 28 patients were treated with a pelvic reconstruction plate (control group). The intraoperative fluoroscopic images of the study group confirmed extra-articular screw placement in all cases. In the control group, intra-articular screw placement was observed intraoperatively in 5 patients (17.86%), and the definitive location of the periarticular hardware could not be determined in 4 patients (14.29%) during the operation. The differences between the two groups were statistically significant ($p = 0.002$). In contrast, the quality of fracture reduction, clinical outcomes, and radiological grading in the study group were not significantly different from those of the control group ($p > 0.05$). The radiographic grade was strongly associated with the clinical outcomes in both the study and control groups ($p < 0.05$).

Conclusion: Reconstruction of posterior wall fractures of the acetabulum using a WAAP can help avoid screw penetration of the hip joint, provide a stable fixation of the posterior wall, and ensure good clinical outcomes.

Editor: Gwendolen Reilly, University of Sheffield, United Kingdom

Funding: The authors have no support or funding to report.

Competing Interests: The authors have declared that no competing interests exist.

* E-mail: dryzzhang@126.com

⁹ These authors contributed equally to this work.

Introduction

Fractures of the posterior wall are the most common type of acetabular fractures, accounting for nearly a third of all fractures of the acetabulum [1,2]. Despite the relative prevalence and simple configuration of fractures of the posterior wall, the outcome may be influenced by various factors. Those beyond the surgeon's control include the injury mechanism, concomitant damage to the femoral head, sciatic nerve injury, frank dislocation, and the patient's age. Critical factors that are within the surgeon's control include the timing of surgery, surgical procedure selection, and a meticulous surgical technique. Intraarticular screw penetration remains the technical error that most influences the clinical outcome [3]. Classically, high quality intraoperative imaging is utilized to avoid screw penetration of the hip joint during surgery [4,5]; and, 3-D navigation can improve the accuracy of screw placement [6,7]. However, navigation technology is only used in a limited number of hospitals. Furthermore, particularly for orthopedic trauma applications, the computed tomography (CT) scanner has limited intraoperative applications [6,7]. Another challenge of acetabular fractures is the fixation of comminuted wall fractures. Although the use of spring plates beneath a buttress plate can be an option for the fixation of comminuted posterior acetabular wall fractures, there is a risk of damage to the articular surface and dificulty of plate positioning [8]. Thus, achieving high quality of posterior wall reductions remains a challenge for orthopedic surgeons.

The purpose of this study is to assess whether the use of a W-shaped acetabular angular plate (WAAP) is helpful in avoiding screw penetration of the hip joint, while providing adequate buttressing to permit stable healing, compared to the conventional standard construct of reconstruction plates.

Methods

A retrospective analysis of posterior wall fractures identified the fractures treated by the senior author at a single level-I trauma center from July 2006 to March 2009. Patients were considered for inclusion if they had a posterior wall fracture of the acetabulum necessitating open reduction and internal fixation (ORIF). This study consisted of any patient with a posterior acetabular fracture treated with a WAAP or pelvic reconstruction plate, during the study period. Exclusion criteria included pathological acetabular fractures, neuropathic arthropathy, dementia and other disease processes which made postoperative compliance unreliable. Patients, who were followed up for less than 24 months, were also excluded.

Preoperative radiographic imaging obtained for each patient consisted of a single standard anteroposterior pelvis film, two 45° oblique Judet views, and a 3-D CT scan. Any patient with a history of dislocation was treated preoperatively with skeletal traction, whereas all others were treated with initial bed rest. Surgery occurred as soon as the general medical condition of the patients permitted. Patients requiring ORIF were assigned alternately to either the study group or control group. A WAAP was assigned to fix the fracture of one patient, and then a reconstruction plate was assigned chronologically to treating the next one.

The Kocher-Langenbeck approach was implemented for all patients. The hip was extended, and the knee was flexed beyond 90 degrees during the retraction of the sciatic nerve. Manual distraction using a proximal femoral pin or bone hook improved the joint visualization, facilitating the removal of intraarticular loose bodies. If marginal impaction of the posterior acetabular wall was present, the impacted segment was elevated until its articular surface was flush with the articular cartilage of the femoral head and then reduced to the adjacent acetabular articular surface. A cancellous bone graft from the greater trochanter was used to fill the defect. An attempt was made to anatomically reduce any posterior wall fragments and hold them temporarily with K-wires. After the reduction, the patients in the study group were fixed using WAAP, whereas the patients in the control group were treated with a pelvic reconstruction plate. The contour and zygomorphy of the WAAP (Figure 1) matched the surface of the posterior column of the acetabulum, and the plate itself can be thought to consist of three regions: the iliac region, the danger zone region, and the ischial tuberosity region. The organization of these regions causes the plate to resemble the English alphabet letter "W". There are two rows of drill holes in the danger zone region. A special safe-angled drilling guide was used to assist in the operation. The angles of the drilling guide were selected in congruence to the contour of the danger zone of the acetabulum, as measured using the MPR CT images[9]. The lower-surface chamber of the safe-angled drilling guide matched the contour of the danger zone aspect of the plate well, and could be assembled and disassembled easily. During the operation, the WAAP with the safe-angled drilling guide was placed along the posterior column from the ilium to the ischial tuberosity, with the outer edge of WAAP parallel to the lateral acetabular brim, and the ischial tuberosity region of the plate was placed on the ischial tuberosity. The angulation of the screw placement in the danger zone was guided by the safe-angled drilling guide. After the appropriate holes of the plate were fixed, the safe-angled drilling guide was removed. Intraoperative fluoroscopic checks, including an anteroposterior view of the hip, a obturator oblique view, an axial veiw of the screw, and a tangential view of the screw, were used to assess the fracture reduction and screw placement in each case. Dynamic fluoroscopy was not employed in the current study. Using the axial and tengential views, whether the screw violated the hip joint was determined. The determinations were made directly from the fluoroscopy monitor. If intrarticular screw penetration was recognised or highly suspected, it was screwed out, and then redrilled through the hole after adjusting the insertion angulation to fix the plate without errant screw placement into the joint.

In the control group, the wall fragments were fixed with interfragmentary screws, and the posterior column was fixed with a long 3.5 mm reconstruction plate from the ilium to ischium. The angulation of the screw placement for the holes of the plate in the danger zone was determined with caution. The intraoperative fluoroscopy at the above-mentioned views was employed frequently to help determine the periacetabular screw location as well as to assess fracture reduction.

The intraoperative fluoroscopic images, postoperative radiographs and a 3-D CT scan were utilized to assess the reduction quality and screw placement (Figure 2). The quality of reduction based on plain radiographs was assessed according to the criteria described by Matta [1]. All patients routinely received intravenous antibiotics, first administered during anesthesia induction and continuing for three days after surgery. Low molecular weight heparin was utilized for thromboprophylaxis. Prevention of heterotopic ossification was used in all patients using a 6 weeks course of Indomethacin. Patients were placed in a continuous passive-motion machine on postoperative day one. By the second postoperative day, active hip movement was encouraged, with progressive resistance of the adductors, quadriceps, and hamstrings. Similar precautions to total hip arthroplasty, such as restricting hip flexion to less than 90° and the prevention of adduction, were taught to all patients. Toe-touch weight-bearing activities with crutches or a walker were allowed for a period of 3 months following which patients were allowed to weight bear unaided.

Each patient was clinically and radiologically assessed at 1, 2, 3, 6 and 12 months, and then annually thereafter. At the final follow-up, the clinical grading was based on the modified Merle d'Aubigne and Postel scoring [1,10]. Heterotopic ossification was graded using the classification system modified by Moed and Smith [11], and avascular necrosis of the hip was classified according to the Ficat and Arlet classification [12]. The radiological and clinical assessments were performed by two independent assessors. The assessor, who performed the clinical assessment, was also blind to the group assignment.

The data was analyzed using SPSS 13.0 (SPSS Inc., Chicago, IL, USA) by an independent biostatistician who was not directly involved with the study. The nonparametric Mann-Whitney *U*-test was used to compare the results of the intraoperative fluoroscopic images and radiographic evaluation of the reduction quality. A parametric Student's *t*-test was used to compare the results of the operative time, blood loss and the clinical outcomes between both of the groups. The Spearman rank correlation was used to compare the relationship between clinical outcomes and associated factors.

Ethics statement

This study has been reviewed and approved by the Institutional Review Board of the Third Hospital of Hebei Medical University. Signed informed consents were obtained from all patient. The clinical investigations have been conducted following the principles expressed in the Declaration of Helsinki.

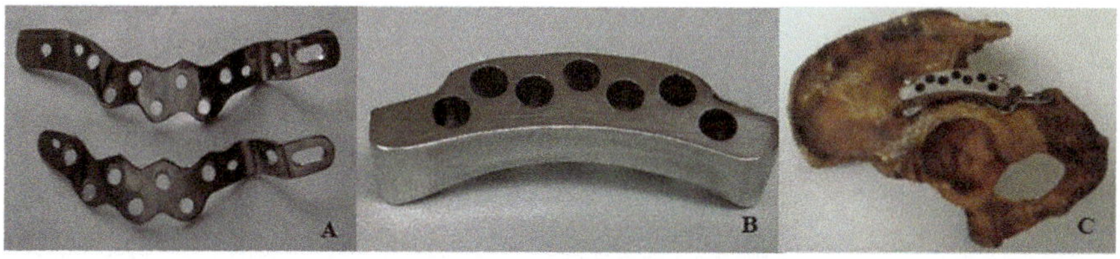

Figure 1. The W-shaped acetabular angular plate (A), the safe-angled drilling guild(B), and both of them assembled(C).

Results

Retrospective analysis of the patient database identified 66 patients who met the inclusion criteria, and of these, 53 patients were followed up for an average of 38 months (range, 25–60 months). The study group consisted of 25 patients treated with WAAP. The control group consisted of 28 patients treated with a pelvic reconstruction plate. There were 47 male and 6 female patients, with a mean age of 35.7 years (range, 18 to 61 years) at the time of injury. There were 31 left fractures and 22 right ones. Marginal posterior impaction of the acetabular wall was present in 25 patients. 42 patients (79.24%) had an associated posterior hip dislocation. Among those patients with a hip dislocation, 32 were reduced within 12 hours after the initial injury, 7 within 12 to 24 hours and 3 after 24 hours. All hip dislocations were treated by closed reduction. Various other concomitant injuries were found in 33 patients (62.26%): 25 had fractures of the lower extremities and 12 (22.64%) had fractures of the upper extremities requiring surgical treatment, 9 (16.98%) had head trauma, 6 (11.32%) had chest injury, 8 (15.09%) had abdominal injury that required laparotomy, and 12 (22.64%) had preoperative sciatic nerve damage. Preoperative radiographic analysis determined that there were 11 single, fragmented fractures and 42 comminuted fractures. The time from injury to operation averaged 7 days (range; 1 to 24 days). Patients in the study group were followed up for 39.40±8.56 months, and 36.75±9.43 months in the control group. The two groups of patients were comparable in sex, age, fracture severity, fractured side, preoperative sciatic nerve damage and follow-up period (Table 1, all $p>0.05$).

Intraoperative fluoroscopic images confirmed extra-articular screw placement in all cases in the study group. In the control group, no intra-articular screw was noted in 19 patients (67.86%), intra-articular screw placement was observed in 5 patients (17.86%), and the definitive location of the periarticular hardware could not be determined in 4 patients (14.29%). The differences between the two groups were statistically significant ($Z=-3.069$, $p=0.002$). The intra-articular and highly-suspected screws in the nine patients of the control group were removed during the operation, and corrective action were taken before completion of the surgical procedure. The operative time and blood loss in the study group were 2.07±0.81 hours and 562.80±212.81 ml, respectively, which were significantly less than the operative time of 2.76±0.75 hours ($t=-3.220$, $p=0.002$) and blood loss of 742.86±234.38 ml ($t=-2.915$, $p=0.005$) in the control group($p<0.05$).

The quality of fracture reduction was graded as anatomical in 19 patients (76.00%), imperfect in 4 (16.00%), and unsatisfactory in 2 (8.00%) in the study group. Among the control group patients, the reduction was graded as anatomical in 18 patients (64.29%), imperfect in 7 (25.00%) and unsatisfactory in 3 (10.71%).There was no significant difference between both groups ($Z=-0.884$, $p=0.377$). The clinical outcomes are summarized in Table 2. In the study group, 76.00 % of the patients had an excellent to good outcome opposed to 60.71% in the control group. No statistically significant differences between both groups were identified ($Z=-1.057$, $p=0.291$).

The most recent follow-up x-rays available were used for the radiological assessment according to the criteria developed by Matta. In the study group, the results were excellent in 10 (40.00%), good in 9 (36.00%), fair in 3 (12.00%) and poor in 3 (12.00%) of the patients, comparable to excellent in 9 (32.14%), good in 8 (28.57%), fair in 7 (25.00%) and poor in 4 (14.29%) of

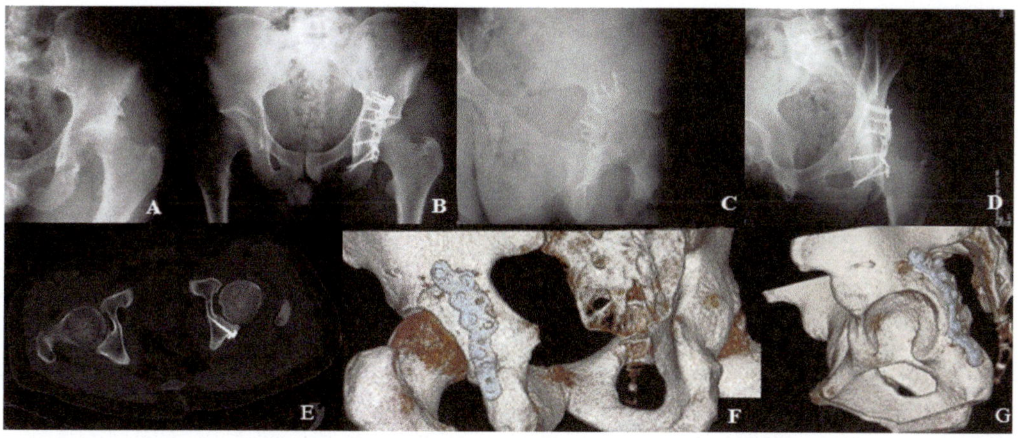

Figure 2. Emergency room radiograph of a 38-year-old man with a posterior wall fracture with posterior dislocation of the femoral head (A). The postoperative radiograph (B, C, D) and CT cut (E) demonstrate the extra-articular screw placement, and the VRT image shows a safe screw insertion into the posterior wall without violation into the joint (F,G).

Table 1. Patient demographics of the WAAP *vs* standard plate groups.

Category	Subcategory	Study Group (n = 25)	Control group (n = 28)	*p*-value
Sex	Male	23	24	0.471
	Female	2	4	
Age (average±SD)		37.2±11.5	34.4±13.9	0.216
Fracture side	Left	16	15	0.442
	Right	9	13	
Fracture severity	Simple, fragmented fracture	3	8	0.138
	Comminuted fracture	22	20	
Hip dislocation		23	19	0.031
Preoperative sciatic nerve damage		7	5	0.378
Follow-up period (average±SD, months)		39.40±8.56	36.75±9.43	0.146

the patients in the control group. No significant difference between the two groups was identified ($Z = -0.905$, $p = 0.366$). Among the five patients with errant screw placement into the hip joint recognised intra-operatively, the results were excellent in 1, good in 1, fair in 2 and poor in 1, comparable to the results of the other 23 patients in the control group ($Z = 1.123$, $p = 0.772$). The Spearman rank correlation showed that the radiographic grade of the reduction was strongly associated with the clinical outcome in both the study group ($r = -0.532$, $p = 0.006$; Table 3) and the control group ($r = -0.765$, $p < 0.000$; Table 4).

Among patients in the study group, the mean functional score at the most recent follow-up was 15.64±2.56. Nine patients were found to have preoperative ipsilateral-associated peroneal nerve injuries. Heterotopic ossification developed in four patients, one of which was grade II and the other three grade I. In addition, four patients developed posttraumatic osteoarthritis, and one patient who demonstrated avascular necrosis of the femoral head and resorption of the fracture fragment exhibited poor results.

In the control group, the mean functional score was 14.75±3.17 at most recent follow-up. One patient had persistent stiffness at his knee that allowed less than 90° of further flexion, and five patients developed heterotopic ossification, two of which were grade II and the other three grade I. Four patients developed posttraumatic osteoarthritis, and avascular necrosis of the femoral head was observed in three patients. No wound infection, iatrogenic neural injury, acetabular nonunion, or pulmonary embolism were noted in either group.

Discussion

A high percentage of long-term satisfactory outcomes can be expected following the anatomic reduction and internal fixation of fractures of the posterior wall [13,14]. Advanced surgical techniques are often required to achieve excellent clinical outcomes, however, especially in the presence of a comminuted fracture [15]. Among posterior acetabular fractures treated operatively, the presence of intraarticular hardware is a serious complication, and has been reported in up to 4% of patients [16–18]. Intraarticular hardware may lead to joint destruction [3], and as such, careful screw insertion and intraoperative fluoroscopy may be necessary to ensure a safe implant location during surgery. It is possible that improvements in the fracture fixation equipment might allow for decreased fluoroscopy time in the operating room, and potentially decreased operative time overall. The uniquely angled design of the drilling guide removes the necessity of evaluating complications, thus facilitating the operation. In the control group, intraoperative fluoroscopy was used frequently in determining the periacetabular screw location, particularly for the axial and tangential views of the screws. Good-quality pelvic fluoroscopy was not always easy to achieve, however, particularly in obese patients. Therefore, the total operative time and blood loss in the control group was more than that observed in the study group. The avoidance of screw placement in the danger zone of the pelvis could minimize the possibility of screw penetration into the hip joint [19]. However, by not placing a screw in the danger zone, the overall stiffness of the internal fixation would be reduced, potentially leading to a loss of fixation in time. According to our experience and the present results, ORIF using WAAP is effective in avoiding screw penetration of the hip joint, especially in the danger zone, thus reducing the operative duration and blood loss.

A variety of methods have been described for posterior acetabular wall fracture fixation. Reconstruction plates, locking reconstruction plates, and buttressing the posterior wall in conjunction with lag screws or spring plates are among the most commonly employed techniques [20]. Results with these methods have not always been good, however, and the presence of comminution of the posterior wall remains one of the most important reasons for this. Failure of fixation of posterior wall

Table 2. Clinical outcomes according to the modified Merle d'Aubigne and Postel score.

Group	Excellent	good	fair	poor	total
Study Group (n (%))	8 (32.00)	11 (44.00)	3 (12.00)	3 (12.00)	25
Control group (n (%))	7 (25.00)	10 (35.71)	5 (17.86)	6 (21.43)	28

Table 3. The clinical outcomes according to reduction quality and radiographic grade in study group.

Fracture reduction		**Clinical outcome**			
		Excellent (n (%))	**Good (n (%))**	**Fair (n (%))**	**Poor (n (%))**
Reduction quality	Anatomical (n = 19)	7 (36.84%)	9 (47.37%)	2 (10.53%)	1 (5.26%)
	Imperfect (n = 4)	1 (25.00%)	2 (50.00%)	0	1 (25.00%)
	Unsatisfactory (n = 2)	0	0	1 (50.00%)	1 (50.00%)
Radiographic grade	Excellent (n = 10)	5 (50.00%)	4 (40.00%)	1 (10.00%)	0
	Good(n = 9)	3 (33.33%)	5(55.56%)	0	1 (11.11%)
	Fair(n = 3)	0	2(66.67%)	1 (33.33%)	0
	Poor (n = 3)	0	0	1 (33.33%)	2 (66.67%)

fractures is a devastating complication that is best prevented by the provision of rigid stability intraoperatively. Inadequate fixation of the fracture - especially in the presence of the high mechanical demands of the hip joint - can lead to a catastrophic loss of fixation, which can in turn result in hip joint instability. Loss of fixation almost inevitably leads to a poor result, and therefore augmentation of the fixation of the posterior wall with some methods has been advocated [21,22]. Ebraheim et al. [21] reported that excellent to good results were achieved in 24 of 32 comminuted posterior wall fractures treated by the buttress technique (fixation with spring plates and reconstruction plates). However, care must be taken in positioning spring plates at the posterior wall, as placement of the plate's teeth into the labrum risks damage to the femoral head cartilage [23]. Comminuted or very peripheral posterior wall fragments also pose a challenge, as it is difficult to reduce and fix every fragment with lag screws, as well as to position the buttress plate effectively in that setting. The "two-level reconstruction" technique for comminuted posterior wall fractures has been advocated by Giannoudis et al. [24]. However, additional operative time is required to ensure extra-articular subchondral screw placement by fluoroscopy prior to definitive fixation of the overlying cortical fragment. Another potential pitfall with this fixation technique is that removal of the subchondral screws is impossible in the setting of postoperative infection or joint erosion. Olson et al. [22] has reported on the use of calcium phosphate to fill incongruous fracture reductions, concluding that it may restore the loading characteristics to near-normal parameters. Further biomechanical and in vivo analyses of this practice are required however, before it can be applied clinically.

The main indication for using WAAP is in the presence of comminution of the posterior wall. In the current study, for those patients who had severe comminution with more than three major fragments, the new device functioned as a splint and provided rigid fixation to the fracture site. 76.00% of the patients had an excellent to good outcome, as opposed to 60.71% in the control group, even though a statistical significance was not determined because of the small sample size. All patients treated using WAAP achieved a congruent reduction, rigid fracture fixation, and sound union within 3 months. Therefore, it is believed that this device can provide a stable fixation of the posterior wall that is amenable to an early range of motion and weight bearing. No loss of reduction, non-union, or residual instability were noted at the final follow-up in any patient.

Limitations to this study include the small sample size and relatively short duration of the follow ups. A correlation between the clinical and radiological outcome and the WAAP could not be determined partially due to the small sample size. Moving forward, long term data with a larger sample size is necessary, and such clinical outcome data will be recorded and presented in the future. Besides, the method of patient allocation is "alternate allocation", which is open to the treating surgeons and has limitations and potential biases. This alllocation method may influence the decision to recruit a patient to ORIF or not. A randomized controlled trial will be required to assess the clinical outcomes of the reconstruction of posterior wall fractures using a WAAP or a reconstruction plate more objectively.

Table 4. Distribution of the clinical outcomes according to reduction quality and radiographic grade in control group.

Fracture reduction		**Clinical coutcome**			
		Excellent (n (%))	Good (n (%))	Fair (n (%))	Poor (n (%))
Reduction quality	Anatomical (n = 18)	5 (27.78%)	9 (50.00%)	2 (11.11%)	2 (11.11%)
	Imperfect (n = 7)	2 (28.57%)	1 (14.29%)	2 (28.57%)	2 (28.57%)
	Unsatisfactory (n = 3)	0	0	1 (33.33 %)	2 (66.67%)
Radiographic grade	Excellent (n = 9)	6 (66.67%)	2 (22.22%)	0	1 (11.11%)
	Good(n = 8)	1 (12.50%)	6 (75.00%)	1 (12.50%)	0
	Fair(n = 7)	0	2 (28.57 %)	3 (42.86%)	2 (28.57%)
	Poor (n = 4)	0	0	1 (25.00%)	3 (75.00%)

Conclusions

Reconstruction of posterior wall fractures of the acetabulum, in particular comminuted fractures, using WAAP has been demonstrated to produce good results. This device helps to avoid intraarticular screw penetration and reduce operative duration and blood loss. The device further provides a stable fixation of the posterior wall that is amenable to early range of motion and weight bearing postoperatively, and results in a good clinical outcome.

Acknowledgments

The authors wish to thank Dr. Xiaolin Zhang, biostatistician, and Dr. Aqin Peng and Pengcheng Wang, Orthopedic surgeons, for their assistance and cooperation in this study.

Author Contributions

Conceived and designed the experiments: YZ QZ WC. Performed the experiments: QZ WC XW YS. Analyzed the data: ZH. Contributed reagents/materials/analysis tools: ZH YS. Wrote the paper: XW QZ WC. Revised the manuscript: ZH YS.

References

1. Matta JM (1996) Fractures of the acetabulum: accuracy of reduction and clinical results in patients managed operatively within three weeks after the injury. J Bone Joint Surg Am 78:1632–1645.
2. Porter SE, Schroeder AC, Dzugan SS, Graves ML, Zhang L, et al. (2008) Acetabular fracture patterns and their associated injuries. J Orthop Trauma 22:165–170.
3. McMaster J, Powell J (2005) Acetabular fractures. Current Orthopaedics 19: 140–154.
4. Norris BL, Hahn DH, Bosse MJ, Kellam JF, Sims SH (1999) Intraoperative fluoroscopy to evaluate fracture reduction and hardware placement during acetabular surgery. J Orthop Trauma 13:414–417.
5. Carmack DB, Moed BR, McCarroll K, Freccero D (2001) Accuracy of detecting screw penetration of the acetabulum with intraoperative fluoroscopy and computed tomography. J Bone Joint Surg Am 83-A:1370–1375.
6. Stockle U, Schaser K, Konig B (2007) Image guidance in pelvic and acetabular surgery—expectations, success and limitations. Injury 38:450–462.
7. Kendoff D, Gardner MJ, Citak M, Kfuri M Jr, Thumes B, et al. (2008) Value of 3D fluoroscopic imaging of acetabular fractures comparison to 2D fluoroscopy and CT imaging. Arch Orthop Trauma Surg 128:599–605.
8. Richter H, Hutson JJ, Zych G (2004) The use of spring plates in the internal fixation of acetabular fractures. J Orthop Trauma 18:179–181.
9. Wu X, Chen W, Zhang Q, Su Y, Guo M, et al. (2010) The study of plate-screw fixation in the posterior wall of acetabulum using computed tomography images. J Trauma 69:423–431.
10. D'Aubigne RM, Postel M (1954) Functional results of hip arthroplasty with acrylic prosthesis. J Bone Joint Surg Am 36-A:451–475.
11. Moed BR, Smith ST (1996) Three-view radiographic assessment of heterotopic ossification after acetabular fracture surgery. J Orthop Trauma 10:93–98.
12. Ficat RP, Arlet J (1980) Necrosis of the femoral head. In: Hungerford DS, editors. Ischemia and necrosis of bone. Baltimore: Williams & Wilkins, pp 171–182.
13. Moed BR (2007) Improving results in posterior wall acetabular fracture surgery. J Trauma 62:S63.
14. Briffa N, Pearce R, Hill AM, Bircher M (2011) Outcomes of acetabular fracture fixation with ten years' follow-up. J Bone Joint Surg Br 93:229–236.
15. Osgood GM (2009) Posterior wall acetabular fractures: update on surgical indications, fixation techniques and outcome measurements. Curr Orthop Pract 20: 511–521.
16. Ebraheim NA, Waldrop J, Yeasting RA, Jackson WT (1992) Danger zone of the acetabulum. J Orthop Trauma 6:146–151.
17. Ruesch PD, Holdener H, Ciaramitaro M, Mast JW (1994) A prospective study of surgically treated acetabular fractures. Clin Orthop Relat Res (305):38–46.
18. Oransky M, Sanguinetti C (1993) Surgical treatment of displaced acetabular fractures: results of 50 consecutive cases. J Orthop Trauma 7:28–32.
19. Gansslen A, Steinke B, Krettek C (2009) [Internal fixation of acetabular posterior wall fractures]. Oper Orthop Traumatol 21:283–295.
20. Tadros AM, O'Brien P, Guy P (2010) Fixation of marginal posterior acetabular wall fractures using locking reconstruction plates and monocortical screws. J Trauma 68:478–480.
21. Ebraheim NA, Patil V, Liu J, Sanford CG Jr, Haman SP (2007) Reconstruction of comminuted posterior wall fractures using the buttress technique: a review of 32 fractures. Int Orthop 31:671–675.
22. Olson SA, Kadrmas MW, Hernandez JD, Glisson RR, West JL (2007) Augmentation of posterior wall acetabular fracture fixation using calcium-phosphate cement: a biomechanical analysis. J Orthop Trauma 21:608–616.
23. Goulet JA, Rouleau JP, Mason DJ, Goldstein SA (1994) Comminuted fractures of the posterior wall of the acetabulum. A biomechanical evaluation of fixation methods. J Bone Joint Surg Am 76:1457–1463.
24. Giannoudis PV, Tzioupis C, Moed BR (2007) Two-level reconstruction of comminuted posterior-wall fractures of the acetabulum. J Bone Joint Surg Br 89:503–509.

Effects of Quadriceps Muscle Fatigue on Stiff-Knee Gait in Patients with Hemiparesis

Julien Boudarham[1]*, Nicolas Roche[1], Didier Pradon[1], Eric Delouf[1], Djamel Bensmail[1], Raphael Zory[1,2]

1 GRCTH, EA4497, CIC-IT 805, CHU Raymond Poincaré, Garches, France, **2** LAMHESS, EA 6309, University of Nice Sophia Antipolis, Nice, France

Abstract

The relationship between neuromuscular fatigue and locomotion has never been investigated in hemiparetic patients despite the fact that, in the clinical context, patients report to be more spastic or stiffer after walking a long distance or after a rehabilitation session. The aim of this study was to evaluate the effects of quadriceps muscle fatigue on the biomechanical gait parameters of patients with a stiff-knee gait (SKG). Thirteen patients and eleven healthy controls performed one gait analysis before a protocol of isokinetic quadriceps fatigue and two after (immediately after and after 10 minutes of rest). Spatiotemporal parameters, sagittal knee and hip kinematics, rectus femoris (RF) and vastus lateralis (VL) kinematics and electromyographic (EMG) activity were analyzed. The results showed that quadriceps muscle weakness, produced by repetitive concentric contractions of the knee extensors, induced an improvement of spatiotemporal parameters for patients and healthy subjects. For the patient group, the increase in gait velocity and step length was associated with i) an increase of sagittal hip and knee flexion during the swing phase, ii) an increase of the maximal normalized length of the RF and VL and of the maximal VL lengthening velocity during the pre-swing and swing phases, and iii) a decrease in EMG activity of the RF muscle during the initial pre-swing phase and during the latter 2/3 of the initial swing phase. These results suggest that quadriceps fatigue did not alter the gait of patients with hemiparesis walking with a SKG and that neuromuscular fatigue may play the same functional role as an anti-spastic treatment such as botulinum toxin-A injection. Strength training of knee extensors, although commonly performed in rehabilitation, does not seem to be a priority to improve gait of these patients.

Editor: Reury F.P. Bacurau, University of Sao Paulo, Brazil

Funding: The authors have no support or funding to report.

Competing Interests: The authors have declared that no competing interests exist.

* E-mail: julien.boudarham@yahoo.fr

Introduction

Stiff-knee-gait (SKG) is characterized by a decrease in peak knee flexion during the swing phase of gait and is frequently observed in patients with hemiparesis following stroke [1,2]. Overactivity of the rectus femoris (RF) muscle related to spasticity causes excessive knee extension moments during swing and has been widely implicated in SKG [3]. This over-activity of the RF is mainly observed in initial pre-swing and may continue in the early and middle swing phases [4,5,6,7]. Spasticity has been defined by Lance (1980) [8] as "a motor disorder characterized by a velocity-dependent increase in the tonic stretch reflex with exaggerated tendon jerks, resulting from hyper-excitability of the stretch-reflex". Spasticity may be the result of intrinsic modifications of the muscle and/or altered reflex properties [9].

Fatigue is another frequent disabling and persistent symptom in chronic neurological diseases such as stroke [10]. There are several definitions of muscle fatigue in the literature. In this study, fatigue is defined as a reduction in the level of the output force produced by muscles during a sustained activity [11]. To our knowledge, the impact of quadriceps fatigue on SKG has never been assessed in patients with hemiparesis. The literature reports paradoxical results regarding the effects of knee extensor muscle fatigue on the gait pattern in healthy subjects. Most studies found no difference in walking speed and stride length after quadriceps muscle fatigue in young healthy subjects [12,13] whereas these parameters were improved in the fatigued state in older adults [12]. Results are also contradictory regarding knee biomechanics after a quadriceps fatigue protocol in young healthy subjects, since some studies report an alteration of kinematic and kinetic parameters and others report no changes [13,14,15]. These examples clearly show that the real impact of quadriceps fatigue on knee kinematics and kinetics during gait is still under debate. Since gait velocity of stroke patients is strongly dependant on the voluntary strength of the knee extensor muscles [16,17], we may hypothesized that quadriceps fatigue would alter biomechanical gait parameters.

The relationship between spasticity and muscle fatigue is a major concern in clinical practice but it is still unclear in the scientific literature. Some studies suggest that there is an interaction between neuromuscular fatigue and stretch reflex amplitude (which is exacerbated in spastic patients). Indeed, some results obtained in healthy subjects show that the amplitude of the stretch reflex decreases in the fatigued state [12,18,19]. This reduction in stretch reflex response might result from an increase in presynaptic inhibition of Ia afferents and/or a decrease in motoneuronal excitability [12,18,19]. Conversely, Biro et al. (2007) [20] showed an enhancement of the gain of the muscle spindle pathways during fatigue when descending drive is low. These results suggest that neuromuscular fatigue may have an effect on spasticity but no study has evaluated this association in patients with neurological disorders such as stroke or multiple

Table 1. Demographic characteristics of subjects.

		Hemiparetic patients (N = 13)	Healthy subjects (N = 11)
		Description of populations	
Gender (M/F)		8/5	8/3
Age (years)		48 (14)	44 (14)
Height (cm)		171 (11)	175 (11)
Weight (kg)		70 (14)	77 (17)
Paretic side (R/L)		7/6	-
Time since stroke (months)		84 (47)	-
ABILOCO (logits)		5.00 (1.59)	-
		Clinical examination	
Spasticity			
MAS	Quadriceps	2[0,2]	-
	Hamstrings	0[0,2]	-
	Triceps surae	1.5[2,2]	-
Strength			
MRC scale	Quadriceps	4[4,5]	-
	Hamstrings	4[3,4]	-
	Triceps surae	3[1,3]	-

For the demographic characteristics of hemiparetic patients and healthy subjects, mean (SD) values are presented. For the clinical examination, median values [1st; 3rd quartiles] are presented. M = male, F = female, R = right, L = left, MAS = Modified Ashworth Scale, MRC = Medical Research Council.

sclerosis. It has been possible to estimate level of spasticity during gait for a few years since the development of musculoskeletal models. Several studies have thus begun to explore the relationship between muscle-tendon stretch velocity and electromyography (EMG) activity of spastic muscles [21,22]. For example, Lampire et al., (2013) [23] showed an increase of maximal RF length and lengthening velocity during the swing phase of gait, one month after injection of botulinum toxin type-A (BoNT-A) in the spastic RF of hemiparetic patients with SKG. They concluded that the improvement of peak knee flexion after BoNT-A injection was mainly due to the decrease in spasticity. These studies suggest that this type of assessment is particularly useful for the estimation of changes in spasticity during gait, after a given treatment.

Therefore, the aim of this study was to evaluate the effects of quadriceps muscle fatigue on biomechanical gait parameters, particularly RF muscle kinematics (length and lengthening velocity) and inappropriate EMG activity, in order to estimate changes in spasticity in stroke patients with SKG caused by RF overactivity. To that end, spatiotemporal parameters, sagittal knee and hip kinematics during swing, RF and VL kinematics and EMG activity were quantified in a population of chronic stroke patients with inappropriate RF activity, before and after an isokinetic fatigue protocol and compared with healthy subjects. We

Table 2. Fatigue protocol parameters.

	Hemiparetic patients (N = 13)		Healthy subjects (N = 11)	
	Fatigue protocol			
maxMVC (N.m)	78.3 (33.9)		173.9 (62.2)†	
Mean total repetitions	64.7 (22.7)		54.8 (17.6)	
Fatigue Index (N.m/rep)	−0.37 (0.30)		−0.62 (0.69)	
RPE after the fatigue protocol	12 [11;13]		12 [12;15]	
	First 3 repetitions	**Last 3 repetitions**	**First 3 repetitions**	**Last 3 repetitions**
RMS RF (μV)	240.6 (186.6)	211.2 (168.3)*	576.2 (220.6)	438.5 (142.2)*
RMS VL (μV)	378.7 (231.8)	354.1 (192.5)	588.1 (219.8)	509.9 (243.5)

For the fatigue protocol parameters mean (SD) values are presented. RPE (rate of perceived exertion) values are expressed as median values [1st; 3rd quartiles]. EMG = electromyography, RF = rectus femoris, VL = vastus lateralis.
†Significant difference between groups ($p<0.05$).
*Significant difference between the beginning and the end of the fatigue protocol ($p<0.05$).

Table 3. Spatio-temporal, kinematic and EMG parameters during gait.

		Hemiparetic patients (N = 13)			Healthy subjects (N = 11)		
		PRE	POST	POST_10	PRE	POST	POST_10
Spatio-temporal parameters							
Velocity (m/s)		0.68 (0.19)	0.75 (0.22)†	0.78 (0.21)*	1.32 (0.22)	1.41 (0.20)†	1.42 (0.23)*
Step length (m)		0.46 (0.08)	0.49 (0.09)†	0.50 (0.08)*	0.67 (0.06)	0.68 (0.08)	0.68 (0.08)
Cadence (step/min)		89.4 (15.5)	92.5 (15.8)†	94.9 (16.6)*	116.0 (10.1)	122.2 (11.4)†	120.8 (11.0)*
Joint kinematics							
Peak hip flexion in swing (°)		36.3 (9.2)	38.8 (8.9)†	37.7 (9.4)*	33.6 (6.8)	33.8 (4.9)	34.4 (6.5)
Peak knee flexion in swing (°)		39.0 (13.8)	43.8 (17.1)†	43.0 (16.7)*	60.2 (4.9)	61.3 (4.6)	61.1 (4.2)
Knee angular velocity at toe off (°/s)		180.9 (96.2)	193.6 (94.2)†	190.5 (98.7)*	314.7 (37.2)	300.5 (39.4)	314.2 (41.4)
Hip angular velocity at toe off (°/s)		101.9 (49.0)	116.4 (54.1)†	114.4 (55.4)*	121.0 (22.1)	130.8 (23.3)	129.7 (22.0)
Muscle kinematics							
Pre-swing	MaxNL RF (mm)	12.9 (8.2)	14.6 (8.4)†	16.4 (9.1)*	21.8 (12.7)	22.4 (13.8)	22.4 (13.4)
	MaxLV RF (m/s)	0.15 (0.09)	0.16 (0.09)†	0.16 (0.11)*	0.24 (0.04)	0.25 (0.02)	0.25 (0.02)
	MaxNL VL (mm)	16.9 (7.1)	17.1 (6.6)	18.4 (7.0)	18.6 (8.2)	19.4 (8.3)	18.6 (7.9)
	MaxLV VL (m/s)	0.20 (0.11)	0.21 (0.11)†	0.22 (0.12)*	0.25 (0.09)	0.26 (0.09)	0.26 (0.09)
Swing	MaxNL RF (mm)	17.0 (13.4)	20.0 (12.6)†	20.1 (13.9)*	37.6 (8.9)	38.1 (8.6)	38.4 (8.6)
	MaxLV RF (m/s)	0.12 (0.10)	0.14 (0.09)†	0.13 (0.10)*	0.24 (0.03)	0.24 (0.03)	0.25 (0.03)
	MaxNL VL (mm)	28.3 (10.4)	30.7 (10.8)†	30.2 (10.8)*	40.3 (16.3)	40.9 (16.4)	40.6 (16.3)
	MaxLV VL (m/s)	0.18 (0.22)	0.22 (0.13)†	0.21 (0.13)*	0.27 (0.10)	0.28 (0.09)	0.28 (0.09)
EMG activity							
Initial Pre-swing	EMG RF (%)	23.9 (8.9)	15.2 (8.7)†	16.6 (8.3)*	15.8 (5.0)	17.6 (8.4)	16.4 (10.9)
	EMG VL (%)	10.8 (6.6)	8.4 (7.5)	9.4 (7.4)	8.9 (4.2)	8.7 (4.5)	6.3 (3.2)
Normal activity	EMG RF (%)	29.1 (10.3)	21.9 (11.1)	25.3 (14.6)	26.0 (11.8)	27.7 16.1)	26.1 (15.6)
	EMG VL (%)	8.9 (6.5)	7.9 (6.0)	9.1 (6.2)	10.9 (6.3)	15.6 (17.0)	11.3 (11.8)
Latter 2/3 of initial swing	EMG RF (%)	31.7 (14.8)	23.9 (14.3)	25.5 (16.8)	22.9 (11.4)	29.7 (19.7)	19.9 (12.1)
	EMG VL (%)	8.5 (6.7)	6.4 (4.1)	7.1 (4.1)	10.5 (5.0)	10.6 (7.4)	11.0 (14.2)
Mid-swing	EMG RF (%)	24.3 (10.7)	18.6 (10.8)	22.7 (17.6)	14.6 (4.0)	13.1 (3.9)	11.3 (3.6)
	EMG VL (%)	11.5 (7.7)	8.5 (5.8)	9.1 (4.4)	7.9 (3.7)	6.9 (4.0)	5.8 (3.3)
Terminal swing	EMG RF (%)	26.2 (9.6)	20.5 (11.1)	21.5 (10.3)	27.3 (5.3)	23.1 (7.8)	21.52 (8.1)
	EMG VL (%)	22.4 (9.5)	15.5 (10.2)	22.6 (15.1)	26.0 (13.0)	23.7 (16.4)	20.6 (14.6)

Mean (SD) spatio-temporal parameters, joint kinematics, muscle kinematics and EMG for the fatigued limb in PRE condition, POST_0 condition and POST_10 condition. MaxNL = Normalized maximal length; MaxLV = maximal lengthening velocity; EMG = electromyography, RF = rectus femoris, VL = vastus lateralis.

†Significant difference between PRE and POST_0 ($p<0.05$).

*Significant difference between PRE and POST_10 ($p<0.05$).

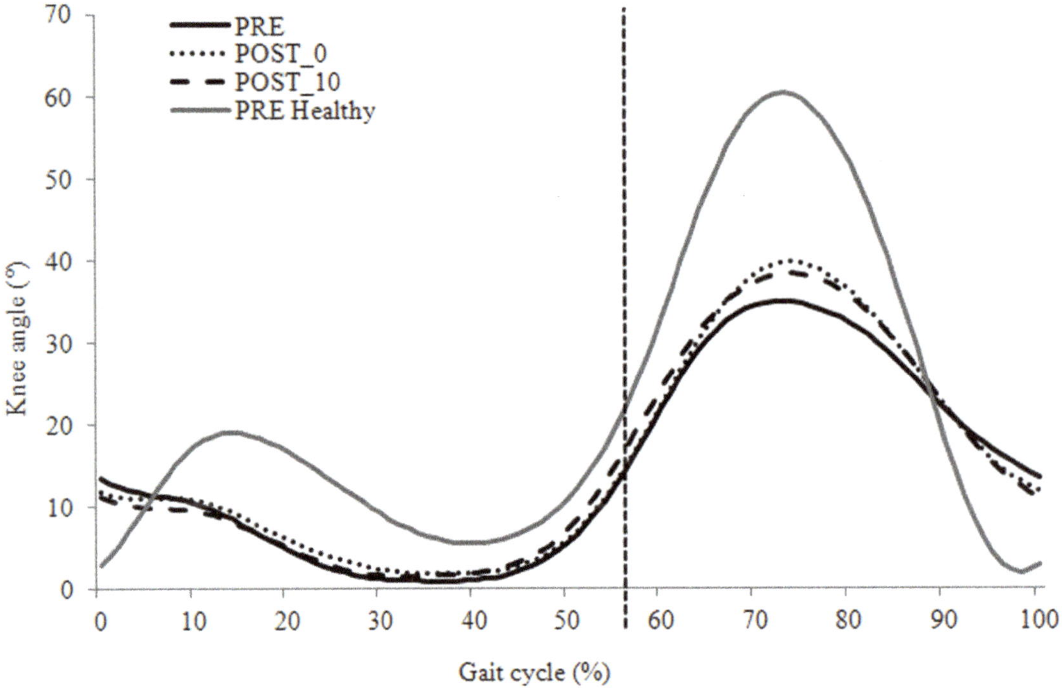

Figure 1. Mean sagittal-plan knee joint angle for the hemiparetic group and the healthy group. The solid black line indicates the PRE condition for the hemiparetic group walking at a mean spontaneous gait velocity of 0.68 m/s, the dotted black line indicates the POST_0 condition for the hemiparetic group walking at a mean spontaneous gait velocity of 0.75 m/s and the dashed black line indicates the POST_10 condition for the hemiparetic group waking at a mean spontaneous gait velocity of 0.78 m/s. The solid gray line indicates the PRE condition for the healthy group walking at a mean spontaneous gait velocity of 1.32 m/s. The vertical solid line represents the beginning of the swing phase of gait.

hypothesized that neuromuscular fatigue of the knee extensor muscles would i) alter spatiotemporal and kinematics gait parameters and ii) increase quadriceps muscle activity and RF stretch reflex at the origin of the SKG.

Materials and Methods

Subjects

Thirteen patients (8 males and 5 females) with chronic hemiparesis following stroke were enrolled in this study (Table 1, age: 48 (14) years; height: 171 (11) cm, mass: 70 (14) kg). Inclusion criteria of patients: over 18 years old, more than 6 months post stroke (chronic-phase), decrease in peak knee flexion in swing, RF EMG activity in mid swing phase, with a score ≥1+ on Modified Ashworth Scale (MAS) [24] for the quadriceps muscle (tested with the hip in extension), ability to walk independently 10 m without walking aids or assistance, no use of anti-spastic medications 6 months before inclusion and no orthopedic surgery in the last 6 months. In addition, eleven healthy subjects without neurological or musculoskeletal pathologies were recruited (8 males and 3 females; 44 (14) years; 175 (11) cm; 77 (17) kg). This study was approved by the local ethics committee, "Comité de Protection des Personnes Ile de France XI", and all subjects provided written informed consent prior to participation in any study-specific procedures.

Procedure

Experimental setup. On their arrival at the laboratory and before the first gait analysis, patients' locomotion ability was assessed using the ABILOCO questionnaire [25]. Next, patients underwent a clinical neurological evaluation. Spasticity and strength of quadriceps, hamstring and triceps surae muscles were evaluated using the Modified Ashworth Scale (MAS) and Medical Research Council (MRC) scale. Then all subjects were equipped with reflective markers and with surface electrodes. Three gait analyses were carried out by participants i) before the quadriceps fatigue protocol (PRE condition), ii) immediately after (POST_0 condition) and iii) after a 10 min seated rest (POST_10 condition). The duration of the rest period was chosen based on previous studies showing that after a few minutes, patients have already recovered a significant portion of their muscle strength [14,26].

Isokinetic fatigue protocol. A ConTrex-MJ isokinetic dynamometer (Contrex, CMV AG, Dübendorf, Switzerland) which allowed recording of instantaneous isokinetic torque was used for the fatigue protocol. Subjects were seated in the chair of the isokinetic dynamometer in a position of 85° of hip flexion with the lower legs hanging over the edge of the seat. The trunk and the paretic lower leg were stabilized using straps across the chest and the waist, and upper thigh, respectively. The contralateral lower limb was also blocked. The axis of the dynamometer was visually aligned with the knee joint axis, which was defined as a line between the medial and lateral condyles of the femur. The distal attachment of the lower limb to the lever of the dynamometer was 3 cm above the lateral malleolus. The passive range of motion designated as acceptable by the patient was determined and used to set the limits of the isokinetic dynamometer. Before the fatigue protocol, calculation of the limb weight was carried out during passive movements in order to remove the gravitational effects of the limb and attachment from each trial. Next, gravity correction was performed with the ConTrex-MJ software (Contrex, CMV AG, Dübendorf, Switzerland).

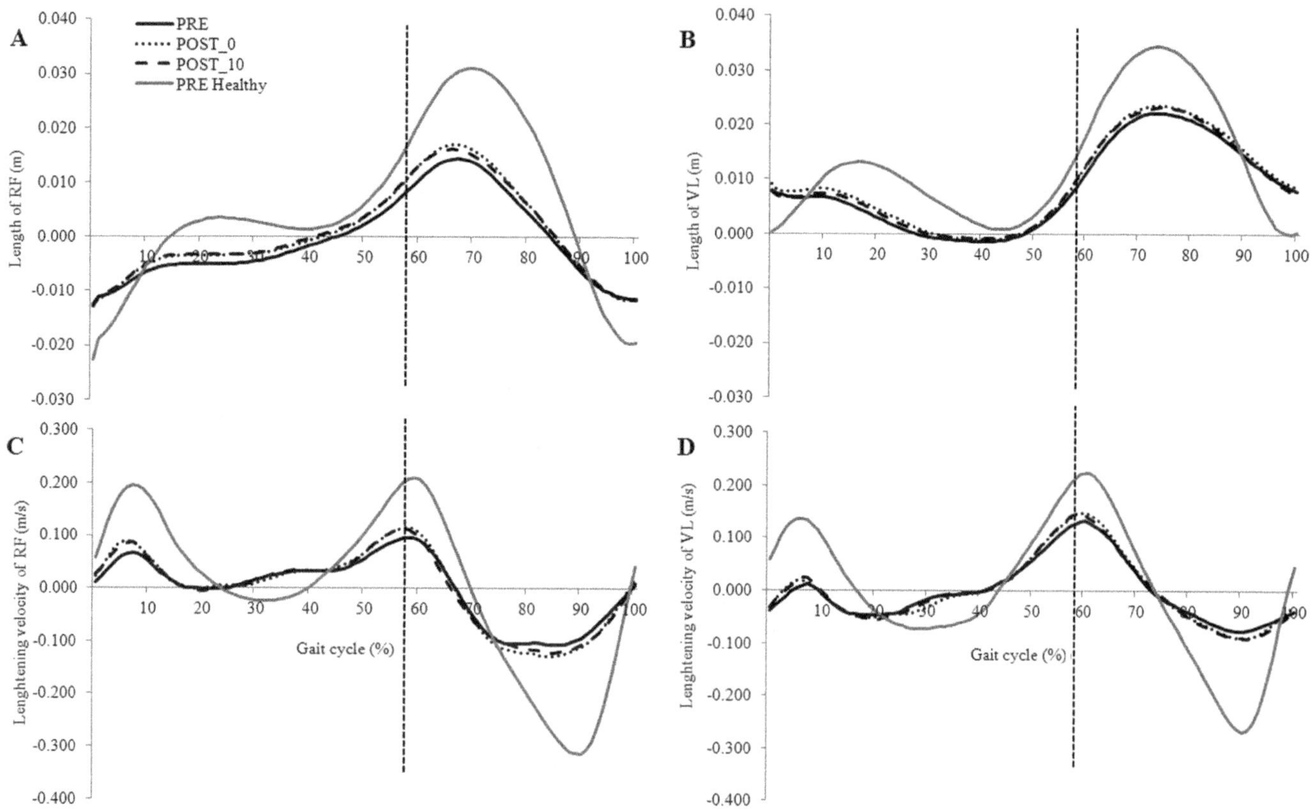

Figure 2. Mean normalized rectus femoris (A) and vastus lateralis length (B), and mean lengthening velocity curve of rectus femoris (C) and vastus lateralis (D). The solid black line indicates the PRE condition for the hemiparetic group walking at a mean spontaneous gait velocity of 0.68 m/s, the dotted black line indicates the POST_0 condition for the hemiparetic group walking at a mean spontaneous gait velocity of 0.75 m/s and the dashed black line indicates the POST_10 condition for the hemiparetic group walking at a mean spontaneous gait velocity of 0.78 m/s. The solid gray line indicates the PRE condition for the healthy group. The vertical solid line represents the beginning of the swing phase of gait. RF = rectus femoris; VL = vastus lateralis.

Participants performed 8 to 12 sub-maximal concentric knee extension repetitions to familiarize themselves with the task. The paretic lower limb for each patient and the non-dominant lower limb for healthy subjects were fatigued. After the warm-up, each subject performed four maximal voluntary contractions (MVC) of the knee extensors at 60°/s. The highest value of torque was taken as maximal torque (maxMVC). The unilateral voluntary isokinetic fatigue protocol consisted of maximal repetitive concentric contractions of the knee extensor muscles at 60°/sec, with a passive return to the initial knee position at 30°/s [10]. Three series were repeated with one minute rest between each. Each series was stopped when the participants reached three consecutive repetitions below 50% of their maxMVC. No limitations were imposed with regard to the number of repetitions. Strong verbal encouragement was given to the subjects during each contraction. Immediately after the end of the fatigue protocol, subjects were asked to estimate rate of perceived exertion on a 6 to 20 Borg scale [27]. After the fatigue protocol, each participant performed the POST_0 condition gait analysis.

Gait analysis. Gait parameters were recorded using 8 optoelectronic cameras (Motion Analysis Corporation, CA, USA) which measured the tridimensional coordinates of 30 reflective markers. Markers were positioned according to the Helen Hays protocol [28]. Nine gait trials were recorded but the three first were removed in order to exclude the adaptation which occurs at the beginning of a gait analysis [29]. Each gait trial was carried out in a 10 m gait corridor. All subjects walked at their self-selected walking velocity. The number of gait cycles recorded was different for the hemiparetic patients and for the healthy subjects (PRE condition: 228 and 95, respectively; POST_0 condition: 212 and 83, respectively; POST_10: condition 199 and 84, respectively). However, in order to make reliable comparison, the number of gait cycles analysed and averaged was significantly similar between the pre and the post fatigue conditions (POST_0 and POST_10), for the two group of subjects. Data were filtered using a fourth-order zero-lag Butterworth low-pass-filter with a cutoff frequency of 6 Hz. Between each gait trial, no rest was allowed and the recording was only stopped between trials while the subjects turned around. The position of the reflective markers was maintained during the whole experiment to limit bias relative to the repositioning of the markers. Ground reaction forces were measured synchronously with the kinematic data using two force-plates (AMTI, Watertown, MA, USA, sampling frequency 1000 Hz) staggered along the walkway.

Electromyographic assessment. Electromyographic (EMG) activities of the RF and vastus lateralis (VL) of the paretic limbs for patients and of the non-dominant leg for healthy subjects were recorded during the gait trials and during each isokinetic session. Two bipolar surface electrodes with built-in pre-amplification (MA311, Motion Lab Systems, LA, USA) were placed directly on the skin, according to SENIAM recommendations [30]. The occurrence of crosstalk (particularly RF and vastus intermedius) cannot be completely excluded, especially during gait that require synergic activation of more than one muscle [31]. The EMG sensors were composed of two circular dry button electrodes (stainless steel) with double-differential preamplifiers. The two active electrodes measured 12 mm in diameter and the inter-electrode distance was 17 mm. All EMG signals were sampled at 1000 Hz, pre-amplified with a gain of 20. Before processing the EMG signal, all signals were band-pass filtered between 3.5 and 350 Hz [32].

Data Analysis

Fatigue assessment. Only data (torque and EMG) from the constant velocity portion of each concentric trial were analyzed because, during acceleration and deceleration phases, data are strongly affected by inertial forces [33]. All isokinetic and EMG data were exported to text files and processed using custom algorithms developed in MatLab version 9.0 (The MathWorks, Inc., MA, USA). The repetitions carried out before the subject to reached 50% of maxMVC were averaged for the 3 sets of fatigue. Peak torque for each repetition and each subject were normalized by his maxMVC. Next, the index of fatigue was calculated as the rate of decline in normalized peak torque represented by the slope of the linear regression, beginning with the highest value of the first 5 consecutive repetitions and ending with the last 5 repetitions [34]. This fatigue index calculation has previously shown to be valid in patients with neurological disorders [35,36]. The RMS values of RF and VL muscles were calculated over a 500 ms period around the occurrence of peak torque (i.e. 250 ms before and 250 ms after) for each repetition and each subject. In addition, the average normalized maximum peak torque and the root mean square (RMS) values of RF and VL EMG was calculated for the first three and the last three repetitions.

SKG assessment. Spatiotemporal and sagittal joint kinematic parameters were computed for each gait cycle, using OrthoTrack 6.5 software (Motion Analysis Corporation, CA, USA). The following spatiotemporal parameters were calculated: gait velocity, step length and cadence. The sagittal hip and knee angles during the swing phase and angular velocity at toe-off were computed for the fatigued limb of both groups [37]. Only the sagittal kinematic plane was evaluated to identify the deviations most frequently described in hemiparetic gait [2,38].

Estimation of RF spasticity during gait. Normal RF muscle activity occurs during the latter half of pre-swing (from final double support to toe-off) and the first third of initial swing. RF muscle activity is considered inappropriate if it occurs during the first half of pre-swing, the latter 2/3 of initial swing, or is present during any portion of mid-swing [2,39]. Hence, inappropriate EMG activity was evaluated during these 3 periods. Mean values of EMG activity of RF and VL muscles were calculated for each sub-phase of gait and each subject. The linear envelope of the EMG signals was calculated according to Shiavi's method (1987) [40]. The amplitude of the linear envelope was normalized with respect to the maximum value recorded across all gait trials in the PRE condition and Mean Amplitude Value (MAV) was calculated as the mean value of the normalized linear envelope over the time interval.

SIMM, (MusculoGraphics, Inc., Santa Rosa, California, USA) modeling software (Delp et al., 1990) was used to calculate the length and lengthening velocity of the musculo–tendinous complex of RF and VL muscles. For a detailed description of the method, see Lampire et al. (2013) [23]. Normalized maximal RF and VL lengths (maxNL) and maximal RF and VL lengthening velocity (maxLV) were calculated during the pre-swing and swing phases.

Statistical Analyses

Kolmogorov-Smirnov tests were conducted before the statistical analysis and confirmed that data were normally distributed. Due to the large difference in baseline values between the two groups, a one-factor ANOVA with repeated measures was used to analyze differences between the three conditions (PRE vs. POST_0 vs. POST_10) for each group separately (hemiparetic patients and healthy subjects) for each gait parameter. Post hoc analysis was performed using the Bonferroni post hoc multiple comparison test. For each parameter where we observed a significant change over time, the percentage of changes for this parameter was compared between the groups using a Student's t test. Comparisons of the several fatigue protocol parameters between the two groups were performed with a Student T-test. The significance level was maintained at $p<0.05$, with Bonferroni adjustments used as appropriate. Values were expressed as mean ± standard deviation. Statistical analysis was performed using Statistica 7 (StatSoft, Inc., Tulsa, OK, USA).

Results

Fatigue Protocol (Table 2)

Post-fatigue, rate of perceived exertion (RPE) on a 6 to 20 point Borg scale was not significantly different between the two groups (Table 2). The maxMVC was significantly higher for healthy subjects compared to patients with hemiparesis (respectively, 173.9 (62.2) N.m and 78.3 (33.9) N.m, $p<0.001$). The number of repetitions to reach 50% of maxMVC, was not different between the two groups (64.7 (22.7) for hemiparetic and 54.8 (17.6) for healthy subjects, $p=0.556$). The magnitude of the slope value (fatigue index) was −0.37 (0.30) and −0.62 (0.69) N.m/rep respectively for the hemiparetic and healthy groups (Table 3), but the difference between the two groups was not significant. The RMS amplitude of the RF muscle was significantly lower in the last three contractions than in the first three, for both the hemiparetic and healthy groups (respectively, 240.6 (186.6) to 211.2 (168.3) µV, $p=0.027$ and 576.2 (220.6) to 438.5 (142.2) µV, $p=0.028$). The RMS amplitude of the VL muscle was not modified by the fatigue protocol (Table 2).

SKG Assessment (Table 3)

For the patients with hemiparesis, gait velocity, step length and cadence of the fatigued limb were significantly greater in POST_0 and POST_10 compared with PRE ($p<0.001$).

Peak hip and knee flexion angles during swing were significantly greater in POST_0 and POST_10 compared with PRE ($p=0.04$ and $p=0.03$, respectively) (Figure 1). Hip and knee angular velocities at toe-off were significantly greater in POST_0 and POST_10 compared with PRE ($p=0.002$ and $p=0.04$, respectively). There were no significant changes in parameters between POST_0 and POST_10.

For healthy subjects, gait velocity and cadence were significantly greater in POST_0 and POST_10 conditions compared with PRE ($p<0.001$). No differences were observed between group for the percentage of changes of these two gait parameters appearing between PRE and POST_0 ($p=0.16$) and between PRE and POST_10 ($p=0.06$). None of the other parameters were significantly modified by the fatigue protocol.

Estimation RF Spasticity during Gait (Table 3)

For the patients with hemiparesis, maxNL of RF ($p=0.003$) and maxLV of VL ($p=0.005$) in pre-swing were greater in POST_0 and POST_10 compared with PRE. In swing, maxNL of RF ($p=0.004$), maxNL of VL ($p=0.004$) and maxLV of VL

($p = 0.003$) were greater in POST_0 and POST_10 compared with PRE (Figure 2). The MAV of RF was lower during initial pre-swing ($p = 0.003$) in POST_0 and POST_10 compared with PRE. No parameters were significantly modified between POST_0 and POST_10.

For the healthy subjects, no change occurred in any muscle kinematic parameter or in the EMG activity.

Discussion

The aim of this study was to evaluate the effects of quadriceps muscle fatigue on biomechanical gait parameters, in hemiparetic patients with SKG. The key finding of this study was that fatigue, produced by repetitive concentric contractions of the knee extensors, induced an improvement in the spatiotemporal parameters of both patients and healthy subjects. For the patient group, the increase in gait velocity and step length was associated with i) an increase of sagittal hip and knee flexion during the swing phase, ii) an increase of the maximal normalized length of the RF and VL and of the maximal VL lengthening velocity during the pre-swing and swing phases, and iii) a decrease in EMG activity of the RF muscle during the initial pre-swing and the latter 2/3 of initial swing phases. These results did not confirm our initial hypothesis.

The number of repetitions to reach 50% of the baseline maxMVC and fatigue index was not statistically different between the two groups, despite different mean values. These results are in contradiction with the literature since, in a recent review, Knorr et al. (2012) [10] showed that muscles of the paretic limb are more fatigue-resistant than muscles of the non-paretic limb or than muscles of healthy subjects. Muscle weakness, deficit of voluntary muscle activation, disordered motor control and/or greater reliance on type I fibers have been proposed to explain the lower peripheral fatigue rate in the paretic limb [10,41]. It seems important to note that the EMG activity (RMS amplitude) of RF muscle decreases, for both groups, between the beginning and the end of the fatiguing exercise when it is not modified for the VL muscle. This result confirm previous studies showing that after an isokinetic fatigue protocol (knee-extensions), fatigue is more pronounced in the RF muscle than in the vastii [42]. Indeed, the bi-articular RF and mono-articular vastii play different functions during seated isokinetic knee-extensions tasks [43].

The present study suggests that specific fatigue of quadriceps muscle improves spatiotemporal gait parameters of both patients and healthy subjects. It should be noted that because of the inclusion criteria (ability to walk independently 10 m without walking aids or assistance), the group of patients presented a good locomotion capacity, explaining the high score on ABILOCO scale. Hence, the results reported in this study are could be only specific to a population of patients with the same clinical characteristics. Our results are consistent with previous studies which highlighted an improvement in gait velocity and step length, in the fatigued state, in older adults [12] and in patients with hemiparesis [44]. However, in the present study, the increase in gait velocity after fatigue occurred via different mechanisms in the healthy subjects and patients, since patients increased both cadence and step length, whereas healthy subjects only increased their cadence. The increase in cadence in the fatigued state has previously been observed in healthy subjects [45]. It is recognized that balance is affected by lower limb fatigue [46]. The concomitant increase in gait speed and cadence may contribute to a better medio-lateral stability due to the decrease in medio-lateral displacement of the center of mass [47,48]. This seems to be a strategy to compensate for impaired balance in the fatigued state.

We can hypothesize that the improvement in step length in the patient group is directly linked with changes in knee and hip flexion of the fatigued limb during the swing phase and thus with the increase in knee and hip angular velocities at toe-off. In order to better understand improvement of walking capacity after fatigue, changes in the non-fatigued limb were also evaluated. Because we observed no significant changes, these results are not presented in this manuscript. After fatigue, the increase in peak hip flexion in the swing phase may be surprising. Indeed, the RF is a bi-articular muscle which acts as hip flexor and knee extensor. Therefore, RF muscle weakening might decrease hip flexion. Granacher et al. (2010) [12] found that the increase in gait velocity after a fatigue protocol induced by isokinetic contractions could be associated with an increase in hip flexion in older adults. They proposed that older adults may have compensated for the fatigue induced decrease in knee extensor strength by increasing hip flexor power during walking. This strategy, frequently observed in older adults to compensate for muscle deficits [49,50], may explain the surprising increase in peak hip flexion, in the swing phase for the patient group. In contrast, this did not occur in healthy subjects since their muscle function is normal.

The analysis of EMG signals and muscle kinematics explains the increase in knee flexion during the swing phase. The EMG activity of the RF muscle during the initial pre-swing phase was significantly lower in the fatigued state, while maxNL and maxLV of RF and VL during the swing phase were significantly higher. During the double support phase of gait, the leg prepares for toe-off, the hip reaches maximum extension and the knee begins to flex. Excessive and prolonged activity of the RF muscle in the pre-swing phase could be induced by the excessive response to muscle stretch, leading to the inappropriate knee extension moment observed in the SKG pattern [51]. In the present study, the fatigue protocol mainly modified the excessive response to RF stretch during the initial pre-swing phase. From these results, it may be hypothesized that the repetition of maximal isokinetic contractions until fatigue is reached affects the stretch reflex loop of this muscle. Granacher et al., (2010) [12] also observed a decline of the functional reflex amplitude in tibialis anterior during gait perturbations, after a similar isokinetic fatigue protocol. A possible explanation could relate to group III and group IV free nerve endings which are sensitive to muscle metabolite accumulation [52,53]. It was reported that the inhibitory effect of group III and group IV muscle afferents reduces the discharge of gamma motoneurons and influences Renshaw inhibition [54]. Their projections on inhibitory interneurones could reduce the excitatory input by presynaptic inhibition of the group-Ia afferents [55,56], predominantly in the extensor muscles [57]. Moreover, Marque et al., (2001) [58] reported that spasticity in the quadriceps muscle can be related to facilitation of the spinal reflex via group-II muscle spindles. Since group-II muscle afferents project on inhibitory interneurones [59], we could hypothesize that metabolite accumulation affecting group III-IV muscle afferents may cause presynaptic inhibition of the group-Ia afferents, and reduce the recruitment of α-motoneurons during the quadriceps stretch. Therefore, the group III and group IV muscle afferents could mediate a reflex which may modulate motoneuron firing rate in a fatigued state [60].

Finally, it seems important to note that the kinematic and EMG improvements, observed in the present study, are very similar to those reported in several studies which evaluated the effects of BoNT-A in the RF to decrease SKG in patients with hemiparesis [6,21,61,62,63]. For example, Lampire et al. (2013) [23] showed that after a BoNT-A injection in the RF of patients with hemiparetic SKG, the increase in knee flexion during swing was correlated with the increase of maxNL of the RF, and associated with an increase in its maximal lengthening velocity. This seems to suggest that the quadriceps fatigue protocol induced a decrease in spasticity which was at the origin of the observed gait improvement, mainly walking velocity. Several studies have shown that the increase of the gait velocity is associated with an increase in knee flexion velocity at toe-off and an increase in peak knee flexion during swing phase of the gait cycle in stroke patients [64,65]. Therefore, we may hypothesize that the kinematic changes observed in the present study are the result of the velocity increase. To answer this question, correlations between the percentage of improvement of RF length or RF maxLV induced by fatigue and the percentage of improvement of the walking velocity have been calculated. No significant correlation was observed. This suggests that the kinematic changes observed in this study are not due to an increase in walking velocity.

The decrease of muscle overactivity after BoNT-A is due to its action on the neuromuscular junction [58] and on the motoneuron γ-intrafusal spindle synapse [66,67,68,69]. Although the BoNT-A injection and the present fatigue protocol seem to have a similar effect on SKG, our study cannot determine whether the physiological causes of these mechanical changes are similar. Therefore, further neurophysiological explorations must be conducted in order to precisely determine the origins of the fatigue induced by this protocol and to estimate the long-term effects of this kind of exercise on spasticity during gait. However, our results may have important implications for designing strength training programs. In clinical practice, spasticity of lower limbs, in patients with hemiparesis, could be managed by combining BoNT-A injection and resistance training. However, the results of the present study clearly show that quadriceps weakness did not alter the gait of hemiparetic patients with SKG. Although the present results were observed after a single session of muscle exertion, they pose the question of the interest of the knee extensors strengthening to improve gait in these patients [70].

This study has several limitations. First, the small number of patients (n = 13) and of healthy subjects (n = 11) included could potentially limit the statistical power of the results. Secondly, our group of patients is relatively young and presents high locomotion ability. So the sample may not be representative of the stroke population. These limitations mean that results must be interpreted with caution and further studies will be conducted in order to confirm our results.

Conclusion

In conclusion, our results clearly show that a specific quadriceps fatigue improved gait velocity in patients with hemiparetic SKG and in healthy subjects. For the patient group, the increase of gait velocity and step length was associated with improvements of peak hip and knee flexion during the swing phase. The decrease in inappropriate activity of RF muscle, initially due to the exaggeration of the stretch reflex in the initial pre-swing phase, seems to show that the increase in knee flexion during swing was due to a decrease in spasticity. With regard to these results, it seems that neuromuscular fatigue may play the same functional role as anti-spastic treatments such as BoNT-A injections during gait of patients with hemiparesis.

Acknowledgments

We thank Johanna Robertson for revision the English in this manuscript.

Author Contributions

Conceived and designed the experiments: JB RZ DB DP. Performed the experiments: JB ED RZ. Analyzed the data: JB ED RZ. Contributed reagents/materials/analysis tools: JB RZ. Wrote the paper: JB NR RZ.

References

1. Kerrigan DC, Gronley J, Perry J (1991) Stiff-legged gait in spastic paresis. A study of quadriceps and hamstrings muscle activity. Am J Phys Med Rehabil 70: 294–300.
2. Perry J (1992) Gait analysis: Normal and pathological function. New Jersey: Slack.
3. Sung DH, Bang HJ (2000) Motor branch block of the rectus femoris: its effectiveness in stiff-legged gait in spastic paresis. Arch Phys Med Rehabil 81: 910–915.
4. Goldberg SR, Ounpuu S, Arnold AS, Gage JR, Delp SL (2006) Kinematic and kinetic factors that correlate with improved knee flexion following treatment for stiff-knee gait. J Biomech 39: 689–698.
5. Reinbolt JA, Fox MD, Arnold AS, Ounpuu S, Delp SL (2008). Importance of preswing rectus femoris activity in stiff-knee gait. J Biomech 41: 2362–2369.
6. Robertson JV, Pradon D, Bensmail D, Fermanian C, Bussel B, et al. (2009) Relevance of botulinum toxin injection and nerve block of rectus femoris to kinematic and functional parameters of stiff knee gait in hemiplegic adults. Gait Posture 29: 108–112.
7. Knuppe AE, Bishop NA, Clark AJ, Alderink GJ, Barr KM, et al. (2013) Prolonged swing phase rectus femoris activity is not associated with stiff-knee gait in children with cerebral palsy: a retrospective study of 407 limbs. Gait Posture 37: 345–348.
8. Lance JW (1980) Spasticity: disordered motor control. Symposium synopsis. 485–494.
9. Mukherjee A, Chakravarty A (2010) Spasticity mechanisms - for the clinician. Front Neurol 17: 149.
10. Knorr S, Rice CL, Garland SJ (2012) Perspective on neuromuscular factors in poststroke fatigue. Disabil Rehabil 34: 2291–2299.
11. Bigland-Ritchie B, Johansson B, Lippold OC, Smith S, Woods JJ (1983) Changes in motoneurone firing rates during sustained maximal voluntary contractions. J Physiol 340: 335–346.
12. Granacher U, Wolf I, Wehrle A, Bridenbaugh S, Kressig RW (2010) Effects of muscle fatigue on gait characteristics under single and dual-task conditions in young and older adults. J Neuroeng Rehabil 7: 56.
13. Murdock GH, Hubley-Kozey CL (2012) Effect of a high intensity quadriceps fatigue protocol on knee joint mechanics and muscle activation during gait in young adults. Eur J Appl Physiol 112: 439–449.
14. Parijat P, Lockhart TE (2008) Effects of quadriceps fatigue on the biomechanics of gait and slip propensity. Gait Posture 28: 568–573.
15. Longpré HS, Potvin JR, Maly MR (2013) Biomechanical changes at the knee after lower limb fatigue in healthy young women. Clin Biomech 28: 441–447.
16. Hsu AL, Tang PF, Jan MH (2003) Analysis of impairments influencing gait velocity and asymmetry of hemiplegic patients after mild to moderate stroke. Arch Phys Med Rehabil 84: 1185–1193.
17. Nakamura R, Watanabe S, Handa T, Morohashi I (1988) The relationship between walking speed and muscle strength for knee extension in hemiparetic stroke patients: a follow-up study. Tohoku J Exp Med 154: 111–113.
18. Moore BD, Drouin J, Gansneder BM, Shultz SJ (2002) The differential effects of fatigue on reflex response timing and amplitude in males and females. J Electromyogr Kinesiol 12: 351–360.
19. Jackson ND, Gutierrez GM, Kaminski T (2009) The effect of fatigue and habituation on the stretch reflex of the ankle musculature. J Electromyogr Kinesiol 19: 75–84.
20. Biro A, Griffin L, Cafarelli E (2007) Reflex gain of muscle spindle pathways during fatigue. Exp Brain Res 177: 157–166.
21. Crenna P (1999) Pathophysiology of lengthening contractions in human spasticity: a study of the hamstring muscles during locomotion. Pathophysiology 5: 283–297.
22. van der Krogt MM, Doorenbosch CA, Becher JG, Harlaar J (2010) Dynamic spasticity of plantar flexor muscles in cerebral palsy gait. J Rehabil Med 42: 656–663.
23. Lampire N, Roche N, Carne P, Cheze L, Pradon D (2013) Effect of botulinum toxin injection on length and lengthening velocity of rectus femoris during gait in hemiparetic patients. Clin Biomech 28: 164–170.
24. Bohannon RW, Smith MB (1987) Interrater reliability of a modified Ashworth scale of muscle spasticity. Phys Ther 67: 206–207.
25. Caty GD, Arnould C, Stoquart GG, Thonnard JL, Lejeune TM (2008) ABILOCO: a Rasch-built 13-item questionnaire to assess locomotion ability in stroke patients. Arch Phys Med Rehabil 89: 284–290.
26. Froyd C, Millet GY, Noakes TD (2013) The development of peripheral fatigue and short-term recovery during self-paced high-intensity exercise. J Physiol. 591: 1339–1346.
27. Borg GA (1982) Psychophysical bases of perceived exertion. Med Sci Sports Exerc 14: 377–381.

28. Kadaba MP, Ramakrishnan HK, Wootten ME (1990) Measurement of lower extremity kinematics during level walking. J Orthop Res 8: 383–392.
29. Boudarham J, Roche N, Pradon D, Bonnyaud C, Bensmail D, et al. (2013) Variations in kinematics during clinical gait analysis in stroke patients. PloS One 8, e66421.
30. Hermens HJ, Freriks B, Disselhorst-Klug C, Rau G (2000) Development of recommendations for SEMG sensors and sensor placement procedures. J Electromyogr Kinesiol 10: 361–374.
31. Byrne CA, Lyons GM, Donnelly AE, O'Keeffe DT, Hermens H, et al. (2005) Rectus femoris surface myoelectric signal cross-talk during static contractions. JElectromyogr Kinesiol 15: 564–575.
32. Merletti R (1999) The standards for reporting EMG data. J Electromyogr Kinesiol 9: 1–4.
33. Knutsson E, Maartensson A (1980) Dynamic motor capacity in spastic paresis and its relation to prime mover dysfunction, spastic reflexes and antagonist co-activation. Scand J Rehabil Med 12: 93–106.
34. Pincivero DM, Gear WS, Sterner RL (2001) Assessment of the reliability of high-intensity quadriceps femoris muscle fatigue. Med Sci Sports Exerc 33: 334–338.
35. Moreau NG, Li L, Geaghan JP, Damiano DL (2009) Contributors to fatigue resistance of the hamstrings and quadriceps in cerebral palsy. Clin Biomech 24: 355–360.
36. Moreau NG, Li L, Geaghan JP, Damiano DL (2008) Fatigue resistance during a voluntary performance task is associated with lower levels of mobility in cerebral palsy. Arch Phys Med Rehabil 89: 2011–2116.
37. Piazza SJ, Delp SL (1996) The influence of muscles on knee flexion during the swing phase of gait. J Biomech. 29: 723–733.
38. Olney SJ, Richards C (1996) Hemiparetic gait following stroke. Part I: Characteristics. Gait Posture 4: 136–148.
39. Annaswamy TM, Giddings CJ, Della Croce U, Kerrigan DC (1999) Rectus femoris: its role in normal gait. Arch Phys Med Rehabil 80: 930–934.
40. Shiavi R, Bugle HJ, Limbird T (1987) Electromyographic gait assessment, Part 2: Preliminary assessment of hemiparetic synergy patterns. J Rehabil Res Dev 24: 24–30.
41. Lukács M, Vécsei L, Beniczky S (2008) Large motor units are selectively affected following a stroke. Clin Neurophysiol 119: 2555–2258.
42. Hu M, Finni T, Alén M, Wang J, Zou L, et al. (2006) Myoelectrical manifestations of quadriceps fatigue during dynamic exercise differ in mono-and bi-articular muscles. Biol Sport 23: 327–339.
43. van Ingen Schenau GJ, Dorssers WM, Welter TG, Beelen A, de Groot G, et al. (1995) The control of mono-articular muscles in multijoint leg extensions in man. J Physiol 484: 247–254.
44. Sibley KM, Tang A, Brooks D, McIlroy WE (2008) Effects of extended effortful activity on spatio-temporal parameters of gait in individuals with stroke. Gait Posture 27: 387–392.
45. Arif M, Ohtaki Y, Nagatomi R, Inooka H (2010) Analysis of the effect of fatigue on walking gait using acceleration sensor placed on the waist. Eng Intell Syst Elec 18: 93–103.
46. Helbostad JL, Sturnieks DL, Menant J, Delbaere K, Lord SR, et al. (2010) Consequences of lower extremity and trunk muscle fatigue on balance and functional tasks in older people: a systematic literature review. BMC geriatrics 10: 56.
47. Orendurff MS, Segal AD, Klute GK, Berge JS, Rohr ES, et al. (2004) The effect of walking speed on center of mass displacement. J Rehabil Res Dev 41: 829–834.
48. Staszkiewicz R, Ruchlewicz T, Forczek W, Laska J (2010) The impact of changes in gait speed and step frequency on the extent of the center of mass displacements. Acta Bioeng Biomech 12: 13–20.
49. Judge JO, Davis RB, Ounpuu S (1996) Step length reductions in advanced age: the role of ankle and hip kinetics. J Gerontol A Biol Sci Med Sci 51: 303–312.
50. Nadeau S, Gravel D, Arsenault AB, Bourbonnais D (1999) Plantarflexor weakness as a limiting factor of gait speed in stroke subjects and the compensating role of hip flexors. Clin Biomech 14: 125–135.
51. Lewek MD, Hornby TG, Dhaher YY, Schmit BD (2007) Prolonged quadriceps activity following imposed hip extension: a neurophysiological mechanism for stiff-knee gait? J Neurophysiol 98: 3153–3162.
52. Gandevia SC (2001) Spinal and supraspinal factors in human muscle fatigue. Physiol Rev 81: 1725–1789.
53. Amann M, Blain GM, Proctor LT, Sebranek JJ, Pegelow DF, et al. (2011) Implications of group III and IV muscle afferents for high-intensity endurance exercise performance in humans. J Physiol 1: 5299–5309.
54. Rossi A, Mazzocchio R, Decchi B (2003) Effect of chemically activated fine muscle afferents on spinal recurrent inhibition in humans. Clin Neurophysiol 114: 279–287.
55. Kalezic I, Bugaychenko LA, Kostyukov AI, Pilyavskii AI, Ljubisavljevic M, et al. (2004) Fatigue-related depression of the feline monosynaptic gastrocnemius-soleus reflex. J Physiol 556: 283–296.
56. Hunter SK, Duchateau J, Enoka RM (2004) Muscle fatigue and the mechanisms of task failure. Exerc Sport Sci Rev 32: 44–49.
57. Martin PG, Smith JL, Butler JE, Gandevia SC, Taylor JL (2006) Fatigue-sensitive afferents inhibit extensor but not flexor motoneurons in humans. J Neurosci 26: 4796–4802.
58. Marque P, Simonetta-Moreau M, Maupas E, Roques CF (2001) Facilitation of transmission in heteronymous group II pathways in spastic hemiplegic patients. J Neurol Neurosurg Psychiatry 70: 36–42.
59. Rudomin P, Schmidt RF (1999) Presynaptic inhibition in the vertebrate spinal cord revisited. Exp Brain Res 129: 1–37.
60. Bigland-Ritchie BR, Dawson NJ, Johansson RS, Lippold OC (1986) Reflex origin for the slowing of motoneurone firing rates in fatigue of human voluntary contractions. J Physiol 379: 451–459.
61. Stoquart GG, Detrembleur C, Palumbo S, Deltombe T (2008) Effect of botulinum toxin injection in the rectus femoris on stiff-knee gait in people with stroke: a prospective observational study. Arch Phys Med Rehabil 9: 56–61.
62. Hutin E, Pradon D, Barbier F, Gracies JM, Bussel B, et al. (2010) Lower limb coordination in hemiparetic subjects: impact of botulinum toxin injections into rectus femoris. Neurorehabil Neural Repair 24: 442–449.
63. Tok F, Balaban B, Yaşar E, Alaca R, Tan AK (2012) The effects of onabotulinum toxin A injection into rectus femoris muscle in hemiplegic stroke patients with stiff-knee gait: a placebo-controlled, nonrandomized trial. Am J Phys Med Rehabil 91: 321–326.
64. Lelas JL, Merriman GJ, Riley PO, Kerrigan DC (2003) Predicting peak kinematic and kinetic parameters from gait speed. Gait Posture 17: 106–112.
65. Hutin E, Pradon D, Barbier F, Bussel B, Gracies JM, et al. (2012) Walking velocity and lower limb coordination in hemiparesis. Gait Posture 36: 205–211.
66. Poulain B, Humeau Y (2003) Mode of action of botulinum neurotoxin: pathological, cellular and molecular aspect. Ann Readapt Med Phys 46: 265–275.
67. Rosales RL, Arimura K, Takenaga S, Osame M (1996) Extrafusal and intrafusal muscle effects in experimental botulinum toxin-A injection. Muscle Nerve 19: 488–496.
68. Stampacchia G, Bradaschia E, Rossi B (2004) Change of stretch reflex threshold in spasticity: effect of botulinum toxin injections. Arch Ital Biol 142: 265–273.
69. Trompetto C, Currà A, Buccolieri A, Suppa A, Abbruzzese G, et al. (2006) Botulinum toxin changes intrafusal feedback in dystonia: a study with the tonic vibration reflex. Mov Disord 21: 777–782.
70. Van der Krogt MM, Delp SL, Schwartz MH (2012) How robust is human gait to muscle weakness? Gait Posture, 36: 113–119.

Identification and Validation of Quantitative Trait Loci (QTL) for Canine Hip Dysplasia (CHD) in German Shepherd Dogs

Lena Fels, Ottmar Distl*

Institute for Animal Breeding and Genetics, University of Veterinary Medicine Hannover, Hannover, Germany

Abstract

Canine hip dysplasia (CHD) is the most common hereditary skeletal disorder in dogs. To identify common alleles associated with CHD, we genotyped 96 German Shepherd Dogs affected by mild, moderate and severe CHD and 96 breed, sex, age and birth year matched controls using the Affymetrix canine high density SNP chip. A mixed linear model analysis identified five SNPs associated with CHD scores on dog chromosomes (CFA) 19, 24, 26 and 34. These five SNPs were validated in a by sex, age, birth year and coancestry stratified sample of 843 German Shepherd Dogs including 277 unaffected dogs and 566 CHD-affected dogs. Mean coancestry coefficients among and within cases and controls were <0.1%. Genotype effects of these SNPs explained 20–32% of the phenotypic variance of CHD in German Shepherd Dogs employed for validation. Genome-wide significance in the validation data set could be shown for each one CHD-associated SNP on CFA24, 26 and 34. These SNPs are located within or in close proximity of genes involved in bone formation and related through a joint network. The present study validated positional candidate genes within two previously known quantitative trait loci (QTL) and a novel QTL for CHD in German Shepherd Dogs.

Editor: William Barendse, CSIRO, Australia

Funding: This study was supported by the Gesellschaft zur Förderung Kynologischer Forschung e.V. (GKF), Bonn, Germany, and the Breeding Associaton of German Shepherd Dogs (Verein für Deutsche Schäferhunde e.V., SV), Augsburg, Germany. The funders had no role in study design, data collection and analysis, decision to publish, or preparation of the manuscript.

Competing Interests: The authors have declared that no competing interests exist.

* E-mail: ottmar.distl@tiho-hannover.de

Introduction

Canine hip dysplasia (CHD) is a common trait in most dog breeds. This orthopedic condition causes instability and subluxation of the hip with secondary signs of osteoarthritis and clinical signs of lameness. Breed prevalences vary widely from 1% to 75% [1]. In German Shepherd Dogs, prevalence of CHD is estimated at 35% [2]. There is strong evidence in support of a genetic predisposition to CHD in German Shepherd Dogs and many other dog breeds. Heritability estimates for German Shepherd Dogs from different European countries were at $h^2 = 0.20$ to 0.35 [2–4]. Results from radiographic screenings for CHD of 48,367 German Shepherd Dogs born in 2001–2007 were used for estimation of heritabilities in threshold and mixed linear-threshold models [4]. In this sample of German Shepherd Dogs, heritability was 0.25 for CHD in the linear model and 0.19–0.27 for binary trait definitions regarding only borderline as CHD-affected and mild to severe CHD cases as CHD-affected versus CHD-free dogs. In a study of 13,124 Australian German Shepherd Dogs born between 1976 and 2005, the heritability of the summed phenotype constructed from nine ordinally-scored British Veterinary Association Hip Traits was 0.30 [5]. Linear models are commonly applied for genetic analyses of CHD as this methodology most correctly reflects the underlying nature of the data [4,5].

Complex segregation analyses demonstrated involvement of a major gene for the German Shepherd Dog [6,7]. Genome-wide linkage studies showed nine genome-wide significant quantitative trait loci (QTL) for CHD in German Shepherd Dogs [8]. A linkage study in a Labrador Retriever-Greyhound crossbred family revealed twelve dog chromosomes (CFA) with chromosome-wide significant markers for CHD [9]. In Portuguese Water Dogs, QTL for signs of CHD were demonstrated on CFA1 and 3 [10,11]. A genome-wide association study (GWAS) for CHD and osteoarthritis (OA) across several dog breeds including Labrador Retriever-Greyhound crosses identified four CHD-associated and two OA-associated SNPs. The CHD-associated SNPs were located on CFA3, 11 and 30 [12], but not within QTL of the Labrador Retriever-Greyhound crossbred linkage study [8]. In 174 Bernese Mountain Dogs, two different CHD-regions were identified on CFA14. A third CHD-associated region was located on CFA37 [13]. A Dutch study on 48 CHD-affected and 30 CHD-free Labrador Retrievers revealed significant SNPs on CFA8 [14] within a previously reported quantitative trait locus (QTL) in German Shepherd Dogs [8]. A 10-bp intronic deletion haplotype within *FBN2* on CFA11 was shown to be associated with CHD [15]. Dogs homozygous for this haplotype had significantly less *FBN2* mRNA in their femoral head articular cartilage [15]. The mutant *FBN2* haplotype was identified in 49 different breeds, but homozygous mutant haplotypes were only prevalent in Labrador and Golden Retrievers [16].

The objective of the present study was to perform a GWAS on 192 dogs to identify SNPs associated with CHD, followed by a validation of CHD-associated SNPs in a stratified sample of 843 dogs. We have chosen the German population of German Shepherd Dogs as this population is well suited for an association study, since this breed represents one of the largest purebred dog populations in Europe with a large phenotypic and genetic variance for CHD and a consistent recording system of CHD including the collection of EDTA-blood samples.

Results

The genome-wide scan using the canine 127K Affymetrix SNP chip (Affymetrix, Santa Clara, CA, USA) revealed five SNPs with $-\log_{10}$P-values>4.3 suggestive for association with CHD (Figure 1). We detected a genome-wide significant CHD-associated SNP on CFA24 in a region which was not significant in a previous linkage study for German Shepherd Dogs (Table S1) [8]. We determined the genome-wide threshold for significance at a $-\log_{10}$P-value > 5.98 which corresponds to a P-value <0.05 after applying the Bonferroni correction for multiple testing. The quantile-quantile (Q-Q) plots illustrated that inflation due to stratification effects had been removed by the mixed linear model employed for CHD (Figure S1).

The validation study included the five most significant SNPs on CFA19, 24, 26 and 34. Two SNPs were located on CFA34 and each one SNP on CFA19, 24 and 26 (Table S2). All these five SNPs were evaluated in 843 German Shepherd Dogs. The minor allele frequencies (MAF) ranged from 0.07 to 0.48 (Table 1). Each one SNP on CFA24, 26 and 34 was significantly associated with CHD in the validation set, whereas the SNP on CFA19 and one SNP on CFA34 did not pass validation (Table 2). The CHD-QTL on CFA24, 26 and 34 were confirmed in the analyses when dogs with the CHD grades C and D were separately compared with all CHD-free dogs (Tables 3–4). The CHD-QTL on CFA24 was also significant for the separate analysis for CHD-E (Table 5). A combined analysis for dogs free from CHD and dogs with CHD-D and CHD-E gave slightly higher $-\log_{10}$P-values compared to the analysis with CHD-A versus CHD-D dogs (data not shown).

The strongest association was found for the SNP on CFA24. In all analyses considering CHD-free German Shepherd Dogs versus mildly to severely CHD-affected dogs (C+D+E or C or D or E or D+E), BICF2S2367279 reached $-\log_{10}$P-values at 10–40. Odds ratios (ORs) were highest for BICF2S2367279 with values at 4.3–5.8. The CHD-associated genotype G/G of BICF2S2367279 on CFA24 occurred in 312/843 dogs and 27/312 were free from CHD and all other 285/312 were CHD-affected. Corresponding figures for BICF2S2367279 on CFA26 were for the CHD-associated genotype A/A were 369/843, 66/369 (CHD-free) and 303/369 (CHD-affected), respectively. The joint genotypes G/G and A/A had a frequency of 222/843 and only 10/222 were free from CHD, whereas 212/222 were CHD-affected.

The proportion of phenotypic variance of CHD explained by the cumulative effects of all five SNPs was 19.6% (all CHD-grades), 21.6% (CHD-A vs C), 31.6% (CHD-A vs CHD-D), 20.7% (CHD-A vs. CHD-E) and 28.0% (CHD-A vs. CHD-D and CHD-E).

Discussion

The present GWAS identified a novel genome-wide significant CHD-QTL on CFA24, which was validated in a large sample of German Shepherd Dogs stratified by sex, age, birth year, CHD-status and ancestry. A slight overestimation of the $-\log_{10}$P-values may be assumed in the detection sample because we used a linear model and not a cumulative logit model. However, the $-\log_{10}$P-value for the SNP on CFA24 was still below the Bonferroni significance threshold of 0.05 (Table S3). Further two QTL from a previous linkage study [8] could be confirmed through a GWAS and a validation study.

In close proximity to the SNP BICF2S2367279 on CFA24, the gene *SRC* (*v-src sarcoma (Schmidt-Ruppin A-2) viral oncogene homolog*) is located. This gene is involved in bone formation mediating cytoskeletal reorganization as well as osteoclast survival in response to RANKL in vitro [17]. Targeted disruption of *src* function in mice caused osteopetrosis, which is characterized by increased bone density due to impairment of osteoclast bone resorbing activity. Osteoclasts from src-null mice failed to form ruffled borders impairing their ability to resorb bone matrix [18].

On CFA26, the SNP BICF2P281364 is located within *KSR2* (*kinase suppressor of ras 2*) which encodes a scaffold protein interacting with members of the RAS/MAPK signalling pathway [19]. KSR2 has been suggested to be involved in activation of

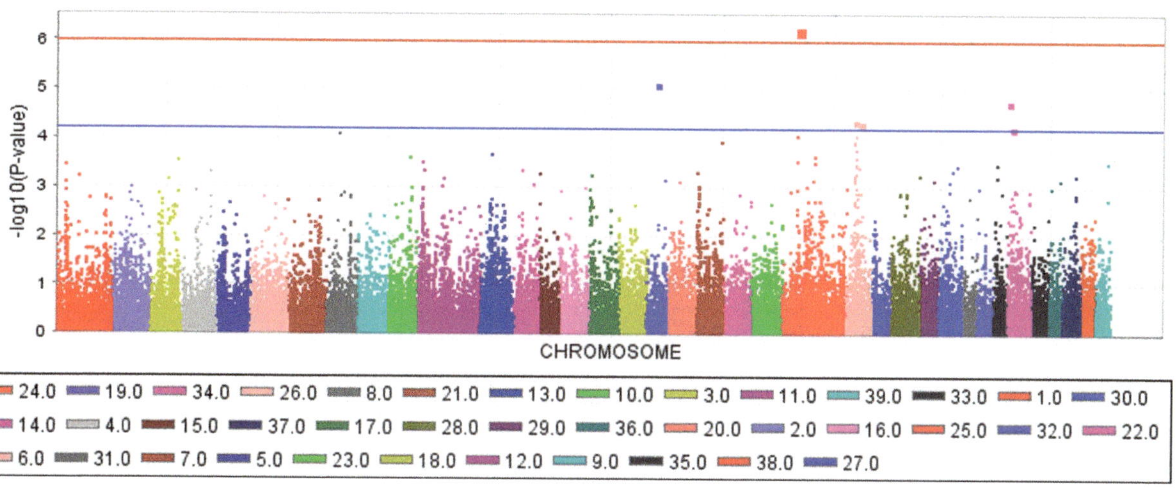

Figure 1. Manhattan plot of $-\log_{10}$P-values of the genome-wide association study for the canine hip dysplasia score in German Shepherd Dogs using a mixed linear model analysis. On the X-axis, the SNPs are given by dog chromosome number. The $-\log_{10}$P-values for each SNP genotype effect are plotted against the SNP position on each chromosome. Chromosomes are differentiated by colors. The color keys are given below the plot. The red line indicates a $-\log_{10}$P-value of 4.3 and the blue line indicates the threshold of the $-\log_{10}$P-values for genome-wide significance after correcting for multiple testing.

Table 1. SNP-IDs of the five SNPs genotyped in the validation set of 843 German Shepherd Dogs, their position on dog chromosome (CFA), their chromosomal position according to CanFam2.0, their minor alleles, their minor allele frequencies (MAF) in all dogs and among 277 unaffected dogs (CHD-grade A) and 566 affected dogs with 349 dogs classified as CHD-grade C, 152 dogs as CHD-grade D and 65 dogs as CHD-grade E.

SNP-ID	CFA	Position	Minor	MAF					
(CanFam2.0)		(Mb)	allele	Total	CHD-A	CHD-C/D/E	CHD-C	CHD-D	CHD-E
TIGRP2P265674	19	35.533	C	0.067	0.070	0.065	0.064	0.060	0.079
BICF2S2367279	24	28.944	G	0.483	0.247	0.607	0.419	0.655	0.587
BICF2P281364	26	17.181	G	0.366	0.506	0.299	0.293	0.305	0.318
BICF2P1086886	34	4.239	T	0.300	0.208	0.344	0.344	0.333	0.365
BICF2P355865	34	39.346	A	0.322	0.287	0.334	0.343	0.332	0.341

Table 2. Odds ratios (OR) of the five SNPs genotyped with their 95% lower (CL) and upper confidence limits (CU), χ^2- and -$\log_{10}$P-values for genotypic, allelic and trend association considering 277 CHD-A German Shepherd Dogs as controls and 566 German Shepherd Dogs classified as CHD-C/D/E as cases.

SNP-ID	CFA	OR	OR-CL	OR-CU	Genotype		Allele		Trend	
					χ^2	-$\log_{10}$P-value	χ^2	-$\log_{10}$P-value	χ^2	-$\log_{10}$P-value
TIGRP2P265674	19	1.01	0.73	1.65	2.96	0.64	0.19	0.18	0.19	0.18
BICF2S2367279	24	4.70	3.72	5.94	130.75	28.39	178.66	40.02	115.71	26.26
BICF2P281364	26	0.42	0.34	0.52	62.04	13.47	65.47	15.22	56.71	13.30
BICF2P1086886	34	1.99	1.55	2.55	29.39	6.38	30.39	7.45	27.39	6.78
BICF2P355865	34	0.78	0.62	0.98	4.65	1.01	4.51	1.47	4.60	1.50

Table 3. Odds ratios (OR) of the five SNPs genotyped with their 95% lower (CL) and upper confidence limits (CU), χ^2-values and -log$_{10}$P-values for genotypic, allelic and trend association considering 277 CHD-A German Shepherd Dogs as controls and 349 German Shepherd Dogs classified as CHD-C as cases.

SNP-ID	CFA	OR	OR-CL	OR-CU	Genotype		Allele		Trend	
					χ^2	-log$_{10}$P-value	χ^2	-log$_{10}$P-value	χ^2	-log$_{10}$P-value
TIGRP2P265674	19	1.11	0.70	1.75	3.57	0.77	0.20	0.19	0.20	0.18
BICF2S2367279	24	4.36	3.37	5.63	105.50	22.91	133.23	30.09	88.47	20.29
BICF2P281364	26	0.41	0.32	0.51	56.35	12.24	56.53	13.26	49.13	11.62
BICF2P1086886	34	1.99	1.53	2.60	26.24	5.70	26.17	6.50	24.24	6.07
BICF2P355865	34	0.77	0.60	0.99	4.51	0.98	4.22	1.40	4.34	1.43

Table 4. Odds ratios (OR) of the five SNPs genotyped with their 95% lower (CL) and upper confidence limits (CU), χ^2- and -log$_{10}$P-values for genotypic, allelic and trend association considering 277 CHD-A German Shepherd Dogs as controls and 152 German Shepherd Dogs classified as CHD-D as cases.

SNP-ID	CFA	OR	OR-CL	OR-CU	Genotype		Allele		Trend	
					χ^2	-log$_{10}$P-value	χ^2	-log$_{10}$P-value	χ^2	-log$_{10}$P-value
TIGRP2P265674	19	1.18	0.66	2.11	2.66	0.58	0.30	0.23	0.31	0.24
BICF2S2367279	24	5.78	4.21	7.93	106.83	23.20	127.20	28.77	87.40	20.05
BICF2P281364	26	0.43	0.32	0.58	32.68	7.10	31.09	7.61	28.64	7.06
BICF2P1086886	34	1.90	1.38	2.63	21.27	4.62	15.47	4.08	14.18	3.78
BICF2P355865	34	0.81	0.60	1.10	1.93	0.42	1.83	0.76	1.83	0.75

Table 5. Odds ratios (OR) of the five SNPs genotyped with their 95% lower (CL) and upper confidence limits (CU), χ^2- and -$\log_{10}$P-values for genotypic, allelic and trend association considering 277 CHD-A German Shepherd Dogs as controls and 65 German Shepherd Dogs classified as CHD-E as cases.

SNP-ID	CFA	OR	OR-CL	OR-CU	Genotype		Allele		Trend	
					χ^2	-$\log_{10}$P-value	χ^2	-$\log_{10}$P-value	χ^2	-$\log_{10}$P-value
TIGRP2P265674	19	0.88	0.42	1.82	0.13	0.15	0.12	0.14	0.13	0.15
BICF2S2367279	24	4.33	2.89	6.51	53.32	11.58	54.71	12.85	41.15	9.85
BICF2P281364	26	0.45	0.30	0.69	15.95	3.46	14.46	3.84	13.92	3.72
BICF2P1086886	34	2.19	1.44	3.33	15.51	3.37	13.70	3.84	13.76	3.68
BICF2P355865	34	0.78	0.51	1.18	1.45	0.31	1.43	0.63	1.45	0.64

molecules like p38 MAPK, cell cycle control proteins and proteins of the ubiquitin proteasome. The p38α and p38β MAPK proteins are important regulators of bone homeostasis controlling expression and activation of transcription factors implicated in osteoblastogenesis like RUNX2 [20,21]. In addition, KSR2 is predicted to mediate PI3K activation. Via PI3K, a RANKL mediated signalling pathway is activated which negatively regulates osteoclast survival [22,23].

On CFA34, the SNP BICF2P1086886 is located approximately 0.7 Mb downstream of the *triple functional domain (PTPRF interacting)* (*TRIO*) gene. The protein encoded by *TRIO* contains three functional domains, a serine/threonine kinase domain and two guanine nucleotide exchange factor (GEF) domains for the family of Rho-like GTPases, specific for Rac1 and RhoA [24]. Rac1 and RhoA act as antagonists, both playing an important role in chondrogenic proliferation and differentiation [25,26]. Chondrocyte-specific deletion of Rac1 in mice leads to dwarfism due to reduced chondrocyte proliferation [27]. Inhibition of Rac1 expression in micromass culture resulted in reduced mRNA levels of the chondrogenic markers collagen II and aggrecan, and decreased accumulation of glycosaminoglycans indicating that Rac1 promotes chondrogenesis [28]. Rac1-deficient chondrocytes had severely reduced levels of inducible nitric oxide synthase protein (iNOS) and nitric oxide production [29]. Mice deficient for iNOS had reduced chondrocyte proliferation and resembled the phenotype of Rac1-deficient growth plates. RhoA overexpression in chondrogenic ATDC5 cells resulted in increased proliferation and a marked delay of hypertrophic differentiation, whereas inhibition of Rho/ROCK signaling inhibited chondrocyte proliferation and accelerates hypertrophic differentiation [30]. Therefore, changing the balance between the GTPases RhoA and Rac1 due to mutations in *trio* will lead to disturbances in cartilage development.

In agreement with previous reports, the CHD-associated regions and the candidate genes identified here, support the key role of enchondral bone formation in the pathogenesis of CHD [8–16]. A candidate region identified in German Shepherd Dogs [8] and Labrador Retrievers [14] on CFA8 at 29 Mb harbours the potential candidate gene *LRR1*. The encoded protein is involved in proteoglycan synthesis through NF-κB signalling transduction and cartilage integrity like iNOS and MAPK proteins [31]. In Bernese Mountain Dogs, *FN1* was identified as a candidate gene for CHD [13]. FN1 had been proposed to have a function in matrix organization of cartilage [32]. In an across-breed GWAS, *EVC* and *EVC2* on CFA3, *PTPRD* on CFA11 and *MFAP1* on CFA30 were suggested as CHD candidate genes [12]. All these genes are highly expressed in cartilage and mutations in these genes can cause chondrodysplasia (*EVC*, *EVC2*), Marfan syndrome (*MFAP1*) or restless legs syndrome (*PTPRD*) [12].

For the candidate genes on CFA24, 26 and 34, we could find a joint network involved in bone formation using GENEMANIA (http://www.genemania.org/). Joint co-expression and physical interactions had been indicated for *TRIO, SRC* and *KSR2*. This may indicate the QTL identified harbour genes contributing to CHD on the same pathways. Using the candidate genes *LRR1*, *FN1*, *PTPRD* and *MFAP1*, we could extend the network for *TRIO, SRC* and *KSR2*, primarily through *RAC1*.

In conclusion, this study identified and corroborated CHD-loci on three different chromosomes for German Shepherd Dogs and is a further step towards elucidation of the genes underlying CHD. The three validated and significantly CHD-associated SNPs are located within or in close proximity to genes which are involved in a joint network regulating bone formation, osteoclast activity, chondrocyte proliferation and differentiation.

Material and Methods

Ethics Statement

All animal work has been conducted according to the national and international guidelines for animal welfare. The dogs in this study were included with the consent of their owners. The blood samples were collected by veterinarians during the routine examination for CHD regarding principles of good veterinary practice. These diagnostic procedures had to be carried out anyway. All blood-sampling of dogs was done in veterinary practices for small animals by trained staff. CHD examinations are compulsory for all dogs intended for breeding and these examinations were performed in veterinary clinics and practices according to the rules for hip screening of the Fédération Cynologique Internationale (FCI). Approval from the ethics committee was not obtained because blood sampling was done during a diagnostic veterinary procedure according to the German Animal Welfare Law (released on 05/18/2006, last changes on 08/07/2013).

Animals

A total of 1035 German Shepherd Dogs had been included in the present association study for CHD. The sample for the GWAS to identify significantly associated SNPs contained 192 dogs and the validation set 834 dogs. First, we selected the dogs for the GWAS and then, the validation sample was collected from available databases and bio-banks. The study population was a stratified sample from all registered and X-rayed dogs of the German population of German Shepherd Dogs born between 2000 and 2005. Dogs had an age at examination of 12–14 months in each cohort. Coancestry among cases and controls as well as within cases and within controls was minimized. In addition, the samples used were stratified by sex, age at radiographic examination, birth year, coancestry and CHD-affection. The pedigree records from eleven generations were employed to calculate relationship coefficients among all dogs using PEDIG software [33]. The study population had mean relationship coefficients among all individual dogs <0.1%. Cases and controls were chosen with equal proportions of sexes and birth cohorts from the years 2000–2005. Dogs were 12–14 months old at radiographic examination. Radiographs and CHD-scores according to the official guidelines of the FCI as well as EDTA-blood samples for parentage testing were collected by the Association for German Shepherd Dogs (SV, Augsburg). Parentage testing is mandatory for all German Shepherd Dogs intended for breeding. For all dogs included in the present study, parentage has been confirmed using an approved set of microsatellites for parentage control. The radiographs were made by veterinarians officially approved by the association of radiographic diagnosis for genetically influenced skeletal diseases of small animals (GRSK) and the German Association for Dog Breeding and Husbandry (VDH) strictly following the requirements for radiographs of hip joints of the FCI. All X-rays were evaluated by a recognized veterinary expert and a subsample of 200 X-rays was re-evaluated by further two experts. Consistency of diagnoses was >99%. These officially recorded CHD-grades were supplied by the SV and used in all subsequent analyses. CHD-A includes dogs with normal hips, CHD-C dogs with slight signs of CHD, CHD-D dogs with moderate signs of CHD and CHD-E dogs with severe signs of CHD using X-rays from both hip joints. Dogs with mild, moderate or severe signs of CHD were defined as CHD-affected. Controls were dogs free from any signs of CHD.

Genome-wide Association Study

A genome-wide screening for polymorphic and CHD-associated SNPs was performed using the canine 127K Affymetrix SNP chip (Affymetrix). This sample included 192 German Shepherd Dogs whereof 96 were free from CHD, 65 mildly, 22 moderately and 9 severely CHD-affected. Cases and controls were balanced by CHD score, sex, birth year, age at veterinary radiographic examination and coancestry. The animals were unrelated at least at the grandparent level. Relationship coefficients with the validation sample were as low as possible and did not exceed 0.1%, on average. The dogs from both data sets, the detection and validation samples, were unrelated at least on the grandparent level. Quality criteria were minor allele frequency (MAF) >0.05, genotyping rate per SNP and animal >0.90 and HWE ($p<0.00001$). After filtering for quality criteria, 47,729 SNPs remained for the final analysis. Data analysis was done for the CHD-score as quasi-continuous target trait. We used a mixed linear model with sex and genotype as fixed effects and a random animal effect through an identity-by-state-kinship (IBS) matrix. A Q-matrix to detect population structure was estimated using principal components (PCAs). We also tested several extended models employing up to five PCAs to show the robustness of the outcome of the GWAS. All these models yielded the same highly significant associated SNP as the final model. Thus, adding principal components for cryptic data structure did not change the results of the final model. Thus, the IBS matrix reflected the genomic relationship matrix among all individuals genotyped and captured the relatedness among animals as well as the cryptic family structure. The analysis was run using TASSEL, version 3.0.164 [34].

Validation Study

Cases and controls were matched by sex, birth year, age at radiographic examination, CHD score and coancestry (Table 6). We edited 843 German Shepherd Dogs out of a group of 12,096 dogs which fitted our study design and had mean relationship coefficients <0.1% with any other individual dog in the sample. The animals were born in 2000–2005 and purebred following the rules of the SV. Distribution of CHD-scores in the 405 males and the 438 females was as follows. In the males, 136 (16.1%) CHD-A, 176 (20.9%) CHD-C, 72 (8.5%) CHD-D and 21 (2.5%) CHD-E; in the females, 141 (16.7%) CHD-A, 173 (20.5%) CHD-C, 80 (9.5%) CHD-D and 44 (5.2%) CHD-E. Dogs scored as CHD-A were treated as unaffected ($n = 277$), dogs scored as CHD-C ($n = 349$), CHD-D ($n = 152$) and CHD-E ($n = 65$) as affected. Association analyses were performed using odds ratios with their 95% confidence limits and χ^2-tests for genotypic and allelic associations and the allelic trend with the CHD status (CHD-A vs. CHD-C/D/E) and with CHD-A versus CHD-C, CHD-D or CHD-E. We tested for the different CHD grades separately to see whether the association is consistent across the different CHD-grades or may be caused by a specific CHD-grade. The CASECONTROL procedure of SAS/Genetics, version 9.3 (Statistical Analysis System, Cary, NC, USA, 2013), was used for these calculations.

DNA Preparation and Genotyping

DNA was isolated from EDTA-blood samples using the NucleoSpin Kit 96 Blood Quick Pure Kit (Macherey-Nagel, Düren, Germany). Five SNPs on CFA19, 24, 26 and 34 were chosen for validation from the GWAS. Genotyping of the validation SNP set consisting of five SNPs was performed using the ABI Prism SNaPshot™ Multiplex System (Life Technologies by Applied Biosystems, Darmstadt, Germany) (Table S2). Single

Table 6. Number of German Shepherd Dogs included in the validation study. Distribution of the 843 dogs by canine hip dysplasia (CHD) score, sex and birth year is given.

Birth year	CHD-A		CHD-C		CHD-D		CHD-E		Total	
	male	female	male	female	male	female	male	female	male	female
2000/2001	35	34	63	58	16	21	10	24	124	137
2002	32	33	31	25	23	18	5	11	91	87
2003	27	27	29	32	14	19	4	4	74	82
2004/2005	42	47	43	58	19	22	2	5	116	132
	136	141	176	173	72	80	21	44	405	438
Total	277		349		152		65		843	

base extension (SBE) primers were designed using online primer design software BatchPrimer3 (http://probes.pw.usda.gov/cgi-bin/batchprimer3/batchprimer3.cgi). According to the manufacturer's instructions, the primer sequences should differ in length by at least four to six nucleotides and should not contain possible extendable hairpin structures. All primers used here had undergone HPLC purification. The primer design was in this way that a difference of seven nucleotides between the SBE primers was achieved by adding non-homologous polynucleotides (poly (dNTP)) at the 5′end. The SBE detection was performed using an ABI Genetic Analyzer 3500 (Life Technologies by Applied Biosystems). Data evaluation was done using GeneMapper, version 4.2 (Life Technologies by Applied Biosystems).

Statistical Analysis

Allele and genotype frequencies of the SNPs were calculated for the different CHD-grades as well as the observed heterozygosity (H_0), the polymorphism information content (PIC) and Hardy-Weinberg equilibrium were estimated using the ALLELE procedure of SAS/Genetics. Association analyses were performed using odds ratios with their 95% confidence limits and χ^2-tests of the CASECONTROL procedure of SAS/Genetics for genotypic and allelic associations and the allelic trend with the CHD status (CHD-A vs. CHD-C/D/E) and with CHD-A versus CHD-C, CHD-D or CHD-E. These four definitions of phenotypes were used for all analyses. A SNP was regarded as genome-wide significantly associated for $-\log_{10}$P-values>5.98 and suggestive for association with $-\log_{10}$P-values>4.3. The same cutoffs were applied for the validation study. A general linear model including all CHD-associated SNPs was used to estimate the proportion of the phenotypic variance explained by these SNPs. Calculations were performed using SAS, version 9.3.

Supporting Information

Figure S1 Q-Q-plot of expected $-\log_{10}$P-values versus observed$-\log_{10}$P-values from the mixed linear model analysis for canine hip dysplasia score in German Shepherd Dogs. Shown are all 47,729 SNPs included in the genome-wide association analysis with the grey line corresponding to the null hypothesis of no association.

Table S1 Results of the genome-wide association study for canine hip dysplasia in 192 German Shepherd Dogs. Given are the SNP-IDs with their locations on the dog chromosome according to CanFam2.0, the minor allele frequencies (MAF) in the sample and $-\log_{10}$P-values (P-MLM) from the mixed linear model analysis. The SNP BICF2S2367279 exceeds the threshold (5.98) for genome-wide significance.

Table S2 Single nucleotide polymorphisms (SNPs) with their chromosomal positions on CanFam2.0, adjacent genes, SBE primers, SBE orientations and SNP motifs genotyped in the validation set including 843 German Shepherd Dogs.

Table S3 Comparison of $-\log_{10}$P-values using a cumulative logit and a linear model for an association analysis of canine hip dysplasia genotyped in the detection sample including 192 German Shepherd Dogs considering 96 CHD-A dogs as controls and 65 mildly, 22 moderately and 9 severely CHD-affected dogs. Shown are the raw $-\log_{10}$P-values of the five highest CHD-associated SNPs for a model with genotype as the sole effect and the overestimation of the raw -$\log_{10}$P-values through a linear model.

Acknowledgments

The authors thank the Associaton of German Shepherd Dogs (Verein für Deutsche Schäferhunde e.V., SV), Augsburg, Germany, for providing the pedigree data, X-rays, the official CHD scores and EDTA-blood samples collected for paternity testing. The authors are grateful to U. Philipp and H. Klippert-Hasberg for expert technical assistance.

Author Contributions

Conceived and designed the experiments: OD. Performed the experiments: LF OD. Analyzed the data: LF OD. Contributed reagents/materials/analysis tools: OD. Wrote the paper: LF OD.

References

1. Janutta V, Distl O (2006) Inheritance of canine hip dysplasia: review of estimation methods and of heritability estimates and prospects on further developments. Dtsch tierärztl Wschr 113: 6–12.
2. Janutta V, Hamann H, Distl O (2008) Genetic and phenotypic trends in canine hip dysplasia in the German population of German shepherd dogs. Berl Münch tierärztl Wschr 121: 102–109.
3. Hamann H, Kirchhoff T, Distl O (2003) Bayesian analysis of heritability of canine hip dysplasia in German shepherd dogs. J Anim Breed Genet 120: 258–268.
4. Stock KF, Klein S, Tellhelm B, Distl O (2011) Genetic analyses of elbow and hip dysplasia in the German shepherd dog. J Anim Breed Genet 128: 219–229.
5. Wilson BJ, Nicholas FW, James JW, Wade CM, Tammen I, et al. (2012) Heritability and phenotypic variation of canine hip dysplasia radiographic traits in a cohort of Australian German shepherd dogs. PLoS One 7(6):e39620.
6. Janutta V, Hamann H, Distl O (2006) Complex segregation analysis of canine hip dysplasia in German shepherd dogs. J Hered 97: 13–20.
7. Mäki K, Janss LLG, Groen AF, Liinamo AE, Ojala M (2004) An indication of major genes affecting hip and elbow dysplasia in four Finnish dog populations. Hered 92: 402–408.
8. Marschall Y, Distl O (2007) Mapping quantitative trait loci for canine hip dysplasia in German shepherd dogs. Mamm Genome 18: 861–870.
9. Todhunter RJ, Mateescu R, Lust G, Burton-Wurster NI, Dykes NL, et al. (2005) Quantitative trait loci for hip dysplasia in a crossbreed canine pedigree. Mamm Genome 16: 720–730.
10. Chase K, Lawler DF, Adler FR, Ostrander EA, Lark KG (2004) Bilaterally asymmetric effects of quantitative trait loci (QTLs): QTLs that affect laxity in the right versus left coxofemoral (hip) joints of the dog (Canis familiaris). Am J Med Genet A 124A: 239–247.
11. Chase K, Lawler DF, Carrier DR, Lark KG (2005) Genetic regulation of osteoarthritis: A QTL regulating cranial and caudal acetabular osteophyte formation in the hip joint of the dog (Canis familiaris). Am J Med Genet A 135: 334–335.
12. Zhou Z, Sheng X, Zhang Z, Zhao K, Zhu L, et al. (2010) Differential genetic regulation of canine hip dysplasia and osteoarthritis. PLoS One 5: e13219.
13. Pfahler S, Distl O (2012) Identification of quantitative trait loci (QTL) for canine hip dysplasia and canine elbow dysplasia in Bernese mountain dogs. PLoS One 7(11): e49782.
14. Lavrijsen IC, Leegwater PA, Martin AJ, Harris SJ, Tryfonidou MA, et al. (2014) Genome wide analysis indicates genes for basement membrane and cartilage matrix proteins as candidates for hip dysplasia in Labrador Retrievers. PLoS One 9(1):e87735.
15. Friedenberg SG, Zhu L, Zhang Z, Foels Wv, Schweitzer PA, et al. (2011) Evaluation of a fibrillin 2 gene haplotype associated with hip dysplasia and incipient osteoarthritis in dogs. Am J Vet Res 72: 530–540.
16. Broeckx BJ, Coopman F, Verhoeven GE, Van Haeringen W, van de Goor L, et al. (2013) The prevalence of nine genetic disorders in a dog population from Belgium, the Netherlands and Germany. PLoS One 8(9):e74811.
17. Boyce BF, Xing L, Yao Z, Yamashita T, Shakespeare WC, et al. (2006) SRC inhibitors in metastatic bone disease. Clinical Cancer Research 12(20 Pt 2): 6291s–5s.
18. Miyazaki T, Tanaka S, Sanjay A, Baron R (2006) The role of c-Src kinase in the regulation of osteoclast function. Mod Rheumatol 16: 68–74.
19. Liu L, Channavajhala PL, Rao VR, Moutsatsos I, Wu L, et al. (2009) Proteomic characterization of the dynamic KSR-2 interactome, a signaling scaffold complex in MAPK pathway. Biochim Biophys Acta 1794: 1485–1495.
20. Chen G, Deng C, Li YP (2012) TGF-β and BMP signaling in osteoblast differentiation and bone formation. Int J Biol Sci 8: 272–288.
21. Thouverey C, Caverzasio J (2012) The p38α MAPK positively regulates osteoblast function and postnatal bone acquisition. Cell Mol Life Sci 69: 3115–3125.
22. Adapala NS, Barbe MF, Langdon WY, Nakamura MC, Tsygankov AY, et al. (2010) The loss of Cbl-phosphatidylinositol 3-kinase interaction perturbs RANKL-mediated signaling, inhibiting bone resorption and promoting osteoclast survival. J Biol Chem 285: 36745–3658.
23. Brennan T, Adapala NS, Barbe MF, Yingling V, Sanjay A (2011) Abrogation of Cbl-PI3K interaction increases bone formation and osteoblast proliferation. Calc Tiss Int 89: 396–410.
24. Debant A, Serra-Pages C, Seipel K, O'Brien S, Tang M, et al. (1996) The multidomain protein Trio binds the LAR transmembrane tyrosine phosphatase, contains a protein kinase domain, and has separate rac-specific and rho-specific guanine nucleotide exchange factor domains. Proc Natl Acad Sci USA 93: 5466–5471.
25. Bellanger JM, Astier C, Sardet C, Ohta Y, Stossel TP, et al. (2000) The Rac1- and RhoG-specific GEF domain of Trio targets filamin to remodel cytoskeletal actin. Nat Cell Biol 2: 888–892.
26. Wang G, Beier F (2005) Rac1/Cdc42 and RhoA GTPases antagonistically regulate chondrocyte proliferation, hypertrophy, and apoptosis. J Bone Min Res 20: 1022–1031.
27. Wang G, Woods A, Agoston H, Ulici V, Glogauer M, et al. (2007) Genetic ablation of Rac1 in cartilage results in chondrodysplasia. Dev Biol 306: 612–623.
28. Woods A, Wang G, Dupuis H, Shao Z, Beier F (2007) Rac1 signaling stimulates N-cadherin expression, mesenchymal condensation, and chondrogenesis. J Biol Chem 282: 23500–23508.
29. Wang G, Yan Q, Woods A, Aubrey LA, Feng Q, et al. (2011) Inducible nitric oxide synthase-nitric oxide signaling mediates the mitogenic activity of Rac1 during endochondral bone growth. J Cell Sci 124: 3405–3413.
30. Wang G, Woods A, Sabari S, Pagnotta L, Stanton LA, et al. (2004) RhoA/ROCK signaling suppresses hypertrophic chondrocyte differentiation. J Biol Chem 279: 13205–13214.
31. Chowdhury TT, Salter DM, Bader DL, Lee DA (2008) Signal transduction pathways involving p38 MAPK, JNK, NFkappaB and AP-1 influences the response of chondrocytes cultured in agarose constructs to IL-1beta and dynamic compression. Inflamm Res 57: 306–313.
32. MacLeod JN, Burton-Wurster N, Gu DN, Lust G (1996) Fibronectin mRNA splice variant in articular cartilage lacks bases encoding the V, III-15, and I-10 protein segments. J Biol Chem 271: 18954–18960.
33. Boichard D (2002) PEDIG: A fortran package for pedigree analysis suited for large populations. Proc 7th WCGALP, Montepellier, France: CD-ROM comm 28–13.
34. Bradbury PJ, Zhang Z, Kroon DE, Casstevens TM, Ramdoss Y, et al. (2007) TASSEL: software for association mapping of complex traits in diverse samples. Bioinformatics 23: 2633–2635.

22

CTXA Hip—An Extension of Classical DXA Measurements Using Quantitative CT

Christopher E. Cann[1,2], Judith E. Adams[3], J. Keenan Brown[1], Alan D. Brett[1]*

1 Mindways Software, Inc., Austin, Texas, United States of America, **2** Department of Radiology, University of California San Francisco, San Francisco, California, United States of America, **3** Department of Clinical Radiology, University of Manchester, Manchester, United Kingdom

Abstract

Bone mineral density (BMD) estimates for the proximal femur using Dual Energy X-ray Absorptiometry (DXA) are currently considered the standard for making a diagnosis of osteoporosis in an individual patient using BMD alone. We have compared BMD results from a commercial Quantitative CT (QCT) BMD analysis system, "CTXA Hip", which provides clinical data for the proximal femur, to results from DXA. We have also used CTXA Hip to determine cortical and trabecular contributions to total BMD. Sixty-nine patients were scanned using 3D QCT and DXA. CTXA Hip BMD measurements for Total Hip and Femoral Neck were compared to DXA results. Twenty-two women were scanned at 0,1,2 years and CTXA Hip and DXA results analyzed for long-term reproducibility. Long-term reproducibility calculated as root-mean-square averages of SDs *in vivo* was 0.012 g/cm^2 (CV = 1.8%) for CTXA Total Hip and 0.011 g/cm^2 (CV = 2.0%) for CTXA Femoral Neck compared to 0.014 g/cm^2 (CV = 2.0%) and 0.016 g/cm^2 (CV = 2.7%), respectively, for DXA. The correlation of Total Hip BMD CTXA vs. DXA was R = 0.97 and for Femoral Neck was R = 0.95 (SEE 0.044 g/cm^2 in both cases). Cortical bone comprised 62±5% (mean ± SD) of total hipbone mass in osteoporotic women. CTXA Hip provides substantially the same clinical information as conventional DXA and in addition provides estimates of BMD in separate cortical and trabecular bone compartments, which may be useful in evaluation of bone strength.

Editor: Hani A. Awad, University of Rochester, United States of America

Funding: The authors have no support or funding to report.

Competing Interests: Christopher Cann and Keenan Brown are stockholders of Mindways Software, Inc. Alan Brett and Keenan Brown are employees of Mindways Software, Inc.

* E-mail: alan@qct.com

Introduction

Osteoporosis is a major public health concern. It is estimated that up to 50% of women and 20% of men in the US are at risk for developing an osteoporosis-related fracture during their lifetime [1]. Bone mineral density (BMD) estimates may be used to test for osteoporotic fracture risk and to make decisions about the initiation of pharmacologic therapy. According to the official positions of the International Society for Clinical Densitometry (ISCD) [2] and the National Osteoporosis Foundation (NOF) [3], central DXA of the lumbar spine and proximal femur is the preferred method for bone mineral density (BMD) testing. Osteoporosis is diagnosed by central DXA in postmenopausal women and in men aged 50 years and older if the T-score of the lumbar spine or hip is −2.5 or less. Low bone mass or osteopenia is classified as a T-score of −1.0 or less [2].

Despite the fracture risk statistics, osteoporosis testing with dual-energy X-ray absorptiometry (DXA) remains underused [4]. However, BMD can also be assessed with other radiologic imaging tools, such as quantitative computed tomography (QCT) that may be available when access to DXA is restricted.

Historically, in spite of QCT having a number of advantages over DXA [5], the use of QCT was limited by a number of factors including the cost and availability of early CT scanners, and the time required for analysis using the first QCT systems. In addition, the original implementations of 2D QCT BMD measurement at the spine tended to show lower precision due to the operator dependence of 2D scan protocols based on tilting a CT gantry, and QCT is associated with a relatively high x-ray dose compared to DXA. However, modern MDCT machines are both fast and widely available, and have allowed the introduction of 3D QCT volumetric scan protocols, reducing operator dependence and enabling CV precision errors of 0.8% [6]. Contemporary low-dose CT techniques directed at focused regions of interest and utilizing Automatic Exposure Control (AEC) can minimize radiation exposure [7].

While DXA of the spine computes an "areal BMD" (aBMD) measurement by the projection of integral (cortical and trabecular) vertebral bone onto a 2D plane, QCT provides a volumetric BMD measure of the trabecular vertebral bone in isolation. This can have an advantage of superior sensitivity due to the higher metabolic rate of turnover of trabecular bone [5]; and can also avoid the confounding effects of joint-space narrowing, osteophytes, aortic calcification and other extra-osseous calcification that can artificially raise a DXA spine BMD measurement [8–11]. However, the measurement of isolated trabecular bone means that QCT vertebral T-scores are somewhat lower than DXA T-scores for the same age [12] and application of the established WHO classification of osteoporosis by DXA T-score is not appropriate. In order to facilitate the interpretation of QCT spine results, the American College of Radiology has in 2008 published guidelines for the performance of QCT [13]; based on these guidelines, volumetric trabecular BMD values from 120 to 80 mg/cm^3 are defined as osteopenic and BMD values below 80 mg/cm^3 as osteoporotic.

In addition to the spine, the hip is an important fracture risk site and therefore an important site for axial BMD measurement [14] and areal BMD measurement at the femoral neck is one of the clinical risk factors included in the WHO FRAX 10-year fracture risk calculation tool [15]. While 3D QCT systems for measurement at the hip have been proposed and developed for research [16], the volumetric BMD measurements from these tools lack the normal comparative data that exists for lumbar spine QCT.

CTXA Hip uses 3D QCT volume data sets to generate bone projection images that visually look like those generated by DXA. CTXA Hip exploits the anatomical detail in the 3D QCT data set to segment bone from surrounding tissues rather than relying on the dual-energy imaging method of DXA. While CTXA Hip and DXA use somewhat different technologies to generate bone projection images of the proximal femur, the projection images from both devices convey the same basic information—total bone mass per projected bone area. This leads to the hypothesis that CTXA Hip BMD estimates provide the same clinical utility as that afforded by DXA. Importantly, the areal BMD measurements and T-scores derived from CTXA Hip may be used with the WHO diagnostic classifications.

This kind of approach has been shown to have excellent correlation with DXA for areal BMD measurement for the Total Hip region [17]. In a previous study using CTXA Hip, Khoo et al compared it with DXA-derived areal bone mineral density and T-scores [18]. However, that study looked at a cohort of elderly patients aged 82.8+/−2.5 years (mean +/− SD) and did not utilize CTXA to derive separate measurement from cortical and trabecular compartments; CTXA Hip may provide more information than DXA from a study due to the greater anatomical detail accessible from the 3D QCT volume data set relative to the information present in the planar projection images intrinsic to DXA.

In this study, we compare CTXA Hip and DXA areal BMD measures at both the femoral neck and total hip regions in a cohort of women between the ages of 20–80 years. We also present cortical and trabecular BMD estimates from standard (DXA) hip ROIs derived using CTXA Hip as additional information available from this method.

Materials and Methods

QCT studies were performed using the QCT Pro calibration phantom and software system with the CTXA Hip analysis module (Mindways Software, Inc., Austin, TX). The Mindways liquid calibration phantom used in this study was based on the original QCT calibration system developed at University of California, San Francisco (UCSF) [19], and mineral density results are reported in terms of equivalent calibrated aqueous potassium phosphate density. The QCT Pro QA phantom included a reference tube that contains aqueous K_2HPO_4 with a concentration of 200.0±0.4 mg/cm^3, and was used within the software both as a cross-calibration reference and for monitoring scanner performance.

Quality assurance (QA) scans were performed once a month according to manufacturer's protocols. In brief, the QA phantom was placed above the calibration phantom and 8–10 axial slices were scanned using the same study protocol used for BMD studies as described below, see Figure 1.

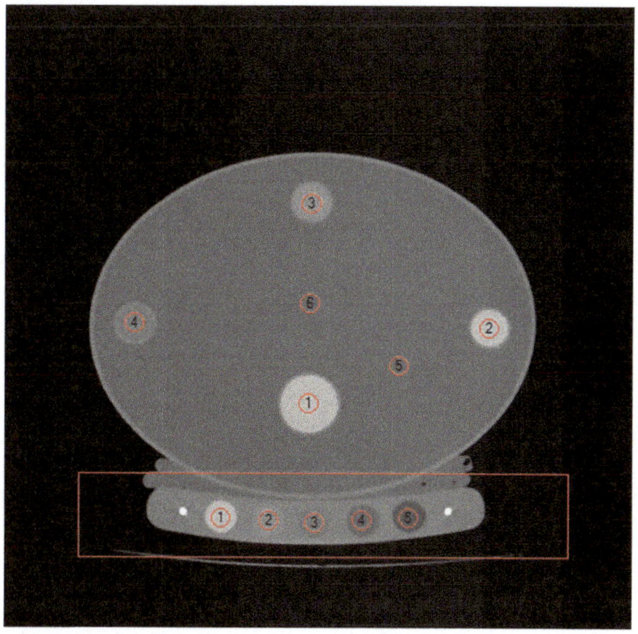

Figure 1. QA study axial image. Completed ROI placement in axial CT slice of quality assurance and CT calibration reference phantoms positioned for QA studies.

Subjects

Precision Study. A total of 22 subjects enrolled as placebo controls in an osteoporosis treatment study at the University of California, San Francisco (UCSF) comprised the precision study group. These "placebo" subjects were all postmenopausal osteoporotic women receiving hormone replacement therapy, calcium and vitamin D, and ranged in age from 55 to 72 years. All women were enrolled in that study by being identified as "osteoporotic" based on a spine or hip BMD T-score by DXA less than −2.5. Hip BMD was measured at yearly intervals for each subject using DXA and QCT. Ten of the 22 women received three hip BMD scans over a two year interval while 12 of the women received four hip BMD scans over a three year interval.

Interobserver Variability. The interobserver variability for BMD estimates using CTXA was estimated by comparing results obtained independently on the same in vivo data set by two trained operators. Data from a single clinical trial site were used for this analysis. Twenty eight studies were analyzed, and the results for estimated BMD of the femoral neck and total hip regions of interest were compared.

CTXA-DXA Comparison

A total of 69 patients having DXA exams for osteoporosis diagnostic testing were recruited from two clinical centers, the University of Manchester, UK, and Schenectady Radiology/Ellis Hospital, Schenectady, NY, for comparison of CTXA Hip and DXA results. Thirty patients were recruited at one center and 39 patients at the other. Seven patients were men and 62 were women. Ages ranged from 20–80 years, but the patients were predominantly postmenopausal women.

Ethics

All subjects involved in this study gave written informed consent, and all research protocols were approved by the Institutional Review Boards at the respective institutions: the

Institutional Review Board of Ellis Hospital, Schenectady, NY, USA; the Committee on Human Research (CHR), the UCSF Institutional Review Board holding Department of Health and Human Services Multiple Project Assurance #M-1169, University of California, San Francisco, USA; and the Ethics Committee of the University of Manchester, Manchester, UK.

Scanning Protocols

CTXA Examinations. CT image data analyzed for these studies using CTXA Hip were acquired using different CT scanner models at the three institutions. At UCSF, a GE9800 (GE Medical Systems, Waukesha, WI) was used, at the University of Manchester a Philips SR4000 (Philips Medical Systems, Best, Netherlands) was used, and at Schenectady Radiology a GE ProSpeed (GE Medical Systems, Waukesha, WI) was used. All CT scanners were maintained as specified by the manufacturers. In addition, all CT systems were further calibrated for QCT using the QCT Pro QA procedures.

Subjects were positioned supine on the CT scanner table, lying on top of a K_2HPO_4 CT calibration phantom and bolus bags so that the calibration phantom extended from the lumbar vertebrae to mid-thigh, to cover the pelvis and proximal femur region. Positioning was used so that the pelvis was as straight as possible and the knees were flat on the scanner table. Subjects were asked to put their feet together and remain still, but the feet were not restrained by a positioner. An anterior-posterior computed radiograph was obtained by the scanner from the iliac crest to mid-thigh, and the top of the femoral head to approximately 1 cm below the inferior extent of the lesser trochanter was defined graphically to define the scanning region. A contiguous series of scans was obtained, 3 mm thick every 3 mm, with a 40 cm display field-of-view (0.781 mm pixel size), and a standard abdomen reconstruction algorithm. Typically 40 images were obtained, with the time to acquire this image set approximately 3.5 minutes on the GE9800 and 1 minute on the Philips and ProSpeed scanners. Scanning parameters varied slightly depending on the capabilities of the CT scanner used and patient size, and were 80 kVp, 240 mAs for the GE9800, and 120 kVp, 100–200 mAs for the Philips and ProSpeed scanners. All subject and QA data were sent to Mindways where analysis was centralized.

DXA Examinations. DXA image data were acquired and analyzed at each site according to standard procedures used at those sites, including daily calibrations for quality control. A single individual at each site was responsible for all DXA analyses. At UCSF, DXA data were acquired using a Hologic QDR1000 (Hologic, Inc., Bedford, MA) scanner, while at the other two sites Hologic QDR4500 scanners were used. The DXA systems were calibrated and maintained in accordance with the manufacturer's specifications. The DXA data were acquired and analyzed according to the manufacturer's instructions.

Data Analysis

QA phantom data for each CT scanner were analyzed using the QCT Pro QA analysis module. Each QA study of 8–10 QA images acquired using the same technique as for subject scans was analyzed to determine CT scanner performance characteristics, and any deviations from expected performance were identified by the software. Any degradation of scanner performance identified by the QA software was resolved before subsequent subject data were analyzed. Subject results were referenced to the appropriate CT scanner QA results.

The QA phantom data is also used by the CTXA Hip software to detect and characterize differences in CT value response and make a correction to the CT calibration slope to compensate for "beam hardening" effects.

CT image data were analyzed in a standardized fashion with the CTXA Hip software, using the left proximal femur unless pathology prevented this. A square box region of interest was centered over the femoral neck as identified on the axial images, and a volumetric region of interest containing the proximal femur was extracted from the CT image data set for analysis. Segmentation of bone from surrounding non-bone tissue was performed using an adaptive algorithm controlled by three parameters. The first parameter defined a threshold below which a pixel could not be classified as bone (default: −250 mg/cm3). The second parameter defined the size of the neighborhood of pixels considered when adaptively modifying the local threshold. A default range corresponds to a neighborhood with a width of approximately five pixels. The third parameter was the initial threshold used to seed the adaptive algorithm, with pixels exceeding the initial threshold tentatively classified as "bone" and the remainder as "not bone" (default: 120 mg/cm3). The result of the segmentation process is a set of voxels identified as "bone" all contained within the outer cortex of the proximal femur. There was no further separation of voxels within this outer envelope as "marrow" vs. "bone" voxels. This 3D data set of bone voxels was then rotated such that the femoral shaft was vertical in the coronal and sagittal planes and the femoral neck was horizontal in the axial plane (Figure 2).

The CTXA Hip software generates a 2-dimensional image similar to a DXA image from the rotated 3D data set by summing all the bone voxels along lines perpendicular to the coronal plane. Each pixel of the resulting image represented the mass of mineral summed along that line, and was further characterized by a known pixel area, and a total volume of bone along the line. Regions of interest representing the common ROIs used for DXA analysis (Total Hip, Femoral Neck, Trochanter, Intertrochanter) were identified automatically on the projected image by the software (Figure 3). The lower extent of the Intertrochanter ROI was set at the lower junction of the lesser trochanter and the femoral shaft. The angle of the femoral neck axis, and the position and size of the femoral neck box ROI, were adjusted by the operator as required.

Results for areal BMD (g/cm^2), volumetric BMD (mg/cm^3), mass (g), area (cm^2) and volume (cm^3) for each of the ROIs were stored in the QCT Pro database and exported as text files for analysis.

In addition to the primary data analysis of total bone in the projected ROIs, the software also allows classification of bone voxels as "cortical" or "trabecular" based on a simple user-defined threshold. A threshold of 350 mg/cm^3 was used to separate "cortical" from "trabecular" bone in these ROIs. This value was chosen empirically as that which compartmentalized the major compressive and tensile trabecular bone groupings as "trabecular" bone. The choice of this threshold also identified higher density endocortical bone as "cortical" even though it was not part of the haversian cortex. The same measurements of area BMD, volumetric BMD, mass, area, and volume were given for each of these compartments. Compartmental analysis of the ROIs was performed for the group of 22 women recruited for the precision study as a homogeneous population of postmenopausal women identified as osteoporotic by DXA.

Statistical Analysis

The precision of area BMD (expressed in g/cm^2) measurements derived with the CTXA Hip was estimated by examining the dispersion of patient measurements acquired at approximately yearly intervals. The mean and standard deviation for the 3 or 4

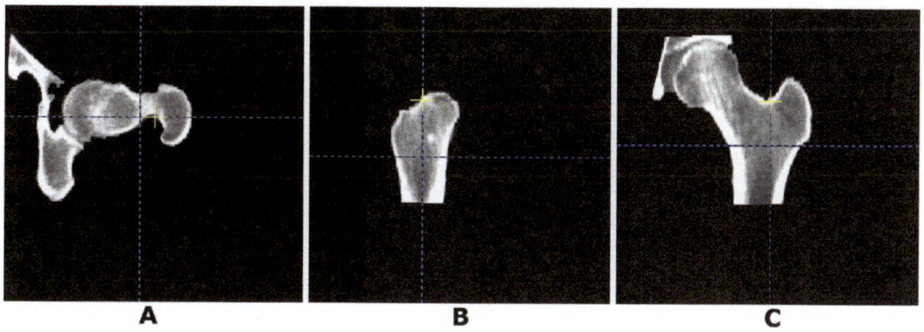

Figure 2. Proximal femur positioning. A) axial, B) sagittal and C) coronal images of segmented bone in proximal femur, rotated into a standard projection.

measurements for each patient were calculated without regard for the rate of bone change. Long-term precision was then estimated by calculating the root-mean-square average of the set of standard deviation estimates for the group of patients [20]. This method provides a conservative estimate of precision, and is justified because the women in this group on average were not losing bone (CTXA Hip Total Hip BMD mean and SEM for baseline, year 1 and year 2, 0.647±0.017, 0.644±0.018, 0.648±0.019 g/cm^2, $p>0.05$ for all comparisons by two tailed t-test).

For interobserver variability, significance of difference of means was tested using a two-tailed t-test.

The accuracy of the CTXA Hip BMD estimates relative to Hologic QDR DXA BMD estimates for the Total Hip and Femoral Neck ROIs was characterized by comparing CTXA Hip and DXA results from the same subject from the two sites using Hologic QDR4500 scanners. Results were first compared by individual site. Similarity of the distributions suggested pooling the results. Pooling of these results was objectively justified based on a two-sample t-test, assuming unequal variances, of the means of the bias distribution for each site. That is, the means of the distribution of patient-specific CTXA Hip minus DXA BMD results determined from paired subject measurements at each of the sites were compared by this method. No inconsistencies in the sample mean comparisons were found either for the total hip or femoral neck data at the 95% confidence level ($p<0.05$).

To ascertain the validity of t-tests, an Anderson-Darling test was used to detect significant deviations from normality in measurement distributions.

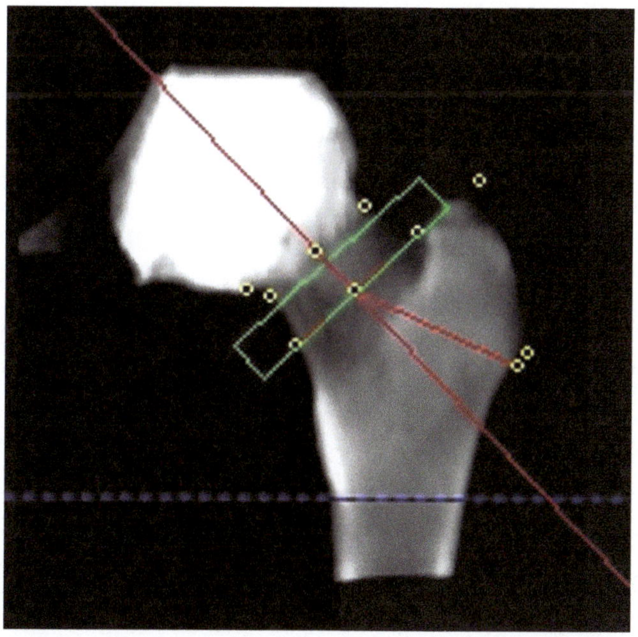

Figure 3. CTXA proximal femur ROI positions. CTXA projected image with standard regions of interest used for BMD calculations (femoral neck, trochanter, intertrochanter, and Total Hip as sum of these three regions). Position of femoral neck box and intertrochanter limit line at base of lesser trochanter, and rotation of femoral neck axis, are adjustable by user. Ward's Triangle ROI is displayed but not used in comparisons.

Results

The results of the long term in vivo precision studies are given in Table 1 (Table S1: "LongTerm In Vivo Precision CTXA vs DXA - Data"), both for precision in terms of the BMD value (g/cm^2) and as the coefficient of variation (CV,%), based on the distribution of the individual patient values. The mean BMD values by CTXA Hip and DXA are also given. There were no significant differences in precision between the CTXA Hip and the DXA results obtained in this study.

Interobserver variability results for CTXA Hip are given in Table 2 (Table S2: "Interobserver Comparison of CTXA BMD Estimates - Data"). The difference in total hip mean BMD estimates was not significant between the two observers at the 95% confidence level ($p = 0.055$), while the femoral neck difference was significant between the two observers at the 95% confidence level ($p = 0.026$). Even though statistically significant, the 1% difference between observers is similar to the 0.9–2.6% obtained using DXA (6,7).

No substantial evidence was found for rejecting the hypothesis that the data measurements are reasonably described by a normal sampling process using the Anderson-Darling test to detect

Table 1. Summary of Long-Term *In Vivo* Precision, CTXA vs. DXA, in Osteoporotic Subjects.

	Total Hip		Femoral Neck	
	CTXA	DXA	CTXA	DXA
Areal Density (g/cm^2)	0.645	0.700	0.551	0.598
Precision (g/cm^2)	0.012	0.014	0.011	0.016
CV (%)	1.8	2.0	2.0	2.7

Table 2. Interobserver Comparison of CTXA BMD Estimates (g/cm²).

	Observer 1	Observer 2	Observer 2 - Observer 1	Observer 2 - Observer 1 (%)
Mean Total Hip BMD	0.668	0.675	0.007	1.0
SD Total Hip BMD	0.142	0.146	0.004	
Mean Femoral Neck BMD	0.585	0.578	−0.007	1.2
SD Femoral Neck BMD	0.121	0.118	−0.003	

significant deviations from normality in measurement distributions.

The correlation between BMD estimates made with CTXA Hip and DXA for total hip and femoral neck regions of interest are given in Table 3 (Table S3: "Correlation of CTXA Hip and DXA BMD results - Data"), for the two clinical sites independently and for pooled results. Figures 4 and 5 show the correlations for total hip and femoral neck graphically. Correlation coefficients of 0.92−0.97 were obtained for femoral neck and total hip ROIs, with Standard Error of the Estimates (SEE) of 0.043−0.047 g/cm².

The segmentation of total bone in the hip into compartments representing "cortical" and "trabecular" bone in DXA-like ROIs differentiates the measurement results of CTXA Hip analysis from DXA. For the study population, the total hip region of interest was found to contain 62.3%±4.8% (mean ± SD) "cortical" bone with the remaining 37.7%±4.8% bone belonging to the "trabecular" bone compartment defined by CTXA Hip. For the femoral neck the proportions were 57.7%±9.5% and 42.3%±9.5%, respectively.

Discussion

The focus on measurements of bone density at the proximal femur as a standard reference [14] has meant DXA has become the gold standard technology used to make these measurements. Theoretically QCT can produce a BMD estimate at the hip in two dimensions that has characteristics similar to DXA, and should give a BMD estimate that is highly correlated with a DXA result. The results of our study show that 2D projected BMD results obtained using the CTXA Hip software correlated highly with results obtained from a common DXA device (QDR4500), and these results are similar to those from other studies. Khoo et al, [18] showed correlation between DXA and CTXA of R = 0.89–0.93 in an older cohort, with a RMS errors of between 0.04–0.06 g/cm². In a comparison of a their own QCT aBMD projection algorithm for Total Hip region, Keyak et al [17] showed a correlation of R = 0.935 with an SEE of 0.046 g/cm².

The results obtained in our study are also similar to the relationship seen between DXA systems from Hologic and Lunar, where a correlation of R = 0.92 and SEE of 0.051 for the Femoral Neck ROI over the same BMD range in a similar population has been reported [21,22].

Long term in vivo precision is an important parameter for clinical practice, and we obtained results for CTXA Hip essentially identical to those from a Hologic QDR1000 system for osteoporotic patients studied under controlled conditions over a 2–3 year period. Our long-term precision in osteoporotic subjects is similar to short-term precision of 2.1–2.9% obtained by other researchers using DXA in similar populations [23,24], indicating that when properly performed QCT methods are just as precise as DXA. Our precision results are consistent with the observations of Khoo et al [18] where CTXA short-term precision estimates that were either non-inferior to or superior to DXA were reported. However, a limitation of the present study is that the results from only two observers where available for the reproducibility analysis.

We observed statistically significant differences in the slope and/or intercept of BMD results from CTXA Hip compared to Hologic DXA. In particular, CTXA Hip BMD estimates for the Total Hip ROI were found to be approximately 0.11 g/cm² lower than QDR 4500 results for the same population. This bias is well modeled by an additive (negative) bias term as shown in Figure 4 where the observed slope in the linear regression analysis was found to be not significantly different from unity. CTXA Hip BMD estimates for the Femoral Neck were also found to be less than the corresponding QDR 4500 results with an average bias of

Table 3. Correlation of CTXA Hip and DXA BMD Results (Site 1, Manchester; Site 2, Schenectady).

Total Hip						
	CTXA BMD	DXA BMD	Slope	Intercept	R	SEE
Site 1 (N = 30)	0.657±0.143	0.766±0.138	0.988	−0.100	0.95	0.046
Site 2 (N = 39)	0.755±0.175	0.851±0.170	0.999	−0.094	0.97	0.043
Site 1+2 (N = 69)	0.712±0.168	0.814±0.161	1.006	−0.106	0.97	0.044
Femoral Neck						
	CTXA BMD	DXA BMD	Slope	Intercept	R	SEE
Site 1 (N = 30)	0.564±0.117	0.645±0.123	0.876	−0.001	0.92	0.047
Site 2 (N = 34)	0.638±0.150	0.713±0.156	0.883	0.004	0.96	0.043
Site 1+2 (N = 64)	0.606±0.141	0.681±0.145	0.888	−0.004	0.95	0.044

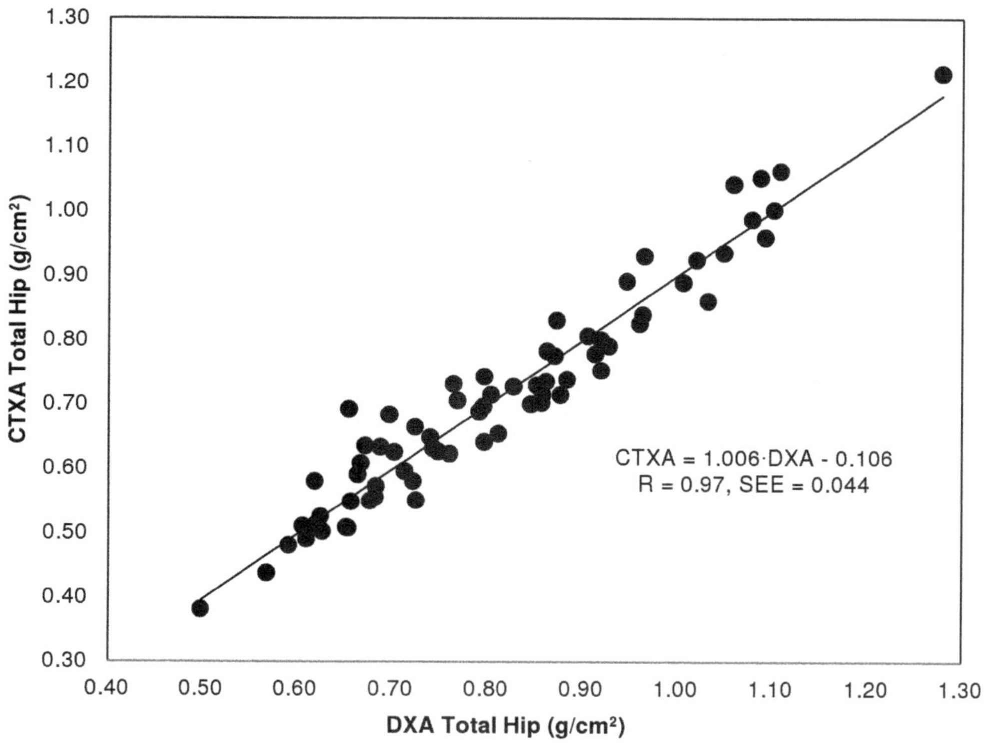

Figure 4. Correlation of area BMD for CTXA and DXA for total hip region of interest.

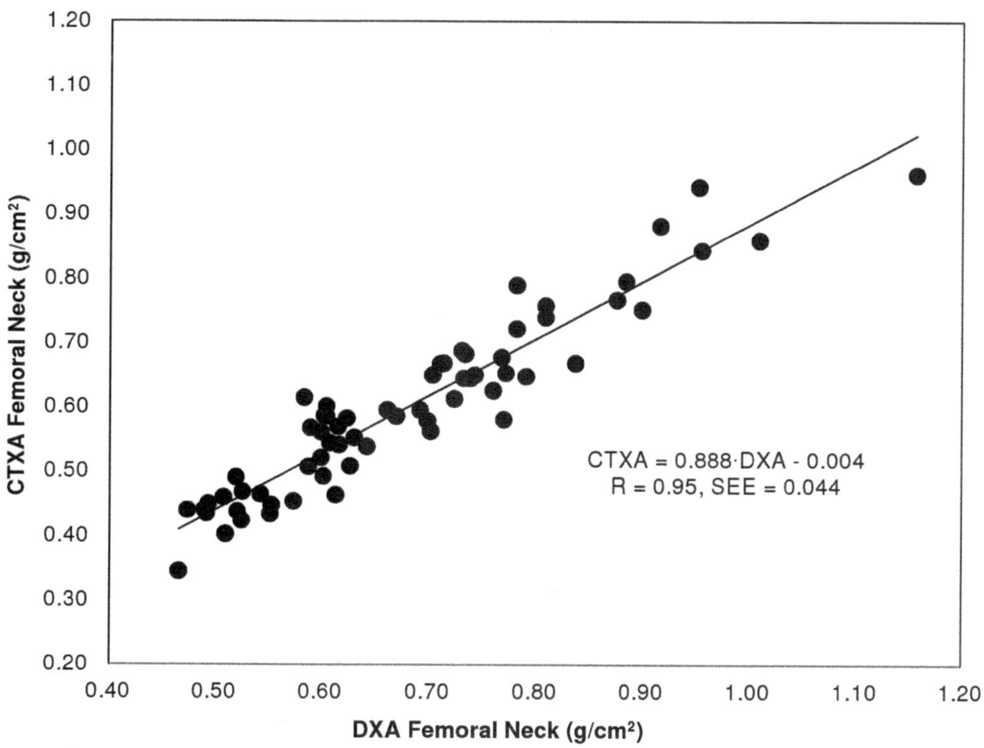

Figure 5. Correlation of area BMD for CTXA and DXA for femoral neck region of interest.

about 0.06 g/cm^2. In this case, however, linear regression analysis indicated the bias was better explained by a model slope significantly different than one with an additive offset not significantly different from zero. As can be seen in Table 1, we also observed statistically significant bias in CTXA Hip and QDR 1000 BMD estimates, with an average bias of about 0.05 g/cm2 at both measurement sites reported here for the osteoporotic patient population comprising our precision study group.

Biases in hip BMD estimates between bone densitometers from various manufacturers have been reported in numerous studies. Biases of the same magnitude we report here have been observed in comparison studies of DXA devices from Hologic, Lunar and Norland [21,22]. As noted by those authors, these differences may be due to technical differences in the way data are acquired and analyzed.

One cause of the differences between QCT (CTXA) aBMD and DXA-derived aBMD relates to the calibration phantoms used [25]. The Hologic DXA scanner uses solid calcium hydroxyapatite (CaHAP) standard for its calibration. QCT uses liquid potassium phosphate (K_2HPO_4) as a mineral standard. Although the mean CaHAP and K_2HPO_4 calibration standards are similar in the trabecular aBMD region, there are slight differences in the calibration slopes, with a propensity for K_2HPO_4 equivalent densities to be slightly lower than corresponding CaHAP equivalent densities. The difference is more pronounced when working at higher densities. Therefore, it is not surprising that QCT-derived mineral mass (BMC) at all corresponding sites of the proximal femur was significantly lower compared to DXA values (Table 1). In addition, the methods used for separating "soft tissue" components of the projection are also very different between QCT and DXA. DXA uses dual energy methods for this and in particular estimates the fat/lean ratio for tissue superimposed with the DXA bone signal. Essentially the soft-tissue component is subtracted in DXA. In CTXA, however, volumetric CT images are segmented into "bone" and "not bone" (mostly soft tissue, air and calibration phantom pixels) pixels using geometric, anatomical and physiological considerations. The "non-bone" pixels are completely removed from the image data prior to generating bone projections and so contribute essentially no signal (and no residual noise) component to the bone projection images and without dependencies on details of the nature and distribution of the surrounding tissue.

Next, DXA standardizes measurement positioning by controlling foot positioning during scanning. While the standard DXA foot positioning does result in turning the femoral neck axis outward such that the femoral neck axis is more nearly orthogonal to the x-ray projection direction, the orthogonality of the femoral neck axis to the projection direction is not what is controlled with DXA. This orthogonality is, however, what is being controlled within CTXA.

Another cause of differences is projection geometry. CTXA uses a parallel beam projection geometry. While older DXA units also use a parallel projection geometry, most DXA units today use fan beam projection geometries that include a depth-dependent magnification attribute. Depending upon DXA unit design, there can also be a residual magnification component related to how far a patient's bone sits above, say, the DXA device table top. In such a situation, DXA BMD estimates can be influenced by patient positioning, including factors that may be difficult to control between DXA scans–such as significant weight loss/gain resulting in an inability to position a patient in the same manner between two scans. All of these are on top of algorithmic variations in core image processing steps used to define various anatomical landmarks and reference lengths used to standardize BMD measurement on a particular device. For example, thresholds of 15% of the maximum BMD across a femoral neck profile to define the lateral margins of the femoral neck (and so the femoral neck width) are likely to be very different in a DXA image, that includes a non-zero, noisy background that is a residual of soft-tissue background subtraction, in comparison to a CTXA image that includes essentially no soft-tissue background and essentially no soft-tissue background noise.

Well-established biases in BMD estimates from different devices are currently handled in clinical densitometry practice by reporting normalized BMD estimates and interpreting normalized proximal-femur BMD scores from all DXA units using the same guidelines. The use of T-scores is the prevalent normalization method in use today [14], although alternative methods for generating "standardized" BMD estimates have been proposed [21,22]. When using the CTXA method, T-scores may be calculated by using conversion equations using the Hologic DXA-acquired NHANES III (National Health and Nutrition Examination Survey III) young normal data with conversion equations for the various anatomical regions [18]. This approach is similar to the adjustment made by DXA equipment manufacturers other than Hologic when using the NHANES III data to calculate T-scores [26]. Alternatively, young normal data may be gathered using the CTXA method in order to calculate T-scores. Although the normal subject data required for standardization of results by the computation of T-scores has been gathered for use with CTXA method and is in current clinical use that is not the subject of the study described here.

Osteoporosis represents a major public health issue, and there is a growing appreciation of the need for wider screening efforts. The recently revised and expanded recommendations by the U.S. Preventive Services Task Force (USPSTF) underscore the need for more screening [27]. The clinical utility of the CTXA hip method is in providing a BMD measurement where DXA may not be available due to space or financial constraints, but an underutilized CT scanner may be used such as in a rural healthcare facility. However, the disadvantage of a higher radiation dose must be considered in particular in younger individuals (e.g., peri-menopausal women).

The higher radiation exposure due to a dedicated QCT exam in comparison to a DXA study can be avoided by the re-use of a CT scan ordered for another reason. The use of QCT for BMD measurement at the lumber vertebrae and hip in conjunction with CT scans ordered for other reasons in the context of improving screening rates, has been explored in a number of studies [28–30] including for CT contrast-enhanced scans [31,32]. For patients undergoing screening CT colonography (CTC), a potential opportunity exists for concurrent BMD screening without the need for any additional imaging, radiation exposure, or patient time [30]. Such dual-use of CT images could increase screening rates or, alternatively, preclude the need for DXA screening in some individuals. Because standard CT colonography exams include the pelvis, CTXA femoral neck measurement rather than lumber spine measurement can be made which provides access to the diagnostic classification using WHO T-scores thresholds and the use of FRAX for fracture risk calculation. The ability of the CTXA method to produce areal BMD and T-scores at the femoral neck which may be used as input to the WHO FRAX tool is particularly important as the field moves away from relying solely on BMD measurement for fracture risk prediction [33].

We have compared a method of deriving DXA-like 2D projections of integral bone from volumetric CT scans to DXA measurements. In principle, there is a large amount of useful 3D information discarded by this approach. In this study, we have presented results from the use CTXA Hip analysis to segment "cortical" and "trabecular" bone compartments which exploits the 3D nature of the acquired 3D image data. In terms of fully 3D analysis of the proximal femur, several methods have been developed [34–39]. Within each anatomic subregion, the density, mass, and volume are computed for the cortical and trabecular components as well as for the integral bone envelope. For trabecular BMD measurements, the precision of these kinds of methods *in vivo* was found to range from 0.6% to 1.1% depending on the volume of interest assessed [34]. Several of these approaches also facilitate geometric and structural analyses of the minimum femoral neck cross section, computing cross-sectional area, estimates of cortical volume and thickness, and moments of inertia for strength estimation. There has also been comparison made of hip structural analysis (HSA) parameters derived by DXA and QCT [40]. However, as has been stated before, the lack of normal data for standardization and the prevailing use of DXA T-scores for diagnostic categorization currently limit these volumetric 3D hip analysis methods to research and clinical trials application.

Conclusion

We hypothesized that CTXA Hip BMD estimates could provide the same clinical utility as that afforded by DXA, and we believe our study results strongly support this hypothesis. High correlation of results from various combinations of DXA devices, along with consistency in measurement precision as characterized by SEE, interobserver variability, and assessment of long-term and short-term measurement precision have been accepted as a basis for using proximal femur results from all commercial DXA devices for clinical decision making within the context of any of numerous national and international clinical densitometry guidelines. Areal BMD and T-scores from CTXA Hip could provide standardized BMD measures from opportunistic osteoporosis screening using CT studies; or a method of osteoporosis screening in areas where DXA is unavailable. The 3D nature of QCT may also provide a more comprehensive estimate of bone strength parameters than similar analyses using DXA data.

Supporting Information

Table S1 Long Term In Vivo Precision CTXA vs DXA - Data.

Table S2 Interobserver Comparison of CTXA BMD Estimates - Data.

Table S3 Correlation of CTXA Hip and DXA BMD results - Data.

Author Contributions

Conceived and designed the experiments: CC JKB JA. Performed the experiments: CC JA. Analyzed the data: CC JKB ADB. Contributed reagents/materials/analysis tools: CC JKB. Wrote the paper: CC JKB JA ADB.

References

1. US Department of Health and Human Services (2004) Bone health and osteoporosis: a report of the Surgeon General. Rockville, MD. doi:10.2165/00002018-200932030-00004.
2. Lewiecki EM, Gordon CM, Baim S, Leonard MB, Bishop NJ, et al. (2008) International Society for Clinical Densitometry 2007 Adult and Pediatric Official Positions. Bone 43: 1115–1121. doi:10.1016/j.bone.2008.08.106.
3. National Osteoporosis Foundation (2013) Clinician's Guide to the Prevention and Treatment of Osteoporosis.
4. Curtis JR, Carbone LD, Cheng H, Hayes B, Laster A, et al. (2008) Longitudinal trends in use of bone mass measurement among older americans, 1999–2005. J Bone Miner Res 23: 1061–1067. doi:10.1359/jbmr.080232.
5. Adams JE (2009) Quantitative computed tomography. Eur J Radiol 71: 415–424. doi:10.1016/j.ejrad.2009.04.074.
6. Prior JC, Vigna YM, Wark JD, Eyre DR, Lentle BC, et al. (1997) Premenopausal ovariectomy-related bone loss: a randomized, double-blind, one-year trial of conjugated estrogen or medroxyprogesterone acetate. J Bone Miner Res 12: 1851–1863. doi:10.1359/jbmr.1997.12.11.1851.
7. Damilakis J, Adams JE, Guglielmi G, Link TM (2010) Radiation exposure in X-ray-based imaging techniques used in osteoporosis. Eur Radiol 20: 2707–2714. doi:10.1007/s00330-010-1845-0.
8. Yu EW, Thomas BJ, Brown JK, Finkelstein JS (2011) Simulated increases in body fat and errors in bone mineral density measurements by DXA and QCT. J Bone Miner Res 27: 119–124. doi:10.1002/jbmr.506.
9. Guglielmi G, Floriani I, Torri V, Li J, van Kuijk C, et al. (2005) Effect of Spinal Degenerative Changes on Volumetric Bone Mineral Density of the Central Skeleton as Measured by Quantitative Computed Tomography. Acta radiol 46: 269–275. doi:10.1080/02841850510012661.
10. Smith JA, Vento JA, Spencer RP, Tendler BE (1999) Aortic calcification contributing to bone densitometry measurement. J Clin Densitom 2: 181–183. doi:10.1385/JCD:2:2:181.
11. Liu G, Peacock M, Eilam O, Dorulla G, Braunstein E, et al. (1997) Effect of osteoarthritis in the lumbar spine and hip on bone mineral density and diagnosis of osteoporosis in elderly men and women. Osteoporos Int 7: 564–569.
12. Faulkner KG, von Stetten E, Miller P (1999) Discordance in patient classification using T-scores. J Clin Densitom 2: 343–350.
13. American College of Radiology (2008) ACR Practice Guideline for the Performance of Quantitative Computed Tomography (QCT) Bone Densitometry.
14. Kanis JA, McCloskey EV, Johansson H, Oden A, Melton LJ, et al. (2008) A reference standard for the description of osteoporosis. Bone 42: 467–475. doi:10.1016/j.bone.2007.11.001.
15. Kanis JA, Johnell O, Oden A, Johansson H, McCloskey E (2008) FRAX and the assessment of fracture probability in men and women from the UK. Osteoporos Int 19: 385–397. doi:10.1007/s00198-007-0543-5.
16. Genant HK, Engelke K, Prevrhal S (2008) Advanced CT bone imaging in osteoporosis. Rheumatology (Oxford) 47 Suppl 4: iv9–16. doi:10.1093/rheumatology/ken180.
17. Keyak JH, Sigurdsson S, Karlsdottir G, Oskarsdottir D, Sigmarsdottir A, et al. (2011) Male-female differences in the association between incident hip fracture and proximal femoral strength: a finite element analysis study. Bone 48: 1239–1245. doi:10.1016/j.bone.2011.03.682.
18. Khoo BCC, Brown JK, Cann CE, Zhu K, Henzell S, et al. (2009) Comparison of QCT-derived and DXA-derived areal bone mineral density and T scores. Osteoporos Int 20: 1539–1545. doi:10.1007/s00198-008-0820-y.
19. Cann CE, Genant HK (1980) Precise measurement of vertebral mineral content using computed tomography. J Comput Assist Tomogr 4: 493–500.
20. Glüer CC, Blake GM, Lu Y, Blunt BA, Jergas M, et al. (1995) Accurate assessment of precision errors: how to measure the reproducibility of bone densitometry techniques. Osteoporos Int 5: 262–270. doi:10.1007/BF01774016.
21. Genant HK, Grampp S, Glüer CC, Faulkner KG, Jergas M, et al. (1994) Universal standardization for dual x-ray absorptiometry: patient and phantom cross-calibration results. J Bone Miner Res 9: 1503–1514. doi:10.1002/jbmr.5650091002.
22. Hui SL, Gao S, Zhou XH, Johnston CC, Lu Y, et al. (1997) Universal standardization of bone density measurements: a method with optimal properties for calibration among several instruments. J Bone Miner Res 12: 1463–1470. doi:10.1359/jbmr.1997.12.9.1463.
23. Wahner HW, Looker A, Dunn WL, Walters LC, Hauser MF, et al. (1994) Quality control of bone densitometry in a national health survey (NHANES III) using three mobile examination centers. J Bone Miner Res 9: 951–960. doi:10.1002/jbmr.5650090621.
24. Slosman DO, Provvedini DM, Meunier PJ, Delmas PD, Sebert JL, et al. (1999) The use of different dual X-ray absorptiometry brands in a multicenter clinical trial: consequences and limits. J Clin Densitom 2: 37–44.
25. Goodsitt MM (1992) Conversion relations for quantitative CT bone mineral densities measured with solid and liquid calibration standards. J Bone Miner Res 19: 145–158.
26. Binkley N, Kiebzak GM, Lewiecki EM, Krueger D, Gangnon RE, et al. (2005) Recalculation of the NHANES database SD improves T-score agreement and reduces osteoporosis prevalence. J Bone Miner Res 20: 195–201. doi:10.1359/JBMR.041115.
27. Nelson H, Haney E, Dana T, Bougatsos C, Chou R (2010) Screening for Osteoporosis: An Update for the US Preventive Services Task Force. Ann Intern Med 153.

28. Papadakis AE, Karantanas AH, Papadokostakis G, Petinellis E, Damilakis J (2009) Can abdominal multi-detector CT diagnose spinal osteoporosis? Eur Radiol 19: 172–176. doi:10.1007/s00330-008-1099-2.
29. Link TM, Koppers BB, Licht T, Bauer JS, Lu Y, et al. (2004) In vitro and in vivo spiral CT to determine bone mineral density: initial experience in patients at risk for osteoporosis. Radiology 231: 805–811. doi:10.1148/radiol.2313030325.
30. Pickhardt PJ, Lee LJ, del Rio AM, Lauder T, Bruce RJ, et al. (2011) Simultaneous screening for osteoporosis at CT colonography: bone mineral density assessment using MDCT attenuation techniques compared with the DXA reference standard. J Bone Miner Res 26: 2194–2203. doi:10.1002/jbmr.428.
31. Bauer JS, Henning TD, Müeller D, Lu Y, Majumdar S, et al. (2007) Volumetric quantitative CT of the spine and hip derived from contrast-enhanced MDCT: conversion factors. AJR Am J Roentgenol 188: 1294–1301. doi:10.2214/AJR.06.1006.
32. Gruber M, Bauer JS, Dobritz M, Beer AJ, Wolf P, et al. (2013) Bone mineral density measurements of the proximal femur from routine contrast-enhanced MDCT data sets correlate with dual-energy X-ray absorptiometry. Eur Radiol 23: 505–512. doi:10.1007/s00330-012-2629-5.
33. Siris ES, Boonen S, Mitchell PJ, Bilezikian J, Silverman S (2012) What's in a name? What constitutes the clinical diagnosis of osteoporosis? Osteoporos Int 23: 2093–2097. doi:10.1007/s00198-012-1991-0.
34. Lang TF, Keyak JH, Heitz MW, Augat P, Lu Y, et al. (1997) Volumetric quantitative computed tomography of the proximal femur: precision and relation to bone strength. Bone 21: 101–108.
35. Kang Y, Engelke K, Kalender WA (2003) A new accurate and precise 3-D segmentation method for skeletal structures in volumetric CT data. IEEE Trans Med Imaging 22: 586–598. doi:10.1109/TMI.2003.812265.
36. Kang Y, Engelke K, Fuchs C, Kalender WA (2005) An anatomic coordinate system of the femoral neck for highly reproducible BMD measurements using 3D QCT. Comput Med imaging Graph 29: 533–541. doi:10.1016/j.compmedimag.2005.05.002.
37. Camp JJ, Karwoski RA, Stacy MC, Atkinson EJ, Khosla S, et al. (2004) System for the analysis of whole-bone strength from helical CT images. In: Amini AA, Manduca A, Proc. SPIE 5369, Medical Imaging 2004: Physiology, Function, and Structure from Medical Images. pp. 74–88. doi:10.1117/12.535745.
38. Lang T, LeBlanc AD, Evans HJ, Lu Y, Genant HK, et al. (2004) Cortical and trabecular bone mineral loss from the spine and hip in long-duration spaceflight. J Bone Miner Res 19: 1006–1012. doi:10.1359/JBMR.040307.
39. Poole KES, Mayhew PM, Rose CM, Brown JK, Bearcroft PJ, et al. (2010) Changing structure of the femoral neck across the adult female lifespan. J Bone Miner Res 25: 482–491. doi:10.1359/jbmr.090734.
40. Khoo BCC, Brown K, Zhu K, Pollock M, Wilson KE, et al. (2012) Differences in structural geometrical outcomes at the neck of the proximal femur using two-dimensional DXA-derived projection (APEX) and three-dimensional QCT-derived (BIT QCT) techniques. Osteoporos Int 23: 1393–1398. doi:10.1007/s00198-011-1727-6.

Interrelationship of Postoperative Delirium and Cognitive Impairment and Their Impact on the Functional Status in Older Patients Undergoing Orthopaedic Surgery: A Prospective Cohort Study

Chih-Kuang Liang[1,2,3], Chin-Liang Chu[1,3,4], Ming-Yueh Chou[1,3,5], Yu-Te Lin[1,2,3]*, Ti Lu[4], Chien-Jen Hsu[6], Liang-Kung Chen[3,7]*

1 Center for Geriatrics and Gerontology, Kaohsiung Veterans General Hospital, Kaohsiung, Taiwan, **2** Division of Neurology, Department of Medicine, Kaohsiung Veterans General Hospital Kaohsiung, Taiwan, **3** Aging and Health Research Center, National Yang Ming University, Taipei, Taiwan, **4** Department of Psychiatry, Kaohsiung Veterans General Hospital, Kaohsiung, Taiwan, **5** Department of Family Medicine, Kaohsiung Veterans General Hospital, Kaohsiung, Taiwan, **6** Department of Orthopaedics, Kaohsiung Veterans General Hospital, Kaohsiung, Taiwan, **7** Center for Geriatrics and Gerontology, Taipei Veterans General Hospital, Taipei, Taiwan

Abstract

Background: The impact of postoperative delirium on post-discharge functional status of older patients remains unclear, and little is known regarding the interrelationship between cognitive impairment and post-operative delirium. Therefore, the main purpose was to evaluate the post-discharge functional status of patients who experience delirium after undergoing orthopaedic surgery and the interrelationship of postoperative delirium with underlying cognitive impairment.

Method: This prospective cohort study, conducted at a tertiary care medical center from April 2011 to March 2012, enrolled all subjects aged over 60 years who were admitted for orthopaedic surgery. The baseline characteristics (age, gender, BMI, and living arrangement), surgery-related factors (ASA class, admission type, type of surgery, and length of hospital stay), results of geriatric assessment (postoperative delirium, cognition, depressive mood, comorbidity, pain, malnutrition, polypharmacy, ADL, and instrumental [I]ADL) and 1–12-month postoperative ADL and IADL functional status were collected for analysis.

Results: Overall, 9.1% of 232 patients (mean age: 74.7±7.8 years) experienced postoperative delirium, which was significantly associated with IADL decline at only 6 and 12 months postoperatively (RR: 6.22, 95% CI: 1.08–35.70 and RR: 12.54, 95% CI: 1.88–83.71, respectively). Delirium superimposed on cognitive impairment was a significant predictor for poor functional status at 6 and 12 months postoperatively (RR: 12.80, 95% CI: 1.65–99.40 for ADL at the 6th month, and RR: 7.96, 95% CI: 1.35–46.99 at the 12th month; RR: 13.68, 95% CI: 1.94–96.55 for IADL at the 6th month, and RR: 30.61, 95% CI: 2.94–318.54 at the 12th month, respectively).

Conclusion: Postoperative delirium is predictive of IADL decline in older patients undergoing orthopaedic surgery, and delirium superimposed on cognitive impairment is an independent risk factor for deterioration of ADL and IADL functional status. Early identification of cognitive function and to prevent delirium are needed to improve functional status following orthopaedic surgery.

Editor: Stephen D. Ginsberg, Nathan Kline Institute and New York University School of Medicine, United States of America

Funding: This work was supported by grants from the Veteran Affairs Commission of Taiwan. The funders had no role in study design, data collection and analysis, decision to publish, or preparation of the manuscript.

Competing Interests: The authors have declared that no competing interests exist.

* Email: ytlin@vghks.gov.tw (YTL); lkchen2@vghtpe.gov.tw (LKC)

Introduction

Delirium is an acute mental disorder that is characterized by rapid onset and a fluctuating course of consciousness disturbance and inattention, possibly leading to further adverse health consequences in the elderly population [1]. Although delirium is a well-recognized geriatric syndrome, it is often overlooked by clinicians and nurses [2,3]. The incidence of delirium following orthopaedic surgery has been reported to be 4–65%. Considerable variation is seen and is dependent on the type of procedure, with the reported incidence being 35–65% in patients undergoing operative treatment of a hip fracture and 9–15% in patients undergoing elective orthopaedic procedures [4,5]. Risk factors for the development of postoperative delirium in older patients include older age, cognitive impairment, depressed mood, poor baseline physical function, comorbid diseases, type of surgery, and institutionalization before admission [6–10]. Although delirium is a common geriatric syndrome, its etiopathogenesis remains unclear. However, preventive strategies focused on early identification and management of risk factors are believed to be superior to strategies that emphasize treatment of delirium after it occurs [10–13].

Delirium subsequent to surgery is associated with higher rates of in-hospital and long-term mortality [14–20], as well as longer hospital stay, longer intensive care unit stay, and higher chance of discharge to nursing facilities [14–16,21]. Although the adverse impact of postoperative delirium has been clearly identified, the impact of postoperative delirium on long-term functional status remains unclear. Dementia or cognitive impairment has been reported as an independent risk factor for delirium [10], and the overall incidence of new delirium was significantly higher among older patients with dementia than among older patients with no dementia [22]. Moreover, pre-fracture cognitive impairment and post-fracture delirium were also strongly associated with higher mortality rate and risk for institutionalization [23,24], and delirium might be an early indicator for post-discharge cognitive decline [25,26]. Although it can result in long-term cognitive decline, postoperative cognitive decline secondary to delirium does not occur in all patients [10]. To date, little is known regarding the interrelationship between delirium and cognitive impairment and their impact on adverse functional status in older patients. Therefore, the purpose of the present study was to evaluate the impact of postoperative delirium, in the presence of underlying cognitive impairment, on changes in the post-discharge functional status of patients who underwent orthopaedic surgery.

Methods

Study design

This prospective cohort study was conducted in a tertiary care medical center in Southern Taiwan. All subjects aged 60 years and older who were admitted for orthopaedic surgery during the period April 2011 to March 2012 were screened for this study. Patients were excluded for the following reasons: (1) medical conditions that prevented comprehensive geriatric assessment (CGA), or admission or transfer to an intensive care unit before enrollment, (2) inability to complete the comprehensive geriatric assessment (CGA), (3) inability to provide informed consent, (4) limited life expectancy less than 6 months such as in cancer and terminal stage heart failure cases, (5) delirium occurring before enrollment or surgery, and (6) incomplete data. The study protocol was approved by the Institutional Review Board of Kaohsiung Veterans General Hospital and written informed consents were obtained from all participants before the study started. During a one-year period, a total of 232 patients were enrolled with mean age of 74.7±7.8 years (range: 60–93). Among them, 28 (12.1%) patients were admitted to the hospital from the emergency department. The incidence of postoperative delirium was 9.1% (21/232).

Preoperative evaluation

Demographic data and surgery characteristics. Two research nurses interviewed all participants to collect the preoperative demographic data (including age, gender, educational level, living arrangement, and body mass index [BMI]), and data on other characteristics including admission type (emergency or elective surgery), type of surgery (including spinal decompression only, spinal surgery with instrumented fusion, total knee arthroplasty, other elective knee surgery, elective total hip arthroplasty [total hip replacement]/bipolar hemiarthroplasty, revision hip surgery, and open reduction and internal fixation [ORIF]/ arthroplasty for hip fracture), ASA (American Society of Anesthesiologists) physical status, and length of hospital stay.

Comprehensive geriatric assessment (CGA). All participants were assessed by trained research nurses using the CGA before preceding the orthopaedic operation, and within the first 24 hours after hospital admission from the outpatient clinics or emergency department. The assessment covered visual and hearing impairments, polypharmacy (defined as currently using >4 prescription drugs for over 2 weeks), depressive symptoms (using the 15-item Chinese Geriatric Depression Scale) [27,28], nutritional status (as determined by the Mini Nutritional Assessment) [29], comorbidity (as evaluated by the Charlson's Comorbidity Index) [30], symptoms of pain (rated on a Visual Analogue Scale) [31], cognitive function (as assessed by the Chinese version of the Mini-Mental State Examination at admission) [32], the Activities of Daily Living (ADL, evaluated by the Barthel Index) [33], and the Lawton-Brody Instrumental ADL (IADL) [34].

Patients were screened for delirium daily by the primary care nurses in the orthopaedic wards after orthopaedic surgery using the Confusion Assessment Method (CAM) [35], and a senior psychiatrist would confirm the diagnosis if the patient was deemed to be confused. The research nurses obtained ADL and IADL scores by conducting telephone interviews of the participating patients or their primary caregivers at 1, 3, 6, and 12 months after hospital discharge.

Statistical analysis

Continuous data are expressed as means ± SD, and categorical data are expressed as percentages. Dichotomous and ordinal variables were compared in those with and without delirium using the Chi-square test or Fisher exact test, and continuous variables were compared using the independent Student *t*-test or Mann-Whitney *U* test when appropriate.

The independent Student *t*-test or Mann-Whitney *U* test were used to compare the ADL or IADL scores between groups based on delirium status at 1, 3, 6, and 12 months. The differences in mean ADL and IADL scores between those with and without delirium at different time points were evaluated using the Analysis of Covariance (ANCOVA) with the inclusion of baseline ADL or IADL scores as covariates. To compare functional changes at 1, 3, 6, and 12 months, ADL or IADL functional decline was defined as lower ADL or IADL score at follow-up than at baseline. Multivariable logistic regression analysis was performed to determine whether delirium was an independent predictor of ADL or IADL decline at follow-up. In this model, age, gender, admission type, type of surgery, hearing impairment, polypharmacy, cognitive impairment, depressive symptoms, BMI, high risk of malnutrition, Charlson's Comorbidity Index (CCI), symptoms of pain, ASA class, and hospital length of stay were entered as explanatory variables.

To evaluate the effect of cognitive problems on long-term functional status (ADL and IADL scores at 1, 3, 6, and 12 months follow-up), four categorical variables representing four groups were defined (no cognitive problem [group A]; cognitive impairment alone indicated by MMSE <24 [group B]; postoperative delirium superimposed on cognitive problems [group C], and delirium only [group D]). ANCOVA was used to compare the mean ADL and IADL scores between these four groups after adjusting for baseline ADL and IADL scores (the covariates). The independent effect of each categorical variable on ADL and IADL outcomes was assessed using multivariable logistic regression

Table 1. Demographic data, functional status, and surgery-related factors in 232 subjects with postoperative delirium or no delirium.

Variables	Total N=232 (% or mean ± SD)	Postoperative delirium N=21 (% or mean ± SD)	No delirium N=211 (% or mean ± SD)	*p* value
Age	74.7±7.8	81.3±5.2	74.1±7.7	<0.001
Educational level	5.8±4.7	6.4±4.6	5.7±4.7	0.522
Gender (male)	108(46.6%)	17(81.0%)	91(43.1%)	0.001
Admission route				0.149
Emergency room	28(12.1%)	5(23.8%)	23(10.9%)	
Outpatient clinic (elective)	204(87.9%)	16(76.2%)	188(89.1%)	
Living				0.035
Alone	32(13.8%)	1(4.8%)	31(14.7%)	
Institutionalized	10(4.3%)	3(14.3%)	7(3.3%)	
With relatives/friends	190(81.9%)	17(81.0%)	173(82.0%)	
BMI	26.5±4.3	23.7±3.2	26.8±4.2	0.001
Polypharmacy (Yes)	106(45.7%)	13(61.9%)	93(44.1%)	0.118
Psychotic drugs (Yes)	36(15.5%)	4(19.0%)	32(15.2%)	0.751
Visual impairment (Yes)	157(67.7%)	18(85.7%)	139(65.9%)	0.064
Hearing impairment (Yes)	38(16.4%)	8(38.1%)	30(14.2%)	0.010
ADL(BI) before admission	94.1±2.3	85.0±19.9	95.0±1.0	0.034
IADL before admission	5.7±1.4	4.4±1.9	5.8±1.3	0.004
Cognitive impairment at admission (MMSE <24)	91(39.2%)	16(76.2%)	75(35.5%)	<0.001
Presence of depressive symptoms (defined by GDS-15>=5)	19(8.2%)	1(4.8%)	18(8.5%)	1.000
Risk of malnutrition (screening by MNA)	19(8.2%)	7(33.3%)	12(5.7%)	<0.001
CCI	0.82±1.07	1.71±1.79	0.73±0.93	0.022
Pain VAS score	4.72±1.58	5.14±1.71	4.68±1.56	0.203
ASA				0.124
ASA 1 and 2	225(97.0%)	19(90.5%)	206(97.6%)	
ASA 3	7(3.0%)	2(9.5%)	5(2.4%)	
Length of hospital stay	8.45±4.46	8.42±4.63	8.76±2.221	0.736
Type of surgery				0.090
Elective spine surgery	60(25.9%)	7(11.7%)	53(88.3%)	
Elective knee surgery	100(43.1%)	6(6.0%)	94(94.0%)	
Elective hip arthroplasty	39(17.7%)	1(2.6%)	38(97.4%)	
ORIF/arthroplasty for hip fracture	33(13.4%)	7(21.2%)	26(78.8%)	

BMI: Body Mass Index; ADL: Activities of Daily Living; BI: Barthel Index; IADL: Instrumental Activities of Daily Living; MMSE: Mini-mental State Examination; GDS: Geriatric Depression Scale; MNA: Mini-nutritional Assessment; CCI: Charlson's Comorbidity Index; VAS: Visual Analogue Scale; ASA: American Society of Anesthesiologists physical status; ORIF: open reduction and internal fixation.
Elective Spine Surgery: Spinal decompression only and Spinal surgery with instrumented fusion.
Elective knee surgery: includes total knee replacement (N=92) and other elective knee surgery (N=8).
Elective hip arthroplasty: includes total hip replacement, bipolar hemiarthroplasty, and revision hip surgery.

analysis after controlling for age, gender, admission type, type of surgery, hearing impairment, polypharmacy, cognitive impairment, depressive symptoms, BMI, high risk of malnutrition, CCI, symptoms of pain, ASA class, and hospital length of stay and baseline IADL or ADL scores as covariates. For all tests, a P value (two-tailed) less than 0.05 was considered statistically significant. All statistical analyses were performed using IBM SPSS version 21 (SPSS Inc., Chicago, IL).

Results

The effect of delirium on functional status

Demographic characteristics of all 232 patients are summarized in Table 1. Fifty of the 232 patients were lost to follow up and therefore excluded from the evaluation of post-discharge functional status. The demographic characteristics of the excluded patients were similar to those of the enrolled patients except for age (77.0±8.7 years vs 74.1±7.4 years, p=0.018) and BMI (25.2±4.5 vs 26.7±4.1 kg/m^2, p=0.015). The number of patients who underwent spinal decompression only, spinal surgery with

Table 2. Comparing the ADL and IADL scores at baseline and 1, 3, 6, and 12 months of follow-up in groups with delirium.

	Time of follow-up (months)								
	Non-adjusted functional status (mean ± SE)					Adjusted baseline functional status by ANCOVA (mean ± SE)			
Outcomes variables	**Baseline**	**1**	**3**	**6**	**12**	**1**	**3**	**6**	**12**
ADL (BI) scores (mean ± SE)									
Delirium (N = 17)	85.9±4.81#	77.9±5.25#	79.4±5.62#	81.8±5.44#	81.8±5.86#	83.0±2.82#	84.5±2.77#	86.9±3.06#	86.4±3.18#
No delirium (N = 165)	95.6±0.80	93.2±0.93	94.9±0.89	95.2±1.00	95.6±0.99	92.7±0.88	94.4±0.87	94.6±0.96	95.2±1.00
IADL scores (mean ± SE)									
Delirium (N = 17)	4.4±0.40#	3.4±0.45#	3.4±0.47#	3.2±0.53#	2.9±0.53#	4.4±0.28#	4.4±0.28#	4.3±0.33#	4.0±0.33#
No delirium (N = 165)	5.8±0.09	5.3±0.11	5.6±0.11	5.6±0.12	5.7±0.12	5.2±0.09	5.5±0.09	5.5±0.10	5.6±0.10

#p<0.05 for comparing groups by delirium status. ANCOVA: Analysis of Covariance.

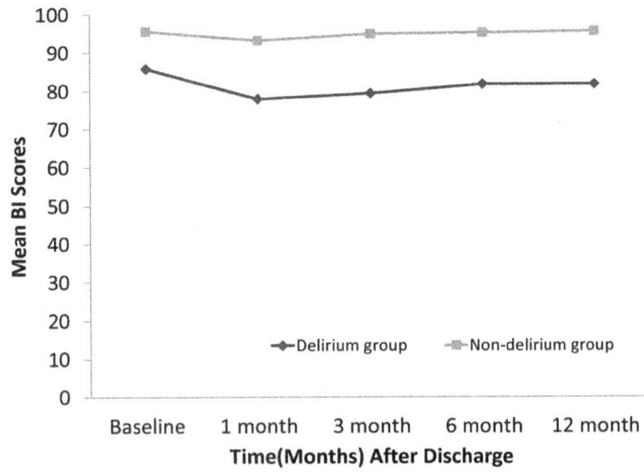

Figure 1. The trend of Barthel Index scores (ADL) (a) and IADL (b) for the delirium and no delirium groups.

instrumented fusion, total knee arthroplasty, other elective knee surgery, elective total hip replacement/bipolar hemiarthroplasty, revision hip surgery, and ORIF/arthroplasty for hip fracture was 7 (3.0%), 53 (22.8%), 92 (39.7%), 8 (3.4%), 31 (13.4%), 8 (3.4%), and 33 (14.2%), respectively. These procedures were grouped into four categories (elective spine surgery, elective knee surgery, elective hip arthroplasty, and ORIF/arthroplasty for hip fracture) for further analysis. Comparing the 50 patients lost to follow up with the 182 included patients, the delirium occurred in a similar proportion of both groups (8.0% [4/50] vs 9.3% [17/182]; data not shown), indicating that delirium did not increase the likelihood of loss to follow up.

At baseline, the 182 enrolled subjects (17 with delirium and 165 without delirium) had an ADL score of 85.9 (standard error [SE] = 4.81) vs 95.6 ([SE] = 0.80) and an IADL score of 4.4 ([SE] = 0.40) vs 5.8 ([SE] = 0.09; Table 2). Figure 1 shows the change in ADL and IADL scores over time after hospitalization for both groups. ADL and IADL scores were significantly different between those who developed post-operative delirium and those who did not. When controlling for baseline ADL, IADL scores remained significantly lower in patients who developed postoperative delirium than in those who did not. Table 3 shows the differences in ADL and IADL decline between the two groups at different follow-up times. Results of univariate logistic regression analysis identified delirium as a predictor of ADL decline at 6 and 12 months (p value: 0.036 vs 0.014), and IADL decline at 3, 6, and 12 months after surgery (p value: 0.033 vs 0.005 vs 0.001). In addition, multivariable logistic regression analysis identified delirium as a predictor of only IADL decline at 6 and 12 months (for IADL at 6 months, adjusted RR: 6.22, 95% CI:1.08–35.70, p value = 0.040; for IADL at 12 months, adjusted RR: 12.54, 95% CI: 1.88–83.71, p value = 0.009).

Impact of combined cognitive problems on functional status

The 182 included patients were divided into four groups based on delirium and cognitive status. The patients in group D (with delirium, but without baseline cognitive impairment) were excluded because of small sample size (N = 4). Baseline ADL and IADL scores were significantly different between patients with no cognitive problems (group A), and those with both baseline cognitive dysfunction and delirium (group C) or with baseline

Table 3. Analysis of the percentage of functional decline and the predicted effect on functional status in groups divided by delirium status using Chi-square test and multivariable logistic regression.

	Percentage of functional decline						Predicted effect on functional decline											
	ADL decline			IADL decline			RR of delirium for ADL decline						RR of delirium for IADL decline					
	Delirium	No delirium		Delirium	No delirium		Unadjusted			Adjusted			Unadjusted			Adjusted		
Follow-up times	N(%)	N(%)	p value	N(%)	N(%)	p value	RR	95% CI	p value	RR	95% CI	p value	RR	95% CI	p value	RR	95% CI	p value
1-month	8/17(47. 1)	46/165(27.9)	0.099	6/13(46.2%)	59/165(35.8)	0.552	2.30	0.84–6.32	0.107	2.45	0.60–9.99	0.210	2.02	0.74–5.52	0.170	1.84	0.47–7.12	0.380
3-month	5/17(29.4)	25/165(15.2)	0.164	6/13(46.2%)	45/165(27.3)	0.045	2.33	0.76–7.20	0.141	1.85	0.36–9.68	0.465	3.00	1.09–8.25	0.033	2.75	0.66–11.47	0.164
6-month	6/15(40.0)	27/160(16.9)	0.040	7/13(53.8)	41/165(24.8)	0.045	3.28	1.08–9.99	0.036	3.68	0.64–21.18	0.144	4.32	1.55–12.08	0.005	6.22	1.08–35.70	0.040
12-month	7/17(41.2)	26/165(15.8)	0.017	8/13(61.5)	39/165(23.6)	0.006	3.74	1.31–10.72	0.014	3.55	0.70–17.91	0.125	5.92	2.06–17.06	0.001	12.54	1.88–83.71	0.009

Covariates after adjusting for ADL: age, gender, admission type, type of surgery, hearing impairment, polypharmacy, MMSE scores, GDS-15 scores, BMI, risk of malnutrition, CCI scores, pain VAS scores, ASA physical status, length of hospital stay, baseline IADL scores.
Covariates after adjusting for IADL: age, gender, admission type, type of surgery, hearing impairment, polypharmacy, MMSE scores, GDS-15 scores, BMI, risk of malnutrition, CCI scores, pain VAS scores, ASA physical status, length of hospital stay, baseline ADL scores.

Table 4. Comparing the ADL and IADL scores at baseline and 1, 3, 6, and 12 months of follow-up in groups divided on the basis of cognitive problems.

	Time of follow-up (months)								
	Non-adjusted functional status (mean ± SE)					Adjusted baseline functional status by ANCOVA (mean ± SE)			
Outcomes variables	Baseline	1	3	6	12	1	3	6	12
ADL (BI) scores (mean ± SE) ^{a,b}									
Non-cognitive problems (A), N=109	$97.2\pm0.71^{\$,*}$	$94.2\pm1.10^{*}$	$95.8\pm1.05^{*}$	$96.3\pm1.00^{*}$	$96.8\pm0.89^{*}$	$93.0\pm1.10^{*}$	$94.5\pm1.08^{*}$	$95.0\pm1.19^{*}$	$95.6\pm1.24^{*}$
Cognitive impairment alone (B), N=56	$92.4\pm1.85^{\$}$	$91.3\pm1.68^{\#}$	$93.2\pm1.62^{\#}$	$92.9\pm2.19^{\#}$	$93.4\pm2.32^{\#}$	$92.6\pm1.53^{\#}$	$94.6\pm1.51^{\#}$	$94.4\pm1.66^{\#}$	$94.8\pm1.72^{\#}$
Delirium superimposed on cognitive impairment (C), N=13	$87.3\pm5.36^{*}$	$77.7\pm6.01^{*,\#}$	$78.5\pm6.76^{*,\#}$	$79.6\pm6.83^{*,\#}$	$79.2\pm7.42^{*,\#}$	$81.8\pm3.21^{*,\#}$	$82.7\pm3.16^{*,\#}$	$84.2\pm3.47^{*,\#}$	$83.3\pm3.61^{*,\#}$
IADL scores (mean ± SE) ^{a,b}									
Non-cognitive problems (A), N=109	$6.1\pm0.09^{*,\$}$	$5.7\pm0.12^{*,\$}$	$5.8\pm0.13^{*,\$}$	$5.9\pm0.14^{*,\$}$	$6.0\pm0.14^{*,\$}$	$5.4\pm0.11^{*}$	$5.5\pm0.11^{*}$	$5.6\pm0.13^{*}$	$5.7\pm0.13^{*}$
Cognitive impairment alone (B), N=56	$5.3\pm0.20^{\#,\$}$	$4.7\pm0.20^{\#,\$}$	$5.0\pm0.21^{\#,\$}$	$5.0\pm0.22^{\#,\$}$	$5.1\pm0.22^{\#,\$}$	$5.0\pm0.15^{\#}$	$5.4\pm0.15^{\#}$	$5.3\pm0.18^{*}$	$5.4\pm0.18^{\#}$
Delirium superimposed on cognitive impairment (C), N=13	$4.3\pm0.47^{*,\#}$	$3.3\pm0.49^{*,\#}$	$3.2\pm0.51^{*,\#}$	$3.1\pm0.60^{*,\#}$	$2.7\pm0.58^{*,\#}$	$4.4\pm0.32^{*,\#}$	$4.4\pm0.32^{*,\#}$	$4.2\pm0.38^{*,\#}$	$3.7\pm0.38^{*,\#}$

$^{*}p<0.05$ for comparing C and A; $^{\#}p<0.05$ for comparing C and B; $^{\$}p<0.05$ for comparing A and B.

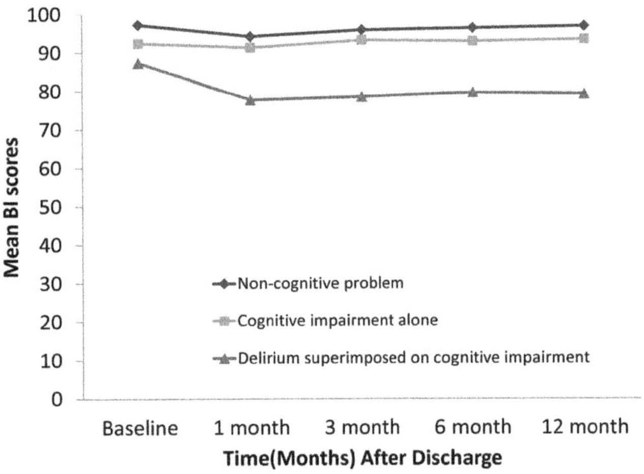

Figure 2. The trend of Barthel Index scores (ADL) (a) and IADL (b) for three groups corresponding to non-cognitive problem, cognitive impairment alone, and delirium superimposed on cognitive impairment.

cognitive dysfunction only (group B; Table 4). In terms of the decline in ADL and IADL scores at 1, 3, 6, and 12 months of follow up, ANCOVA (after adjustment for baseline ADL and IADL values) found significant ADL and IADL decline only in group C (Figure 2). After controlling for confounders (Table 5), multivariable logistic regression still showed the tendency for ADL and IADL to decline in patients in group C at 6 and 12 months (Adjusted RR for ADL at 6 months: 12.80, 95% CI: 1.65–99.40; Adjusted RR for ADL at 12 months: 7.96, 95% CI: 1.35–46.99; Adjusted RR for IADL at 6 months: 13.68, 95% CI: 1.94–96.55; Adjusted RR for IADL at 12 months: 30.61, 95% CI: 2.94–318.54).

Discussion

This prospective study investigated the effects of postoperative delirium on functional status (defined as decline in ADL and IADL scores) in patients who underwent orthopaedic surgery, and examined the interrelationship between underlying cognitive impairment and post-operative delirium. Postoperative delirium was an important predictor for poor IADL but not for poor ADL results. Moreover, delirium superimposed on cognitive problems was a stronger predictor of poor post-discharge functional status than cognitive impairment alone. The risk factors for the development of postoperative delirium identified in this study were in agreement with those identified by previous studies [6–10]. However, the incidence of postoperative delirium was lower in the present study than in previous studies, and the difference might be attributed to the higher percentage of elective surgery patients in our study (elective vs emergency surgery: 87.9% vs 12.1%). Moreover, patients in critical condition and unable to give their informed consent, such as some demented patients, were excluded from our study, thereby reducing the incidence of postoperative delirium.

Postoperative delirium had a strong adverse impact on IADL score after controlling for common geriatric problems, comorbidity, polypharmacy, and surgery-related conditions. A previous study reported that delirium had no significant effect on ADL score 6 months after surgery and attributed the relationship between delirium and mortality to some significant underlying medical problems [36]. An association between postoperative

Table 5. Multivariable logistic regression analysis of the predicted effect on functional status at the 6 and 12-month follow-up in groups divided on the basis of cognitive problems.

	ADL decline								IADL decline							
	at 6 months				at 12 months				at 6 months				at 12 months			
	Unadjusted		Adjusted		Unadjusted		Adjusted		Unadjusted		Adjusted		Unadjusted		Adjusted	
Independent variables	**RR**	**95% CI**	**RR**	**95% CI**	**RR**	**95% CI**	**RR**	**95% CI**	**RR**	**95% CI**	**RR**	**95% CI**	**RR**	**95% CI**	**RR**	**95% CI**
Cognitive impairment only (B) vs non-cognitive problem (A)	1.44	0.62–3.36	1.50	0.52–4.39	1.04	0.43–2.50	0.99	0.32–3.06	1.54	0.73–3.20	1.95	0.79–4.78	1.5	0.71–3.14	1.88	0.76–4.66
Delirium superimposed on cognitive impairment (C) vs non-cognitive problem (A)	6.75[&]	1.84–24.78	12.80[*]	1.65–99.40	6.31[&]	1.89–21.11	7.96[*]	1.35–46.99	4.13[*]	1.27–13.46	13.68[&]	1.94–96.55	5.98[&]	1.79–20.03	30.61[&]	2.94–318.54

[*]$p<0.05$, [&]$p<0.01$.
Covariates after adjusting for ADL: age, gender, admission type, type of surgery, hearing impairment, polypharmacy, GDS-15 scores, BMI, risk of malnutrition, CCI scores, pain VAS scores, ASA physical status, length of hospital stay, baseline IADL scores.
Covariates after adjusting for IADL: age, gender, admission type, type of surgery, hearing impairment, polypharmacy, GDS-15 scores, BMI, risk of malnutrition, CCI scores, pain VAS scores, ASA physical status, length of hospital stay, baseline ADL scores.

delirium and change in functional status at the time of hospital discharge and/or during follow up has also been shown in past studies [37–39]. However, the focus of most of these studies is short-term functional status. Although Vida et al. reported that delirium had an adverse effect on long-term IADL functional status 18 months after hospitalization, the effect disappeared after controlling for confounders [40]. In contrast to our results showing a relationship of postoperative delirium to IADL functional decline, those of Edelstein et al. demonstrated that decline in basic ADL but not IADL at 1-year follow-up was more likely in hip fracture surgery patients with postoperative delirium [41]. All the patients in the study by Edelstein et al. underwent hip fracture surgery, which has a greater impact on postoperative delirium and functional status than elective orthopaedic surgery. Furthermore, our study placed more emphasis on geriatric problems as confounders, e.g., malnutrition, polypharmacy, mood status, and symptoms of pain, which impact the risk of postoperative delirium as well as postoperative function. To the best of our knowledge, this is the first study to demonstrate the adverse impact of postoperative delirium on post-discharge ADL and IADL functional status after controlling for most geriatric problems considered as potential confounders. The adverse impact of postoperative delirium in this study was more profound on the IADL than ADL score. The baseline ADL scores for patients developing postoperative delirium and not developing postoperative delirium (85.9±4.81 and 95.6±0.80, respectively) indicated only mild impairment. It implied that the adverse effect of postoperative delirium might be reduced in robust elderly patients. Moreover, the predictive effect of delirium on IADL functional status was only noted 6 and 12 months after surgery. Therefore, factors other than delirium might have a greater effect on short-term functional status of elderly patients undergoing orthopaedic surgery.

Although delirium alone is not predictive for ADL decline during follow-up (after adjusting for confounders such as MMSE), delirium superimposed on cognitive impairment was significantly associated with ADL and IADL decline after surgery. In addition, postoperative delirium was more likely to develop in patients with severe cognitive impairment than in patients with moderate cognitive impairment (mean MMSE scores: group A 26.7±1.8 vs group B 19.8±3.8 vs group C 16.0±4.2). Underlying cognitive impairment (MMSE score <24) alone was not associated with postoperative ADL and IADL decline. The effects of severe cognitive impairment and postoperative delirium were highly interactive. Recovery from postoperative functional impairment by elderly patients undergoing orthopaedic surgery was dependent on the cognitive ability to adhere to rehabilitation programs. Givens et al. reported that each additional cognitive or mood disorder was associated with a greater risk of poor functional status [42]. Therefore, the results of this current study not only confirm the need to identify patients at risk for postoperative delirium, but also the highly interactive nature of the effects of baseline cognitive impairment and superimposed delirium on both ADL and IADL decline.

Despite the effort put into it, this study has several limitations. First, 21.6% (50/232) of the study subjects did not complete follow-up interviews. It has been reported that patients who experience delirium are more likely to miss follow-up appointments [43]. Although the incidence of delirium and the demographic data were similar between patients who completed follow-up and those who did not, there may still be a high risk of systematic attrition bias. Followed-up patients may have poorer clinical outcomes, therefore, the impact of delirium on long-term functional status may be underestimated in these patients. Second, the incidence of postoperative delirium was lower in our study than in previously published studies. Though delirium in this study was detected by the CAM and confirmed by a senior psychiatrist, who avoided overestimation, underestimation was still possible because we excluded patients who were admitted or transferred to ICU or unable to give informed consent, e.g., demented patients. Third, although the baseline cognitive function (assessed on admission before orthopaedic surgery) may be influenced by fracture or pain and lead to overestimation of cognitive impairment, it was not a predictor of ADL and IADL decline in our studies. Fourth, use of a wide range of procedures (performed within a single anatomic region) will impact both the risk of delirium as well as postoperative functional status. Because there were few patients undergoing operations, such as spinal decompression only, other elective knee surgery, and revision hip surgery, we treated similar types of surgery as single covariates, grouping them into four categories (elective spine surgery, elective knee surgery, elective hip arthroplasty, and ORIF/arthroplasty for hip fracture). Further work is needed to investigate the link between postoperative delirium and functional status in patients undergoing orthopaedic surgery at single operative site.

In conclusion, this prospective study evaluated the impact of different cognitive factors on ADL and IADL decline in elderly people undergoing orthopaedic surgery, and it was noted that delirium superimposed on cognitive impairment strongly affects both long-term ADL and IADL functional status. Early identification of patients with baseline cognitive impairment and implementation of strategies to prevent delirium may reduce the likelihood of functional decline following orthopaedic surgery in older patients. Further study is needed to confirm this.

Acknowledgments

Our local Institutional Review Board approved the present study protocol. The study was supported by the Veteran Affairs Commission of Taiwan. All authors declare no conflicts of interest.

The authors would like to thank all staff in the Orthopaedic Department for their valuable assistance in collecting the delirium symptom data. We also wish to thank Mr. Zhao-Rong Li, Associate Professor, Department of Business Management, National Kaohsiung Normal University, for his statistical assistance.

Author Contributions

Conceived and designed the experiments: CKL CLC YTL LKC. Performed the experiments: CKL CLC MYC TL CJH. Analyzed the data: CKL CLC LKC. Contributed reagents/materials/analysis tools: CLC MYC TL CJH. Wrote the paper: CKL YTL LKC.

References

1. Inouye SK (2006) Delirium in older persons. N Engl J Med 354: 1157–1165.
2. Élie M, Rousseau F, Cole M, Primeau F, McCusker J, et al. (2000) Prevalence and detection of delirium in elderly emergency department patients. CMAJ 163(8): 977–981.
3. Inouye SK, Foreman MD, Mion LC, Katz KH, Cooney LM Jr (2001) Nurses' recognition of delirium and its symptoms: comparison of nurse and researcher ratings. Arch Intern Med 161(20): 2467–2473.
4. Rudolph JL, Marcantonio ER (2011) Review articles: postoperative delirium: acute change with long-term implications. Anesth Analg 112: 1202–1211.
5. Gustafson Y, Berggren D, Brännström B, Bucht G, Norberg A, et al. (1988) Acute confusional states in elderly patients treated for femoral neck fracture. J Am Geriatr Soc 36: 525–530.
6. Schor JD, Levkoff SE, Lipsitz LA, Reilly CH, Cleary PD, et al. (1992) Risk factors for delirium in hospitalized elderly. JAMA 267: 827–831.

7. Levkoff SE, Evans DA, Liptzin B, Cleary PD, Lipsitz LA, et al. (1992) Delirium. The occurrence and persistence of symptoms among elderly hospitalized patients. Arch Intern Med 152: 334–340.
8. Wu CH, Chang CI, Chen CY (2012) Overview of studies related to geriatric syndrome in Taiwan. J Clin Gerontol Geriatr 3: 14–20.
9. Pompei P, Foreman M, Rudberg MA, Inouye SK, Braund V, et al. (1994) Delirium in hospitalized older persons: outcomes and predictors. J Am Geriatr Soc 42: 809–815.
10. Sanders RD, Pandharipande PP, Davidson AJ, Ma D, Maze M (2011) Anticipating and managing postoperative delirium and cognitive decline in adults. BMJ 343: d4331.
11. Chu CL, Liang CK, Lin YT, Chow PC, Pan CC, et al. (2011) Biomarkers of delirium: Well evidenced or not? J Clin Gerontol Geriatr 2: 100–104.
12. Inouye SK, Bogardus ST Jr, Charpentier PA, Leo-Summers L, Acampora D, et al. (1999) A multicomponent intervention to prevent delirium in hospitalized older patients. N Engl J Med 340: 669–676.
13. Marcantonio ER, Flacker JM, Wright RJ, Resnick NM (2001) Reducing delirium after hip fracture: a randomized trial. J Am Geriatr Soc 49: 516–522.
14. Rudolph JL, Jones RN, Rasmussen LS, Silverstein JH, Inouye SK, et al. (2007) Independent vascular and cognitive risk factors for postoperative delirium. Am J Med 120: 807–813.
15. Norkiene I, Ringaitiene D, Misiuriene I, Samalavicius R, Bubulis R, et al. (2007) Incidence and precipitating factors of delirium after coronary artery bypass grafting. Scand Cardiovasc J 41: 180–185.
16. Marcantonio ER, Flacker JM, Michaels M, Resnick NM (2000) Delirium is independently associated with poor functional recovery after hip fracture. J Am Geriatr Soc 48: 618–624.
17. Robinson TN, Raeburn CD, Tran ZV, Angles EM, Brenner LA, et al. (2009) Postoperative delirium in the elderly: risk factors and outcomes. Ann Surg 249: 173–178.
18. Koster S, Hensens AG, van der Palen J (2009) The long-term cognitive and functional outcomes of postoperative delirium after cardiac surgery. Ann Thorac Surg 87: 1469–1474.
19. Gottesman RF, Grega MA, Bailey MM, Pham LD, Zeger SL, et al. (2010) Delirium after coronary artery bypass graft surgery and late mortality. Ann Neurol 67: 338–344.
20. Lundstrom M, Edlund A, Bucht G, Karlsson S, Gustafson Y (2003) Dementia after delirium in patients with femoral neck fractures. J Am Geriatr Soc 51: 1002–1006.
21. Witlox J, Eurelings LS, de Jonghe JF, Kalisvaart KJ, Eikelenboom P, et al. (2010) Delirium in elderly patients and the risk of postdischarge mortality, institutionalization, and dementia: a meta-analysis. JAMA 304: 443–451.
22. Fick DM, Steis MR, Waller JL, Inouye SK (2013) Delirium superimposed on dementia is associated with prolonged length of stay and poor outcomes in hospitalized older adults. J Hosp Med 8: 500–505.
23. Steiner JF, Kramer AM, Eilertsen TB Kowalsky JC (1997) Development and validation of a clinical prediction rule for prolonged nursing home residence after hip fracture. J Am Geriatr Soc 45: 1510–1514.
24. Holmes J, House A (2000) Psychiatric illness predicts poor outcome after surgery for hip fracture: A prospective cohort study. Psychol Med 30: 921–929.
25. Francis J, Kapoor WN (1992) Prognosis after hospital discharge of older medical patients with delirium. J Am Geriatr Soc 40: 601–606.
26. Koponen H, Stenbäck U, Mattila E, Soininen H, Reinikainen K, et al. (1989) Delirium among elderly persons admitted to a psychiatric hospital: clinical course during the acute stage and one-year follow-up. Acta Psychiatr Scand 79: 579–585.
27. Liao YC, Yeh TL, Ko HC, Luoh CM, Lu HF (1995) Geriatric depression scale (GDS) – a preliminary report of reliability and validity for Chinese version. Changhua Med J 1; 11–17. (in Chinese)
28. Nyunt MS, Fones C, Niti M, Ng TP (2009) Criterion-based validity and reliability of the Geriatric Depression Screening Scale (GDS-15) in a large validation sample of community-living Asian older adults. Aging Ment Health 13: 376–382.
29. Kaiser MJ, Bauer JM, Ramsch C, Uter W, Guigoz Y, et al. (2009) Validation of the Mini Nutritional Assessment Short-Form (MNA-SF): a practical tool for identification of nutritional status. J Nutr Health Aging 13: 782–788.
30. Charlson ME, Pompei P, Ales KL, MacKenzie CR (1987) A new method of classifying prognostic comorbidity in longitudinal studies: development and validation. J Chronic Dis 40: 373–383.
31. Huskisson EC (1974) Measurement of pain. Lancet 2(7889): 1127–1131.
32. Folstein MF, Folstein SE, McHugh PR (1975) Mini-mental status: a practical method for grading the cognitive state of patients for the clinical use. J Psychiatr Res 12: 189–198.
33. Collin C, Wade DT, Davies S, Horne V (1988) "The Barthel ADL Index: a reliability study." Int Disability Study 10: 61–63.
34. Lawton MP, Brody EM (1969) Assessment of older people: Self-maintaining and instrumental activities of daily living. The Gerontologist 9: 179–186.
35. Inouye SK, Van Dyck CH, Alessi CA, Balkin S, Siegal AP, et al. (1990) Clarifying confusion: the confusion assessment method. A new method for detection of delirium. Ann Intern Med 113: 941–948.
36. Francis J, Kapoor WN (1990) Delirium in hospitalized elderly. J Gen Intern Med 5: 65–79.
37. Inouye SK, Rushing JT, Foreman MD, Palmer RM, Pompei P (1998) Does delirium contribute to poor hospital outcomes? A three-site epidemiologic study. J Gen Intern Med 13: 234–242.
38. Marcantonio ER, Flacker JM, Michaels M, Resnick NM (2000) Delirium is independently associated with poor functional recovery after hip fracture. J Am Geriatr Soc 48: 618–624.
39. Quinlan N, Rudolph JL (2011) Postoperative delirium and functional decline after noncardiac surgery. J Am Geriatr Soc 59 Suppl 2: S301–304.
40. Vida S, Galbaud du Fort G, Kakuma R, Arsenault L, Platt RW, et al. (2006) An 18-month prospective cohort study of functional outcome of delirium in elderly patients: activities of daily living. Int Psychogeriatr 18: 681–700.
41. Edelstein DM, Aharonoff GB, Karp A, Capla EL, Zuckerman JD, et al. (2004) Effect of postoperative delirium on outcome after hip fracture. Clin Orthop Relat Res (422): 195–200.
42. Givens JL, Sanft TB, Marcantonio ER (2008) Functional recovery after hip fracture: the combined effects of depressive symptoms, cognitive impairment, and delirium. J Am Geriatr Soc 56: 1075–1079.
43. Rudolph JL, Marcantonio ER, Culley DJ, Silverstein JH, Rasmussen LS, et al. (2008) Delirium is associated with early postoperative cognitive dysfunction. Anaesthesia 63: 941–947.

24

Risk Factors for Periprosthetic Joint Infection after Total Hip Arthroplasty and Total Knee Arthroplasty in Chinese Patients

Chuanlong Wu, **Xinhua Qu**, **Fengxiang Liu, Huiwu Li, Yuanqing Mao*, Zhenan Zhu***

Department of Orthopaedics, Shanghai Ninth People's Hospital, Shanghai Jiaotong University School of Medicine, Shanghai, People's Republic of China

Abstract

Purpose: The purpose of this hospital-based case–control study was to evaluate the risk factors for periprosthetic joint infection (PJI) of total hip arthroplasty (THA) and total knee arthroplasty (TKA) in Chinese patients.

Method: From January 2000 to December 2012, 45 patients undergoing THA and TKA who developed PJI were recruited for case subjects; controls were 252 without PJI, matched by year of index for surgery and type of surgery. Conditional logistic regressions were run to compute odds ratios (ORs) and 95% confidence intervals (CIs).

Results: Demographic factors and comorbid conditions associated with an increased adjusted risk of PJI (in decreasing order of significance) were diabetes (OR = 5.47, 95% CI: 1.77–16.97; $p = 0.003$), age (65–75 vs. 45–65 years) (OR = 3.36, 95% CI: 1.30–8.69; $p = 0.013$), BMI (≥28 vs. 18.5–28 kg/m^2) (OR = 2.77, 95% CI: 1.20–6.40; $p = 0.017$), place of residence (rural) (OR = 2.63, 95% CI: 1.13–6.10; $p = 0.025$) and alcohol abuse (OR = 2.95, 95% CI: 1.06–8.23; $p = 0.039$).

Conclusion: Patients with diabetes, older age, BMI of ≥28 kg/m^2 and alcohol abuse or living in rural areas, had increased PJI risk. Additional systematic large-scale studies are needed to verify these results.

Editor: Lyle L. Moldawer, University of Florida College of Medicine, United States of America

Funding: This work was supported by grants from the National Natural Science Foundation of China (No. 81171729 and No. 81301590), Major Basic Research of Science and Technology Commission of Shanghai Municipality (Grant No. 11DJ1400303), and Fund for Key Disciplines of Shanghai Municipal Education Commission (J50206). The funders had no role in study design, data collection and analysis, decision to publish, or preparation of the manuscript.

Competing Interests: The authors have declared that no competing interests exist.

* E-mail: 13761360486@163.com (YM); zhenan_zhu@126.com (ZZ)

These authors contributed equally to this work.

Introduction

The techniques of total hip arthroplasty (THA) and total knee arthroplasty (TKA) are highly successful procedures and have become conventional methods for improving quality of life and reducing pain in patients with joint diseases. Despite this, periprosthetic joint infection (PJI), a common complication of total joint arthroplasty (TJA), can have catastrophic consequences. PJI rates can reach as high as 3% following primary THA [1], and can occur in up to 2% of uncomplicated TKA cases [2].

Several demographic factors and comorbid conditions are risk factors for PJI after THA and TKA, including age [3,4], sex [5–8], race [7], diabetes, obesity, alcohol abuse, preoperative diagnosis, tobacco use, congestive heart failure, chronic pulmonary disease, chronic liver disease, renal disease, preoperative anemia, oncologic disease, bone cancer, metastatic tumor, and neurologic disease [5,6,8–16]. Poultsides et al. [7] found that race was an important risk factor for PJI; compared with whites, other races had an increased risk of PJI. Namba et al. [6,11], however, indicated that Asians (vs. whites) had no significant difference in PJI risk. To our knowledge, data on the risk factors for PJI in Asian populations is very scarce. Therefore, this study aimed to evaluate the risk factors for PJI after THA and TKA in Chinese patients.

Methods

Ethics statement

This case–control study is a hospital-based retrospective investigation conducted at the Shanghai Ninth People's Hospital in Shanghai, China. This study was approved by the Ethics Committee of Shanghai Ninth People's Hospital, and all participants provided written informed consent.

Study population

From January 2000 to December 2012, patients undergoing THA or TKA who developed PJI were enrolled for cases group. Controls were patients undergoing THA or TKA without PJI, matched by year of index surgery and type of surgery. Each case was matched with 5 controls. The case and control groups did not differ significantly in terms of demographic or clinical characteristics (retrieved from patients' medical records).

Data collection

We collected data through clinical records, including operative notes, inpatient charts, and discharge summaries. The demographic characteristics of patients included age, sex, and place of residence. To investigate the influence of age on PJI, age was stratified into 4 groups (<45 years, 45–65 years, 65–75 years, and >75 years) [7]. Place of residence was categorized as "urban" and "rural." Because body mass index (BMI) criteria vary by country, we used the official Chinese guidelines and divided subjects into the following 2 groups: overweight (18.5–28 kg/m^2) and obese (≥28 kg/m^2).

The preoperative diagnosis for which THA or TKA was collected included osteoarthritis, femoral head necrosis, developmental dysplasia of the hip, fracture, rheumatoid arthritis, and other. The comorbid conditions of patients included tobacco use, alcohol abuse, diabetes, treatment of diabetes (insulin), hypertension, cardiovascular event, chronic pulmonary disease, chronic liver disease, renal disease, preoperative anemia, prostatic disorder, substance abuse, cerebral infarction, oncologic disease, neurologic disease, history of tuberculosis, gout, and ankylosing spondylitis. These comorbid conditions were chosen based on the specific diseases used to determine the composite Charlson Comorbidity Index [17] as well as other diseases used as comorbidity measures for administrative databases, which are associated with increased length of hospital stay, hospital charges, complications, and mortality [18]. Furthermore, pre-existing diseases identified as risk factors for PJI in clinical studies were also included [14]. We also collected data on dental procedures performed within 6 months before TJA. These data were collected through patients' medical records.

At the same time, we collected and reviewed previous studies examining the risk factors for PJI or surgical site infection (SSI) in patients who underwent joint arthroplasty.

Definition of PJI

PJI in our study is present when one of the following occurs: (1) a sinus tract communicates with the prosthesis; (2) positive culture results from 2 or more tissue or fluid samples from the affected prosthesis; or (3) 4 of the following 6 criteria are present: (a) elevated serum C-reactive protein level and erythrocyte sedimentation rate, (b) elevated synovial white blood cell count, (c) high synovial polymorphonuclear (PMN) leukocyte percentage, (d) presence of purulence in the joint, (e) positive culture result from one sample from the affected joint, and (f) PMN leukocyte count of more than 5 per high-powered field in 5 high-powered fields on histologic analysis at 400× magnification.

Statistical analysis

The distributions of demographic characteristics and comorbid conditions between cases and controls were compared using chi-squared tests. Pearson's chi-squared test was used for qualitative variable analysis, and Fisher's exact test was used when n (number of data) was less than 20 or when any value was less than 5. We systematically assessed the influence of each characteristic on the risk of PJI. All tests were 2-sided. We used conditional logistic regression to calculate odds ratios (ORs) and 95% confidence intervals (CIs) to estimate the effect of each factor on the risk of PJI. All variables were regressed on PJI with adjustment for patient characteristics. All analyses were conducted using SPSS version 18.0 (IBM Corporation, Armonk, NY) with significance set at the 5% level.

Results

Patient characteristics

Fifty-two cases were identified but 7 were later excluded due to incomplete data. Our final sample comprised 45 case patients (average age, 67 years; range, 41–85 years) and 252 controls (average age, 63 years; range, 24–93 years).

Table 1 presents the distributions of 45 cases and 252 controls according to age, sex, place of residence, type and diagnosis. By design, cases and controls had similar distribution by type ($p = 0.492$). Cases had a lower proportion of subjects aged 45–65 years (28.9% vs. 44.8%), living in an urban area (60.0% vs. 73.8%), and with a preoperative diagnosis of fracture (24.4% vs. 34.9%), but a higher proportion of subjects aged 65–75 years (42.2% vs. 27.0%) with a preoperative diagnosis of rheumatoid arthritis (22.2% vs. 10.7%). There was no significant difference in the distribution of sex between groups ($p = 0.843$).

Risk factors for PJI

Table 2 shows distribution of cases and controls according to patient characteristics. The case group had a higher prevalence of diabetes (37.8% vs. 9.5%, $p<0.001$), prevalence of diabetes treatment (insulin) (17.8% vs. 2.4%, $p<0.001$), prevalence of alcohol abuse (33.3% vs. 13.5%, $p = 0.001$), and proportion of patients with a BMI≥28 kg/m^2 (57.8% vs. 36.1%, $p<0.001$). The differences of distribution according to other characteristics were not statistically significant ($p>0.05$).

Table 3 examines the ORs of the independent risk factors for PJI through multivariate regression analysis. Demographic factors and comorbid conditions associated with increased adjusted risk of PJI (in decreasing order of significance) were diabetes (OR = 5.47;

Table 1. Patient demographics and other characteristics according to occurrence of PJI.

	Periprosthetic joint infection		
	Yes (n = 45)	No (n = 252)	P*
Age, y			0.107
<45	2 (4.4)	19 (7.5)	
45–65	13 (28.9)	113 (44.8)	
65–75	19 (42.2)	68 (27.0)	
≥75	11 (24.4)	52 (20.6)	
Sex			0.843
Male	20 (44.4)	108 (42.9)	
Female	25 (55.6)	144 (57.1)	
Place of residence			0.058
Rural	18 (40.0)	66 (26.2)	
Urban	27 (60.0)	186 (73.8)	
Type			0.492
THA	28 (62.2)	170 (67.5)	
TKA	17 (37.8)	82 (32.5)	
Diagnosis			0.237
Osteoarthritis	8 (17.8)	54 (21.4)	
Femoral head necrosis	8 (17.8)	30 (11.9)	
Developmental dysplasia of the hip	6 (13.3)	40 (15.9)	
Fracture	11(24.4)	88 (34.9)	
Rheumatoid arthritis	10 (22.2)	27 (10.7)	
Other	2 (4.4)	13 (5.2)	

All values are expressed as n (%).
*According to chi-square test.
Abbreviations: THA, total hip arthroplasty; TKA, total knee arthroplasty.

Table 2. Patient comorbidities according to occurrence of PJI.

	Periprosthetic joint infection		
	Yes	**No**	**P***
Body mass index, kg/m²			**<0.001**
<18.5	1 (2.2)	5 (2.0)	
18.5–28	18 (40.0)	156 (61.9)	
≥28	26 (57.8)	91 (36.1)	
Diabetes	17 (37.8)	24 (9.5)	**<0.001**
Treatment of diabetes (insulin)	8 (17.8)	6 (2.4)	**<0.001**
Alcohol abuse	15 (33.3)	34 (13.5)	**0.001**
Anemia	3 (6.7)	31 (12.3)	0.274
Dental procedure with antibiotic	5 (11.1)	18(7.1)	0.359
Neurologic disease	1 (2.2)	13 (5.2)	0.392
Oncologic disease	1 (2.2)	12 (4.8)	0.443
Dental procedure	8 (26.7)	35 (13.9)	0.495
Ankylosing spondylitis	1 (2.2)	11 (4.4)	0.501
Tobacco use	5 (11.1)	37 (14.7)	0.527
Hypertension	9 (20.0)	60 (23.8)	0.577
Cardiovascular event	5 (11.1)	31 (12.3)	0.822
Chronic pulmonary disease	7 (15.6)	36 (14.3)	0.824
Chronic liver disease	4 (8.9)	20 (7.9)	0.829
Prostatic disorder	4 (8.9)	25 (9.9)	0.830
Cerebral infarction	3 (6.7)	15 (6.0)	0.853
Substance abuse	4 (8.9)	24 (9.5)	0.893
Renal disease	6 (13.3)	32 (12.7)	0.907
Gout	3 (6.7)	16 (6.3)	0.936
History of tuberculosis	2 (4.4)	11 (4.4)	0.981

All values are expressed as n (%).
*According to the chi-square test.

95% CI, 1.77–16.97; $p = 0.003$), age (65–75 years; OR = 3.36; 95% CI, 1.30–8.69; $p = 0.013$), BMI (≥28 kg/m^2; OR = 2.77; 95% CI, 1.20–6.40; $p = 0.017$), place of residence (rural; OR = 2.63; 95% CI, 1.13–6.10; $p = 0.025$), and alcohol abuse (OR = 2.95; 95% CI, 1.06–8.23; $p = 0.039$). Dental procedures had an OR of 1.71 (95% CI, 0.38–7.70; $p = 0.487$), while dental procedures with antibiotic prophylaxis had an OR of 1.38 (95% CI, 0.20–9.54; $p = 0.743$) (Table 3). No meaningful differences were found in the other factors.

Table 3. Independent risk factors for PJI after multivariate regression analysis.

Patient demographics/comorbid conditions	Odds ratio	95% CI	P
Diabetes	5.47	1.77–16.97	**0.003**
Age (65–75 y vs. 45–65 y)	3.36	1.30–8.69	**0.013**
BMI (≥28 kg/m² vs. 18.5–28 kg/m²)	2.77	1.20–6.40	**0.017**
Place of residence (rural)	2.63	1.13–6.10	**0.025**
Alcohol abuse	2.95	1.06–8.23	**0.039**
Age (>75 y vs. 45–65 y)	2.54	0.83–7.79	0.103
Treatment of diabetes (insulin)	3.69	0.63–21.69	0.148
Chronic pulmonary disease	2.35	0.68–8.15	0.177
Hypertension	0.55	0.19–1.61	0.279
Substance abuse	1.80	0.45–7.21	0.408
Cerebral infarction	0.46	0.07–3.12	0.426
Dental procedure	1.71	0.38–7.70	0.487
Renal disease	1.43	0.43–4.80	0.559
Gout	1.51	0.32–7.10	0.600
Cardiovascular event	1.32	0.39–4.52	0.654
Chronic liver disease	1.34	0.36–5.04	0.663
Anemia	0.74	0.17–3.26	0.688
Tobacco use	1.29	0.35–4.76	0.703
Ankylosing spondylitis	0.62	0.05–7.43	0.704
BMI (<18.5 kg/m² vs. 18.5–28 kg/m²)	1.55	0.12–20.16	0.740
Dental procedure with antibiotic	1.38	0.20–9.54	0.743
THA (vs. TKA)	0.89	0.37–2.12	0.789
Male (vs. female)	0.95	0.40–2.21	0.899
Age (<45 y vs. 45–65 y)	0.91	0.15–5.40	0.919
Prostatic disorder	0.94	0.23–3.87	0.930
Oncologic disease	0.90	0.08–10.69	0.936
Neurologic disease	0.94	0.10–8.95	0.958
History of tuberculosis	1.02	0.16–6.44	0.980
Diagnosis			
Rheumatoid arthritis (vs. osteoarthritis)	2.81	0.69–11.47	0.151
Femoral head necrosis	2.02	0.52–7.89	0.314
Developmental dysplasia of the hip	1.54	0.40–5.89	0.527
Other	1.72	0.19–15.13	0.626
Fracture	0.83	0.24–2.89	0.772

Abbreviations: BMI, body mass index; CI, confidence interval; THA, total hip arthroplasty; TKA, total knee arthroplasty.

Discussion

This study provides the first evidence that diabetes, age of 65–75 years, BMI≥28 kg/m^2, rural place of residence, and alcohol abuse were independently associated with increased risk of PJI for TJA patients in a Chinese population.

Demographic factors

Age. We found that patients aged 65–75 years had 3.36-fold higher risk of PJI compared with patients aged 45–65 years. Similarly, Ridgeway et al. [3] reported that patients aged 75–79 years and >80 years had a 1.56- and 1.66 -fold increased risk of PJI, respectively, compared with patients aged <65 years after all types of hip replacement. In general, older patient age would seem to coincide with poorer nutritional status and weakened immunity, resulting in elevated risk of infection.

In contrast, a single-center analysis of 8,494 joint arthroplasties, including both hip and knee procedures, showed that younger age was associated with increased risk of infection [4]. The authors explained that younger patients are generally more active than older patients; thus, younger patients potentially subject their implants to greater numbers of use cycles, leading to wear, potential revision surgery, and possibility of infection. Their study is limited, however, due to the small number of cases (43 patients). Another study[7] reported that patients aged <45 years had a 1.70-fold higher risk of PJI compared with patients aged 45–65 years. Their explanation was that this specific age group includes those undergoing TJA for inflammatory diseases (rheumatoid arthritis, systemic lupus), and those with suppressed immune systems, posttraumatic osteoarthritis after open/complex fractures necessitating multiple prior surgeries, and/or hemophilia. Other studies have reported that age had no significant effect on risk of PJI [5–8,11,19] (**Table 4 and Table 5**). More trials are needed to research the mechanism between age and PJI.

Place of residence. To our knowledge, no study has specifically reported place of residence to be a risk factor associated with incidence of PJI. We found that compared with urban patients, those living in rural areas had a 2.63-fold increased risk of PJI. This may be due to more activities, delay in diagnosing the underlying disease, irregular treatment, or difficulty paying medical expenses in some rural areas. The difference between city and rural areas also may be explained in terms of social status and education. The specific reasons for increased risk in patients living in rural require further elucidation.

Comorbid conditions

Diabetes. In the current study, patients with diabetes had an increased risk of PJI (adjusted OR = 5.47; 95% CI, 1.77–16.97) compared with patients without diabetes. Similarly, a case–control study focusing on primary hip and knee arthroplasties, conducted by Lai et al. [12], showed that PJI incidence was 3.91 times higher in patients reporting a history of diabetes. Jamsen et al. [13] analyzed the one-year incidence of PJI in a single-center series of 7,181 patients with primary hip and knee replacements, conducted between 2002 and 2008, and found that diabetes more than doubled the risk of PJI, independent of obesity (adjusted OR = 2.3; 95% CI, 1.1–4.7). Several studies have also suggested that diabetes increases the risk of postoperative infection in TJA patients [6,7,9,10] (**Table 4 and Table 5**).

Previous literature has suggested several mechanisms behind the relationship between diabetes and PJI, but no definite conclusions have been made. On one hand, Joshi et al. reported that diabetes seems to increase the likelihood of infection caused by certain bacteria, such as *Staphylococcus aureus* [20], which is a susceptible bacteria for PJI. On the other hand, whether adaptive immune responses are affected by diabetes is still controversial [21,22]. Finally, multiple factors have been cited as affecting the risk of PJI in diabetic patients, including type of hyperglycemia treatment, glycemic control, occurrence of diabetes-related complications, and postoperative hyperglycemia [23–26]. In contrast, some studies have reported that diabetes has no effect on PJI risk [5,15,27,28] (**Table 4 and Table 5**). In summary, more research, particularly looking at the molecular mechanisms of diabetes affecting PJI risk, is urgently needed.

BMI. Our data showed that patients with a BMI greater than 28 kg/m^2 had a 2.77 -fold higher risk of PJI compared with patients with a BMI between 18.5 and 28 kg/m^2. Likewise, in 2013, Bozic et al. [5] found that obesity independently increased the risk of PJI by 2.12 times after reviewing 587 patients who underwent THA. In another study examining the Medicare sample claims database of 40,919 patients who underwent primary THA, obesity was associated with a 1.73 -fold increased risk of PJI [15]. Several other studies also support our results regarding the effect of BMI on PJI risk [6,9,11,14,15]. Reduced immunity and increased susceptibility of obese individuals to infection may explain why obese patients more easily develop PJI [29]. In contrast, Poultsides et al. [7] indicated that obesity was associated with a 0.87-times-fold decreased risk of PJI in patients who underwent primary hip and knee arthroplasties. The authors explained that the reason for this may be that readmission data were not captured and these patients may present more commonly after discharge from the hospital, especially since the length of stay is now 3–4 days (or less) for most TJAs.

Alcohol. Our data showed alcohol abuse to carry a 2.95-fold higher risk of PJI. Very few studies have found alcohol abuse to be associated with an increased risk of infection in TJA patients. In a 10-year study of patients who underwent primary hip and knee arthroplasties, Poultsides et al. [7] found that alcohol abuse carried a 1.57-fold higher risk of PJI. Excessive alcohol consumption plays an important role in the development of cirrhosis, which shows an increased incidence of bacterial infection [30]. Impaired phago-

Table 4. Data from previous studies examining risk factors for periprosthetic joint infection (PJI) or surgical site infection (SSI) in patients who underwent THA and TKA.

Author	Year	Country	Research type	Total number of patients	Position	Statistical method
Bozic et al.	2013	USA	Case–control	587	THA-PJI	Multivariate Cox regression
Namba et al.	2013	USA	Cohort study	56,216	TKA-SSI	Multivariate Cox regression
Everhart at al.	2013	USA	Cohort study	1,891	TJA-SSI	Logistic regression
Poultsides et al.	2012	USA	Cohort study	1,196,691	Hip and knee arthroplasty-PJI	Logistic regression
Namba et al.	2012	USA	Cohort study	30,491	THA-SSI	Multivariate Cox regression
Dale et al.	2012	Norway	Cohort study	432,168	THA-PJI	Multivariate Cox regression
Bozic et al.	2012	USA	Cohort study	40,919	THA-PJI	Multivariate Cox regression
Bozic et al.	2012	USA	Cohort study	83,011	TKA-PJI	Multivariate Cox regression
Song et al.	2012	Republic of Korea	Cohort study	6,848	THA,TKA-SSI	Logistic regression
Peel et al.	2011	Australia	Case–control	189	Hip and knee arthroplasty-PJI	Logistic regression
Pulido et al.	2008	USA	Cohort study	9,245	Hip and knee arthroplasty-PJI	Logistic regression
Babkin et al.	2007	Israel	Case-control	180	TKA-SSI	Logistic regression
Kasteren et al.	2007	Holland	Cohort study	1,922	THA-SSI	Logistic regression
Lai et al.	2007	Canada	Case-control	52	Hip and knee arthroplasty-PJI	Logistic regression
Ridgeway et al.	2005	UK	Cohort study	24,808	Hip arthroplasty-SSI	Logistic regression

Abbreviations: THA, total hip arthroplasty; TKA, total knee arthroplasty; TJA, total joint arthroplasty.

Table 5. Data from previous studies examining risk factors (positive results in this article) for periprosthetic joint infection or surgical site infection in patients who underwent THA and TKA, in detail.

Literatures	Patient demographics/ comorbid conditions	Age, y	BMI, kg/m²	Diabetes	Alcohol abuse
Bozic et al. (2013)	HR (95% CI), P-value	**≤44 vs. >75:** 0.47 (0.13–1.70), 0.25; **45–54 vs. >75**: 1.01 (0.43–2.36), 0.99; **55–64 vs. >75**: 1.22 (0.59–2.54), 0.59; **65–74 vs. >75**: 0.90 (0.40–2.00), 0.80	**Obesity**: 2.12 (1.08–4.16), 0.03	1.11 (0.53–2.30), 0.79	
Namba et al. (2013)	HR (95% CI), P-value	**1-year increment**: 0.99 (0.98–1.00), 0.17	**≥35 vs. <35**: 1.47 (1.17–1.85), 0.01	1.28 (1.03–1.60), 0.03	
Everhart et al. (2013)	OR (95% CI), P-value		**≥50**: 5.28 (1.38–17.1), 0.01	1.83 (1.02–3.27), 0.05	
Poultsides et al. (2013)	OR (95% CI), P-value	**0–44 vs. 45–64**: 1.70 (1.48–1.95), 0.01; **65–74 vs. 45–64**: 0.90 (0.83–0.97), 0.01; **≥75 vs. 45–64**: 0.98 (0.90–1.06), 0.23	**Obesity**: 0.87 (0.78–0.97), 0.01	**Uncomplicated diabetes**: 0.95 (0.86–1.04), 0.28 **Complicated diabetes**: 1.54 (1.22–1.94), 0.01	1.57 (1.23–2.00), 0.01
Namba et al. (2012)	HR (95% CI), P-value	**1-year increment**: 1.00 (0.98–1.01), 0.72	**<18.5 vs. 18.5–30**: 2.88 (0.89–9.23), 0.08; **30–35 vs. 18.5–30**: 1.56 (1.03–2.37), 0.04; **≥35 vs. 18.5–30**: 2.37 (1.55–3.61), <0.01	1.25 (0.85–1.83), 0.26	
Dale et al. (2012)	HR (95% CI), P-value	**40–51 vs. <40**: 1.1 (0.8–1.5), 0.6; **60–69 vs. <40**: 1.1 (0.8–1.5), 0.7; **70–79 vs. <40**: 1.1 (0.8–1.5),0.6; **80–89 vs. <40**: 0.9 (0.7–1.3), 0.8; **≥90 vs. <40**: 0.7 (0.4–1.4), 0.3			
Bozic et al. -THA(2012)	HR (95% CI), P-value		**Obesity**: 1.73 (1.35–2.22), 0.01	1.31 (1.12–1.53), 0.06	1.72 (0.98–3.01), 0.06
Bozic et al. -TKA (2012)	HR (95% CI), P-value		**Obesity**: 1.22 (1.03–1.44), 0.02	1.19 (1.06–1.34), 0.01	1.11 (0.63–1.97), 0.71
Song et al. (2012)	OR (95% CI), P-value			**TKA and THA**: 1.56 (1.10–2.21), >0.05 **THA**: 1.97 (1.20–3.22), >0.05	
Peel et al. (2011)	OR (95% CI), P-value			**Knee replacement**: 1.5 (0.9–2.7), 0.2; **Hip replacement**: 1.4 (0.8–2.2), 0.2; **Hip and knee replacements**: 1.4 (0.9–2.1), 0.06	
Pulido et al. (2008)	OR (95% CI), P-value		**≥40**: 3.23 (1.6–6.5), 0.01		
Kasteren et al. (2007)	OR (95% CI), P-value	**Per 10-year increase**: 1.4 (1.0–2.1), 0.08			
Lai et al. (2007)	OR (95% CI), P-value		**Obesity (BMI>30)**: NS	3.91 (1.06–14.44), 0.04	
Ridgeway et al. (2005)	OR (95% CI), P-value	**65–74 vs. <65**: 1.13 (0.85–1.50), <0.01; **75–79 vs.** <65: 1.56 (1.16–2.10), <0.01; **≥80 vs. <65**: 1.66 (1.24–2.21), <0.01			

Abbreviations: BMI, body mass index; HR, hazard ratio; NS, not significant; OA, osteoarthritis; OR, odds ratio; THA, total hip arthroplasty; TKA, total knee arthroplasty; RR, relative risk.

cytic function may be another important reason [31]. In addition, studies have shown that alcohol affects both branches of the immune system on multiple levels and disrupts many immune mechanisms [32].

Dental procedures. Bacteremia from distant infectious foci may cause prosthesis contamination through a hematogenic route. Dental is one of the primary foci most frequently reported in the worldwide literature. The association of dental procedures with risk of PJI has been actively debated for many years. Compared with dental procedure without antibiotic prophylaxis, we found that dental procedure with antibiotic prophylaxis had a lower risk of PJI, but that both dental procedure with or without antibiotic prophylaxis were not significant risk factors for PJI (p>0.05). The new "American Academy of Orthopedic Surgeons (AAOS) and

American Dental Association (ADA) Clinical Practice Guideline on Prevention of Orthopaedic Implant Infection in Patients Undergoing Dental Procedures" [33] indicates that dental procedures are not risk factors for subsequent total hip or knee infection. The use of antibiotic prophylaxis prior to dental procedures did not decrease the risk of subsequent total hip or knee infection [34]. Our results support the guideline.

Previous studies have found that TKA (vs. THA) [14], male (vs. female) sex [5–8], femoral head necrosis (vs. osteoarthritis) [6,8], rheumatic disease [10,15], hip fracture [8], posttraumatic arthritis [6], inflammatory disease [8], tobacco use [9], congestive heart failure [7,10], chronic pulmonary disease [7,10], chronic liver disease [7], renal disease [7,10], preoperative anemia [10,15], oncologic disease [7], bone cancer [9], metastatic tumor [10], and neurologic disease [7] are significant increased risk factors for PJI, and that male (vs. female) sex [11] significantly decreases the risk of PJI (**Table S1**). However, we did not find these conditions to be significantly associated with PJI risk after controlling for all clinical and demographic factors in our study ($p>0.05$). Different circumstances, races, study designs, and statistical analyses may explain the discrepancies between various studies. Our findings are of significant importance to Chinese individuals.

Strengths and limitations of this study

Our study has several strengths over previous studies on this topic. First, to the best of our knowledge, this is the first case–control study to investigate the effect of patient factors on PJI risk in a Chinese population. Compared with whites, Chinese individuals use more antibiotics when they have a common cold or other diseases. Therefore, we believe it is very significant to investigate the risk factors for infection in the Chinese population. Second, we found that patients living in rural areas had an increased risk of PJI compared with urban patients. This is a warning for rural patients and local government. Third, we confirmed the point of the new "AAOS-ADA Clinical Practice Guideline on Prevention of Orthopaedic Implant Infection in Patients Undergoing Dental Procedures."

Nevertheless, this study has some limitations. First, more than 90% of individuals with diabetes had the type 2 variant, which is believed to have multiple causes (including obesity). We were unable to discriminate between type 1 and type 2 diabetes in our analyses; hence, we could not analyze the association between diabetes subtype and PJI risk. Second, the number of patients with PJI was rather low, which may have reduced the generalizability of our conclusions. Finally, because of the low number of study subjects, we did not distinguish between high-risk and low-risk dental procedures. This may have affected the accuracy of the influence of dental procedure on PJI risk.

Conclusion

In conclusion, patients with diabetes, age of 65–75 years, BMI≥28 kg/m^2, alcohol abuse, or residence in rural areas had increased risk of PJI in this Chinese population. Further systematic studies evaluating the risk factors for PJI in Asian populations are needed to confirm these findings.

Supporting Information

Table S1 Data from previous studies examining risk factors(others) for periprosthetic joint infection or surgical site infection in patients who underwent THA and TKA, in detail.

Author Contributions

Conceived and designed the experiments: CW XQ FL YM ZZ. Performed the experiments: CW XQ FL HL YM ZZ. Analyzed the data: CW XQ FL HL YM ZZ. Contributed reagents/materials/analysis tools: CW XQ FL HL YM ZZ. Wrote the paper: CW XQ YM ZZ.

References

1. Bozic KJ, Ries MD (2005) The impact of infection after total hip arthroplasty on hospital and surgeon resource utilization. J Bone Joint Surg Am 87: 1746–1751.
2. Sculco TP (1993) The economic impact of infected total joint arthroplasty. Instr Course Lect 42: 349–351.
3. Ridgeway S, Wilson J, Charlet A, Kafatos G, Pearson A, et al. (2005) Infection of the surgical site after arthroplasty of the hip. J Bone Joint Surg Br 87: 844–850.
4. Malinzak RA, Ritter MA, Berend ME, Meding JB, Olberding EM, et al. (2009) Morbidly obese, diabetic, younger, and unilateral joint arthroplasty patients have elevated total joint arthroplasty infection rates. J Arthroplasty 24: 84–88.
5. Bozic KJ, Ward DT, Lau EC, Chan V, Wetters NG, et al. (2013) Risk Factors for Periprosthetic Joint Infection Following Primary Total Hip Arthroplasty: A Case Control Study. J Arthroplasty.
6. Namba RS, Inacio MC, Paxton EW (2013) Risk factors associated with deep surgical site infections after primary total knee arthroplasty: an analysis of 56,216 knees. J Bone Joint Surg Am 95: 775–782.
7. Poultsides LA, Ma Y, Della Valle AG, Chiu YL, Sculco TP, et al. (2013) In-hospital surgical site infections after primary hip and knee arthroplasty—incidence and risk factors. J Arthroplasty 28: 385–389.
8. Dale H, Fenstad AM, Hallan G, Havelin LI, Furnes O, et al. (2012) Increasing risk of prosthetic joint infection after total hip arthroplasty. Acta Orthop 83: 449–458.
9. Everhart JS, Altneu E, Calhoun JH (2013) Medical Comorbidities Are Independent Preoperative Risk Factors for Surgical Infection After Total Joint Arthroplasty. Clin Orthop Relat Res.
10. Bozic KJ, Lau E, Kurtz S, Ong K, Berry DJ (2012) Patient-related risk factors for postoperative mortality and periprosthetic joint infection in medicare patients undergoing TKA. Clin Orthop Relat Res 470: 130–137.
11. Namba RS, Inacio MC, Paxton EW (2012) Risk factors associated with surgical site infection in 30,491 primary total hip replacements. J Bone Joint Surg Br 94: 1330–1338.
12. Lai K, Bohm ER, Burnell C, Hedden DR (2007) Presence of medical comorbidities in patients with infected primary hip or knee arthroplasties. J Arthroplasty 22: 651–656.
13. Jamsen E, Nevalainen P, Eskelinen A, Huotari K, Kalliovalkama J, et al. (2012) Obesity, diabetes, and preoperative hyperglycemia as predictors of periprosthetic joint infection: a single-center analysis of 7181 primary hip and knee replacements for osteoarthritis. J Bone Joint Surg Am 94: e101.
14. Pulido L, Ghanem E, Joshi A, Purtill JJ, Parvizi J (2008) Periprosthetic joint infection: the incidence, timing, and predisposing factors. Clin Orthop Relat Res 466: 1710–1715.
15. Bozic KJ, Lau E, Kurtz S, Ong K, Rubash H, et al. (2012) Patient-related risk factors for periprosthetic joint infection and postoperative mortality following total hip arthroplasty in Medicare patients. J Bone Joint Surg Am 94: 794–800.
16. Song KH, Kim ES, Kim YK, Jin HY, Jeong SY, et al. (2012) Differences in the risk factors for surgical site infection between total hip arthroplasty and total knee arthroplasty in the Korean Nosocomial Infections Surveillance System (KONIS). Infect Control Hosp Epidemiol 33: 1086–1093.
17. Charlson ME, Pompei P, Ales KL, MacKenzie CR (1987) A new method of classifying prognostic comorbidity in longitudinal studies: development and validation. J Chronic Dis 40: 373–383.
18. Elixhauser A, Steiner C, Harris DR, Coffey RM (1998) Comorbidity measures for use with administrative data. Med Care 36: 8–27.
19. van Kasteren ME, Mannien J, Ott A, Kullberg BJ, de Boer AS, et al. (2007) Antibiotic prophylaxis and the risk of surgical site infections following total hip arthroplasty: timely administration is the most important factor. Clin Infect Dis 44: 921–927.
20. Joshi N, Caputo GM, Weitekamp MR, Karchmer AW (1999) Infections in patients with diabetes mellitus. N Engl J Med 341: 1906–1912.
21. Eibl N, Spatz M, Fischer GF, Mayr WR, Samstag A, et al. (2002) Impaired primary immune response in type-1 diabetes: results from a controlled vaccination study. Clin Immunol 103: 249–259.
22. Pozzilli P, Gale EA, Visalli N, Baroni M, Crovari P, et al. (1986) The immune response to influenza vaccination in diabetic patients. Diabetologia 29: 850–854.
23. Marchant MH Jr, Viens NA, Cook C, Vail TP, Bolognesi MP (2009) The impact of glycemic control and diabetes mellitus on perioperative outcomes after total joint arthroplasty. J Bone Joint Surg Am 91: 1621–1629.

24. Pedersen AB, Mehnert F, Johnsen SP, Sorensen HT (2010) Risk of revision of a total hip replacement in patients with diabetes mellitus: a population-based follow up study. J Bone Joint Surg Br 92: 929–934.
25. Meding JB, Reddleman K, Keating ME, Klay A, Ritter MA, et al. (2003) Total knee replacement in patients with diabetes mellitus. Clin Orthop Relat Res: 208–216.
26. Yurgin N, Secnik K, Lage MJ (2007) Antidiabetic prescriptions and glycemic control in German patients with type 2 diabetes mellitus: a retrospective database study. Clin Ther 29: 316–325.
27. Dowsey MM, Choong PF (2008) Obesity is a major risk factor for prosthetic infection after primary hip arthroplasty. Clin Orthop Relat Res 466: 153–158.
28. Chesney D, Sales J, Elton R, Brenkel IJ (2008) Infection after knee arthroplasty a prospective study of 1509 cases. J Arthroplasty 23: 355–359.
29. Hegde V, Dhurandhar NV (2013) Microbes and obesity–interrelationship between infection, adipose tissue and the immune system. Clin Microbiol Infect 19: 314–320.
30. Mendenhall CL, Seeff L, Diehl AM, Ghosn SJ, French SW, et al. (1991) Antibodies to hepatitis B virus and hepatitis C virus in alcoholic hepatitis and cirrhosis: their prevalence and clinical relevance. The VA Cooperative Study Group (No. 119). Hepatology 14: 581–589.
31. Gomez F, Ruiz P, Schreiber AD (1994) Impaired function of macrophage Fc gamma receptors and bacterial infection in alcoholic cirrhosis. N Engl J Med 331: 1122–1128.
32. Gamble L, Mason CM, Nelson S (2006) The effects of alcohol on immunity and bacterial infection in the lung. Med Mal Infect 36: 72–77.
33. Jevsevar DS, Abt E (2013) The New AAOS-ADA Clinical Practice Guideline on Prevention of Orthopaedic Implant Infection in Patients Undergoing Dental Procedures. J Am Acad Orthop Surg 21: 195–197.
34. Berbari EF, Osmon DR, Carr A, Hanssen AD, Baddour LM, et al. (2010) Dental procedures as risk factors for prosthetic hip or knee infection: a hospital-based prospective case-control study. Clin Infect Dis 50: 8–16.

25

Are Subject-Specific Musculoskeletal Models Robust to the Uncertainties in Parameter Identification?

Giordano Valente[1]*, Lorenzo Pitto[1], Debora Testi[2], Ajay Seth[3], Scott L. Delp[3,4], Rita Stagni[5], Marco Viceconti[6], Fulvia Taddei[1]

1 Medical Technology Laboratory, Rizzoli Orthopaedic Institute, Bologna, Italy, **2** BioComputing Competence Centre, SCS s.r.l., Bologna, Italy, **3** Department of Bioengineering, Stanford University, Stanford, California, United States of America, **4** Department of Mechanical Engineering, Stanford University, Stanford, California, United States of America, **5** Department of Electrical, Electronic and Information Engineering, University of Bologna, Bologna, Italy, **6** Department of Mechanical Engineering and INSIGNEO Institute for *In Silico* Medicine, University of Sheffield, Sheffield, United Kingdom

Abstract

Subject-specific musculoskeletal modeling can be applied to study musculoskeletal disorders, allowing inclusion of personalized anatomy and properties. Independent of the tools used for model creation, there are unavoidable uncertainties associated with parameter identification, whose effect on model predictions is still not fully understood. The aim of the present study was to analyze the sensitivity of subject-specific model predictions (i.e., joint angles, joint moments, muscle and joint contact forces) during walking to the uncertainties in the identification of body landmark positions, maximum muscle tension and musculotendon geometry. To this aim, we created an MRI-based musculoskeletal model of the lower limbs, defined as a 7-segment, 10-degree-of-freedom articulated linkage, actuated by 84 musculotendon units. We then performed a Monte-Carlo probabilistic analysis perturbing model parameters according to their uncertainty, and solving a typical inverse dynamics and static optimization problem using 500 models that included the different sets of perturbed variable values. Model creation and gait simulations were performed by using freely available software that we developed to standardize the process of model creation, integrate with OpenSim and create probabilistic simulations of movement. The uncertainties in input variables had a moderate effect on model predictions, as muscle and joint contact forces showed maximum standard deviation of 0.3 times body-weight and maximum range of 2.1 times body-weight. In addition, the output variables significantly correlated with few input variables (up to 7 out of 312) across the gait cycle, including the geometry definition of larger muscles and the maximum muscle tension in limited gait portions. Although we found subject-specific models not markedly sensitive to parameter identification, researchers should be aware of the model precision in relation to the intended application. In fact, force predictions could be affected by an uncertainty in the same order of magnitude of its value, although this condition has low probability to occur.

Editor: Monica Soncini, Politecnico di Milano, Italy

Funding: This study was supported by the EU-funded NMS Physiome project (FP7-ICT-248189), and supported in part by the EU-funded VPHOP project (FP7-ICT-223865). The funders had no role in study design, data collection and analysis, decision to publish, or preparation of the manuscript. Co-author Debora Testi is employed by BioComputing Competence Centre, SCS s.r.l. BioComputing Competence Centre, SCS s.r.l. provided support in the form of salary for author DT, but did not have any additional role in the study design, data collection and analysis, decision to publish, or preparation of the manuscript. The specific roles of these authors are articulated in the 'author contributions' section.

Competing Interests: Debora Testi is affiliated to the BioComputing Competence Centre, SCS s.r.l. commercial company.

* Email: valente@tecno.ior.it

Introduction

Advances in computing power and numerical methods for modeling and simulation of movement are expanding the use of computational models of the musculoskeletal system in research and clinical applications [1,2]. Calculation of muscle and joint forces represent a challenging modeling application [3,4]. Because musculoskeletal geometry and tissue properties can vary markedly among individuals, the accuracy of generic models has been questioned [5,6], particularly when studying musculoskeletal disorders [7,8]. Conversely, subject-specific models allow inclusion of individual musculoskeletal anatomy and properties, providing an alternative approach to calculating muscle moment arms [9,10], muscle and joint forces [11,12], bone and cartilage stresses [13,14].

In general, analyses of musculoskeletal dynamics require the use of musculoskeletal models and the application of rigid body dynamics and optimization methods to calculate muscle forces [2,15]. Until now, the creation of subject-specific musculoskeletal models and simulations of movement has represented a time-consuming process, and there has been limited modeling software available to standardize the process and make musculoskeletal modeling more efficient. Consequently, few attempts have been made to create subject-specific models and study musculoskeletal pathological conditions (e.g., [16–18]). In fact, model creation requires data collections from different technology (e.g., MRI, gait analysis), and processing the data to create a model of musculoskeletal dynamics. The process involves the definition and calculation of subject-specific modeling parameters from imaging data, including the identification of: tissue volumes and densities to calculate body inertial properties; body landmark positions to define joint reference frames and constraints; muscle attachment points to define the geometry of muscles; and muscle architecture parameters to calculate muscle force-generating capacities.

Independent of the software used, there are unavoidable uncertainties in parameter identification during the process of model creation. These uncertainties have different sources: they can be operator-dependent (e.g., when a user identifies body landmark positions and point positions of musculotendon actuators), or related to the unavailability of measurements *in vivo*, such as maximum muscle tension and musculotendon architecture parameters (e.g., muscle physiological cross-sectional area, fiber length and tendon slack length). Sensitivity analyses to different parameters have been performed to assess variations in model predictions and determine which parameters have the most influence (e.g., [19–21]). However, these analyses have not assessed how the uncertainties associated with the creation of subject-specific musculoskeletal models, and their combined effect, may affect model predictions.

Therefore, the aim of the present study is to analyze the sensitivity of subject-specific model predictions (i.e., joint angles, joint moments, muscle and joint contact forces) during walking to the uncertainties in the values for model parameters. To achieve this aim, we first created a musculoskeletal model of the lower limbs from MRI of a healthy subject. We then performed a Monte-Carlo probabilistic analysis accounting for the uncertainties associated with the creation of the model, including body landmark positions, maximum muscle tension and musculotendon geometry. The analysis was performed by using freely available musculoskeletal modeling software that we developed in an effort to standardize subject-specific model creation and generate accurate models using an efficient workflow. The modeling software integrates with OpenSim [22], a widely used multi-body-dynamics solver adopted in musculoskeletal applications (e.g., [19,23,24]).

Materials and Methods

Ethics statement

This study was approved by the Bioethical Committee of the University of Bologna, Italy (July 7, 2012). Written informed consent was obtained from the participant.

Experimental data

One healthy subject (male; age: 31 years; height: 183 cm; weight: 70.5 kg) volunteered to participate in this study. The experimental data collection included lower-body MRI scans and gait analysis data, freely available at the dedicated SimTK.org project page (https://simtk.org) and described as follows.

Pelvis and lower limbs were imaged using a 1.5 T MR scanner (Intera, Koninklijke Philips N.V., The Netherlands). Four series of images were obtained at different resolutions: a full lower-body scan (T1-weighted Magnetization Transfer, 5 mm slice thickness, 5.5 mm slice spacing, resolution of 512×512 pixels), and three higher resolution acquisitions at the hip (T1-weighted High Resolution Turbo Spin Echo, 5 mm slice thickness, 5.5 mm slice spacing, resolution of 864×864 pixels), at the knee (T1-weighted Turbo Spin Echo, 3 mm slice thickness, 3.3 mm slice spacing, resolution of 560×560 pixels) and at the ankle (T1-weighted Turbo Spin Echo, 3 mm slice thickness, 3.3 mm slice spacing, resolution of 1024×1024 pixels) joint regions.

The subject was assessed by means of gait analysis. The experiment was carried out using a stereophotogrammetric system (SMART-D BTS, Milano, Italy) and two force platforms (Bertec Corporation, USA). Twenty-nine retro-reflective markers were attached to the pelvis, thighs, shanks and feet of the analyzed subject. A trial of level walking at self-selected speed was carried out. Joint neutral position was collected from a standing posture, as well as joint flexion position from a seated posture. All data were collected at 200 samples per second. Relevant anatomical landmarks [25] were calibrated in standing and flexed posture using the pointer technique illustrated in Cappozzo et al. [26]. Segmental kinematics of the pelvis and lower limbs was reconstructed via a C.A.S.T. approach [26] with double calibration [27] to minimize soft tissue artifact propagation.

Workflow of subject-specific musculoskeletal modeling

We investigated the robustness of model predictions to the uncertainties in the identification of the parameters needed to create an image-based musculoskeletal model of the lower limbs, using MRI and gait data (Figure 1). To the purpose, freely available software that we developed, i.e., NMSBuilder and the Probabilistic Musculoskeletal Modeling module (PMM), was used to create the baseline subject-specific model and perform probabilistic simulations of gait, leveraging OpenSim. Additional details on the software system can be found in the Appendix S1. All of the software is available at the dedicated SimTK.org project page (https://simtk.org).

Baseline subject-specific model

The model used in this study was defined as a 7-segment, 10-degree-of-freedom (DOF) articulated system, actuated by 84 musculotendon units, and referred to as the baseline model. The seven rigid bodies included pelvis, thighs, shanks and feet. Each body volume was derived from the MR images, and the inertial properties (mass, center of mass and moments of inertia) were calculated assuming each body composed of two parts, the bone and soft tissue, having uniform densities of 1.42 g/cm^3 and 1.03 g/cm^3 [28], respectively. Each hip was modeled as a 3 DOF ball-and-socket joint, each knee and ankle as a 1 DOF hinge joint. Body and joint coordinate systems were identified according to the ISB standards [29]. The hip joint was defined at the center of the femoral head, the knee axis of rotation was defined as the trans-epcondylar line [30], and the ankle axis of rotation was defined as the trans-malleolar line [31]. The number and paths of the musculotendon actuators were defined according to the generic model proposed by Delp and co-workers [32]. The model includes one or more lines of action per muscle, acting between origin points on the proximal body and insertion points on the distal body. Intermediate via-points are included to model the paths of muscles wrapping over underlying structures. The maximum isometric force (F_{max}) of each musculotendon unit (i) was estimated, assuming muscle fiber length proportional to musculotendon length [33], as:

$$F_{\max i}=(PCSA)_i\cdot\sigma=\left(\frac{Vol}{l_0}\right)_i\cdot\sigma=\left(\frac{Vol}{l_0^{(gen)}\cdot\frac{l_{MT}}{l_{MT}^{(gen)}}}\right)_i\cdot\sigma \qquad (1)$$

where $PCSA$ is the muscle physiological cross-sectional area, Vol is the muscle volume calculated from MRI, l_0 and l_{MT} are the optimal fiber length (unknown) and the musculotendon length (calculated from MRI) for the subject-specific model, respectively, $l_0^{(gen)}$ and $l_{MT}^{(gen)}$ are the corresponding quantities for the generic model [32], and σ is the maximum muscle tension set to 61 N/cm^2 [34].

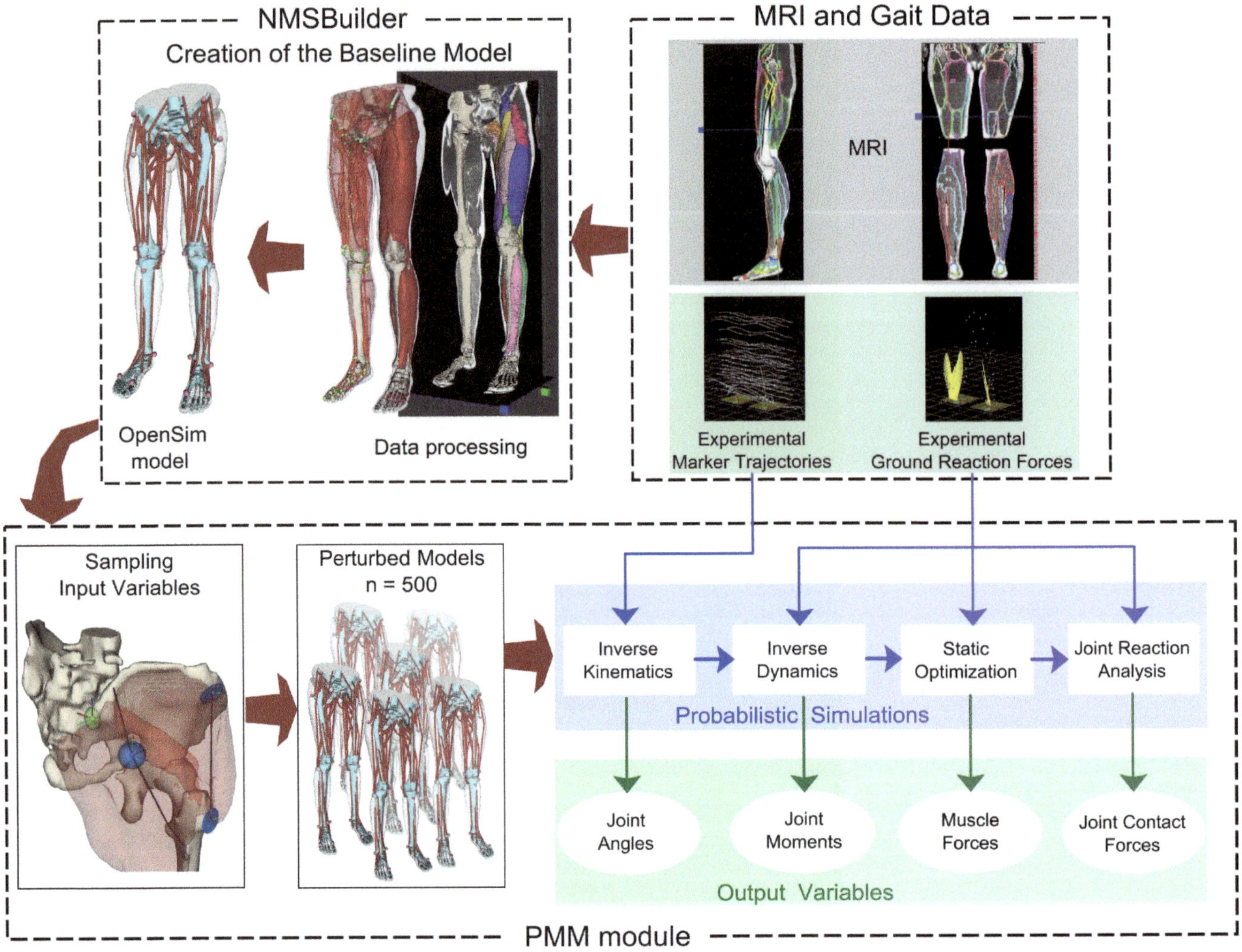

Figure 1. Workflow of subject-specific musculoskeletal modeling. The modeling software systems were applied to study the sensitivity of model predictions to the uncertainties in parameter identification. Lower-body MRI and gait analysis data were acquired for a healthy subject. NMSBuilder was used to create the baseline subject-specific model leveraging OpenSim. The Probabilistic Musculoskeletal Modeling module (PMM) was used to create probabilistic simulations of gait through a Monte-Carlo analysis, by interfacing Matlab and OpenSim. The input variables were perturbed according to their uncertainties, and the corresponding OpenSim models were created that included the different sets of perturbed variables. Using each model and the recorded gait analysis data, simulations of gait were run to calculate the stochastic output variables.

To create the baseline model, bone and soft tissue meshes (pelvis, thighs, shanks and feet) were segmented semi-automatically using Amira (Visage Imaging, Berlin, Germany). NMSBuilder was then used to create the subject-specific musculoskeletal model. The segmented surfaces were imported in NMSBuilder as STL files, and were divided into seven body districts, each made of bone and soft tissue parts [35]. The data were organized into a hierarchical structure. Different density values were then assigned to each part as metadata attributes, to calculate the inertial properties of each body. The necessary anatomical landmarks were virtually palpated [36] on the body surfaces with the help of the superimposed MR images. Subsequently, the landmark positions were used to define the reference frames of each body and the joint positions and orientations (in the parent and child bodies). The positions of musculotendon origin, via and insertion points were assigned as close as possible to those in the generic model [32]. This was done by applying an affine registration based on the body landmarks to initialize the musculotendon point positions, and then adjusting the points according to a centroid approach [37] and visually comparing their positions in the MR images. Next, the values of maximum isometric muscle force were assigned to each musculotendon unit as metadata attributes. Finally, the C++ commands of the OpenSim application programming interface (API) were generated and compiled to create the baseline OpenSim model.

Probabilistic simulations of gait

A probabilistic study was performed to analyze the sensitivity of model predictions to the uncertainties associated with the creation of the baseline model, given the specific articulated linkage actuated by musculotendon units represented by line segments. Therefore, three categories of variable parameters were defined (Figure 2), resulting in a total of 312 stochastic input variables:

1. Body landmark positions. The x-, y- and z-coordinates of the 21 landmarks in each corresponding body reference frame were assumed as normally distributed variables. The standard deviations of each variable (Table 1) were calculated via an experimental study. In this experiment, five expert modelers used NMSBuilder to virtually palpate the landmarks on the bone

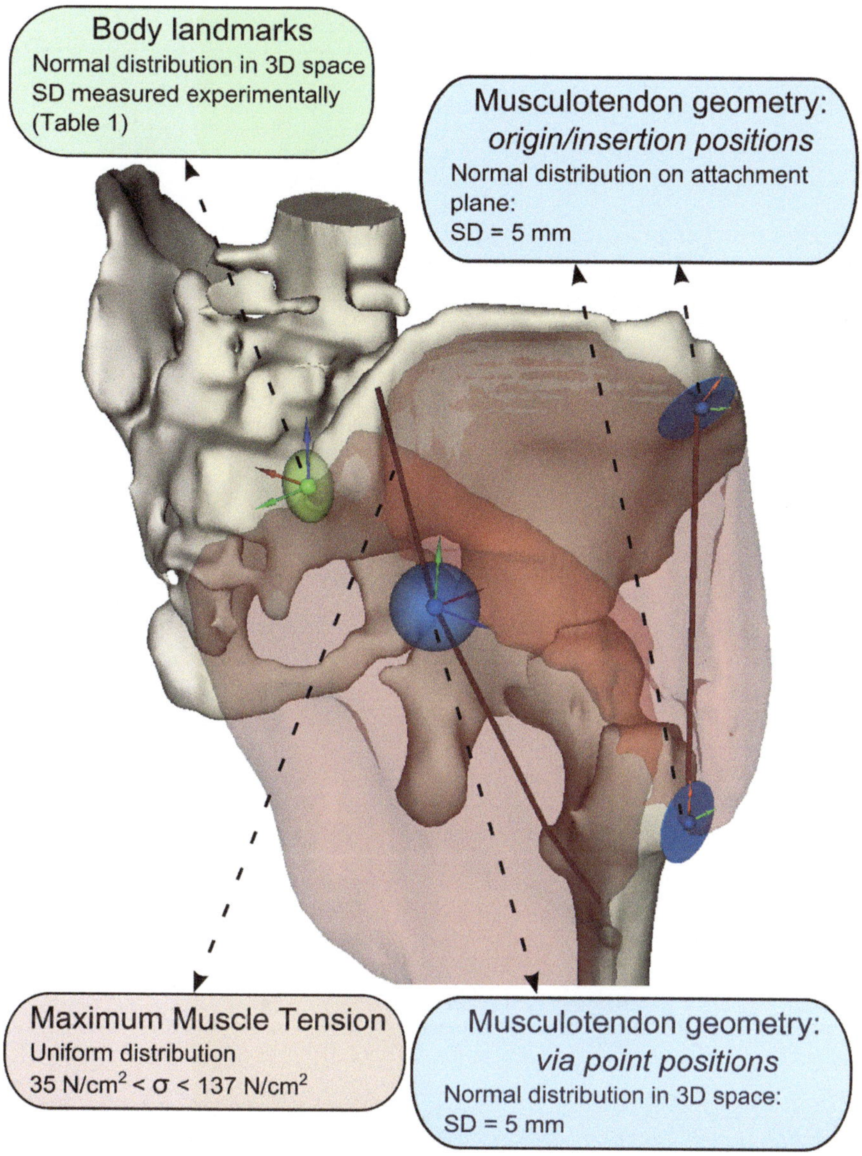

Figure 2. Schematic of statistical perturbation of the input variables. To analyze the sensitivity of model predictions to the uncertainties in parameter values, three categories of stochastic input variables were identified (for a total of 312 input variables): body landmark positions (affecting position and orientation of body reference frames and joints, inertial tensors and joint kinematics), musculotendon geometry (position of origin/insertion and via points defining musculotendon paths and affecting muscle moment arms) and maximum muscle tension (affecting maximum force-generating capacity of the muscles). Each variable was assumed as normally or uniformly distributed, and a Latin Hypercube Sampling strategy was applied to efficiently sample the variables from their distribution.

surfaces three times within a time interval of two weeks. Landmark positions affect calculation of body reference frames, inertial tensors, joint positions and orientations, and joint kinematics.

2. Musculotendon geometry. The positions of the 89 points of the musculotendon paths affecting moment arm lengths were assumed as normally distributed variables. The points included origins, pseudo-origins (most distal via point on the proximal body), pseudo-insertions (most proximal via point on the distal body), and insertions, according to the definition of the different musculotendon paths. A plane approximating each musculotendon attachment area was calculated, so that each origin and insertion point position could be perturbed along two directions on the plane. Points belonging to attachment areas with large length/width ratio were approximated by a line and perturbed along one direction only. Conversely, each position of pseudo-origin and pseudo-insertion points was perturbed along the three directions of the body reference frame. Therefore, a total of 209 normally distributed variables were defined. Mean values were assumed those of the baseline model and standard deviations were set to 5 mm, as derived from the error in locating muscle attachment points from the measurement of surface landmarks [38].

3. Maximum muscle tension. The maximum muscle tension (σ) was assumed as a uniformly distributed variable, ranging from 35 N/cm^2 to 137 N/cm^2 [39]. Consequently, the maximum isometric force of each musculotendon unit was calculated, using equation (1), as:

Table 1. Standard deviations of the body landmark positions measured experimentally.

		Standard Deviation (mm)		
		X	Y	Z
Body landmarks	SACRUM	0.7	0.6	1.8
	RASIS	1.6	0.4	2.6
	RPSIS	0.8	0.3	2.1
	LASIS	1.2	0.6	2.3
	LPSIS	0.9	0.4	2.8
	RGT	1.0	1.4	1.1
	RME	0.4	0.7	1.3
	RLE	0.6	1.6	1.3
	RHC	0.6	0.8	1.5
	RHF	2.2	0.8	0.3
	RTT	3.5	1.3	4.2
	RLC	0.7	3.5	1.2
	RMC	0.5	1.5	0.6
	RMM	1.6	0.9	0.5
	RLM	0.7	0.5	0.3
	RCA	1.1	1.0	0.3
	RFM	0.8	1.6	0.1
	RSM	0.8	0.7	1.0
	RVM	0.7	0.7	0.4
	RPAI	0.6	1.4	0.1
	RPAII	0.6	0.5	0.0

Values were measured through virtual palpation using NMSBuilder by 5 operators in 3 trials each. X, Y and Z indicate antero-posterior, cranio-caudal and medio-lateral directions of the body reference frames, respectively. Body landmark acronyms indicate: sacrum (SACRUM), right anterior superior iliac spine (RASIS), right posterior superior iliac spine (RPSIS), left anterior superior iliac spine (LASIS), left posterior superior iliac spine (LPSIS), right great trochanter (RGT), right medial epicondyle (RME), right lateral epicondyle (RLE), right hip center (RHC), right head of fibula (RHF), right tibial tuberosity (RTT), right lateral tibial condyle (RLC), right medial tibial condyle (RMC), right medial malleolus (RMM), right lateral malleolus (RLM), right calcaneus (RCA), right first metatarsus (RFM), right second metatarsus (RSM), right fifth metatarsus (RVM), right superior plantar aspect of calcaneus (RPAI), right inferior plantar aspect of calcaneus (RPAII).

$$F_{\max i,j} = \left(\frac{Vol}{l_0^{(gen)} \cdot \frac{l_{MT}}{l_{MT}^{(gen)}}} \right)_i \cdot \sigma_j \qquad (2)$$

where i is the musculotendon unit and j the sample of muscle specific tension within the specified range.

Uncertainties introduced by volume segmentation were not included, being segmentation a time-consuming process and hence performed by a single operator. The stance phase of one gait cycle was selected to be included in the analysis, as it is the most interesting phase from the musculoskeletal loading standpoint. PMM allowed us to perform a Monte-Carlo analysis that included kinematic and dynamic simulations of the stance phase of gait (Figure 1), leveraging the OpenSim API. The baseline model was opened in PMM, and a Latin Hypercube Sampling (LHS) strategy [40,19] was applied to generate an efficient sampling of the input variables from their distribution. This made possible the generation of OpenSim models that included the different sets of perturbed variable values. Using each model, Inverse Kinematics, Inverse Dynamics, Static Optimization (minimizing the sum of muscle activations squared and neglecting the force-length-velocity relationships of muscle [41]) and Joint Reaction analysis were run to calculate the following stochastic output variables: joint angles, joint moments, muscle forces and joint contact forces. A convergence criterion was defined as a stopping rule for the Monte-Carlo simulations. Five-hundred simulations ensured that the output variables reached convergence. Specifically, over the last 10% of the simulations, the means and standard deviations of each output variable were within the 2% of each final mean and standard deviation [11,19,20]. A perturbed simulation was considered unsuccessful if joint dynamic equilibrium could not be achieved. Specifically, unsuccessful simulations occurred if the use of reserve actuators on any joint DOF exceeded 5% of the peak joint moment [24] in at least one frame of the stance phase. Preliminary analysis of the results showed that the 0.8% of the simulations run was unsuccessful, suggesting that muscle forces were generally able to generate the required joint moments. The unsuccessful simulations were excluded from the subsequent data analysis.

Data analysis

The analysis was focused on joint angles, joint moments, major muscle forces, i.e. gluteus medius anterior (*GMedA*), middle (*GMedM*) and posterior (*GMedP*), gluteus maximus anterior (*GMaxA*), tensor fascia latae (*TFL*), *psoas*, *iliacus*, semimbranosus (*Semimem*), rectus femoris (*Rec Fem*), vastus medialis (*Vas Med*), lateralis (*Vas Lat*) and intermedius (*Vas Int*), medial (*Med Gas*) and

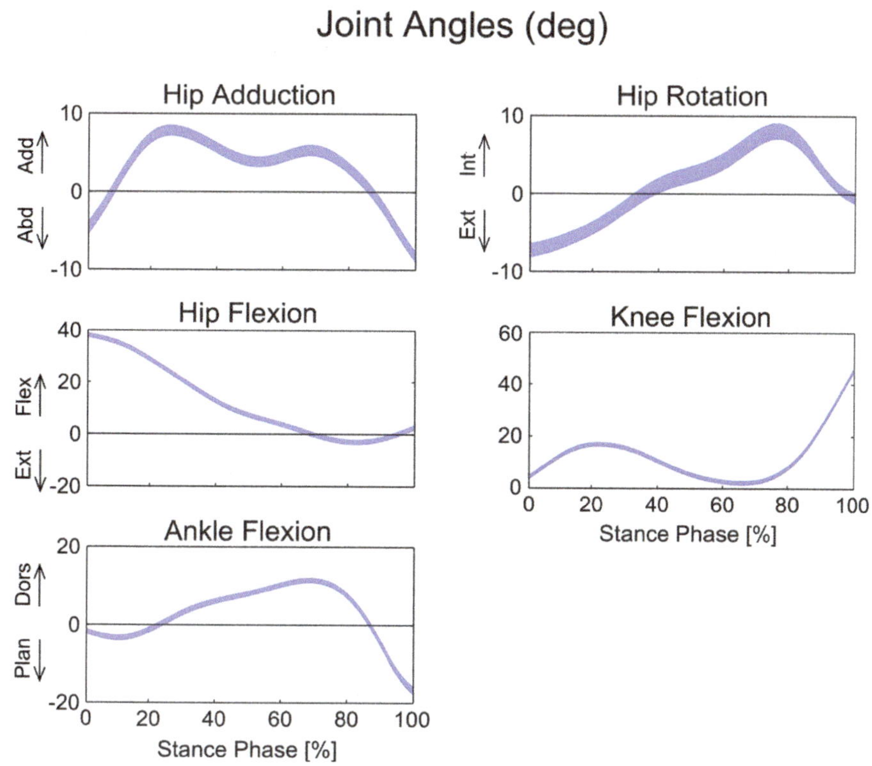

Figure 3. Variability in joint angles due to the perturbation of model variables. Bands represent mean values ±1 standard deviation (in degrees) during the stance phase of gait.

lateral (*Lat Gas*) gastrocnemius, *soleus*, tibialis anterior (*Tib Ant*), and joint contact forces, i.e. hip, knee and ankle force magnitude. First, all quantities were expressed in percentage of the stance phase, and the force values were normalized to the subject body-weight and thus expressed in multiples of body-weight (BW). The data were then post-processed to evaluate the statistical variability

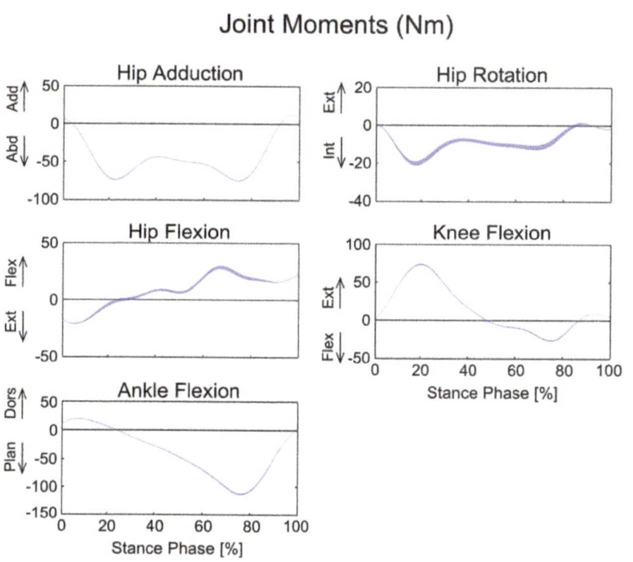

Figure 4. Variability in net joint moments due to the perturbation of model variables. Bands represent mean values ±1 standard deviation (in Nm) during the stance phase of gait.

in the output variables and the correlations between output and input variables. The variability was analyzed as maximum and mean standard deviation (among the output samples at each time step), and range (difference between maximum and minimum values at each time step) during the stance phase of gait. A correlation analysis was performed that evaluated the statistically significant ($p<0.001$) coefficients of determination (R^2) between all output and input variables.

Results

The joint angles and joint moments were relatively insensitive to the expected variation in musculoskeletal parameters. We found that the maximum standard deviation among joint angles during the stance phase of gait was only 1°, and the maximum range was 7° (Figure 3). Similarly, the maximum standard deviation among joint moments from perturbation of model parameters was only 1.4 Nm, and the maximum range was 9.1 Nm (Figure 4). Joint contact forces and muscle forces presented a more marked variability compared to joint angles and joint moments. Joint contact forces showed a maximum standard deviation of 0.26 BW and a maximum range of 2.14 BW at the knee (Figure 5, Table 2). Although the standard deviations of joint contact forces were 10 times smaller than the corresponding force values, the maximum ranges presented the same order of magnitude. Muscle forces showed larger variability in *Soleus*, *Med Gas*, *Rec Fem* and *Psoas* (Figure 6, Table 2), resulting in a maximum standard deviation of 0.23 BW and a maximum range of 1.54 BW in *Soleus*.

Given the relatively small variability in joint kinematics and kinetics, we analyzed only the correlations between joint contact forces and input variables during the stance phase of gait. Among these correlations, only 6.3% showed significant R^2 ($p<0.001$). In

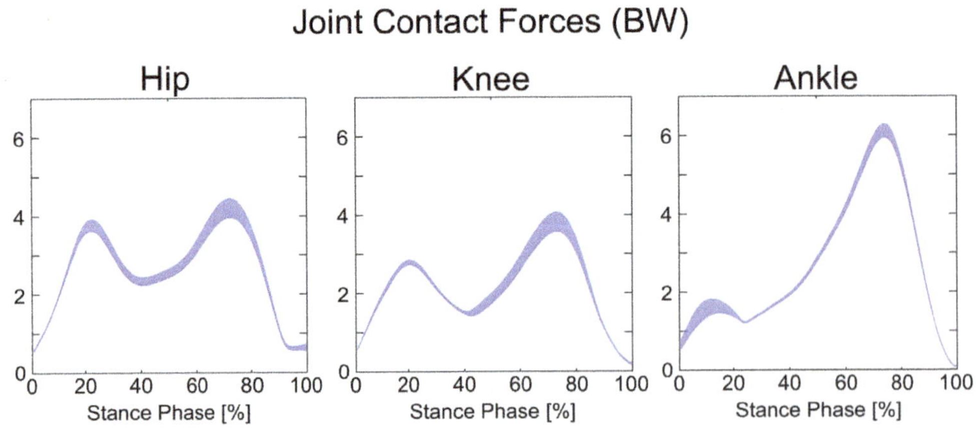

Figure 5. Variability in joint contact forces due to the perturbation of model variables. Bands represent mean values ±1 standard deviation (in BW) during the stance phase of gait.

addition, 1.3% showed significant R^2 greater than 0.2 and never exceeding 0.7, where only seven input variables out of 312 were involved (Figure 7). The hip contact force mostly correlated with the point positions defining the geometry of *GMedA*, *Iliacus* and *Psoas*, and with the maximum muscle tension in the early stance phase. The knee contact force mostly correlated with the geometric definition of *Vas Lat*, *Iliacus* and *GMedA*, and with that of *Med Gas*, *Rec Fem* and *Soleus* for a less extended portion of stance phase. The ankle contact force mostly correlated with the geometric definition of *Soleus* and with the maximum muscle tension for a less extended portion of stance phase. The significant R^2 between joint contact forces and body landmark positions were all less than 0.1 during the stance phase. These results (Figure 7) showed a weak correlation between output and input variables,

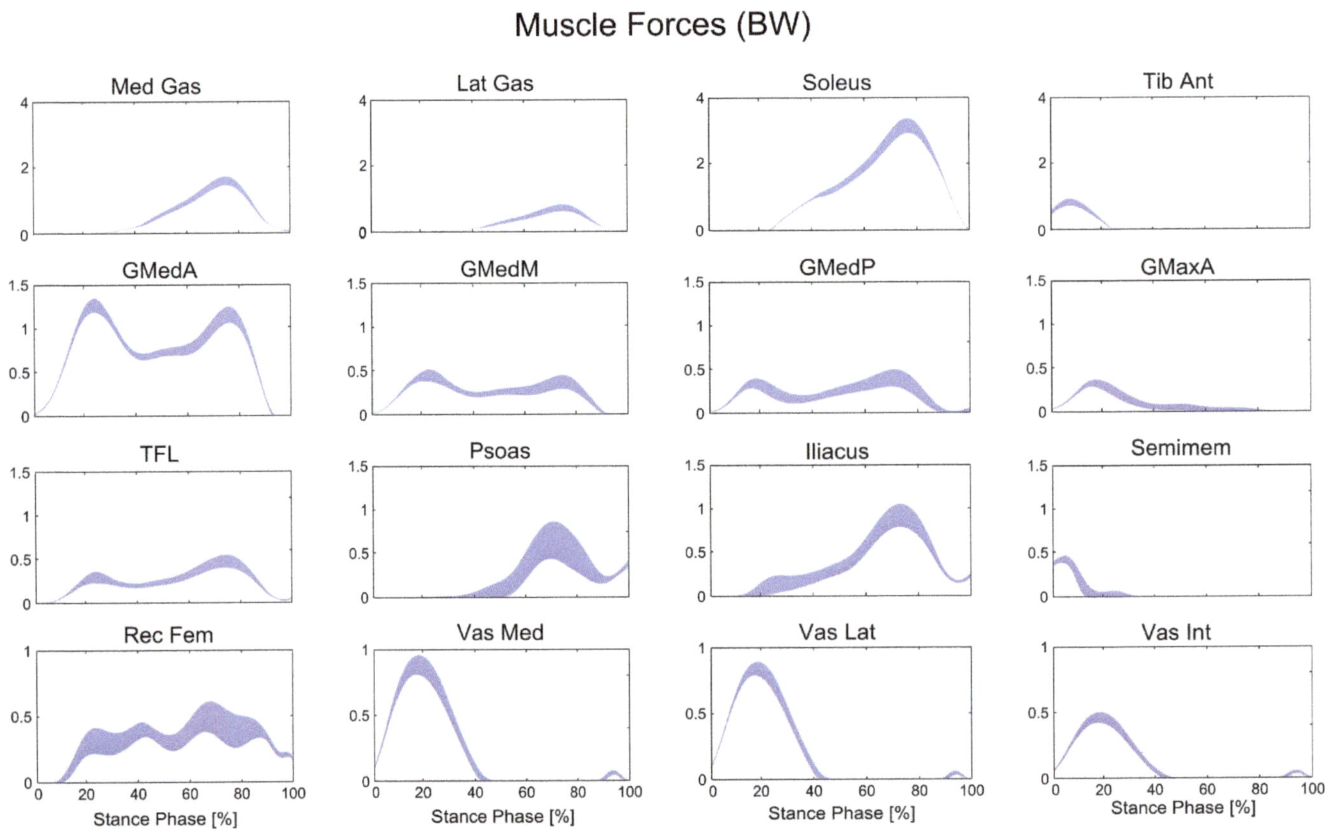

Figure 6. Variability in the major muscle forces due to the perturbation of model variables. Bands represent mean values ±1 standard deviation (in BW) during the stance phase of gait. Muscles shown are: medial (*Med Gas*) and lateral (*Lat Gas*) gastrocnemius, soleus, tibialis anterior (*Tib Ant*), gluteus medius anterior (*GMedA*), middle (*GMedM*) and posterior (*GMedP*), gluteus maximus anterior (*GMaxA*), tensor fascia latae (*TFL*), psoas, iliacus, semimembranosus (*Semimem*), rectus femoris (*Rec Fem*), vastus medialis (*Vas Med*), lateralis (Vas Lat) and intermedius (*Vas Int*).

Table 2. Variability in joint contact and muscle forces.

		Standard Deviation (BW)		Range (BW)	
		Mean	Max	Mean	Max
Joint Contact Forces	Hip	0.13	0.25	0.75	1.51
	Knee	0.11	0.26	0.84	2.14
	Ankle	0.10	0.23	0.62	1.58
Muscle Forces	Med Gas	0.05	0.14	0.33	0.95
	Lat Gas	0.03	0.10	0.21	0.67
	Soleus	0.08	0.23	0.54	1.54
	Tib Ant	0.02	0.10	0.11	0.68
	GMedA	0.05	0.09	0.32	0.66
	GMedM	0.04	0.08	0.25	0.51
	GmedP	0.05	0.10	0.31	0.59
	GMaxA	0.03	0.06	0.17	0.40
	TFL	0.01	0.03	0.08	0.17
	Psoas	0.05	0.15	0.33	0.89
	Iliacus	0.07	0.13	0.42	0.79
	Semimem	0.01	0.03	0.04	0.19
	Rec Fem	0.07	0.14	0.44	0.88
	Vas Med	0.01	0.04	0.07	0.24
	Vas Lat	0.02	0.07	0.11	0.35
	Vas Int	0.01	0.02	0.04	0.13

Standard deviations and ranges of the magnitudes of joint contact forces and the major muscle forces are reported as mean and maximum values across the stance phase of gait.

without a marked influence of specific input variables. The sampled input variables and the complete set of post-processed output variables are available at the dedicated SimTK.org project page (https://simtk.org).

Discussion

In this study, we analyzed the sensitivity of the predictions of an MRI-based musculoskeletal model (i.e., joint angles, joint moments, muscle and joint contact forces) during walking to the unavoidable uncertainties in parameter identification, i.e., body landmark positions, maximum muscle tension and musculotendon geometry (Figure 1).

Overall, the unavoidable uncertainties in parameter identification during the process of model creation have a moderate effect on model predictions during gait. In fact, we found that the main outcomes of model predictions, i.e., joint contact forces and muscle forces, had a maximum standard deviation of 0.26 BW across the stance phase of gait (Figure 5 and 6, Table 2). In addition, there were no critical parameters that markedly affected model predictions. We performed a correlation analysis between joint contact forces and input variables (Figure 7), and found few significant R^2, whose values never exceeded 0.7. The input variables involved were the point positions defining the geometry of few musculotendon actuators that presented larger force-generating capacities and the maximum muscle tension in limited portions of the stance phase.

Although we found that subject-specific models are not markedly sensitive to the uncertainties in parameter identification, there is no conclusive answer to the robustness of subject-specific models. In fact, the precision of model predictions should be evaluated with regards to specific applications. For example, we found ranges (differences between maximum and minimum of the predicted value) that reached 2.1 BW in joint contact forces at the knee during the gait cycle (Table 2). In this case, the result could be affected by an uncertainty in the same order of magnitude of its value, although this condition has low probability to occur. Therefore, one should be aware of the uncertainty in musculoskeletal force predictions according to their intended application (e.g., investigation of risk of bone fracture and bone stress distribution).

To our knowledge, this is the first study investigating how the combined effect of the uncertainties in model parameters affects the predictions of a subject-specific musculoskeletal model, using a probabilistic approach. Therefore, this represents the most extended sensitivity analysis of musculoskeletal modeling predictions, providing an overall scenario of robustness of subject-specific musculoskeletal models to the uncertainties in parameter identification. Consequently, only partial or indirect comparisons with the literature were possible. We found an effect of anatomical landmark positions on predicted joint moments weaker than that showed in a previous probabilistic study limited to inverse dynamics results [21]. The uncertainties that we assigned to the landmark positions (Table 1) were lower than those in the prior study (i.e., standard deviations of 2 mm for all landmarks in each direction). We evaluated experimentally the standard deviations of the distribution by using an accurate method for landmark virtual palpation [36] implemented in NMSBuilder, which allowed us to

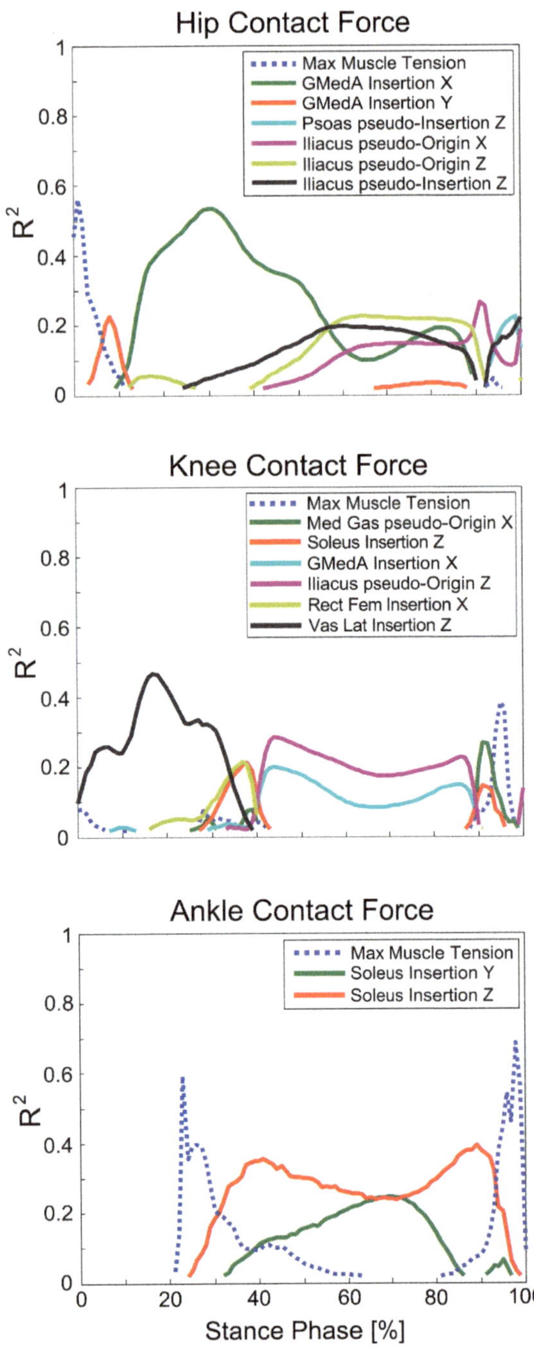

Figure 7. Significant R^2 between joint contact forces and input variables during the stance phase of gait. Correlations between hip, knee and ankle joint contact forces and input variables: only statistically significant ($p<0.001$) R^2 exceeding 0.2 at least in one frame during the stance phase of gait are plotted.

improve the uncertainty in the identification of landmark positions. Similarly, we found a weaker effect of musculotendon geometry on predicted muscle forces compared to a previous study [42] that used a fixed-size perturbation (±10 mm) applied to each musculotendon point position along each direction of the local reference frames. Differently from that study, we assigned an uncertainty (standard deviation of 5 mm) derived from the range of landmark location errors [38], we adopted a probabilistic approach to analyze all possible configurations of musculotendon point positions, and we constrained the muscle attachment points to vary on the bone surfaces. In addition, our results generally confirm the weak influence of maximum muscle tension on the calculated muscle forces, when minimizing a cost function in static optimization problems [20,43,44]. We additionally found that the maximum muscle tension played a more relevant role on joint contact forces during transient phases of the gait cycle (Figure 7). Differently from previous studies, our approach explored the range of maximum muscle tension found in the literature [39] using a uniform distribution, rather than an arbitrary-size perturbation of a baseline value. However, the portions of stance phase showing larger correlations were not biomechanically relevant, as most muscles were inactive or exerted low forces.

The results of our study are affected by some limitations. We limited the study to a healthy subject and we investigated only the task of level walking as the most common daily activity. Model robustness might be different in pathological conditions and for other motor tasks such as sit-to-stand, stair ascent or descent. Although further investigations might extend our findings, the healthy subject included in this study can be considered representative of physiological conditions, and adding greater complexity was beyond the aim of the study. We did not include musculotendon parameters describing force-length-velocity relationships (i.e., optimal fiber length, tendon slack length and pennation angle). Changes in these parameters, and particularly in tendon slack length of some muscles, can markedly affect model dynamics predictions [20,44]. However, measurements and corresponding uncertainties of these parameters are difficult to obtain *in vivo* and even by dissection studies [2]; in addition, the lack of implementation of musculotendon force-length-velocity relationships has a small influence on force predictions during walking [41]. Further, we did not consider the uncertainty introduced by representing the musculotendon units by deformable line segments in the model. However, our aim was to analyze the effect of the uncertainties in the parameters identifying a specific state-of-the art model, and including more accurate muscle path representation (e.g., [45]) would have introduced large computational costs and additional uncertainty not compatible with our analysis.

This study has relevant potentials within the computational biomechanics community. We assessed robustness of musculoskeletal models to the uncertainties in parameter identification using a probabilistic approach. Although in presence of the limitation regarding the impossibility to validate muscle forces, our results confirm that musculoskeletal models represent a promising tool that is heading towards clinical applicability, particularly to improve treatment of orthopaedic and neurological diseases [1,15]. The analysis has been facilitated by the use of an efficient workflow (Figure 1), whose software tools allowed us to reduce time and effort. The freely available modeling software may provide a marked contribution to create subject-specific models and simulations of movement more efficiently, saving time and effort, and without necessarily requiring high skilled expertise.

In summary, our study revealed that the uncertainties in parameter identification of subject-specific musculoskeletal models have a moderate effect on model predictions, and there are not specific parameters considered crucial for the degree of model robustness. However, the precision of model predictions should be considered carefully with regards to the intended application. In fact, model predictions such as joint contact forces may present maximum ranges of variability that are in the same order of magnitude of their values.

Supporting Information

Appendix S1 Musculoskeletal modeling software.

Author Contributions

Conceived and designed the experiments: GV LP FT. Performed the experiments: GV LP. Analyzed the data: GV LP FT. Wrote the paper: GV. Contributed software design and development: GV LP DT AS SLD MV FT. Produced gait analysis data: RS. Edited the manuscript: GV LP DT AS SLD RS MV FT.

References

1. Fregly BJ, Besier TF, Lloyd DG, Delp SL, Banks SA, et al. (2012) Grand Challenge Competition to Predict In Vivo Knee Loads. Journal of Orthopaedic Research 30: 503–513.
2. Pandy MG, Andriacchi TP (2010) Muscle and joint function in human locomotion. Annu Rev Biomed Eng 12: 401–433.
3. Fregly BJ (2009) Design of Optimal Treatments for Neuromusculoskeletal Disorders using Patient-Specific Multibody Dynamic Models. Int J Comput Vis Biomech 2: 145–155.
4. Fernandez JW, Pandy MG (2006) Integrating modelling and experiments to assess dynamic musculoskeletal function in humans. Experimental physiology 91: 371–382.
5. Wagner DW, Stepanyan V, Shippen JM, DeMers MS, Gibbons RS, et al. (2013) Consistency Among Musculoskeletal Models: Caveat Utilitor. Annals of Biomedical Engineering 41: 1787–1799.
6. Scheys L, Spaepen A, Suetens P, Jonkers I (2008) Calculated moment-arm and muscle-tendon lengths during gait differ substantially using MR based versus rescaled generic lower-limb musculoskeletal models. Gait & posture 28: 640–648.
7. Correa TA, Schache AG, Graham HK, Baker R, Thomason P, et al. (2012) Potential of lower-limb muscles to accelerate the body during cerebral palsy gait. Gait & posture 36: 194–200.
8. Lenaerts G, Bartels W, Gelaude F, Mulier M, Spaepen A, et al. (2009) Subject-specific hip geometry and hip joint centre location affects calculated contact forces at the hip during gait. Journal of Biomechanics 42: 1246–1251.
9. Scheys L, Desloovere K, Suetens P, Jonkers I (2011) Level of subject-specific detail in musculoskeletal models affects hip moment arm length calculation during gait in pediatric subjects with increased femoral anteversion. Journal of Biomechanics 44: 1346–1353.
10. Valente G, Martelli S, Taddei F, Farinella G, Viceconti M (2012) Muscle discretization affects the loading transferred to bones in lower-limb musculoskeletal models. Proceedings of the Institution of Mechanical Engineers, Part H: Journal of Engineering in Medicine 226: 161–169.
11. Martelli S, Valente G, Viceconti M, Taddei F (2014). Sensitivity of a subject-specific musculoskeletal model to the uncertainties on the joint axes location. Comput Methods Biomech Biomed Engin Jun 25:1–9 [Epub ahead of print].
12. Lenaerts G, Mulier M, Spaepen A, Van der Perre G, Jonkers I (2009) Aberrant pelvis and hip kinematics impair hip loading before and after total hip replacement. Gait & posture 30: 296–302.
13. Besier TF, Gold GE, Beaupre GS, Delp SL (2005) A Modeling Framework to Estimate Patellofemoral Joint Cartilage Stress In Vivo. Medicine & Science in Sports & Exercise 37: 1924–1930.
14. Jonkers I, Sauwen N, Lenaerts G, Mulier M, Van der Perre G, et al. (2008) Relation between subject-specific hip joint loading, stress distribution in the proximal femur and bone mineral density changes after total hip replacement. Journal of Biomechanics 41: 3405–3413.
15. Erdemir A, McLean S, Herzog W, van den Bogert AJ (2007) Model-based estimation of muscle forces exerted during movements. Clinical Biomechanics (Bristol, Avon) 22: 131–154.
16. Taddei F, Martelli S, Valente G, Leardini A, Benedetti MG, et al. (2012) Femoral loads during gait in a patient with massive skeletal reconstruction. Clinical Biomechanics (Bristol, Avon) 27: 273–280.
17. Correa TA, Baker R, Graham HK, Pandy MG (2011) Accuracy of generic musculoskeletal models in predicting the functional roles of muscles in human gait. Journal of Biomechanics 44: 2096–2105.
18. Gerus P, Sartori M, Besier TF, Fregly BJ, Delp SL, et al. (2013) Subject-specific knee joint geometry improves predictions of medial tibiofemoral contact forces. Journal of Biomechanics 46: 2778–2786.
19. Valente G, Taddei F, Jonkers I (2013) Influence of weak hip abductor muscles on joint contact forces during normal walking: probabilistic modeling analysis. Journal of Biomechanics 46: 2186–2193.
20. Ackland DC, Lin Y-C, Pandy MG (2012) Sensitivity of model predictions of muscle function to changes in moment arms and muscle–tendon properties: A Monte-Carlo analysis. Journal of Biomechanics 45: 1463–1471.
21. Langenderfer JE, Laz PJ, Petrella AJ, Rullkoetter PJ (2008) An efficient probabilistic methodology for incorporating uncertainty in body segment parameters and anatomical landmarks in joint loadings estimated from inverse dynamics. Journal of Biomechanical Engineering 130: 014502.
22. Delp SL, Anderson FC, Arnold AS, Loan P, Habib A, et al. (2007) OpenSim: open-source software to create and analyze dynamic simulations of movement. IEEE Transactions on Biomedical Engineering 54: 1940–1950.
23. Crossley KM, Dorn TW, Ozturk H, van den Noort J, Schache a G, et al. (2012) Altered hip muscle forces during gait in people with patellofemoral osteoarthritis. Osteoarthritis and cartilage 20: 1243–1249.
24. van der Krogt MM, Delp SL, Schwartz MH (2012) How robust is human gait to muscle weakness? Gait & posture 36: 113–119.
25. Benedetti MG, Catani F, Leardini A, Pignotti S, Giannini S (1998) Data management in gait analysis for clinical applications. Clinical Biomechanics (Bristol, Avon) 13: 204–215.
26. Cappozzo A, Catani F, Della Croce U, Leardini A (1995) Position and orientation in space of bones during movement: anatomical frame definition and determination. Clinical Biomechanics (Bristol, Avon) 10: 171–178.
27. Cappello A, Stagni R, Fantozzi S, Leardini A (2005) Soft Tissue Artifact Compensation in Knee Kinematics by Double Anatomical Landmark Calibration: Performance of a Novel Method During Selected Motor Tasks. IEEE Transaction on Biomedical Engineering 52: 992–998.
28. Dumas R, Aissaoui R, Mitton D, Skalli W, Guise JAD (2005) Personalized Body Segment Parameters From Biplanar Low-Dose Radiography. IEEE Transactions on Biomedical Engineering 52: 1756–1763.
29. Wu G, Siegler S, Allard P, Kirtley C, Leardini A, et al. (2002) ISB recommendation on definitions of joint coordinate system of various joints for the reporting of human joint motion—part I: ankle, hip, and spine. Journal of Biomechanics 35: 543–548.
30. Churchill DL, Incavo SJ, Johnson CC, Beynnon BD (1998) The transepicondylar axis approximates the optimal flexion axis of the knee. Clinical Orthopaedics and Related Research 356: 111–118.
31. Lundberg A, Svenson OK, Nemeth G, Selvik G (1989) The axis of rotation of the ankle joint. Journal of Bone and Joint Surgery 71: 94–99.
32. Delp SL, Loan JP, Hoy MG, Zajac FE, Topp EL, et al. (1990) An interactive graphics-based model of the lower extremity to study orthopaedic surgical procedures. IEEE Transactions on Biomedical engineering 37: 757–767.
33. Correa TA, Pandy MG (2011) A mass-length scaling law for modeling muscle strength in the lower limb. Journal of Biomechanics 44: 2782–2789.
34. Arnold EM, Ward SR, Lieber RL, Delp SL (2010) A model of the lower limb for analysis of human movement. Annals of biomedical engineering 38: 269–279.
35. Clauser CE, McConville JT, Young JW (1969) Weight, volume, and center of mass of segments of the human body. AMRL-TR-69-70 Wright Patterson Air Force Base, Ohio.
36. Taddei F, Ansaloni M, Testi D, Viceconti M (2007) Virtual palpation of skeletal landmarks with multimodal display interfaces. Medical informatics and the Internet in medicine 32: 191–198.
37. Scheys L, Jonkers I, Loeckx D, Maes F, Spaepen A, et al. (2006) Image based musculoskeletal modeling allows personalized biomechanical analysis of gait. Lecture notes in computer science 4072: 58–66.
38. Pal S, Langenderfer JE, Stowe JQ, Laz PJ, Petrella AJ, et al. (2007) Probabilistic modeling of knee muscle moment arms: effects of methods, origin-insertion, and kinematic variability. Annals of biomedical engineering 35: 1632–1642.
39. Buchanan TS, Lloyd DG, Manal K, Besier TF (2004) Neuromusculoskeletal modeling: estimation of muscle forces and joint moments and movements from measurements of neural command. Journal of applied biomechanics 20: 367–395.
40. McKay MD, Beckman RJ, Conover WJ (1979) Comparison of Three Methods for Selecting Values of Input Variables in the Analysis of Output from a Computer Code. Technometrics 21: 239–245.
41. Anderson FC, Pandy MG (2001) Static and dynamic optimization solutions for gait are practically equivalent. Journal of Biomechanics 34: 153–161.
42. Carbone V, van der Krogt MM, Koopman HFJM, Verdonschot N (2012) Sensitivity of subject-specific models to errors in musculo-skeletal geometry. Journal of Biomechanics 45: 2476–2480.
43. Xiao M, Higginson J (2010) Sensitivity of estimated muscle force in forward simulation of normal walking. J Appl Biomech 26, 142–149.
44. De Groote F, Van Campen A, Jonkers I, De Schutter J (2010) Sensitivity of dynamic simulations of gait and dynamometer experiments to Hill muscle model parameters of knee flexors and extensors. Journal of Biomechanics 43: 1876–1883.
45. Blemker SS, Delp SL (2005) Three-dimensional representation of complex muscle architectures and geometries. Annals of biomedical engineering 33: 1433–1437.

Feasibility of Progressive Strength Training Implemented in the Acute Ward after Hip Fracture Surgery

Lise Kronborg[1,2]*, Thomas Bandholm[1,2,3,4], Henrik Palm[4], Henrik Kehlet[5], Morten Tange Kristensen[1,2,4]

1 Physical Medicine and Rehabilitation Research – Copenhagen (PMR-C), Copenhagen University Hospital, Hvidovre, Denmark, **2** Department of Physical Therapy, Copenhagen University Hospital, Hvidovre, Denmark, **3** Clinical Research Centre, Copenhagen University Hospital, Hvidovre, Denmark, **4** Department of Orthopedic Surgery, Copenhagen University Hospital, Hvidovre, Denmark, **5** Section for Surgical Pathophysiology, Rigshospitalet, Copenhagen University, Copenhagen, Denmark

Abstract

Importance: Patients with a hip fracture lose more than 50% knee-extension strength in the fractured limb within one week of surgery. Hence, immediate progressive strength training following hip fracture surgery may be rational, but the feasibility unknown.

Objective: To examine the feasibility of in-hospital progressive strength training implemented in the acute ward following hip fracture surgery, based on pre-specified criteria for feasibility.

Design, Setting and Patients: A prospective cohort study conducted in an acute orthopedic hip fracture unit at a university hospital. A consecutive sample of 36 patients, 18 with a cervical and 18 with a trochanteric hip fracture (27 women and 9 men, mean (SD) age of 79.4 (8.3) years) were included between June and December 2012.

Intervention: A daily (on weekdays) program of progressive knee-extension strength training for the fractured limb, using ankle weight cuffs in 3 sets of 10 repetition maximum loadings.

Main outcomes and Measures: The primary outcome was the change in training load (kg) during the knee-extension strength training. The secondary outcomes were changes in hip fracture-related pain and maximal isometric knee-extension strength.

Results: The strength training was commenced at a mean of 2.4 (0.7) days after surgery. The training loads (kilograms lifted) increased from 1.6 (0.8) to 4.3 (1.7) kg over 4.3 (2.2) training sessions ($P<.001$). The maximal isometric knee-extension strength of the fractured limb increased from 0.37 (0.2) to 0.61 (0.3) Nm/kg ($P<.001$), while the average strength deficit in the fractured limb decreased from 50% to 32% (% non-fractured, $P<.001$). Only 3 of 212 sessions were not performed because of severe hip fracture-related pain.

Conclusion and Relevance: Progressive knee-extension strength training of the fractured limb commenced in the acute ward seems feasible, and may reduce strength asymmetry between limbs without hip pain interfering. The clinical efficacy needs confirmation in a randomized controlled design.

Trial Registration: ClinicalTrials.gov ID: NCT01616030

Editor: Amir A. Zadpoor, Delft University of Technology (TUDelft), Netherlands

Funding: This study was funded by grants from the Danish Physical Therapy Association, the IMK foundation and the Capital Region of Copenhagen, the Hvidovre Hospital's Research Fund, and the Lundbeck foundation (UCSF), Denmark. The funding agencies had no influence on the study design, methods, subjects, data collection, analyses or manuscript. The funders had no role in study design, data collection and analysis, decision to publish, or preparation of the manuscript.

Competing Interests: The authors have declared that no competing interests exist.

* E-mail: lisekronborg@hotmail.com

Introduction

Factors affecting the functional prognosis after hip fracture surgery are multiple [1], and patients are at risk of decreased physical function [2–4], new injurious falls and fractures [5,6], and increased need of supportive care [7]. Despite the fact that patients follow a multimodal fast-track program [8], a loss of knee-extension strength in the fractured limb of more than 50% (% of non-fractured) occurs during the first week after hip fracture surgery and is associated with impaired physical function [9]. Corresponding deficits are also reported within 2–3 weeks following hip fracture surgery [10,11]. Patients with trochanteric fractures seem to experience greater knee-extension strength deficits, perform worse in functional parameters, and experience more fracture-related pain compared to patients with cervical fractures [9,12–15], which indicates fracture type-specific patho-physiology.

With respect to recovery after a hip fracture, early mobilization [16–18] and extended physical therapy including strength training implemented 6 weeks after fracture seem to promote recovery of physical function [19]. Still, "current guidelines do not include detailed recommendations about exercise after hip fracture" [20] and no study has yet succeeded in a full recovery of the early loss of knee-extension strength [10,11,21,22] or function [22,23]. In theory, physical therapy including strength training should optimally be implemented in the acute ward immediately following surgery, where the deficits are greatest, to avoid further functional decline and to substantially enhance recovery after a hip fracture. However, only two studies [10,22] have investigated strength training shortly (2 weeks) following the fracture. Although elective surgery and hip fractures are not the same, preliminary evidence suggests that strength training implemented immediately following total hip [24] and knee [25] arthroplasty is feasible and does not appear to exacerbate postoperative symptoms. If this is also true for patients following a hip fracture is currently unknown.

The primary aim of this study was to examine the feasibility of in-hospital progressive strength training implemented immediately following hip fracture surgery, based on pre-specified criteria for feasibility. We decided that feasibility was indicated if: 1) the absolute training loads increased progressively, 2) fracture-related pain during strength training did not increase during the program, and 3) more than 80% of the planned training sessions were completed.

Methods

Design and Setting

The study was a prospective cohort study performed as a feasibility study [26] in an acute orthopedic hip fracture unit at a university hospital. The main purpose was to indicate the feasibility of the strength training intervention prior to the confirmatory study registered at clinicaltrials.gov (NCT00848913). The protocol for this trial and supporting CONSORT checklist are available as supporting information; see Checklist S1 and Protocol S1.

After written informed consent, patients were to strength train their knee extensors in the fractured limb progressively on all weekdays throughout their hospitalization. The same skilled physical therapist, who was blinded to all baseline data until end of study, allocated all eligible patients for the present study and supervised all test and training sessions, except for one test (1% of tests) and four (2%) training sessions. The study was approved by the Capital Region's Research Ethics Committee (H-A-2007-0127), registered at clinicaltrials.gov (NCT01616030), and conducted according to the principles expressed in the Declaration of Helsinki. The reporting of the study adheres to the STROBE guidelines for cohort studies [27], (Please see Checklist S1).

Patients

A total of 185 consecutive patients admitted with an acute hip fracture between 6th of June 2012 and 6th of December 2012 were assessed for eligibility. The inclusion criteria were: age ≥65 years, ability to speak and understand Danish, able to give written informed consent no later than by the 3rd postoperative day, and home residing with an independent pre-fracture ability to walk indoor, according to a modified and reliable [14,28] New Mobility Score (NMS) [29] of 2 or more. The exclusion criteria were: postoperative weight bearing restrictions, multiple fractures, postoperative medical complications, terminal illness, neurological impairment, alcoholic addiction and comprehensive co-morbidity. Ninety-seven patients did not meet our inclusion criteria, 4 declined to participate while 44 patients were excluded due to other reasons (Fig. 1). Baseline data for age, sex, body weight, prefracture function (the Functional Recovery Score [30,31] and the modified NMS [14]), Mental status (Mini Mental State Examination, MMSE) [32], the American Society of Anesthetists (ASA) score [33] and type of fracture were collected from medical records or clinical evaluation of patients.

All patients followed a multimodal fast-track program that included a daily regular physical therapy program (without strength training) at postoperative day 1–3 (weekends included) and 2–5 times per week (weekends not included) hereafter. The regular physical therapy that consisted of 12 specific "hip-related" exercises (repetitions and intensity not standardized) was combined with training of basic mobility activities, such as walking and stair climbing. The program was progressed from actively assisted bed exercises to transfers in and out of bed; sit to stand from a chair, and to more specific and hip-related weight-bearing exercises. Gait reeducation and balance exercises were performed both at the bedside and in a gym located within the hip fracture ward. Walking aids were changed according to the patient's level of independent mobility. The program did not include progressive strength training of the knee extensors. The number of regular physical therapy sessions and their duration (minutes) were recorded for all patients.

Intervention

The progressive fractured-limb knee-extension strength training program was conducted once every weekday, and each session consisted of 3 sets of 10 repetitions performed with an intensity of 10 repetition maximum (RM), defined as ±2 RM [34]. Training loads were adjusted on a set-by-set basis and 1-minute pauses separated the sets. The exercise intervention is documented in table 1, according to the study protocol (Please see Protocol S1 and Protocol S2) and descriptors by Toigo & Boutellier [34] and the recommendations from the CONSORT extension for non-pharmacologic treatment [35].

1. The patient was seated on the bedside, hips and knees in 90° flexion, hands placed on the mattress for support, no contact between the patient's fractured limb and the floor. The foot of the non-fractured limb resting on a low stool.
2. As a warm-up exercise, the patient performed 5 knee-extensions for each limb separately, without any training loads applied.
3. A weight-cuff matching the patient's level of 10RM was attached around the patient's ankle of the fractured limb.
4. The patient's lower leg was assisted to full knee-extension to allow the first voluntary contraction to be eccentric. The patient held the knee extended for approximately 2 sec before lowering the lower leg into vertical position within 3 sec. and repeated the concentric extension with a duration of 3 sec. (Table 1)
5. The patient kept repeating this exercise for as many repetitions as possible at the required rate until fatigue, defined as not being able to perform a full knee-extension or maintain the rate. The patient was verbally motivated to reach state of fatigue. The exercise was stopped at 15 repetitions without fatigue and the load was increased for the following set.

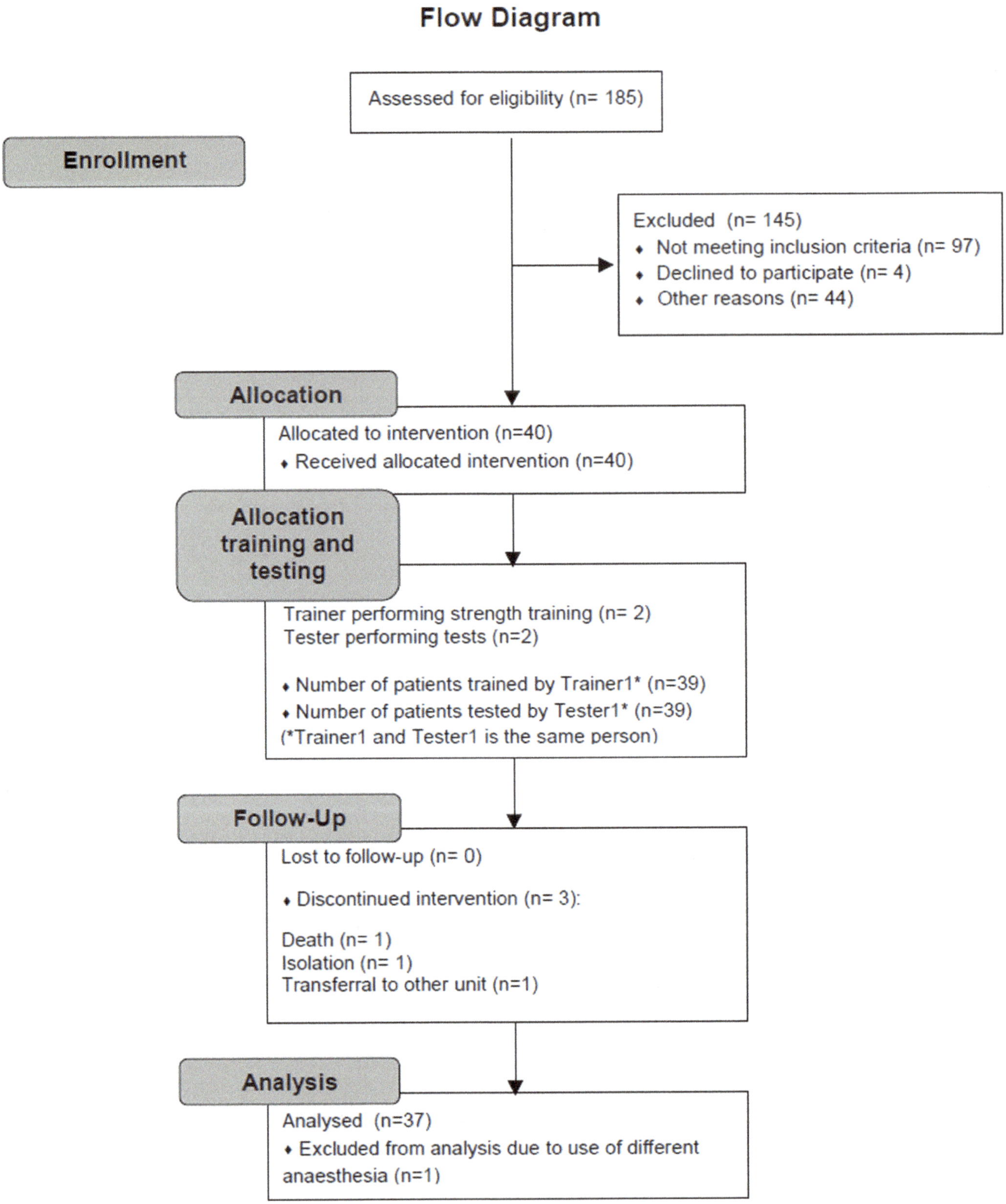

Figure 1. Flowchart of patient enrollment.

Safety Precautions

A senior orthopedic consultant cleared all patients for enrolment in the study, and the intervention was stopped in case of any adverse events related to the strength training or any complications that contraindicated further participation in

Table 1. Strength training descriptors [32].

Variable	Knee-extension exercise
Load, repetition maximum	10
Repetitions per set	10
Sets per session	3
Rest between sets, seconds	120
Sessions per week	5
Contraction modes, seconds	2 Isometric, 3 Eccentric, 3 Concentric
Rest between repetitions, seconds	0
Time under tension, seconds	240
Contraction failure in each set	Yes
Range of motion, degrees	90°
Rest between training sessions, hours	24
Anatomical definition of the exercise (exercise form)	Yes

the study. All potentially adverse events or complications were recorded.

Outcome Measures

Training Load

The absolute load (kg) corresponding to 10 RM was recorded for each set at each training session, with the load used in the last of three sets recorded. For each patient, the load used at the last set in the first, middle and last training session was used as data point. Completing less than 2 sets of 10 repetitions in each planned session was defined as a session failure. All causes of session failure were recorded.

Knee-extension Strength

Maximal isometric knee-extension strength was assessed at a knee joint angle of 90° at the day of inclusion and the day before discharge, using a reliable strap-fixated handheld dynamometer [36–38]. Patients, unable to be tested at Day 1 after surgery, were tested the following day, or at the latest at Day 3 post-surgery.

The patients were seated as described for the strength training, with the center of the resistance pad placed 4 cm above the lateral malleolous. The patients performed 1 sub maximal knee-extension followed by 4 maximal knee-extensions for each limb (non-fractured first) with strong and standardized verbal encouragement. The contractions were separated by 1-minute pauses. Maximal isometric knee-extension strength in each leg was subsequently expressed as the maximal voluntary torque per kilo body mass, using the lever arm (distance from the lateral epicondyle of the femur to the center of the resistance pad) and body mass of each patient [25]. The greatest value was identified for each leg and used as data points. These two data points were also used to calculate a strength deficit of the fractured limb as a percentage of the non-fractured limb, and used as the strength deficit data point.

Hip Fracture-related Pain

Hip fracture-related pain was assessed once before (at rest) and once during all strength training sets and testing sessions, in addition to all functional performance tests using a five-point Verbal Ranking Scale (VRS 0–4 points; 0 = none, 1 = light, 2 = moderate, 3 = severe and 4 = intolerable pain.) The VRS has proved superior to other pain scales [39], and used in previous hip fracture studies [9,12,15]. The highest pain level reported from each assessment was used as data points.

Functional Assessment

During the daily regular physical therapy sessions, the patients were evaluated on their basic mobility capacity by the reliable [40] Cumulated Ambulation Score (CAS) [18,41]. The post-surgery day of independent ambulation was used as data point [42].

Upon discharge, all patients with an independent walking ability performed the reliable [43] Timed Up and Go test (TUG) [44] 3 times [45] (the fastest of 3 assessments used), and the 10 m fast speed walking test (10 MWT) [46] 1 time, using a rollator as a standardized walking aid in both tests [47]. The 3-step (0–30 s) Tandem test [48] of static balance was recorded as seconds of unsupported stance, while fear of falling was assessed by the Short Falls Efficacy Scale International (FES-I, 7–28 points, high scores indicating fear of falling) [49].

Statistical Analysis

The most fundamental principle of progressive strength training [50] is to progressively overload the exercising muscle as it becomes stronger [51]. This can be accomplished by progressively increasing the training load (kilograms lifted), while the exercise intensity is kept constant, e.g. 10 RM as in the present study. So, the sample size of the present study was determined based on the primary outcome (change in training loads) and a definition of the smallest clinically relevant increase in training load as being 1.5 kilograms (SD of 2.0) over 5 training sessions. In a fast-track surgery setting, 5 training sessions seems realistic, given an average hospitalization of 12 days, and no training at weekends. To be able to establish this effect, 16 patients needed to be included, using a standard of 80% power and type 1 error rate of 5%. To allow for a fracture type-specific indication of feasibility and an overall dropout rate of 20%, a total of 40 patients were included (20 patients with trochanteric and 20 patients with cervical fractures). We report all analyses related to the feasibility of the intervention – other than that of the training load - using descriptive statistics, and these analyses were considered primary [26]. All analyses related to the secondary outcomes were considered explorative.

All data were examined for normality of distribution (Kolmogorov-Smirnoff and Q-Q plots). Differences between cervical and trochanteric fractures were examined using the chi-square or Fisher exact tests for categorical data, the Students t-test or the Mann Whitney-U test for continuous data, as appropriate, while Paired *t* tests were used to examine changes in maximal isometric knee-extension strength for both limbs, and fractured as % of non-fractured. Repeated measures ANOVAs, in addition to a General Linear Mixed Model (adjusted for fracture type and number of training sessions) with Bonferroni adjustments were used to examine for changes in training loads over time (first, middle and last strength training session). Assumptions for these analyses were evaluated and found valid. Further, the eta-squared statistical analysis for independent-sample t-test ($t^2/(t^2+N1+N2-2)$) was used to examine the effect size of changes in training loads and in the fractured limb maximal isometric knee-extension strength, according to guidelines proposed by Cohen [52]. According to Cohen's classification, effect size above .01 indicates small effect,.06 moderate effect, and .14 large effect size. Data are presented as means (1 SD) when normally distributed, otherwise as medians (first-third quartile), or as numbers with percentages. The level of significance was set at *P* less than .05. All analyses were conducted with SPSS statistical (version 19; SPSS inc. Chicago, Illinois, USA).

Results

Descriptive Characteristics

Characteristics, participation, and outcomes for the 36 patients (18 with a cervical and 18 with a trochanteric hip fracture) who completed the full test and training program between June and December 2012 (9 men and 27 women with a mean age of 79.4 (8.3) years) are presented in table 2 and figure 1. No significant between-fracture type differences in baseline characteristics (Table 2) or in the day of the first or last strength training session existed (Table 3, $P>.11$).

Training Loads

The absolute loads (the kilograms that were lifted) increased progressively from a mean of 1.6 (0.8) to 4.3 (1.7) kilograms (t (48.1) = −8.66, $P<.001$, eta squared = .52) (Fig. 2A), over a mean of 4.3 (2.2) training sessions. The General Mixed Model showed no significant interaction between type of fracture and progression of training loads over time, ($P=.121$, partial eta squared = .12), while there was a substantial progression in training loads for both fracture types (within-subjects analysis, $P<.001$, partial eta squared = .38). The main effect between fracture type groups comparing progression of training loads was not significant, (between-subjects analysis, $P=.862$, partial eta squared = .001).

Adherence to Program

The initial strength test was postponed to Day 2 in 11 patients due to nausea (n = 4), tiredness (n = 4), pain (n = 2) and delirium (n = 1) and to Day 3 in 1 patient due to tiredness. Strength training was initiated at a mean of 2.4 (0.7) days post-surgery and ended at day 8.6 (4.2) (Day 0 = day of surgery) (Table 3). One hundred-eighty three (86%) out of 212 possible training sessions were completed, and 16 patients completed all planned sessions with no adverse events related to the strength training. Reasons for session failure were mainly related to exhaustion (55%) and nausea (24%), while only 3 sessions (2 patients with a trochanteric fracture) of a total of 212 sessions were not started or completed, due to a VRS pain score of 3 (severe pain) (Table 3).

Hip fracture related pain. More than 80% of the patients reported no or light pain during strength training and with the same number of patients reporting moderate or severe hip pain during the first (6 patients) and last (1 patient) training session (Fig. 2B). Similarly, more than 85% (n = 31) reported no or light pain during the baseline test of knee-extension strength. Upon discharge, all patients completing the program (n = 36) reported no or light pain at rest, while 32 (89%) patients reported no or light pain during the strength test. No patients reported intolerable pain (VRS = 4) during any of the above-mentioned sessions or outcome assessments.

Strength deficit. The fractured limb knee-extension strength increased significantly from a mean of .37 (0.2) to .61 (0.8) Nm/Kg (t (70) = −3.97, $P<.001$, eta squared = .18, Fig. 2C), while deficits decreased from an average of 50% (34) at baseline to 32% (26) at discharge ($P<.001$, Fig. 2D), and was more pronounced at discharge in patients with a trochanteric fracture (43%), compared to those with a cervical fracture (20%, $P=.004$, Table 2).

Functional Outcomes

No significant between fracture-type differences were found for the 10 MWT, TUG and Tandem test or in scores of the short FES-I questionnaire upon discharge from hospital (Table 2, $P>.14$).

Discussion

The main finding of the present study was that physical therapy including progressive strength training (10 RM) implemented in the acute ward immediately after hip fracture surgery seems feasible. That is, we found that the training load increased substantially, and more than that defined as the smallest effect worth detecting, while hip fracture-related pain was low to moderate and adherence high. The results also support that this type of physical therapy exercise might establish efficacy in reducing the knee-extension strength deficits of the fractured limb.

Training Load

The absolute training loads of the fractured limb increased progressively by an average of 188% from the first to the last training session, demonstrating a large observed effect size.

This underlines the importance of adjusting training loads on a set-by-set basis, when implementing this exercise modality clinically. Our increase in training load corresponds well to that reported in a fast-track total knee arthroplasty program with immediate progressive strength training of the knee extensors [25]. In the current study, the increase in training load was achieved with high adherence as reflected in less than one training session failure per patient, and with the 4 (10%) dropouts unrelated to the strength training or other assessments.

Hip Fracture-related Pain

Pain during the knee-extension strength training was generally low, even though we used the highest pain value recorded in each session as data points. Similarly, pain did not appear to influence the muscle strength testing, in accordance with that previously reported [25]. This is, however, in contrast to previous reports of hip fracture-related pain influencing in-hospital functional performances, such as walking with weight bearing on the operated leg, shortly after hip fracture surgery [12,15], and lower than that previously reported by Sherrington et al. at a later time-point [11]. The reason may be that both the test of muscle strength and training were performed using an open kinetic chain, where the foot is not fixed in space, as opposed to a closed kinetic chain exercise or task, where the foot is fixed in space (e.g. rise from a chair). So, even though the quadriceps muscle is loaded heavily during the strength training exercise, little compressive or shear

Table 2. Characteristics and results of patients following an in-hospital strength training program.

Variable	Total group (n = 36)	Cervical (n = 18)	Trochanteric (n = 18)	*P* Value
Age, mean (SD), years	79.4 (8.3)	78.9 (7.5)	80.4 (9.3)	.75
Men, number (%)	9 (25)	3 (33)	6 (67)	.25
Women, number (%)	27 (75)	15 (56)	12 (44)	
Body weight, mean (SD), kg	65.1 (15.0)	62.6 (16.5)	66.4 (13.3)	.34
NMS, median (IQR), 0–9 score	9 (4.5–9)	9 (5–9)	9 (4.5–9)	.66
ASA, median (n = 1/2/3/4 score)	2 (8/19/9/0)	2 (4/9/5/0)	2 (4/10/4/0)	.81
Hindsoe, median (IQR), 0–9 score	9 (8–9)	9 (7.75–9)	9 (7.75–9)	.68
FRS, median (IQR), 0–100 points	97 (72–100)	94.5 (71.25–100)	97 (70.25–99)	.87
MMSE, median (IQR), 0–30 points	26 (4.4)	25.56 (5.1)	26.4 (3.6)	.58
Knee-extension strength outcomes				
MVT f % nf at training start, mean (SD)	50.3 (33.6)	61.5 (40.0)	38.9 (21.4)	.04
MVT f % nf at discharge, mean (SD)	68.2 (25.2)	80.0 (21.8)	56.5 (23.3)	.004
MVT nf at start, mean (SD), Nm/kg	0.87 (0.4)	0.79 (0.4)	0.95 (0.4)	.19
MVT f at start, mean (SD), Nm/kg	0.37 (0.2)	0.41 (0.2)	0.33 (0.2)	.19
MVT nf at discharge, mean (SD), Nm/kg	0.95 (0.4)	0.87 (0.3)	1.03 (0.5)	.22
MVT f at discharge, mean (SD), Nm/kg	0.61 (0.3)	0.69 (0.3)	0.54 (0.3)	.14
Functional outcomes				
Independent in basis mobility (CAS = 6), number (%)	29 (81)	16 (55)	13 (45)	.21
Day of independence in basic mobility, mean (SD)	6.2 (2.3)	6.1 (3.0)	6.4 (2.0)	.73
10 MWT, m/s, mean (SD), (n = 28[a])	0.59 (0.3)	0.61 (0.3), (n = 14)	0.57 (0.3), (n = 14)	.79
TUG, s, mean (SD), (n = 27[a])	30.9 (20.3)	29.5 (18.6), (n = 14)	32.4 (22.7), (n = 13)	.72
Tandem, s, mean (SD), (0–30 s), (n = 29[b])	17.7 (10.2)	19.1 (10.5), (n = 15)	16.3 (10.1), (n = 14)	.47
Short FES-I (7–28 points), mean (SD), (n = 32[c])	15.9 (10.2)	14.1 (5.1), (n = 15)	17.5 (7.6), (n = 17)	.14

Abbreviations: NMS; New Mobility Score. ASA; American Society of Anaesthesiologists physical classification system. Hindsoe Test: Test of memory. FRS: Functional Recovery Score. MMSE: Mini Mental State Examination. Post-opr.: Post-operative. MVT; maximal voluntary torque. f: fractured limb. nf: non-fractured limb. CAS: Cumulated Ambulation Score. 10 MWT: 10 m fast speed walking test, TUG: Timed up and go test using standardized aid (rollator), Tandem: Tandem test of balance. Short FES-I: Falls Efficacy Scale –International.

[a]Functional tests were only performed in patients with an independent walking ability with a rollator at discharge.

[b]Balance test was only performed in patients able to stand without support.

[c]Four missing tests due to lack of time since discharge test was performed on the actual day of discharge (n = 3) or delirium (n = 1).

forces are likely to occur in the operated hip, as opposed to those occurring during rising from a chair, where substantial hip extensor power is generated [53]. Another explanation may be that the multimodal analgesia regimen consisting of postoperative continuous epidural analgesia (96 hours postoperatively), paracetamol, NSAID and supplied by opioids if needed [54], may differ from that used in e.g. the study by Sherrington et al [11].

Strength Deficit

The fractured limb knee-extension strength deficit decreased with approximately 18% when calculated as a mean of the 2 fracture type groups. However, greater deficits were seen for patients with a trochanteric as compared to those with a cervical fracture, and neither group reached the level of the non-fractured limb. With respect to discharge status, the deficit was reduced to 32% in the present study, as compared to 53% in a previous study, in which patients followed the same multimodal fast-track program, but did not undergo strength training [9]. This suggests that this type of exercise implemented immediately following surgery may be effective in reducing the strength deficit of the fractured limb, as a large effect size for changes in maximal isometric knee-extension strength was found, but needs experimental verification in a randomized controlled study design. Supporting a likely effect, Mitchell et al [10] found good compliance with a 6-week progressive quadriceps strength training program implemented in an inpatient rehabilitation setting shortly (median of 15 days post-surgery) after hip fracture. These authors found that the fractured leg extensor power increased significantly by 157% in the strength training group, compared to 63% in the control group at the 6-week follow up [10]. This was obtained although the exercise intensity was started at 50% of 1 RM (equal to >15 RM) and first increased to 80% of 1 RM (equal to 7 RM) in the last two of the six weeks of training, as opposed to an intensity of 10 RM (equal to 75% of 1 RM) from day 1 in the present study. These findings are supported by a newly published 6-week progressive strength training program (twice weekly, and training loads adjusted on a set-to-set basis) by Overgaard and Kristensen [22], conducted in an outpatient municipality setting. The later study included home-dwelling patients at a mean of 17.5 (5.7) days after hip fracture surgery, and reported an increase in fractured limb knee extension strength by 67%, while the fractured limb strength deficit (% non-fractured) was reduced from 40% to 17% at end of the program.

To that, a randomized controlled study by Binder et al [21] with a strength training intervention started after ceased standard physical therapy (average of 14 weeks post hip fracture surgery) in community dwelling elderly participants, reported effect of the

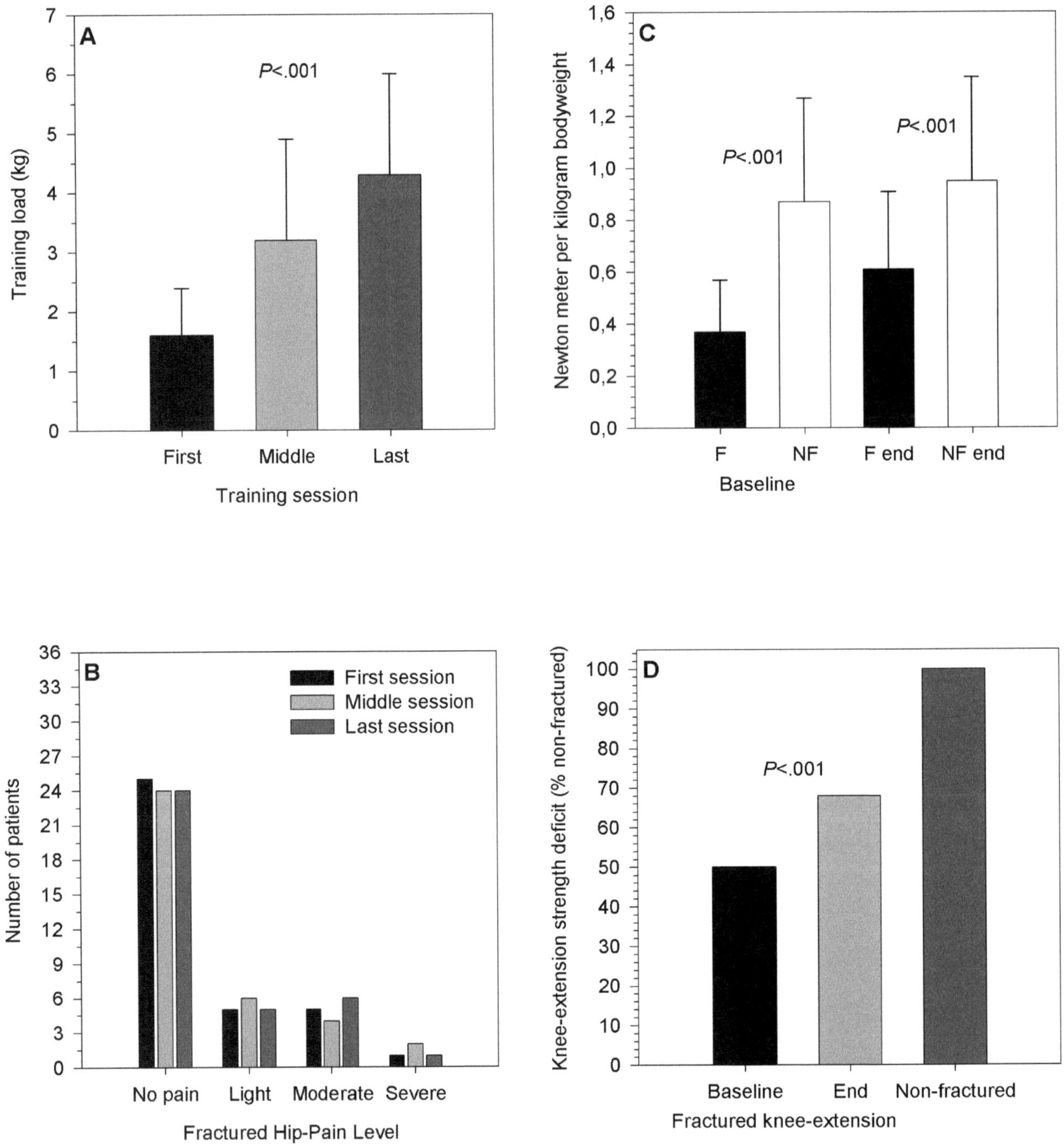

Figure 2. Outcomes on training load, hip-pain and knee-extension strength. A) Progression of training loads (kg) during the first, middle and last training session. B) Hip fracture-related pain during the first, middle and last strength training session. C) Knee-extension strength (Nm/kg), fractured (F) and non-fractured (NF) limb at baseline and discharge (end). D) Fractured limb knee-extension strength (% non-fractured) before and after training.

intervention. Further, Sherrington et al [11] reported in a 2-week inpatient rehabilitation program, that both patients who followed a weight-bearing and a non-weight-bearing exercise program improved markedly on strength and functional performances.

Finally, the same overall effect in favor of strength training after hip fracture was found by Singh et al [55], who implemented a 1-year community-based strength training program 6–8 weeks after the fracture and found a positive effect on ADL dependency, reduced nursing home admissions and mortality, when compared to usual care. On the contrary, a yearlong low-intensity home exercise intervention program showed no significant between-group differences for functional performances [56].

Nonetheless, although an increasing number of studies provide evidence for strength training as an important intervention after

Table 3. Program timeline, Adherence to programme and detailed physical therapy applied at unit according to regular regime.

Variable	Total group (n = 36)	Cervical (n = 18)	Trochanteric (n = 18)	*P* Value
Strength training				
First session day, mean (SD), Post-opr.	2.4 (0.7)	2.4 (0.7)	2.4 (0.7)	.81
Last session day, mean (SD), Post-opr.	8.6 (4.2)	7.4 (4.2)	9.7 (4.1)	.11
Day of discharge, mean (SD), Post-opr.	12.3 (6.6)	10.0 (4.6)	14.5 (7.5)	.04
Possible sessions, mean (SD)	5.1 (2.6)	4.2 (2.5)	6.0 (2.4)	.03
Training sessions conducted, mean (SD)	4.3 (2.2)	3.6 (2.0)	4.9 (2.2)	.06
Adherence to strength program				
No. (%) of possible training sessions	212	86 (41)	126 (59)	.07
No. (%) of training sessions conducted	183 (86)	75 (41)	108 (59)	.03
No. (%) of patients missing sessions	20 (56)	8 (40)	12 (60)	.18
No. (%) of strength sessions failure due to				
Exhaustion	16 (55)	6 (38)	10 (62)	.01
Nausea	7 (24)	4 (57)	3 (43)	.66
Hip fracture-related pain	3 (10)	0	3 (100)	
Logistics	2 (7)	0	2 (100)	
Cognitive dysfunction	1 (4)	1 (100)	0	
Regular physiotherapy without strength training				
Sessions, median (IQR), days	6 (4–7)	5 (3–6.25)	6 (6–7.5)	.02
Total time, mean (SD), min	126 (56)	109 (47)	144 (61)	.07
Time per session, mean (SD), min	22 (7)	21 (7)	22 (7)	.56
Total functional therapy time, mean (SD), min	74 (47)	66 (45)	84 (47)	.19
Total exercise therapy time, mean (SD), min	52 (30)	43 (28)	60 (31)	.18

hip fracture, none has so far succeeded in eliminating the fracture limb strength deficit, and none has started the intervention in the acute ward and exercised daily as in the present study. Hence, a care trajectory with progressive strength training implemented in the acute ward shortly following surgery, and continued on an outpatient basis after discharge is indicated to be effective towards several outcomes.

Functional Outcomes

No significant difference between fracture type groups was found in any of the functional performances, which is in contrast to that previously reported, at the same time point after hip fracture surgery in patients who did not undergo strength training [42,57]. The explanation hereto is probably lack of power, as the present study was not powered to investigate this specifically. Mitchell et al [9] reported a mean gait speed of 0.38 m/s 10 weeks after intervention in a comparable population, which is considerably lower than the 0.59 m/s found in this study at discharge from the acute ward. Compared to cut-points for severe mobility limitation, a gait speed of 0.59 m/s is still way below the cut-point of 1.22 m/s measured in well-functioning older adults [58], and should be addressed in rehabilitation after a hip fracture. Nonetheless, according to a recent systematic review [59], most of the patients included in the present study will be able to walk outside their house after discharge.

Study Weaknesses and Strengths

The included patients had a relatively high cognitive and prefracture functional level, which restricts our findings to patients with similar characteristics. Still, this is in accordance with previous studies [8–10;14], and the intervention is considered feasible within the study population. In general, the same physical therapist supervised all training and testing, which might have influenced results. However, we kept baseline data inaccessible to the tester until the study was completed, to minimize this influence. Finally, the promising results could to some extent be argued related to the regular physical therapy applied in the ward or spontaneous recovery. The greatest strength of our study is the well-described and simple intervention, making it realistic and low in cost to implement as a part of routine practice in the acute ward.

Conclusion

Physical therapy including progressive strength training (10 RM) implemented in the acute ward immediately after hip fracture surgery seems feasible. That is, we found that the training load increased substantially, and more than that defined as the smallest clinically relevant increase, while hip fracture-related pain was low to moderate and adherence high. The findings suggest that progressive strength training may reduce the knee-extension strength deficits of the fractured limb, but the intervention and the clinical efficacy need confirmation in a randomized controlled design.

Supporting Information

Protocol S1 Complete study trial protocol as approved by ethics committee, English version.

Protocol S2 Complete study trial protocol as approved by ethics committee, original language.

Checklist S1 STROBE checklist of items that should be included in reports of cohort studies.

Acknowledgments

Additional contribution: We thank all of the patients participating in this study for their valuable contribution. A special thank to the participating physical therapists, Maria Svennergren (B. Pt.), Kirsten Aunskjær Pedersen (Pt.), Kirsten Juel Nielsen (Pt.), Maria StokholmVan (B. Pt.) og Sanne Busk Stie (B. Pt.), nurse staff and doctors from the Hip Fracture Unit and the Department of Orthopedic Surgery at Hvidovre Hospital, whom provided essential cooperative assistance with the study without any compensation.

Author Contributions

Conceived and designed the experiments: MTK TB HP HK. Performed the experiments: MTK LK. Analyzed the data: MTK TB LK. Contributed reagents/materials/analysis tools: MTK TB. Wrote the paper: LK MTK TB. Critical revision of the manuscript for important intellectual content: MTK TB LK HP HK. Obtained funding: MTK TB LK HK. Study supervision: MTK TB HP HK.

References

1. Kristensen MT (2011) Factors affecting functional prognosis of patients with hip fracture. Eur J Phys Rehabil Med 47: 257–264. R33112514 [pii].
2. Rosell PA, Parker MJ (2003) Functional outcome after hip fracture. A 1-year prospective outcome study of 275 patients. Injury 34: 529–532.
3. Salpakoski A, Portegijs E, Kallinen M, Sihvonen S, Kiviranta I, et al. (2011) Physical inactivity and pain in older men and women with hip fracture history. Gerontology 57: 19–27. 000315490 [pii];10.1159/000315490 [doi].
4. Ariza-Vega P, Jimenez-Moleon JJ, Kristensen MT (2013) Change of residence and functional status within three months and one year following hip fracture surgery. Disabil Rehabil. 10.3109/09638288.2013.813081 [doi].
5. Egan M, Jaglal S, Byrne K, Wells J, Stolee P (2008) Factors associated with a second hip fracture: a systematic review. Clin Rehabil 22: 272–282. 0269215507081573 [pii];10.1177/0269215507081573 [doi].
6. Bischoff-Ferrari HA, Dawson-Hughes B, Platz A, Orav EJ, Stahelin HB, et al. (2010) Effect of high-dosage cholecalciferol and extended physiotherapy on complications after hip fracture: a randomized controlled trial. Arch Intern Med 170: 813–820. 170/9/813 [pii];10.1001/archinternmed.2010.67 [doi].
7. Portegijs E, Buurman BM, Essink-Bot ML, Zwinderman AH, de Rooij SE (2012) Failure to Regain Function at 3 months After Acute Hospital Admission Predicts Institutionalization Within 12 Months in Older Patients. J Am Med Dir Assoc. S1525-8610(12)00093-X [pii];10.1016/j.jamda.2012.04.003 [doi].
8. Kehlet H (2011) Fast-track surgery-an update on physiological care principles to enhance recovery. Langenbecks Arch Surg 396: 585–590.
9. Kristensen MT, Bandholm T, Bencke J, Ekdahl C, Kehlet H (2009) Knee-extension strength, postural control and function are related to fracture type and thigh edema in patients with hip fracture. Clin Biomech (Bristol, Avon) 24: 218–224. S0268-0033(08)00295-7 [pii];10.1016/j.clinbiomech.2008.10.003 [doi].
10. Mitchell SL, Stott DJ, Martin BJ, Grant SJ (2001) Randomized controlled trial of quadriceps training after proximal femoral fracture. Clin Rehabil 15: 282–290.
11. Sherrington C, Lord SR, Herbert RD (2003) A randomised trial of weight-bearing versus non-weight-bearing exercise for improving physical ability in inpatients after hip fracture. Aust J Physiother 49: 15–22.
12. Foss NB, Kristensen MT, Palm H, Kehlet H (2009) Postoperative pain after hip fracture is procedure specific. Br J Anaesth 102: 111–116. aen345 [pii];10.1093/bja/aen345 [doi].
13. Cornwall R, Gilbert MS, Koval KJ, Strauss E, Siu AL (2004) Functional outcomes and mortality vary among different types of hip fractures: a function of patient characteristics. Clin Orthop Relat Res 64–71. 00003086-200408000-00009 [pii].
14. Kristensen MT, Kehlet H (2012) Most patients regain prefracture basic mobility after hip fracture surgery in a fast-track programme. Dan Med J 59: A4447. A4447 [pii].
15. Kristensen MT (2013) Hip fracture-related pain strongly influences functional performance of patients with an intertrochanteric fracture upon discharge from the hospital. PM R 5: 135–141. S1934-1482(12)01634-6 [pii];10.1016/j.pmrj.2012.10.006 [doi].
16. Oldmeadow LB, Edwards ER, Kimmel LA, Kipen E, Robertson VJ, et al. (2006) No rest for the wounded: early ambulation after hip surgery accelerates recovery. ANZ J Surg 76: 607–611. ANS3786 [pii];10.1111/j.1445-2197.2006.03786.x [doi].
17. Siu AL, Penrod JD, Boockvar KS, Koval K, Strauss E, et al. (2006) Early ambulation after hip fracture: effects on function and mortality. Arch Intern Med 166: 766–771. 166/7/766 [pii];10.1001/archinte.166.7.766 [doi].
18. Foss NB, Kristensen MT, Kehlet H (2006) Prediction of postoperative morbidity, mortality and rehabilitation in hip fracture patients: the cumulated ambulation score. Clin Rehabil 20: 701–708.
19. Auais MA, Eilayyan O, Mayo NE (2012) Extended exercise rehabilitation after hip fracture improves patients' physical function: a systematic review and meta-analysis. Phys Ther 92: 1437–1451. ptj.20110274 [pii];10.2522/ptj.20110274 [doi].
20. Sherrington C, Tiedemann A, Cameron I (2011) Physical exercise after hip fracture: an evidence overview. Eur J Phys Rehabil Med 47: 297–307. R33112524 [pii].
21. Binder EF, Brown M, Sinacore DR, Steger-May K, Yarasheski KE, et al. (2004) Effects of extended outpatient rehabilitation after hip fracture: a randomized controlled trial. JAMA 292: 837–846. 10.1001/jama.292.7.837 [doi];292/7/837 [pii].
22. Overgaard J, Kristensen MT (2013) Feasibility of progressive strength training shortly after hip fracture surgery. World J Orthop 4: 248–258. 10.5312/wjo.v4.i4.248 [doi].
23. Hung WW, Egol KA, Zuckerman JD, Siu AL (2012) Hip fracture management: tailoring care for the older patient. JAMA 307: 2185–2194. 1167293 [pii];10.1001/jama.2012.4842 [doi].
24. Suetta C, Magnusson SP, Rosted A, Aagaard P, Jakobsen AK, et al. (2004) Resistance training in the early postoperative phase reduces hospitalization and leads to muscle hypertrophy in elderly hip surgery patients–a controlled, randomized study. J Am Geriatr Soc 52: 2016–2022. JGS52557 [pii];10.1111/j.1532-5415.2004.52557.x [doi].
25. Jakobsen TL, Husted H, Kehlet H, Bandholm T (2012) Progressive strength training (10 RM) commenced immediately after fast-track total knee arthroplasty: is it feasible? Disabil Rehabil 34: 1034–1040. 10.3109/09638288.2011.629019 [doi].
26. Arain M, Campbell MJ, Cooper CL, Lancaster GA (2010) What is a pilot or feasibility study? A review of current practice and editorial policy. BMC Med Res Methodol 10: 67. 1471-2288-10-67 [pii];10.1186/1471-2288-10-67 [doi].
27. von EE, Altman DG, Egger M, Pocock SJ, Gotzsche PC, et al. (2007) The Strengthening the Reporting of Observational Studies in Epidemiology (STROBE) statement: guidelines for reporting observational studies. Lancet 370: 1453–1457. S0140-6736(07)61602-X [pii];10.1016/S0140-6736(07)61602-X [doi].
28. Kristensen MT, Bandholm T, Foss NB, Ekdahl C, Kehlet H (2008) High inter-tester reliability of the new mobility score in patients with hip fracture. J Rehabil Med 40: 589–591. 10.2340/16501977-0217 [doi].
29. Parker MJ, Palmer CR (1993) A new mobility score for predicting mortality after hip fracture. J Bone Joint Surg Br 75: 797–798.
30. Zuckerman JD, Koval KJ, Aharonoff GB, Hiebert R, Skovron ML (2000) A functional recovery score for elderly hip fracture patients: I. Development. J Orthop Trauma 14: 20–25.
31. Zuckerman JD, Koval KJ, Aharonoff GB, Skovron ML (2000) A functional recovery score for elderly hip fracture patients: II. Validity and reliability. J Orthop Trauma 14: 26–30.
32. Folstein MF, Folstein SE, McHugh PR (1975) "Mini-mental state". A practical method for grading the cognitive state of patients for the clinician. J Psychiatr Res 12: 189–198. 0022-3956(75)90026-6 [pii].
33. American Society of Anesthesiologists (1963) New classification of physical status. Anesthesiology 24: 111.
34. Toigo M, Boutellier U (2006) New fundamental resistance exercise determinants of molecular and cellular muscle adaptations. Eur J Appl Physiol 97: 643–663. 10.1007/s00421-006-0238-1 [doi].
35. Boutron I, Moher D, Altman DG, Schulz KF, Ravaud P (2008) Extending the CONSORT statement to randomized trials of nonpharmacologic treatment: explanation and elaboration. Ann Intern Med 148: 295–309. 148/4/295 [pii].
36. Roy MA, Doherty TJ (2004) Reliability of hand-held dynamometry in assessment of knee extensor strength after hip fracture. Am J Phys Med Rehabil 83: 813–818. 00002060-200411000-00001 [pii].
37. Schaubert KL, Bohannon RW (2005) Reliability and validity of three strength measures obtained from community-dwelling elderly persons. J Strength Cond Res 19: 717–720. R-15954 [pii];10.1519/R-15954.1 [doi].
38. Sherrington C, Lord SR (2005) Reliability of simple portable tests of physical performance in older people after hip fracture. Clin Rehabil 19: 496–504.
39. Leino KA, Kuusniemi KS, Lertola KK, Olkkola KT (2011) Comparison of four pain scales in patients with hip fracture or other lower limb trauma. Acta Anaesthesiol Scand 55: 495–502. 10.1111/j.1399-6576.2010.02373.x [doi].
40. Kristensen MT, Andersen L, Bech-Jensen R, Moos M, Hovmand B, et al. (2009) High intertester reliability of the cumulated ambulation score for the evaluation of basic mobility in patients with hip fracture. Clin Rehabil 23: 1116–1123. 0269215509342330 [pii];10.1177/0269215509342330 [doi].

41. Kristensen MT, Jakobsen TL, Nielsen JW, Jorgensen LM, Nienhuis RJ, et al. (2012) Cumulated Ambulation Score to evaluate mobility is feasible in geriatric patients and in patients with hip fracture. Dan Med J 59: A4464. A4464 [pii].
42. Kristensen MT, Foss NB, Ekdahl C, Kehlet H (2010) Prefracture functional level evaluated by the New Mobility Score predicts in-hospital outcome after hip fracture surgery. Acta Orthop 81: 296–302. 10.3109/17453674.2010.487240 [doi].
43. Kristensen MT, Henriksen S, Stie SB, Bandholm T (2011) Relative and absolute intertester reliability of the timed up and go test to quantify functional mobility in patients with hip fracture. J Am Geriatr Soc 59: 565–567. 10.1111/j.1532-5415.2010.03293.x [doi].
44. Podsiadlo D, Richardson S (1991) The timed "Up & Go": a test of basic functional mobility for frail elderly persons. J Am Geriatr Soc 39: 142–148.
45. Kristensen MT, Ekdahl C, Kehlet H, Bandholm T (2010) How many trials are needed to achieve performance stability of the Timed Up & Go test in patients with hip fracture? Arch Phys Med Rehabil 91: 885–889. S0003-9993(10)00091-2 [pii];10.1016/j.apmr.2010.01.021 [doi].
46. Watson M (2002) Refining the ten-metre walking test for use with neurologically impared people. Physiotherapy 88: 386–397.
47. Kristensen MT, Bandholm T, Holm B, Ekdahl C, Kehlet H (2009) Timed up & go test score in patients with hip fracture is related to the type of walking aid. Arch Phys Med Rehabil 90: 1760–1765. S0003-9993(09)00421-3 [pii];10.1016/j.apmr.2009.05.013 [doi].
48. Rossiter-Fornoff JE, Wolf SL, Wolfson LI, Buchner DM (1995) A cross-sectional validation study of the FICSIT common data base static balance measures. Frailty and Injuries: Cooperative Studies of Intervention Techniques. J Gerontol A Biol Sci Med Sci 50: M291–M297.
49. Kempen GI, Yardley L, van Haastregt JC, Zijlstra GA, Beyer N, et al. (2008) The Short FES-I: a shortened version of the falls efficacy scale-international to assess fear of falling. Age Ageing 37: 45–50. afm157 [pii];10.1093/ageing/afm157 [doi].
50. Delorme TL (1945) Restoration of muscle power by heavy-resistance exercises. J Bone Joint Surg Am 27: 645–67.
51. American College of Sports Medicine (2009) American College of Sports Medicine position stand. Progression models in resistance training for healthy adults. Med Sci Sports Exerc 41: 687–708. 10.1249/MSS.0b013e3181915670 [doi].
52. Cohen JW (1988) Statistical power analysis for the behavorial sciences. Hillsdale, N.J.: Lawrence Erlbaum Associates.
53. Hwang S, Kim Y, Kim Y (2009) Lower extremity joint kinetics and lumbar curvature during squat and stoop lifting. BMC Musculoskelet Disord 10: 15. 1471-2474-10-15 [pii];10.1186/1471-2474-10-15 [doi].
54. Foss NB, Kristensen MT, Kristensen BB, Jensen PS, Kehlet H (2005) Effect of postoperative epidural analgesia on rehabilitation and pain after hip fracture surgery: a randomized, double-blind, placebo-controlled trial. Anesthesiology 102: 1197–1204. 00000542-200506000-00020 [pii].
55. Singh NA, Quine S, Clemson LM, Williams EJ, Williamson DA, et al. (2012) Effects of high-intensity progressive resistance training and targeted multidisciplinary treatment of frailty on mortality and nursing home admissions after hip fracture: a randomized controlled trial. J Am Med Dir Assoc 13: 24–30. S1525-8610(11)00273-8 [pii];10.1016/j.jamda.2011.08.005 [doi].
56. Orwig DL, Hochberg M, Yu-Yahiro J, Resnick B, Hawkes WG, et al. (2011) Delivery and outcomes of a yearlong home exercise program after hip fracture: a randomized controlled trial. Arch Intern Med 171: 323–331. 171/4/323 [pii];10.1001/archinternmed.2011.15 [doi].
57. Kristensen MT, Foss NB, Kehlet H (2009) Factors with independent influence on the 'timed up and go' test in patients with hip fracture. Physiother Res Int 14: 30–41. 10.1002/pri.414 [doi].
58. Manini TM, Visser M, Won-Park S, Patel KV, Strotmeyer ES, et al. (2007) Knee extension strength cutpoints for maintaining mobility. J Am Geriatr Soc 55: 451–457. JGS1087 [pii];10.1111/j.1532-5415.2007.01087.x [doi].
59. Salbach NM, O'Brien K, Brooks D, Irvin E, Martino R, et al. (2013) Speed and distance requirements for community ambulation: A systematic review. Arch Phys Med Rehabil. S0003-9993(13)00475-9 [pii];10.1016/j.apmr.2013.06.017 [doi].

The Hip Lag Sign - Prospective Blinded Trial of a New Clinical Sign to Predict Hip Abductor Damage

Alexander Kaltenborn[1,2,3*§], Catherine M. Bourg[1§], Andreas Gutzeit[4,5], Fabian Kalberer[1]

1 Department of Orthopedic Surgery, Kantonsspital Winterthur, Winterthur, Switzerland, 2 Department of Trauma and Orthopedic Surgery, Federal Armed Forces Hospital Westerstede, Westerstede, Germany, 3 Department of General, Visceral and Transplant Surgery, Hannover Medical School, Hannover, Germany, 4 Department of Radiology, Kantonsspital Winterthur, Winterthur, Switzerland, 5 Department of Radiology, Paracelsus Medical University Salzburg, Salzburg, Austria

Abstract

This study introduces and validates the Hip Lag Sign, a new clinical parameter to determine hip abductor damage, which appears to be one major cause for greater trochanteric pain syndrome. 26 patients who underwent standardized MRI-examination were prospectively enrolledbetween October 2009 and March 2012. A standard physical examination of the hip was performed, including the Hip Lag Sign as it is defined for the first time in this work. Hip Lag Sign results were statistically compared toMR images, to pain levels measured with the visual analogue scale and to results of the modified Harris Hip Score as a universal and well established diagnostic tool for the hip. Chi^2- and Mann-Whitney-U-analysis were applied. Diagnostic accuracy was tested with 2×2-table-calculations.Kappa statistics were used to analyze inter-observer variability. A positive Hip Lag Sign is significantly associated with MRI-proven hip abductor damage ($p<0.001$). The Hip Lag Sign has a sensitivity of 89.47% and a specificity of 96.55%. The positive and negative predictive values are 94.44%, resp. 93.33%. Its diagnostic Odds Ratio is 239.000 ($p<0.001$; 95%-CI: 20.031-2827.819). The number needed to diagnose was 1.16.Inter-observer consistency was 98.1% and kappa statistics for inter-observer variability were 0.911. The Hip Lag Sign is specific and sensitive, easy and fast to perform and allows a reliable assessment on the hip abductors' status, especially when there is no access to further diagnostic devices such as MRI for example due to restricted resources like in developing countries. Thus, we recommend the inclusion of the Hip Lag Sign into everyday hip examinations, especially dealing with patients suffering from greater trochanteric pain syndrome.

Editor: Jason Mulvenna, Queensland Institute of Medical Research, Australia

Funding: The authors have no support or funding to report.

Competing Interests: The authors have declared that no competing interests exist.

* E-mail: alexander.kaltenborn@gmail.com

§ These authors contributed equally to this work.

Introduction

10–25% of the general populationsuffer from greater trochanteric pain syndrome, characterised by persistent pain and tenderness over the greater trochanter [1]. Greater trochanteric pain syndrome is generally underestimated and underdiagnosed, resulting in a chronic undertreatment of these patients, not to forget the social and economic fallout that comes with chronic pain and limitation of mobility. Although a great variety of causes, e.g. trochanteric bursitis, iliotibial tract friction or coxa vara, are known to be attributed to greater trochanteric pain syndrom, we place our focus on lesions of the hip abductors as one of the primary causes of pain in the lateral hip region [2–4].

The major hip abductors are the gluteus medius and minimus muscles which are essential for gait and balance, seeing as they ensure hip stability throughout the whole gait process [5]. For this particular reason, comparable to the rotator cuff in the shoulder, lesions of these muscles are often referred to as 'rotator cuff tears of the hip' [6–8], which are currently best diagnosed using magnetic resonance imaging (MRI) [9]. But MR examination is also strongly dependent from technical dependencies and the experience of the radiologists [10]. Unfortunately, hip abductor damages are often missed by physicians or even misdiagnosed as bursitis which leads to wrong treatments and prolonged pain [11]. Unnecessary infiltrations or injections of corticosteroids increase the risk of adverse events such as infections and further harm the patient [12]. If patients with greater trochanteric pain syndrome do not respond to conservative treatment, gluteal tendon pathologies definitely represent one of the most important differential diagnoses which should not be clinically missed [2].

Considering this, the paucity of research on hip abductor damage and the lack of a reliable clinical sign are surprising. Especially in times of optimizing quality and resource management against the backdrop of struggling healthcare systems, cutting down unnecessary, expensive MRI-examinations seems to be reasonable. Moreover, physicians in rural areas or developing countries who depend on physical examinations are in need of a reliable clinical sign to safely diagnose hip abductor damages [13].

This is the reason why it is imperative to look for new diagnostic tools and why we investigate the Hip Lag Sign. Aim of this study is to clarify, if the Hip Lag Sign is a reliable parameter to clinically diagnose hip abductor damage.

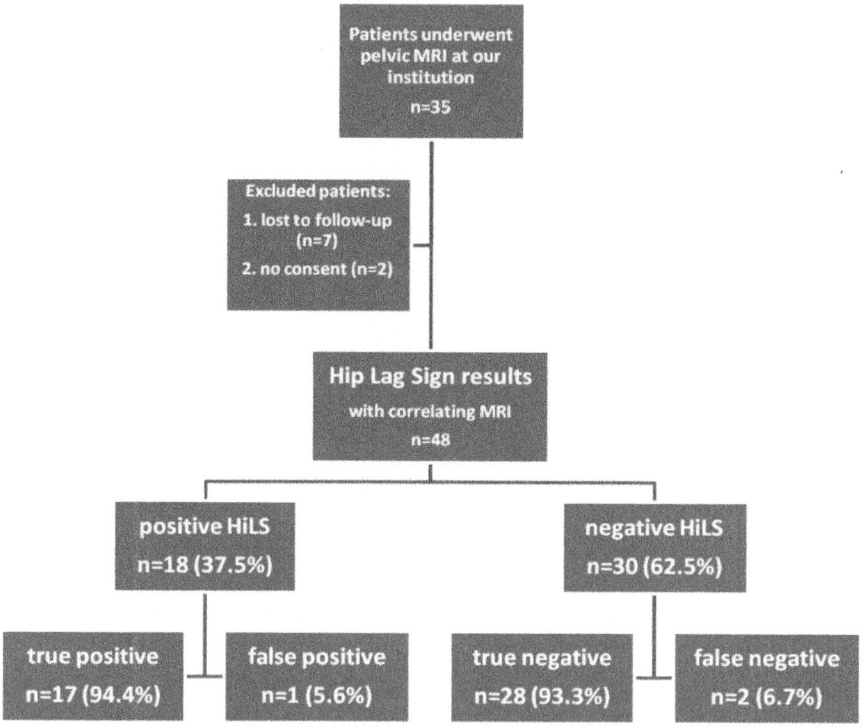

Figure 1. Flow Chart. Shown is the flow of patients through the Hip Lag Sign-study according to STARD-Guidelines.

Patients and Methods

This is a blinded, prospective, single-centre study with 26 patients who underwent MRI-examination at our institution between October 2009 and March 2012. MR images were statistically compared to Hip Lag Sign results, to pain levels measured with the visual analogue scale and to results of the modified Harris Hip Score as a universal and well established diagnostic tool for the hip [14,15]. The flow of the patients through this study according to the *Standard for Reporting of Diagnostic Accuracy* (STARD) – Guidelines is pictured in Figure 1 [16].The local institutional review board approved the study protocol. Written informed consent was obtained from all patients prior to examination and inclusion.

Inclusion and exclusion criteria

Both patients with and without total hip arthroplasty in their history were included (23 hip replacements in 16 patients [61.54%]). Excluded were cases where abductor tendon insertion was not visible on MR-imaging due to metal artefacts induced by total hip arthroplasty (n = 0), paediatric patients defined as younger than 18 years (n = 0), patients who were lost to follow-up (n = 7), and patients without informed consent (n = 2).One-sided MRI-studies were performed for 4 patients. The cases where no correlating MRI was available were excluded from statistical analysis. The participating patients' characteristics are listed in Table 1.

MR imaging

For MR imaging of the study population a 1.5 T MRI scanner (Achieva, Philips Healthcare, Best, Netherlands) was used. All MRI examinations were done in standardized supine position on the examination table and images were acquired with a 16 channel XL torso coil (Philips Healthcare, Best, Netherlands). MR imaging was used to proof hip abductor damage defined as partial or complete rupture of the gluteus minimus and/or gluteus medius tendon, tendinosis, and/or gluteus minimus/medius atrophy. MRI was analyzed by a board examined radiologist with 12 years of experience in musculoskeletal diseases.

Physical Examination

To test for the Hip Lag Sign, the patient has to lie in a lateral, neutral position with the affected leg being on top. The examiner then positions one arm under this leg to have good hold and control over the relaxed extremity, whereas the other hand stabilizes the pelvis. The next step is to passively extend to 10° in the hip, abduct to 20° and rotate internally as far as possible, while the knee remains in a flexed position of 45°. After the patient is asked to hold the leg actively in this position, the examiner releases the leg. The Hip Lag Sign is considered positive if the patient is not able to keep the leg in the aforementioned abducted, internally rotated position and the foot drops more than 10 cm. To ensure an accurate result, the test should be repeated three times (see Fig. 2).

The two clinical examiners who tested the study population for the hip lag sign were both tutored by the head of hip surgery unit at our institution immediately before the beginning of this study to allow a standardised and well executed physical examination.

They both examined the patients independently and filed their test results on an anonymous study examination sheet, which was marked with an identification number. After testing for the Hip Lag Sign on both sides, the patient was asked for her/his symptoms, any history of specific treatment or total hip arthroplasty, and a modified Harris Hip Score was evaluated. Finally the test results were compared to the MRI results of the patient.

Table 1. Shown are the patients' characteristics of all included cases.

	Sex	Age	BMI	Hip Abductor Damage	Hip Lag Sign	cl. Hip Lag Sign	mHHS	VAS	THA
1	♀	69	33.7	gluteus medius PR	+	–	89	3	+
2	♀	74	28.3	gluteus medius/minimus R right & left	+	–	53	6	+
3	♀	75	23.8	ri: gluteus medius / minimus R le: gluteus medius / minimus atrophy	+	+	52	8	+
4	♀	79	20.2	gluteus medius / minimus R	+	–	93	1	–
5	♂	49	27.9	nil	–	–	84	3	+
6	♀	78	22.0	gluteus minimus R / medius atrophy right & left	+	+	76	3	–
7	♀	62	26.4	gluteus medius / minimus atrophy	+	–	71	7	+
8	♂	57	27.8	nil	–	–	83	6	+
9	♂	60	28.1	nil	–	–	93	7	–
10	♀	27	18.4	nil	–	–	96	2	–
11	♀	48	21.4	nil	–	–	73	5	+
12	♀	74	23.9	nil	–	–	63	7	+
13	♂	78	26.9	gluteus minimus / medius PR	+	–	71	5	–
14	♀	77	24.6	gluteus medius / minimus atrophy	+	–	50	7	–
15	♀	71	25.5	gluteus medius / minimus atrophy	+	–	80	4	+
16	♀	68	28.7	gluteus minimus PR / medius tendinosis	+	–	100	6	+
17	♀	76	33.7	gluteus minimus / medius tendinosis	+	–	55	8	+
18	♀	43	38.3	nil	–	–	73	5	–
19	♀	66	28.0	gluteus minimus / medius PR	+	–	49	7	–
20	♂	24	24.2	nil	–	+	84	7	–
21	♂	80	24.7	nil	–	–	89	1	+
22	♀	75	20.6	gluteus medius atrophy	+	–	67	7	+
23	♀	76	22.7	partial gluteus medius atrophy	+	–	95	0	+
24	♂	58	24.2	gluteus minimus degeneration and PR	–	–	96	5	+
25	♀	72	24.2	gluteus medius PR	+	–	30	9	–
26	♀	66	26.2	nil	–	–	72	3	–

(BMI = Body Mass Index; Hip Lag Sign = Hip Lag Sign; cl Hip Lag Sign = contralateral Hip Lag Sign; mHHS = modified Harris Hip Score; VAS = visual analogue scale; PR = partial rupture; R = rupture).

Both examiners did not know the patient or the patient's case file beforehand. At the time of physical examination, the examiner had no knowledge which side was affected by abductor damage.

Statistical analysis

Sensitivity, specificity and number needed to diagnose of the Hip Lag Sign were calculated using a 2×2-table (see Tabl. 2). Significance of correlations was determined with the Chi^2-Test and the Mann-Whitney-U-Test. Furthermore, we calculated a positive and negative predictive value as well as diagnostic Odds Ratios and Likelihood Ratios according to *STARD*-guidelines [16]. Kappa statistics were used to analyze inter-observer variability.

For all statistical tests a p-value <0.05 was defined as significant. The IBM SPSS statistics software version 20.0 (IBM, Somers, NY, USA) was used to perform statistical analysis.

Results

A total of 52 Hip Lag Signs were performed on 26 patients (7 males, 19 females; 27%, 73%, respectively) with a mean age of 64.4 years (median 71.5 years, range: 24–80 years) who fulfilled the inclusion and exclusion criteria at the time of physical examination. The average Body Mass Index defined as body weight in kg divided by height in m squared was 25.87 (median 24.65, range: 18.4–38.3).

23 of 48 examined hips (47.92%) have been treated with total hip arthroplasty, which has no statistically significant effect on the Hip Lag Sign results (p = 0.565).

There were no MR images available for four hips. Therefore, we excluded these cases and 48 Hip Lag Sign results remain for further statistical analysis. 18 Hip Lag Signs (37.5%) werepositive, which is defined as the case cohort. Thus, 30 Hip Lag Signs (62.5%) were tested negative and are representing the control group. After comparing the Hip Lag Sign results with the MR images, 17 out of 18 positive Hip Lag Signs can be confirmed true positive (94.4%) and only 2 of the 30 negative results (6.7%) must be considered as false negative (see Table 2).

Taking these results into account, we evaluated a sensitivity of 89.47% (95%-CI: 66.82%–98.39%) corresponding with a specificity of 96.55% (95%-CI: 82.17%–99.42%). The positive predictive value of the Hip Lag Sign is 94.44% (95%-CI: 72.63%–99.07%); the negative predictive value was calculated at 93.33% (95%-CI: 77.89%–98.99%). 1.16 patients have to be tested with the Hip Lag Sign to identify one case of hip abductor damage (number needed to diagnose = 1/[sensitivity-(1-specificity)] = 1.16).

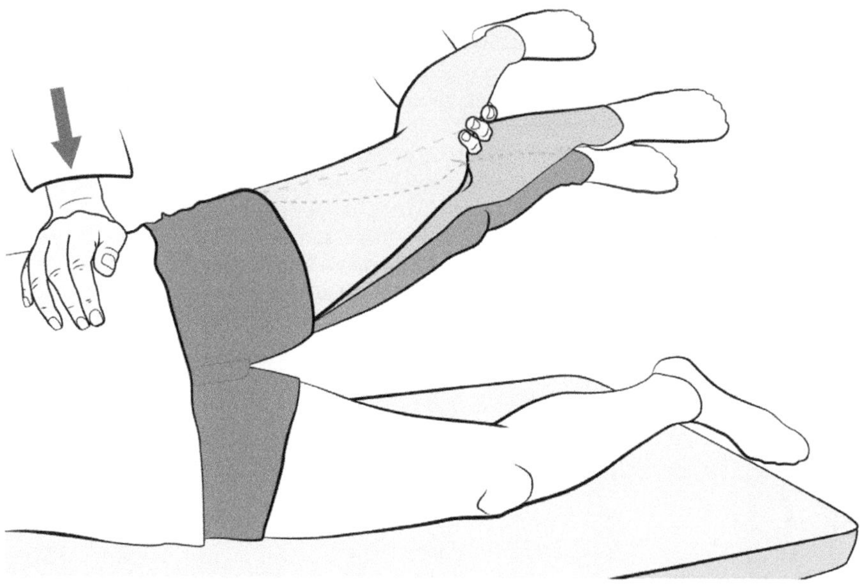

Figure 2. The Hip Lag Sign. Shown is the Hip Lag Sign as it is defined in this work: To test for the Hip Lag Sign, the patient has to lie in a lateral, neutral position with the affected leg being on top. The examiner then positions one arm under this leg to have good hold and control over the relaxed extremity, whereas the other hand stabilizes the pelvis. The next step is to passively extend to 10° in the hip, abduct and rotate internally as far as possible, while the knee remains in a flexed position of 45°. After the patient is asked to hold the leg actively in this position, the examiner releases the leg. The Hip Lag Sign is considered positive, if the patient is not able to keep the leg in the aforementioned abducted, internally rotated position and the foot drops more than 10 cm.

Table 2. Shown is the 2×2-table to execute calculations for sensitivity, specificity, as well as positive and negative predictive value.

Hip abductor damage				
Hip Lag Sign		yes (n = 19)	no (n = 29)	
	positive (n = 18)	17 (94.4%)	1 (5.6%)	**PPV 94.44%**
	negative (n = 30)	2 (6.7%)	28 (93.3%)	**NPV 93.33%**
		Sensitivity 89.47%	**Specificity 96.55%**	

(Chi^2-test: ***p<0.001***; Mann-Whitney-U-test: *p<0.001*).
(PPV = positive predictive value; NPV = negative predictive value).

A positive Hip Lag Sign result is significantly associated with MRI-proven hip abductor damage as it is defined above ($p<0.001$; Chi^2- and Mann-Whitney-U-test).

As a measure of the effectiveness of a diagnostic test, the calculated diagnostic Odds Ratio is 238.000 ($p<0.001$; 95%-CI: 20.031–2827.819). Positive Likelihood Ratio can be reported at 25.95 (95%-CI: 3.76–179.14) and negative Likelihood Ratio at 0.11 (95%-CI: 0.03–0.41).

All but one Hip Lag Sign result were consistent between the two examiners; the non-consistent case was seen wrong positive by one physician. Thus, the inter-observer consistency is 98.1% and kappa statistics for inter-observer variability are 0.911. The Hip Lag Sign results reported in the manuscript are with the aforementioned wrong positive test included.

The mean modified Harris Hip Score in the study population is 74.04 (median: 74.50; range: 30–100). Visual analogue scale levels range from zero to nine with a mean level of 5.25 (median: 6.00).

Neither modified Harris Hip Score results ($p = 0.326$) nor visual analogue scale-pain level ($p = 0.491$) are significantly associated with positive Hip Lag Sign results. Categorization of the study

Table 3. Shown is the categorisation of the study population in four outcome subgroups regarding the modified Harris Hip Score.

	Modified Harris Hip Score Outcome Subgroup			
	Poor (<70)	**Fair (70–79)**	**Good (80–89)**	**Excellent (90–100)**
Number of Patients	6 (23.1%)	6 (23.1%)	6 (23.1%)	8 (30.8%)
Abductor Damage	4	2	3	7
Positive Hip Lag Sign result	3 (1 false negative)	3 (1 false positive)	3	6 (1 false negative)

There is no significant clustering ($p = 0.195$ [Chi^2] for abductor damage; $p = 0.701$ [Chi^2] for Hip Lag Sign result).

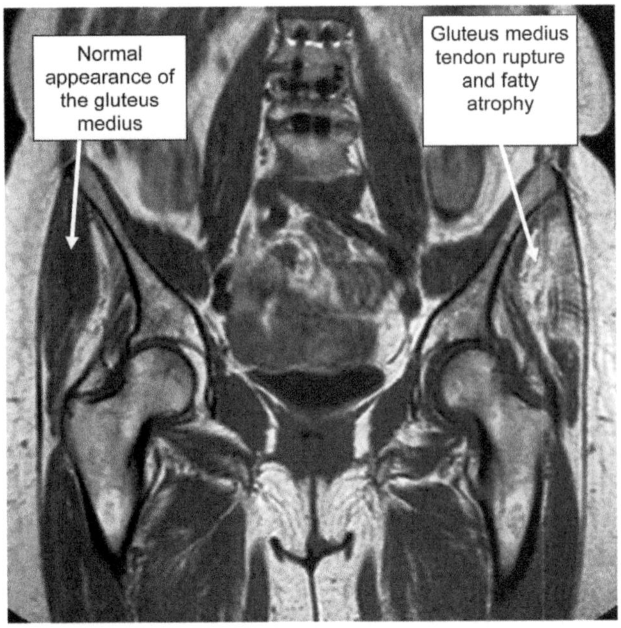

Figure 3. Hip abductor damage on MRI. Shown is the coronal T1-weighted MR-image at the level of the greater trochanter of a 72 year old female patient, complaining of severe lateral hip pain on the left side, radiating down to the knee. The greater trochanter is very tender on palpation and the patient presents with a reduced walking distance and difficulties during the gait cycle. The Hip Lag Sign was positive on the left side.

population into the fourmodified Harris Hip Scoreoutcome subgroups is summarized in Table 3.

Discussion

Hip pain represents a common cause of consultation in the orthopaedic departments around the world. Unfortunately the aetiology is often unknown or can only be confirmed by conducting expensive, time-consuming diagnostic tests, e.g. MRI (see Fig. 3). Our study demonstrates that the Hip Lag Sign is a very accurate test to predict hip abductor damage, which is one of the major causes of hip pain and greater trochanteric pain syndrome [2,3]. It has a high sensitivity and specificity and therefore presents a viable diagnostic option that takes less than a minute and is very easy to perform while bringing no extra costs to a struggling healthcare system.All used statistical tests were able to show a significant correlation of Hip Lag Signresults and hip abductor damage ($p<0.001$). The Hip Lag Sign's simplicity and concurrent accuracy especially advocates its use in rural areas or developing countries where no access to further technical diagnostics such as MRI is available.

The specificity of Hip Lag Sign being 96.55% nicely demonstrates that if negative, the patient, with a high probability, does not have hip abductor damage and the physician can focus his often restricted resources on other reasons for hip pain. Moreover, a positive predictive value of 94.44% signifies that at least 94 out of 100 patients tested are true positive, meaning that they are diagnosed correctly.For these patients, inappropriate and potentially harming treatments such as corticosteroid injections should be prevented. Since tendinosis as well as partial and full thickness gluteus tendon tears can be repaired endoscopically with good results regarding pain relief and function, the Hip Lag Sign-positive patient should be transferred to an experienced hip surgeon for further therapy [17,18].

Our findings suggest that the modified Harris Hip Score and the visual analogue scale do not correlate with the Hip Lag Sign or the MRI results in a statistically significant manner.

Strikingly, compared to the usually performed Trendelenburg test to examine the hip abductors, for which a sensitivity of only 72.7% and a specificity of only 76.9% are reported, we could show that the Hip Lag Sign is a more reliable clinical sign for this entity [19]. However, comparison of the widely used Trendelenburg's test with the new Hip Lag Sign needs to be investigated further in the future.

There are limitations ofthis study. The number of participants was rather small, and this naturally influences the statistical outcome. This also explains why the diagnostic Odds Ratio had such a wide-ranging confidence interval. Nevertheless, a diagnostic Odds Ratio of 238 means that if a patient has a positive Hip Lag Sign, the probability that he/she has hip abductor damage is significantly 238 times higher than if tested negative ($p<0.001$).

If this were a multi-centre, randomized controlledtrial, the number of cases would have been much higher, and the statistical analysis more precise. Thus, we suggest conducting a study with a higher evidence-level to confirm the promising results reported in this manuscript.

In conclusion, we find that the Hip Lag Sign is a very accurate, new way of looking for hip abductor damage and we recommend its inclusion into the common physical examination of the hip.

Acknowledgments

The authors would like to thank Dr. M. Pisan for infrastructural support, Dr. H. Schrem for editorial support during preparation of this manuscript, and C. Winschel for essential technical support.

Author Contributions

Conceived and designed the experiments: AK CMB AG FK. Performed the experiments: AK CMB AG FK. Analyzed the data: AK CMB AG FK. Contributed reagents/materials/analysis tools: AK CMB AG FK. Wrote the paper: AK CMB AG FK.

References

1. Strauss EJ, Nho SJ, Kelly BT (2010)Greater trochanteric pain syndrome. Sports Med Arthroscl8: 113–119.
2. Aepli-Schneider N, Treumann T, Müller U, Schmid L (2012). [Degenerative rupture of the hip abductors. Missed diagnosis with therapy-resistant trochanteric pain of the hips and positive Trendelenburg sign in elderly patients]. Z Rheumatol 71: 68–74.
3. Kingzett-Taylor A, Tirman PF, Feller J, et al. (1999) Tendinosis and tears of gluteus medius and minimus muscles as a cause of hip pain: MR imaging findings. AJR Am J Roentgenol173: 1123–1126.
4. Klauser AS, Martinoli C, Tagliafico A, et al. (2013) Greater trochanteric pain syndrome. Semin Musculoskelet Radiol 17: 43–48.
5. Gottschalk F, Kourosh S, Leveau B (1989) The functional anatomy of tensor fasciae latae and gluteus medius and minimus. J Anat 166: 179–189.
6. Lachiewicz PF (2011) Abductor tendon tears of the hip: evaluation and management. J Am Acad Orthop Surg 19: 385–391.
7. Jeanneret L, Kurmann PT, van Linthoudt D (2008) [Rotator cuff tear of the hip]. Rev Med Suisse 14: 1226–1229.
8. Bunker TD, Esler CN, Leach WJ (1997) Rotator-cuff tear of the hip. J Bone Joint Surg Br 79: 618–620.
9. Cvitanic O, Henzie G, Skezas N, Lyons J, Minter J (2004) MRI diagnosis of tears of the hip abductor tendons (gluteus medius and gluteus minimus). AJR Am J Roentgenol 182: 137–143.
10. Sutter R, Kalberer F, Binkert CA, Graf N, Pfirrmann CW, et al. (2013) Abductor tendon tears are associated with hypertrophy of the tensor fasciae latae muscle. Skeletal Radiol 42: 627–633.

11. Cormier G, Berthelot JM, Maugars Y; SRO (Société de Rhumatologie de l'Ouest) (2006)Gluteus tendon rupture is underrecognized by French orthopedic surgeons: results of a mail survey. Joint Bone Spine 73: 411–413.
12. Bard H (2009) [Tendinopathy of the gluteus medius tendon]. Rev Prat 59: 463–468.
13. Kaltenborn A, Schrem H, Becker HP (2013) Military medicine needs reliable clinical signs and tests to guide prognosis and management. Mil Med 178: 937–938.
14. Harris WH (1969) Traumatic arthritis of the hip after dislocation and acetabular fractures: treatment by mold arthroplasty. An end-result study using a new method of result evaluation. J Bone Joint Surg Am 51: 737–755.
15. Marchetti P, Binazzi R, Vaccari V, et al. (2005) Long-term results with cementlessFitek (or Fitmore) cups. J Arthroplasty 20: 730–737.
16. Bossuyt PM, Reitsma JB, Bruns DE, et al. (2003) Standards for Reporting of Diagnostic Accuracy. Towards complete and accurate reporting of studies of diagnostic accuracy: the STARD initiative. BMJ 326: 41–44.
17. Domb BG, Nasser RM, Botser IB (2010) Partial-thickness tears of the gluteus medius: rationale and technique for trans-tendinous endoscopic repair. Arthroscopy 26: 1697–1705.
18. Voos JE, Rudzki JR, Shindle MK, Martin H, Kelly BT (2007) Arthroscopic anatomy and surgical techniques for peritrochanteric space disorders in the hip. Arthroscopy 23: 1246.e1–5.
19. Bird PA, Oakley SP, Shnier R, Kirkham BW (2001) Prospective evaluation of magnetic resonance imaging and physical examination findings in patients with greater trochanteric pain syndrome. Arthritis Rheum 44: 2138–2145.

Permissions

All chapters in this book were first published in PLOS ONE, by The Public Library of Science; hereby published with permission under the Creative Commons Attribution License or equivalent. Every chapter published in this book has been scrutinized by our experts. Their significance has been extensively debated. The topics covered herein carry significant findings which will fuel the growth of the discipline. They may even be implemented as practical applications or may be referred to as a beginning point for another development.

The contributors of this book come from diverse backgrounds, making this book a truly international effort. This book will bring forth new frontiers with its revolutionizing research information and detailed analysis of the nascent developments around the world.

We would like to thank all the contributing authors for lending their expertise to make the book truly unique. They have played a crucial role in the development of this book. Without their invaluable contributions this book wouldn't have been possible. They have made vital efforts to compile up to date information on the varied aspects of this subject to make this book a valuable addition to the collection of many professionals and students.

This book was conceptualized with the vision of imparting up-to-date information and advanced data in this field. To ensure the same, a matchless editorial board was set up. Every individual on the board went through rigorous rounds of assessment to prove their worth. After which they invested a large part of their time researching and compiling the most relevant data for our readers.

The editorial board has been involved in producing this book since its inception. They have spent rigorous hours researching and exploring the diverse topics which have resulted in the successful publishing of this book. They have passed on their knowledge of decades through this book. To expedite this challenging task, the publisher supported the team at every step. A small team of assistant editors was also appointed to further simplify the editing procedure and attain best results for the readers.

Apart from the editorial board, the designing team has also invested a significant amount of their time in understanding the subject and creating the most relevant covers. They scrutinized every image to scout for the most suitable representation of the subject and create an appropriate cover for the book.

The publishing team has been an ardent support to the editorial, designing and production team. Their endless efforts to recruit the best for this project, has resulted in the accomplishment of this book. They are a veteran in the field of academics and their pool of knowledge is as vast as their experience in printing. Their expertise and guidance has proved useful at every step. Their uncompromising quality standards have made this book an exceptional effort. Their encouragement from time to time has been an inspiration for everyone.

The publisher and the editorial board hope that this book will prove to be a valuable piece of knowledge for researchers, students, practitioners and scholars across the globe.

List of Contributors

Baohui Yang, Haopeng Li, Xijing He, Guoyu Wang and Siyue Xu
Department of Orthopaedic Surgery, The 2nd Affiliated Hospital of Medical College, Xi'an Jiaotong University, Xi'an, Shaanxi Province, People's Republic of China

Judith Cohen-Bittan
Université Pierre et Marie Curie (UMRS 956, UMRS 1158), Paris, France

Jacques Boddaert and Marc Verny
Université Pierre et Marie Curie (UMRS 956, UMRS 1158), Paris, France
Department of Geriatrics, Groupe hospitalier (GH) Pitié-Salpêtrière, Assistance Publique Hôpitaux de Paris (APHP), Paris, France

Frédé ric Khiami
Department of Orthopedic Surgery and Trauma, GH Pitié-Salpêtrière, APHP, Paris, France

Yannick Le Manach
Departments of Anesthesia & Clinical Epidemiology and Biostatistics, Michael DeGroote School of Medicine, Faculty of Health Sciences, McMaster University, Hamilton, Ontario, Canada

Mathieu Raux
Université Pierre et Marie Curie (UMRS 956, UMRS 1158), Paris, France
Department of Anesthesiology and Critical Care, GH Pitié-Salpêtrière, APHP, Paris, France
Institut national de la santé et de la recherche médicale (UMRS 956, UMRS 1158, UMR 689), Paris, France

Jean-Yves Beinis
Department of Rehabilitation, Groupe Hospitalier Charles Foix, APHP, Ivry-sur-Seine, France,

Bruno Riou
Université Pierre et Marie Curie (UMRS 956, UMRS 1158), Paris, France
Department of Emergency Medicine and Surgery, GH Pitié-Salpêtrière, APHP, Paris, France
Institut national de la santé et de la recherche médicale (UMRS 956, UMRS 1158, UMR 689), Paris, France

Maria Luisa Cristina, Anna Maria Spagnolo, Marina Sartini, Donatella Panatto, Roberto Gasparini, Paolo Orlando, Gianluca Ottria and Fernanda Perdelli
Department of Health Sciences, University of Genoa, Genoa, Italy

J. Christiaan Keurentjes and Rob G. Nelissen
Department of Orthopaedic Surgery, Leiden University Medical Center, Leiden, The Netherlands

David Blane
Department of Primary Care and Public Health, Imperial College London, London, United Kingdom

Melanie Bartley
Department of Epidemiology and Public Health, University College London, London, United Kingdom

Johan J. B. Keurentjes
Department of Information Management, Kadaster/ Dutch Land Registry Office, Apeldoorn, The Netherlands

Marta Fiocco
Department of Medical Statistics and BioInformatics, Leiden University Medical Center, Leiden, The Netherlands

J. Christiaan Keurentjes, Thea P. M. Vliet Vlieland and Rob G. Nelissen
Department of Orthopaedic Surgery, Leiden University Medical Center, Leiden, The Netherlands

Marta Fiocco
Department of Medical Statistics and BioInformatics, Leiden University Medical Center, Leiden, The Netherlands

Cynthia So-Osman
Department of Research and Development, Sanquin Blood Supply South West Region, Leiden, The Netherlands

Ron Onstenk
Department of Orthopaedic Surgery, Groene Hart Hospital, Gouda, The Netherlands

Ankie W. M. M. Koopman- Van Gemert
Department of Anaesthesiology, Albert Schweitzer Hospital, Dordrecht, The Netherlands

Ruud G. Pöll
Department of Orthopaedic Surgery, Slotervaart Hospital, Amsterdam, The Netherlands

Herman M. Kroon
Department of Radiology, Leiden University Medical Center, Leiden, The Netherlands

Feng Liu, Zhefeng Chen, Yanqing Gu, Qing Wang, Weiding Cui and Weimin Fan
Department of Orthopedics, the First Affiliated Hospital with Nanjing Medical University, Nanjing, China

Ineke C. M. Lavrijsen, Peter A. J. Leegwater, Marianna A. Tryfonidou, Henri C. M. Heuven and Herman A. W. Hazewinkel
Department of Clinical Sciences of Companion Animal, Faculty of Veterinary Medicine, Utrecht University, Utrecht, The Netherlands

Alan J. Martin and Stephen J. Harris
Waltham Centre for Pet Nutrition, Leicestershire, United Kingdom

David N. Gumieiro and Gilberto J. C. Pereira
Surgery and Orthopedic Department, Botucatu Medical School, UNESP - Univ Estadual Paulista, Botucatu, Brazil

Bruna P. M. Rafacho, Andrea F. Gonçalves, Priscila P. Santos, Paula S. Azevedo, Leonardo A. M. Zornoff, Luiz S. Matsubara, Sergio A. R. Paiva and Marcos F. Minicucci
Internal Medicine Department, Botucatu Medical School, UNESP – Univ Estadual Paulista, Botucatu, Brazil

Naveen K. Kadri, Bernt Guldbrandtsen, Peter Sørensen and Goutam Sahana
Centre for Quantitative genetics and Genomics, Department of Molecular Biology and Genetics, Aarhus University, Aarhus, Denmark

Rea Rodriguez-Raecke, Kristin Ihle and Arne May
Department of Systems Neuroscience, University Medical Center Hamburg Eppendorf, Hamburg, Germany

Andreas Niemeier and Wolfgang Ruether
Department of Orthopaedics, University Medical Center Hamburg Eppendorf, Hamburg, Germany

Kenneth E. S. Poole and Paul M. Mayhew
Department of Medicine, University of Cambridge, Cambridge, Cambridgeshire, United Kingdom

Graham M. Treece and Andrew H. Gee
Department of Engineering, University of Cambridge, Cambridge, Cambridgeshire, United Kingdom

Jan Vaculík and Pavel Dungl
Department of Orthopaedics, Faculty of Medicine, Charles University Prague and Bulovka Hospital, Prague, Czech Republic

Martin Horák
Department of Radiology, Homolka Hospital, Prague, Czech Republic

Jan J. Štěpán
Department of Rheumatology, Faculty of Medicine 1, Charles University Prague and Institute of Rheumatology, Prague, Czech Republic

Chih-Yu Chang
Department of Emergency Medicine, Changhua Christian Hospital, Changhua, Taiwan
Department of Biological Science and Technology, National Chiao Tung University, Hsinchu, Taiwan
Institute of Bioinformatics and Systems Biology, National Chiao Tung University, Hsinchu, Taiwan

Yan-Ren Lin
Department of Emergency Medicine, Changhua Christian Hospital, Changhua, Taiwan
Department of Biological Science and Technology, National Chiao Tung University, Hsinchu, Taiwan
School of Medicine, Chung Shan Medical University, Taichung, Taiwan
School of Medicine, Taipei Medical University, Taipei, Taiwan

Mei-Chueh Yang
Department of Emergency Medicine, Changhua Christian Hospital, Changhua, Taiwan

Wen-Liang Chen and Hua-Chin Lee
Department of Biological Science and Technology, National Chiao Tung University, Hsinchu, Taiwan

Hui-Ling Huang and Shinn-Ying Ho
Department of Biological Science and Technology, National Chiao Tung University, Hsinchu, Taiwan
Institute of Bioinformatics and Systems Biology, National Chiao Tung University, Hsinchu, Taiwan

Yi-Fan Liou and Li-Ping Ciou
Institute of Bioinformatics and Systems Biology, National Chiao Tung University, Hsinchu, Taiwan

Chih-Chi Ke
Institute of Multimedia Engineering, National Chiao Tung University, Hsinchu, Taiwan

Chu-Chung Chou
Department of Emergency Medicine, Changhua Christian Hospital, Changhua, Taiwan
School of Medicine, Chung Shan Medical University, Taichung, Taiwan
School of Medicine, Taipei Medical University, Taipei, Taiwan

Zhao Haien, Ma Baoan, Guo Mingjun and Fan Qingyu
Department of Orthopaedic Surgery, Tangdu Hospital, The Fourth Military Medical University, Xi'an, China

Jiang Yong
Department of Orthopaedic Surgery, Hong Hui Hospital, Xi'an Jiaotong University College of Medicine, Xi'an, China

Lorenzo Moja
Department of Biomedical Sciences for Health, University of Milan, Milan, Italy
Clinical Epidemiology Unit, IRCCS Galeazzi Orthopedic Institute, Milan, Italy

Giuseppe Banfi
University of Milan, Milan, Italy
Clinical Epidemiology Unit, IRCCS Galeazzi Orthopedic Institute, Milan, Italy

Valentina Pecoraro
University of Milan, Milan, Italy

Cristian Ricci and Luca Germagnoli
Clinical Epidemiology Unit, IRCCS Galeazzi Orthopedic Institute, Milan, Italy

Alessandra Piatti
Epidemiological Observatory, ASL Milano, Milan, Italy

Gianni Virgili
Department of Oto Specialised Surgical Sciences, University of Florence, Florence, Italy

Georgia Salanti
Clinical and Molecular Epidemiology Unit and Clinical Trials and Evidence-Based Medicine Unit Department of Hygiene and Epidemiology, School of Medicine, University of Ioannina, Ioannina, Greece,

Alessandro Liberati
Department of Oncology, Hematology and Respiratory Diseases, University of Modena and Reggio Emilia, Modena, Italy

Bente Holm
The Lundbeck Centre for Fast-track Hip and Knee Arthroplasty, Copenhagen University Hospital, Hvidovre, Denmark
Department of Physical Therapy, Physical Medicine and Rehabilitation Research - Copenhagen (PMR-C), Copenhagen University Hospital, Hvidovre, Denmark

Kristian Thorborg
Department of Physical Therapy, Physical Medicine and Rehabilitation Research - Copenhagen (PMR-C), Copenhagen University Hospital, Hvidovre, Denmark
Arthroscopic Centre Amager, Copenhagen University Hospital, Amager, Copenhagen, Denmark
Department of Orthopedic Surgery, Copenhagen University Hospital, Hvidovre, Denmark

Henrik Husted
The Lundbeck Centre for Fast-track Hip and Knee Arthroplasty, Copenhagen University Hospital, Hvidovre, Denmark,
Department of Orthopedic Surgery, Copenhagen University Hospital, Hvidovre, Denmark

Henrik Kehlet
The Lundbeck Centre for Fast-track Hip and Knee Arthroplasty, Copenhagen University Hospital, Hvidovre, Denmark
Section for Surgical Pathophysiology, Copenhagen University Hospital, Rigshospitalet, Copenhagen, Denmark

Thomas Bandholm
Department of Physical Therapy, Physical Medicine and Rehabilitation Research - Copenhagen (PMR-C), Copenhagen University Hospital, Hvidovre, Denmark
Department of Orthopedic Surgery, Copenhagen University Hospital, Hvidovre, Denmark
Clinical Research Centre, Copenhagen University Hospital, Hvidovre, Copenhagen, Denmark

Sophia Pfahler and Ottmar Distl
Institute for Animal Breeding and Genetics, University of Veterinary Medicine Hannover, Hannover, Germany

Zhang Yang, Wang Jian, Li Zhi-han, Xiao Jun, Zhao Liang, Yan Ge and Shi Zhan-jun
Department of Orthopaedic Surgery, Nanfang Hospital, Southern Medical University, Guangzhou, Guangdong, China

Shizue Masuki
Department of Sports Medical Sciences, Shinshu University Graduate School of Medicine, Matsumoto, Japan

Yutaka Morishima
Department of Sports Medical Sciences, Shinshu University Graduate School of Medicine, Matsumoto, Japan
Department of Rehabilitation, Hamamatsu University School of Medicine, Hamamatsu, Japan

Takashi Mizushima and Katsuya Yamauchi
Department of Rehabilitation, Hamamatsu University School of Medicine, Hamamatsu, Japan

Mayuko Morikawa and Hiroshi Nose
Jukunen Taiikudaigaku Research Center, Matsumoto, Japan

Qi Zhang, Wei Chen, Yanling Su, Zhiyong Hou and Yingze Zhang
1 Department of Orthopaedic Surgery, The Third Hospital of Hebei Medical University, Shijiazhuang, Hebei, P.R. China

Xiaobo Wu
Department of Orthopaedic Surgery, The Second Hospital of Tangshan, Tangshan, Hebei, P.R. China

Julien Boudarham, Nicolas Roche, Didier Pradon, Eric Delouf and Djamel Bensmail
GRCTH, EA4497, CIC-IT 805, CHU Raymond Poincaré, Garches, France

Raphael Zory
GRCTH, EA4497, CIC-IT 805, CHU Raymond Poincaré, Garches, France
LAMHESS, EA 6309, University of Nice Sophia Antipolis, Nice, France

Lena Fels and Ottmar Distl
Institute for Animal Breeding and Genetics, University of Veterinary Medicine Hannover, Hannover, Germany

J. Keenan Brown1, Alan D. Brett
Mindways Software, Inc., Austin, Texas, United States of America

Christopher E. Cann
Mindways Software, Inc., Austin, Texas, United States of America
Department of Radiology, University of California San Francisco, San Francisco, California, United States of America

Judith E. Adams
Department of Clinical Radiology, University of Manchester, Manchester, United Kingdom

Chih-Kuang Liang and Yu-Te Lin
Center for Geriatrics and Gerontology, Kaohsiung Veterans General Hospital, Kaohsiung, Taiwan
Division of Neurology, Department of Medicine, Kaohsiung Veterans General Hospital Kaohsiung Taiwan
Aging and Health Research Center, National Yang Ming University, Taipei, Taiwan

Chin-Liang Chu
Center for Geriatrics and Gerontology, Kaohsiung Veterans General Hospital, Kaohsiung, Taiwan
Aging and Health Research Center, National Yang Ming University, Taipei, Taiwan
Department of Psychiatry, Kaohsiung Veterans General Hospital, Kaohsiung, Taiwan

Ming-Yueh Chou
Center for Geriatrics and Gerontology, Kaohsiung Veterans General Hospital, Kaohsiung, Taiwan
Aging and Health Research Center, National Yang Ming University, Taipei, Taiwan
Department of Family Medicine, Kaohsiung Veterans General Hospital, Kaohsiung, Taiwan

Ti Lu
Department of Psychiatry, Kaohsiung Veterans General Hospital, Kaohsiung, Taiwan

Chien-Jen Hsu
Department of Orthopaedics, Kaohsiung Veterans General Hospital, Kaohsiung, Taiwan

Liang-Kung Chen
Aging and Health Research Center, National Yang Ming University, Taipei, Taiwan,
Center for Geriatrics and Gerontology, Taipei Veterans General Hospital, Taipei, Taiwan

Chuanlong Wu, Xinhua Qu, Fengxiang Liu, Huiwu Li, Yuanqing Mao and Zhenan Zhu
Department of Orthopaedics, Shanghai Ninth People's Hospital, Shanghai Jiaotong University School of Medicine, Shanghai, People's Republic of China

Giordano Valente, Lorenzo Pitto and Fulvia Taddei
Medical Technology Laboratory, Rizzoli Orthopaedic Institute, Bologna, Italy

Debora Testi
BioComputing Competence Centre, SCS s.r.l., Bologna, Italy

Ajay Seth
Department of Bioengineering, Stanford University, Stanford, California, United States of America

Scott L. Delp
Department of Bioengineering, Stanford University, Stanford, California, United States of America
Department of Mechanical Engineering, Stanford University, Stanford, California, United States of America

Rita Stagni
Department of Electrical, Electronic and Information Engineering, University of Bologna, Bologna, Italy

Marco Viceconti
Department of Mechanical Engineering and INSIGNEO Institute for In Silico Medicine, University of Sheffield, Sheffield, United Kingdom

Thomas Bandholm
Physical Medicine and Rehabilitation Research - Copenhagen (PMR-C), Copenhagen University Hospital, Hvidovre, Denmark
Department of Physical Therapy, Copenhagen University Hospital, Hvidovre, Denmark
Clinical Research Centre, Copenhagen University Hospital, Hvidovre, Denmark
Department of Orthopedic Surgery, Copenhagen University Hospital, Hvidovre, Denmark

Morten Tange Kristensen
Physical Medicine and Rehabilitation Research - Copenhagen (PMR-C), Copenhagen University Hospital, Hvidovre, Denmark
Department of Physical Therapy, Copenhagen University Hospital, Hvidovre, Denmark
Department of Orthopedic Surgery, Copenhagen University Hospital, Hvidovre, Denmark

Lise Kronborg
Physical Medicine and Rehabilitation Research - Copenhagen (PMR-C), Copenhagen University Hospital, Hvidovre, Denmark
Department of Physical Therapy, Copenhagen University Hospital, Hvidovre, Denmark

Henrik Palm
Department of Orthopedic Surgery, Copenhagen University Hospital, Hvidovre, Denmark

Henrik Kehlet
Section for Surgical Pathophysiology, Rigshospitalet, Copenhagen University, Copenhagen, Denmark

Catherine M. Bourg and Fabian Kalberer
Department of Orthopedic Surgery, Kantonsspital Winterthur, Winterthur, Switzerland

Alexander Kaltenborn
Department of Orthopedic Surgery, Kantonsspital Winterthur, Winterthur, Switzerland
Department of Trauma and Orthopedic Surgery, Federal Armed Forces Hospital Westerstede, Westerstede, Germany
Department of General, Visceral and Transplant Surgery, Hannover Medical School, Hannover, Germany

Andreas Gutzeit
Department of Radiology, Kantonsspital Winterthur, Winterthur, Switzerland
Department of Radiology, Paracelsus Medical University Salzburg, Salzburg, Austria

Index